KIDNEY PROTECTION

KIDNEY PROTECTION

Strategies for Renal Preservation

EDITED BY

VIJAY LAPSIA

BERNARD G. JAAR

A. AHSAN EJAZ

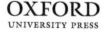

OXFORD
UNIVERSITY PRESS

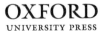

OXFORD
UNIVERSITY PRESS

Oxford University Press is a department of the University of Oxford. It furthers
the University's objective of excellence in research, scholarship, and education
by publishing worldwide. Oxford is a registered trade mark of Oxford University
Press in the UK and certain other countries.

Published in the United States of America by Oxford University Press
198 Madison Avenue, New York, NY 10016, United States of America.

© Oxford University Press 2019

CIP data is on file at the Library of Congress
ISBN 978-0-19-061162-0

1 3 5 7 9 8 6 4 2

Printed by Webcom Inc., Canada

To my parents, my wife Varsha, and son Neil for their love and support.
—Vijay Lapsia

To my parents, my wife Dora, my children Stephanie and
Gabriel for their unyielding support.
—Bernard G. Jaar

To my mother whose vision and love of knowledge has inspired me
and through me the students I teach. To Andrea and Noel for
their unwavering support.
—A. Ahsan Ejaz

CONTENTS

PREFACE

Today, kidney disease affects approximately 10% of the population worldwide. More than 2.6 million individuals are estimated to be receiving renal replacement therapy, with the majority residing in high-income countries. Chronic kidney disease (CKD) is fast becoming a major public health issue even in resource poor settings, with some estimates predicting a disproportionate increase in countries such as China and India.

In almost every recent paper dealing with the implications of CKD, the disease is referred to as an important public health problem. The Global Burden of Disease study data not only support the claims that CKD as currently defined is a global health problem but also that death rates due to CKD are increasing. In addition, hospital- and population-based reports in North America and Europe suggest a dramatic increase in the incidence of acute kidney injury (AKI). As populations age, similar trends are being reported in low- and middle-income countries. Many strategies have been proposed to reduce this growing burden of kidney disease at a population level. While early identification and improving equity of access to renal replacement therapies (RRT) by itself are important, they are unlikely to solve this enormous problem. In addition to better availability of RRT and transplantation on demand, it is important that efforts continue to be focused on primary prevention, protection, and slowing progression of kidney disease as much as possible.

In today's complex clinical environment, contending with the challenges and realizing the yet untapped potential of technological and biomedical research innovations requires that a provider stay abreast of the ever-changing knowledge base. Over the past decades, better understanding of the mechanisms that cause disease has improved the ability to prevent, diagnose, and treat common afflictions such as diabetes and heart disease, major causes of end-stage kidney failure. High-quality research evidence is now available to guide and shape the practice of kidney protection.

Unfortunately, the number of journal articles, technology assessments, and practice guidelines that any provider must read to stay current is well beyond human capacity, and the rapid evolution of care practices and availability of many therapeutic alternatives compound this already overwhelming body of information available to guide clinical decision-making. The first edition of this book, therefore, is an endeavor to assemble this information in a concise and lucid format with the goal of helping the clinician at the bedside intent on protecting the kidneys whether that is in critical care, perioperatively, or in the outpatient setting.

The book would be of interest to not only the practicing nephrologist but also any clinician interested in renal preservation. For that matter, the book has been divided into 6 sections with the first 2 sections focusing on understanding and assessing kidney disease followed by a section on general concepts in protecting renal function. The rest of the sections consist of chapters focusing on major themes such as drugs or systemic illnesses impacting renal function.

Finally, I am grateful to the authors and editors who diligently help compile the overwhelming body of information into thorough thoughtful concise reviews. I am also grateful to the publisher, designers, and copy editors for making this book possible. I sincerely hope that you find this book to be a comprehensive and accessible summary of the resources available to protect the kidneys in everyday clinical scenarios.

Vijay Lapsia

CONTRIBUTORS

Ala Abudayyeh, MD
Associate Professor
Section of Nephrology
The University of Texas MD
Anderson Cancer Center
Houston, TX

Anjali Acharya
Medicine
Jacobi Medical Center
Bronx, NY
Renal Division
Jacobi Medical Center
Bronx, NY

Ayub Akbari, MD, FRCPC, Msc
Associate Professor
Division of Nephrology
Department of Medicine
University of Ottawa
ON, Canada

Muhammad S. Akhter, MD
Nephrology Fellow
Mount Sinai Beth
Israel

Nada Alachkar, MD
Department of Medicine,
Division of Nephrology
The Johns Hopkins University School of
   Medicine
Baltimore, MD

Abdo M. Asmar, MD, FACP
Associate Professor of Medicine and Medical
   Education
Department of Internal Medicine
University of Central Florida,
College of Medicine
Orlando, FL

Serena M. Bagnasco, MD
Associate Professor of Pathology
Directory, Renal Biopsy Service
The Johns Hopkins Hospital
Baltimore, MD

Joanne M. Bargman, MD, FRCPC
Professor, Department of Medicine
University of Toronto
Toronto, CA

David P. Basile
Department of Cellular & Integrative Physiology
Indiana University School of Medicine
Indianapolis, IN

Uyanga Batnyam, MD
Medical Resident
Department of Internal Medicine
University of Central Florida, College of
   Medicine
Orlando, FL

Sahar Bayat, MD, PhD
University of Rennes, EHESP Rennes,
   Sorbonne Paris Cité
Rennes, France

Julie Belliere, MD, PhD
Department of Nephrology and Organ
   Transplantation
CHU Rangueil
Toulouse, France

Giampaolo Bianchi, MD
Full Professor
Department of Urology
University of Modena & Reggio Emilia
Modena, Italy

Kirk N. Campbell, MD
Associate Professor of Medicine
Division of Nephrology, Department of
    Medicine
Icahn School of Medicine at Mount Sinai
New York, NY

Lili Chan, MD
Instructor
Division of Nephrology, Department of
    Medicine
Icahn School of Medicine at Mount Sinai
New York, NY

Fouad T. Chebib
Division of Nephrology and Hypertension,
    Department of Internal Medicine
Mayo Clinic
Rochester, MN

Michael J. Choi
Division of Nephology
Johns Hopkins University School of Medicine
Baltimore, MD

Cécile Couchoud, MD, PhD
REIN registry
Agence de la biomédecine
Saint Denis La Plaine, France

Bhagwan Dass, MD
Clinical Associate Professor
Department of Medicine
University of Florida
Gainesville, FL

Priya Deshpande
Icahn School of Medicine at Mount Sinai
New York, NY

Miten J. Dhruve
Division of Nephrology
Michael Garron Hospital
Toronto, ON

Joseph DiNorcia, MD
Assistant Professor of Surgery
Division of Liver, Pancreas, and Intestine
    Transplantation, Department of Surgery
David Geffen School of Medicine, University of
    California
Los Angeles, CA

Thomas Dowling, PharmD, PhD
Assistant Dean and Professor
Director Office of Research and Sponsored
    Programs
Ferris State University
Big Rapids, MI

François Durand, MD
Hepatology and Liver Intensive Care
Hospital Beaujon
Clichy, France
University Paris Diderot
Paris, France

A. Ahsan Ejaz, MD
Professor of Medicine
Division of Nephrology, Hypertension and
    Renal Transplantation
University of Florida
Gainesville, FL

Stanislas Faguer, MD, PhD
Professor
Department of Nephrology and Organ
    Transplantation
CHU Rangueil
Toulouse, France

Samira Farouk
Instructor
Division of Nephrology, Department of
    Medicine
Icahn School of Medicine at Mount Sinai
New York, NY

David A. Ferenbach
Department of Renal Medicine
Royal Infirmary of Edinburgh
Edinburgh, Scotland, UK
MRC Centre for Inflammation Research,
    Queen's Medical Research Institute
University of Edinburgh
Edinburgh, UK

Nancy Ferrari, MD
Department of Urology
University of Modena & Reggio Emilia
Modena, Italy

Claire Francoz, MD, PhD
Hepatology and Liver Intensive Care
Hospital Beaujon
Clichy
Paris, France
Service d'Hepatologie
Clichy, France

Duvuru Geetha, MD, MRCP (UK)
Associate Professor of Medicine
Division of Nephrology, Department of
    Medicine
Johns Hopkins University
Baltimore, MD

Yuri S. Genyk, MD
Professor of Clinical Surgery, Surgical Director
Liver Transplant Program, Division of
  Hepatobiliary, Pancreas, and Abdominal
  Organ Transplant, Department of Surgery
Keck School of Medicine, University of Southern
  California
Los Angeles, CA

Jonathan M. Gleadle
School of Medicine
Flinders University
Adelaide, Australia
Department of Renal Medicine, Flinders
  Medical Centre
Adelaide, Australia

Ilias P. Gomatos, MD, PhD
Division of Nephrology, Department of Medicine
Icahn School of Medicine at Mount Sinai
New York, NY

Ramnika Gumber, MD
Division of Nephrology, Department of
  Medicine
University of Pennsylvania
Philadelphia, PA

William Hahn, BS
Research Assistant
Division of Nephrology, Hypertension &
  Transplantation
University of Florida
Gainesville, FL

Ryan W. Haines, MBBS, MRCP
Clinical Research Fellow in Adult Critical Care
  Unit
The Royal London Hospital, Barts Health NHS
  Trust
London, UK

Ramy M. Hanna, MD
Division of Nephrology, Department of
  Medicine
David Geffen School of Medicine
University of California
Los Angeles, CA

Nikolas B. Harbord, MD
Division Chief, Nephrology, Mount Sinai Beth
  Israel, Assistant Professor of Medicine
Icahn School of Medicine at Mount Sinai
New York, NY

John Cijiang He
Icahn School of Medicine at Mount Sinai
New York, NY

Swapnil Hiremath, MD, MPH, FASN
Assistant Professor
Division of Nephrology, Department of
  Medicine
University of Ottawa
Ontario, Canada

Jonathan J. Hogan, MD
Division of Nephrology, Department of
  Medicine
University of Pennsylvania
Philadelphia, PA

Wael F. Hussein
Departments of Nephrology and Internal
  Medicine
University Hospital Limerick
Ireland
Graduate Entry Medical School, University of
  Limerick
Ireland

Bernard G. Jaar, MD, MPH
Division of Nephrology, Department of
  Medicine
Nephrology Center of Maryland, Johns Hopkins
  School of Medicine
Department of Epidemiology
Johns Hopkins Bloomberg School of
  Public Health
Welch Center for Prevention, Epidemiology and
  Clinical Research
Johns Hopkins Medical Institutions
Baltimore, MD

Navin Jaipaul, MD, MHS
Professor of Medicine
Division of Nephrology, Department of
  Medicine
Loma Linda University School of Medicine
Chief of Nephrology
VA Loma Linda Healthcare System
Loma Linda, CA

Nassim Kamar, MD, PhD
Professor
Department of Nephrology and Organ
  Transplantation
Université Paul Sabatier, CHU Toulouse
Toulouse, France

Hania Kassem, MD
Division of Nephrology and Hypertension,
    Department of Medicine
University of Texas Medical Branch
Galveston, TX

Lewis Kaufman, MD
Associate Professor
Division of Nephrology
Icahn School of Medicine at Mount Sinai
New York, NY

Tonia Kim, MD
Associate Professor
Division of Nephrology, Department of
    Medicine
Icahn School of Medicine at Mount Sinai
New York, NY

Joshua D. King, MD
Division of Nephrology, Department of
    Medicine
University of Virginia School of Medicine
Charlottesville, VA

Daphne Knicely
Division of Nephology
Johns Hopkins University School of Medicine
Baltimore, MD

Abhilash Koratala, MD
Assistant Professor of Medicine
Division of Nephrology, Hypertension and
    Renal Transplantation
University of Florida
Gainesville, FL

Vijay Lapsia, MD
Associate Professor
Department of Medicine
Icahn School of Medicine at Mount Sinai
New York, NY

Timothy S. Larson, MD
Mayo Clinic
Rochester, MN

Susan Lerner, MD
Associate Professor of Surgery
Kidney/Pancreas Transplantation Program
Icahn School of Medicine at Mount Sinai
New York, NY

Nelson Leung, MD
Division of Nephrology and Hypertension
Mayo Clinic
Rochester, MN

John Manllo-Dieck, MD
Department of Medicine, Division of
    Nephrology
The Johns Hopkins University School of
    Medicine
Baltimore, MD

Sandhya Manohar, MBBS
Division of Nephrology and Hypertension
Mayo Clinic
Rochester, MN

Annette L. Mazzone
School of Medicine, Flinders University
Adelaide, Australia
Cardiac Surgery Research and Perfusion
Cardiac and Thoracic Surgical Unit
Flinders Medical Centre
Adelaide, Australia

Madhav C. Menon, MD
Assistant Professor
Division of Nephrology, Department of
    Medicine
Icahn School of Medicine at Mount Sinai
New York, NY

Joseph A. Messana, MD
Renal Division
Perelman School of Medicine, University of
    Pennsylvania
Philadelphia, PA

Alain Meyrier MD, PhD
Professor of Medicine Emeritus
Université Paris-Descartes Medical School
Paris, France

Salvatore Micali
Associate Professor
Department of Urology
University of Modena & Reggio Emilia
Modena, Italy

Rajesh Mohandas, MD
Associate Professor
Division of Nephrology, Hypertension &
    Transplantation
University of Florida
Gainesville, FL

Jose Manuel Monroy-Trujillo, MD
Assistant Professor of Medicine
Division of Nephrology, Department of
    Medicine
Johns Hopkins University School of Medicine
Baltimore, MD

Mitra K. Nadim, MD, FASN
Professor of Clinical Medicine
Division of Nephrology and Hypertension,
    Department of Medicine
Keck School of Medicine, University of Southern
    California
Los Angeles, CA

Timothy Nguyen, PharmD, BCPS, FASCP
Associate Professor of Pharmacy
Long Island University (LIU Pharmacy—
    Arnold & Marie Schwartz College of
    Pharmacy and Health Sciences)
New York, NY

Eoin D. O'Sullivan
Department of Renal Medicine
Royal Infirmary of Edinburgh
Edinburgh, Scotland, UK

Babu J. Padanilam
Department of Cellular & Integrative
    Physiology
University of Nebraska Medical Center

Rulan S. Parekh, MD
Department of Pediatrics and Medicine,
    Hospital for Sick Children
University Health Network and University of
    Toronto
Toronto, Canada

Marie D. Philipneri
Professor of Internal Medicine
Department of Internal Medicine, Division of
    Nephrology
Saint Louis University School of Medicine
St. Louis, MO

María Pilar Ricard Andres, MD, PhD
Departamento de Hematología
Universidad Autónoma de Madrid
Madrid, Spain

Martine Pollack-Zollman, MD
Assistant Professor
Division of Nephrology, Department of
    Medicine
Icahn School of Medicine at Mount Sinai
New York, NY

John R. Prowle, MD, FFICM, FRCP
Senior Lecturer in Intensive Care Medicine
William Harvey Institute, Barts and the London
    School of Medicine and Dentistry, Queen
    Mary University of London
London, UK
Honorary Consultant Intensivist and
    Nephrologist
Adult Critical Care Unit and Department of
    Renal and Transplant Medicine
The Royal London Hospital, Barts Health NHS
    Trust
London, UK

Stefano Puliatti, MD
Department of Urology
University of Modena & Reggio Emilia
Modena, Italy

Anjay Rastogi, MD, PhD
Division of Nephrology, Department of
    Medicine
David Geffen School of Medicine, University of
    California, Los Angeles
Los Angeles, CA

Katia López Revuelta, MD, PhD
Departamento de Nefrología
Universidad Autónoma de Madrid
Madrid, Spain

Bernardo Rocco, MD
Associate Professor
Department of Urology
University of Modena & Reggio Emilia
Modena, Italy

Claudio Ronco, MD
Department of Nephrology, Dialysis and
    Transplantation
International Renal Research Institute (IRRIV)
San Bortolo Hospital
Vicenza, Italy

Edward A. Ross, MD
Professor and Chair
Department of Internal Medicine
University of Central Florida, College of
    Medicine
Orlando, FL

Sara Samoni, MD
Institute of Life Sciences, Sant'Anna School of
  Advanced Studies
Pisa, Italy
International Renal Research Institute (IRRIV)
Department of Nephrology, Dialysis and
  Transplantation
San Bortolo Hospital
Vicenza, Italy

Paul G. Schmitz
Professor of Internal Medicine
Department of Internal Medicine,
  Division of Nephrology
Saint Louis University School of Medicine
St. Louis, MO

Umut Selamet, MD
Division of Nephrology, Department of
  Medicine
David Geffen School of Medicine, University of
  California, Los Angeles
Los Angeles, CA

Akash Sethi, DO
Division of Nephrology, Department of
  Medicine
University of Pennsylvania
Philadelphia, PA

Sapna Shah, MD
Renal Transplant Fellow
Department of Medicine
Icahn School of Medicine at Mount Sinai
New York, NY

Aisha Shaikh, MD
Icahn School of Medicine at Mount Sinai
New York, NY

Shuchita Sharma
Icahn School of Medicine at Mount Sinai
New York, NY

Girish Singhania
Assistant Professor of Medicine
Division of Nephrology
University of Utah Hospital
Salt Lake City, UT

Rupinder K. Sodhi
Assistant Professor of Internal Medicine
Department of Internal Medicine, Division of
  Nephrology
Saint Louis University School of Medicine
St. Louis, MO

Austin G. Stack
Departments of Nephrology and Internal
  Medicine
University Hospital Limerick
Ireland
Graduate Entry Medical School, University of
  Limerick
Ireland
Health Research Institute, University of Limerick,
  Limerick
Ireland

Larisa G. Tereshchenko, MD, PhD
Knight Cardiovascular Institute, Oregon Health
  and Science University
Portland, OR
Cardiovascular Division, Department of
  Medicine
School of Medicine, Johns Hopkins University
Baltimore, MD

Sumeska Thavarajah
Division of Nephology
Johns Hopkins University School of Medicine
Baltimore, MD

Vicente E. Torres
Division of Nephrology and Hypertension,
  Department of Internal Medicine
Mayo Clinic
Rochester, MN

Raymond R. Townsend, MD
Renal Division
Perelman School of Medicine, University of
  Pennsylvania
Philadelphia, PA

Tran Tran, PharmD, BCPS
Associate Professor
Midwestern University, Chicago College of
  Pharmacy

Joseph A. Vassalotti, MD
Associate Clinical Professor
Division of Nephrology, Department of
  Medicine
Icahn School of Medicine at Mount Sinai
New York, NY

Jonathan W. Waks, MD
Division of Cardiovascular Medicine
Beth Israel Deaconess Medical Center,
  Harvard Medical School
Boston, MA

Jonathan Winston, MD
Professor
Division of Nephrology, Department of
  Medicine
Icahn School of Medicine at Mount Sinai
New York, NY

Christina M. Wyatt, MD
Icahn School of Medicine at Mount Sinai
New York, NY

David C. Wymer, MD
Associate Professor Medicine and Radiology,
  Associate Chair Radiology
Department of Radiology
University of Florida
Gainesville, FL

David T. G. Wymer, MD
Department of Radiology
Mount Sinai Medical Center
Miami Beach, FL

Samuel Mon-Wei Yu
Medicine
Jacobi Medical Center
Bronx, NY

SECTION I

Understanding Kidney Disease

Epidemiology and Etiology of Kidney Disease

CÉCILE COUCHOUD AND SAHAR BAYAT

Over 10% of the world population is affected by chronic kidney disease (CKD), as defined by international guidelines, and is at higher risk of cardiovascular events, acute kidney injury (AKI) episodes, progression to end-stage renal disease (ESRD), and death. This emphasizes the utmost importance of CKD prevention and kidney function protection. In recent years, more and more data are available on these patients thanks to cohort studies and registries in high- and middle-income countries. However, information on low-income countries is still lacking.

AN EVOLUTIVE PRAGMATIC DEFINITION OF CKD

A major step forward for research in kidney disease epidemiology was made in 2002 when a clear definition of CKD was proposed in the Kidney Disease Outcomes Quality Initiative guidelines.[1] CKD was defined based on the presence of kidney damage and level of kidney function (glomerular filtration rate [GFR]), irrespective of diagnosis. This allowed promoting many studies on CKD prevalence, incidence, and outcomes, independently of its cause. In 2012, the guidelines for CKD evaluation, classification, and management were updated by the Kidney Disease/Improving Global Outcomes (KDIGO) CKD Work Group.[2] It recommended that CKD should be classified based on cause, GFR and albuminuria (CGA staging: cause, GFR category, and albuminuria category). The preferred equation to calculate the estimated GFR (eGFR) is the one proposed by the Chronic Kidney Disease Epidemiology Collaboration research group that takes into account sex, age, ethnic origin, and serum creatinine level.[2] Albuminuria is assessed by using the urinary albumin-to-creatinine ratio.

VARIOUS RISK FACTORS OF KIDNEY DISEASES OCCURRENCE

Risk factors of kidney disease occurrence may directly cause the nephropathy (e.g., a genetic defect) or may contribute to kidney damage. They can be intrinsic in a "patient at risk," such as the presence of diabetes, or they can be related to a "situation at risk," such as analgesic abuse. Primary prevention among the identified risk groups must be organized to decrease the risk of kidney disease appearance. Moreover, many risk factors also contribute to kidney damage progression in patients with CKD, and, therefore, they also are the target of secondary prevention.[3]

Diabetes and hypertension are the leading CKD causes in all developed and many developing countries, whereas glomerulonephritis and unknown causes are more common in countries of Asia and sub-Saharan Africa.[4] Infectious diseases, herbal medicines, and environmental toxins also contribute to CKD burden in low-income countries.[5] Nevertheless, data on comparisons between countries must be considered with caution because of the heterogeneity in the access to renal biopsy or other specific diagnostic tools, disease stage at the time of diagnosis, and classification in the absence of standard definitions.

Besides the known risk factors, recent studies have focused on metabolic syndrome, genetic aspects, nondirect medical factors, and low birth weight as major risk factors of CKD occurrence. According to the American Heart Association, metabolic syndrome (MetS) is a cluster of 3 or more of the following medical conditions: central obesity, elevated triglyceride levels, low high-density lipoprotein amount, hypertension, and elevated fasting glucose.[6] MetS and all its individual components are among the main medical risk factors of CKD in the general population.[7-11] They also affect renal allograft survival.[12,13] In addition, observational studies have highlighted the development of MetS in patients with established CKD,[14] suggesting a bidirectional relationship between MetS and CKD. The mechanisms of kidney injury in patients with MetS are multiple and not completely understood. Insulin resistance is a very important MetS-related etiological factor of CKD.[14,15] Obesity causes renal injuries through several mechanisms, particularly hypertension, hyperglycemia, and dyslipidemia. Moreover, obesity is, on its own, a CKD risk factor.[16,17] Indeed, the prevalence of obesity-related glomerulopathy is increasing concomitantly with the obesity epidemic. Obesity also contributes to CKD progression in other glomerulopathies, especially in diabetic and immunoglobulin A nephropathies.[18]

There are also several genetic causes of CKD, such as congenital anomalies of the kidney and urinary tract and autosomal dominant polycystic disease. Moreover, the Framingham Heart Study (in a community-based population) showed that serum creatinine and GFR levels are heritable and suggested that there is a genetic component in CKD development.[19] A recent meta-analysis of genome-wide association studies on eGFR confirmed that 53 loci are associated with eGFR.[20] However, the genetic risk score, derived from the Framingham Heart Study, to predict the risk of incident stage 3 CKD does not improve disease discrimination beyond the known clinical risk factors (including hypertension and diabetes).[21]

Among nondirect medical factors, race, poverty, or low birth weight also are associated with CKD incidence. The burden of CKD and ESRD is different among the various racial and ethnic groups. According to the US Renal Data System,[22] in 2014, the adjusted ESRD incidence rate ratios for blacks/African Americans, Native Americans and Asians/Pacific Islanders, compared with whites, were 3.1, 1.2, and 1.2, respectively. The rate ratio for Hispanics versus non-Hispanics was 1.3. Compared with whites, ESRD prevalence in 2014 was about 3.7, 1.4, and 1.5 times higher in blacks, Native Americans, and Asians, respectively. A recent ancillary study within the Multi-Ethnic Study of Atherosclerosis, which included older black and white people, showed no difference in the measured GFR between these groups.[23] This suggests that other factors, such as faster GFR decline, must contribute to the higher ESRD incidence in older black people. Neighborhood socioeconomic disadvantage has been associated with higher incidence rates of renal replacement therapy (RRT) in Australia.[24] In the United States, in all sex/race groups, the incidence of ESRD caused by all primary renal diseases was highest among people with the lowest socioeconomic status and progressively decreased with higher socioeconomic status.[25] A higher incidence rate of RRT was observed in rural areas of Australia compared to major cities[26] and in rural counties of South Carolina compared to urban counties.[27] Finally, low birth weight and prematurity are associated with a lower nephron number and, consequently, with increased lifelong risk of hypertension, proteinuria, and kidney disease.[28] This subject is covered in greater detail in Chapter 4.

HIGH INCIDENCE AND PREVALENCE OF CKD

CKD Incidence: More Than 30% of the World Population Will Develop CKD During Their Life

Based on data from 9 general population cohorts and 8 high-risk cohorts (patients with diabetes, hypertension, or cardiovascular disease), the Chronic Kidney Disease Prognosis Consortium estimated that the incidence rate of progressive CKD in people without CKD at baseline is 2 events per 1,000 person-years in general population cohorts and 5.5 in high-risk cohorts.[29] Based on the National Health and Nutrition Examination Survey in the United States, at birth, the estimated lifetime risk of stage 3a+, 3b+, 4+ CKD and ESRD is 59.1%, 33.6%, 11.5%, and 3.6%, respectively.[30] In comparison, the estimated lifetime risk of developing diabetes for individuals born in 2000 in the United States is 32.8% for males and 38.5% for females. Another study showed that the predicted residual lifetime incidence of CKD for US adults aged 30 to 49, 50 to 64, and 65 years or older without CKD at baseline is 54%, 52%, and 42%, respectively.[31] Similarly, using data from the Framingham Offspring Study, it was calculated that the residual lifetime risk of CKD in participants without CKD (eGFR $\geq$60 mL/min/1.73 m^2) at the age of 50 years is 41.3% (95% confidence interval [CI] 38.5–44.0).[32] The risk is higher for people with risk factors at baseline, for instance, diabetes (52.6%, 95% CI 44.8–60.4), hypertension (50.2%, 95% CI 46.1–54.3), and obesity (46.5%, 95% CI 41.1–52.0). For individuals without risk factors at baseline, the lifetime risk of CKD is lower (34.2%, 95% CI 29.4–39.0) compared with participants with 1, 2, or 3 risk factors (45.0%, 51.5%, and 56.1%, respectively; P <0.01 for all compared with those without risk factors).

CKD Prevalence: More Than 10% of the World Population Live with CKD

A systematic review estimated that in 2010, the age-standardized global prevalence of CKD (stages 1–5) in adults aged ≥20 and older was 10.4% in men (95% CI 9.3–11.9%) and 11.8% in women (95% CI 11.2–12.6%) worldwide.[33] When countries were divided according to the income, the prevalence was 8.6% in men (95% CI 7.3–9.8%) and 9.6% in women (95% CI 7.7–11.1%) from high-income countries, and 10.6% in men (9.4–13.1%) and 12.5% in women (95% CI 11.8–14.0%) from low- and middle-income countries. Various cross-sectional studies on CKD prevalence in the general population have shown important variations across countries. In Europe, the sex- and age-adjusted prevalence of CKD (stages 1–5) varies between 3% in Norway and 17% in northeast Germany.[34] CKD prevalence was 5.5% in Morocco for the 2009–2011 period,[35] 7.9% in Korea for 2011–2012,[36] 10.3% in China in 2006,[37] 13% in the United States in 1999–2004,[38] and 13.9% in sub-Saharan Africa.[39] Moreover, CKD prevalence increases with age and is higher in high-risk groups, such as people with diabetes, hypertension, or obesity. Nevertheless, these data have to be considered with caution because of the heterogeneity in the methods used to measure creatinine and albuminuria and to calculate eGFR as well as in the sample selection criteria.[40]

In comparison, the worldwide prevalence of high blood pressure (>140/90 mmHg) is 24.1% (CI 95% 21.4–27.1) in men and 20.1% (95% CI 17.8–22.5) in women,[41] the prevalence of adult diabetes is 9.0% (95% CI 7.2–11.1) in men and 7.9% (95% CI 6.4–9.7) in women,[42] and the prevalence of adults with a body mass index ≥25 (overweight/obesity) is 36.9% (95% CI 36.3–37.4) in men and 38.0% (95% CI 37.5–38.5) in women.[43]

HUGE GEOGRAPHICAL VARIATIONS OF INCIDENCE AND PREVALENCE OF END-STAGE RENAL DISEASE

Most high-income countries have put in place ESRD registries for patients on RRT that allow the accurate assessment of the number and characteristics of patients on dialysis or with a functioning graft. Such registries are now progressively developing also in low-income countries in association with RRT implementation.[44] The incidence rate of treated ESRD varied from 455 per million general population (PMP) in Taiwan to 49 PMP in Bangladesh in 2014.[22] Many factors may explain such variation, including not only the disease and risk factor burden, but also the variable access to RRT, depending on

resources, healthcare expenditure and supply, place of conservative care, medical practice patterns (e.g., time of RRT start).[4,45–49] The prevalence rate of treated ESRD, which is the result of incidence rate and mortality, varied from 3,219 PMP in Taiwan to 113 PMP in Bangladesh in 2014. Low prevalence rates may be due to low incidence of ESRD or to high mortality rates for treated patients. All those indicators have to be interpreted together to have a comprehensive view of the problem. Less information is available on patients with ESRD not treated by RRT.[50] Restricted treatment funding or more conservative approaches explain these geographical variations.[51]

AKI AND CKD: A BIDIRECTIONAL RELATIONSHIP

In a systematic review that pooled 147 studies (3,212,925 patients) using a KDIGO-equivalent definition of AKI, the overall pooled incidence rate of AKI in adults was 21.0% (95% CI 18.7–23.6) and the pooled AKI-associated mortality was 23.3% (95% CI 21.3–25.5).[52] The Chronic Kidney Disease Prognosis Consortium estimates that the incidence rate for an AKI code at hospitalization discharge in patients without CKD at baseline is 1 event per 1,000 person-years in general population cohorts and 1.5 in high-risk cohorts.[29] Several studies suggest that AKI incidence is increasing in both high-income and low-income countries.[53,54] Nevertheless, these data must be considered with caution due to the differences and trends in patients' identification, AKI definition, and cause of kidney injury, which vary among clinical settings and socioeconomic environments. Concerning AKI causes, sepsis, hypovolemia, drugs, and ischemia are common in both high- and low-income countries. Moreover, traditional herbal treatments, less strictly regulated use of nonprescription medicines, environmental toxins, tropical infectious diseases, natural disasters, and obstetric AKI (related to nonoptimal antenatal care and abortion management) are also reported as AKI causes in low-income countries.[55,56]

Many studies have shown an association between AKI and CKD. In a systematic review of 13 cohort studies, Coca et al.[57] have estimated that patients with AKI are at higher risk of CKD (hazard ratio [HR], 8.8 [3.1–25.5]), ESRD (HR 3.1 [1.9–5.0]), and death (HR 2.0 [1.3–3.1]) compared with patients without AKI. In these cohorts, the pooled rates of CKD and ESRD were 25.8 per 100 person-years (range 3.4–72.2) and 8.6 per 100 person-years (range 0.63–28.1), respectively. On the other hand, the Chronic Kidney Disease Prognosis Consortium reported that reduced eGFR and increased albumin/creatinine ratio are strong risk factors for AKI[58] in people with or without diabetes or hypertension.[59] AKI incidence rate in people with CKD at baseline varies from 4 to 110 events per 1,000 person-years, according to the GFR and albuminuria.[29] This bidirectional relationship is still debated and needs further investigations.[60,61] AKI may be a marker that identifies higher-risk patients with CKD who are more likely to progress rapidly or who have more comorbid conditions that increase the risk of exposure to nephrotoxic procedures or drugs. This subject is covered in greater details in Chapter 3.

SEVERE OUTCOMES OF CKD

CKD Outcomes: Beware of Competing Risk Factors

Lower eGFR and higher albuminuria are risk factors for ESRD, AKI, and progression of CKD in both general and high-risk populations independently of each other and of cardiovascular risk factors. The Kidney Failure Risk Equation includes several ESRD risk factors, such as age, sex, eGFR, calcium, and phosphate concentrations to predict the risk of ESRD in patients with CKD with high discrimination and adequate calibration.[62,63] In addition, lower eGFR and higher albuminuria also are each independently associated with all-cause mortality[64] or cardiovascular mortality[65,66] in both women and men,[67] with or without diabetes,[68] and with or without hypertension.[69] Mortality rates in patients with CKD vary from 6.7 to 320 per 100 person-years according to age and renal function.[70] Older patients have a lower relative risk of mortality but higher absolute risk.[70] CKD and cardiovascular diseases share common risk factors. Patients with CKD are among the highest risk groups for cardiovascular events.[71] In the Chronic Renal Insufficiency Cohort Study, the composite outcome event rate of congestive heart failure, myocardial infarction, and stroke was 2.1 and 5.9 per 100 person-years in nondiabetic and diabetic patients, respectively.[72] These outcomes must be considered together because they act as competing risks.

ESRD Outcomes: The Issue of Unequal Access to Treatment

ESRD registries give an accurate image of the outcomes, particularly on the access to renal transplantation and survival, for patients on RRT. Access to kidney transplantation varies greatly among countries with kidney transplantation rates ranging from 0.6 PMP in Bangladesh to 60.3 PMP in Jalisco, Mexico. The highest prevalence of patients with ESRD and a functioning kidney transplant is found in Norway (657 PMP, which represents 72% of all patients with ESRD). Various factors affect the access to renal transplantation, including national health policies on organ donation and transplantation and local factors, such as type of patients with ESRD and waiting list practices.[73,74]

Mortality is higher among people with ESRD. The 5-year relative survival of patients on dialysis is lower than that reported for many cancers in Italy.[75] The 5-year survival rate after RRT start is 49% in Europe but decreases to 22% for patients older than 75 years at initiation.[76] Geographical variability on mortality rates is strongly influenced by the heterogeneity of patients starting RRT and, more important, by inequalities in access to dialysis or transplantation. Indeed, in low-income countries, most patients with ESRD who start dialysis discontinue the treatment and die because of the unaffordable cost.[77]

A PROMINENT PLACE AMONG OTHER CHRONIC DISEASES

The Global Burden of Disease Study has recently published several articles that provide information on CKD incidence, prevalence, disability, and mortality.[78,79] Although these studies have several limitations in terms of quality of the data sources and classifications, they give important information by comparing the burden, geographical patterns, and temporal trends of many different chronic diseases. The age-standardized death rates due to CKD increased by 36.9% between 1990 and 2013, mainly due to diabetes mellitus-associated nephropathy, while the cancer and cardiovascular disease death rates decreased by 14.7% and 22%, respectively, during the same period. In 1990, CKD was ranked 36 among the 50 causes of global years of life lost. In 2013, it moved up to position 19. CKD is among the top 10 causes of global years of life lost in Singapore, Greece, Israel, many Latin America, Oceania, North Africa, and Middle East countries. In 2013, the number of years lived with disability, worldwide, was $12,347 \times 10^3$ for

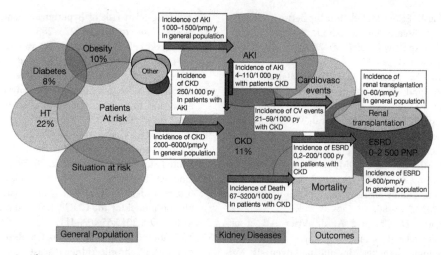

FIGURE 1.1 Incidence and prevalence of chronic kidney disease, acute kidney injury, and end-stage renal disease. The estimated prevalence rate is indicated in the circle. The estimated incidence rate is shown under the corresponding arrow. py = person-year. pmp/y = per million population – year. CV = cardiovascular. HT = hypertension.

CKD, while it was $29,518 \times 10^3$ for diabetes mellitus, $6,763 \times 10^3$ for neoplasm, and $21,177 \times 10^3$ for cardiovascular disease.[78] Due to population growth and aging, CKD rate increased by 49.5% between 1990 and 2013, but decreased by 2.8% after adjusting for age.

CONCLUSION

Kidney diseases are poorly known outside expert circles and often considered as silent; however, frequently they strongly affect patients' life. Over 30% of people will develop CKD during their life. The main data discussed in this chapter are summarized in Fig. 1.1.

REFERENCES

1. National Kidney Foundation. K/DOQI clinical practice guidelines for chronic kidney disease: evaluation, classification, and stratification. *Am J Kidney Dis.* 2002;39:S1–S266.
2. Kidney Disease: Improving Global Outcomes (KDIGO) CKD Work Group. KDIGO 2012 clinical practice guideline for the evaluation and management of chronic kidney disease. *Kidney Int. Suppl.* 2013;3(1): 1–150.
3. McClellan WM, Flanders WD. Risk factors for progressive chronic kidney disease. *J Am Soc Nephrol.* 2003;14:S65–S70.
4. Jha V, Garcia-Garcia G, Iseki K, et al. Chronic kidney disease: global dimension and perspectives. *Lancet.* 2013;382:260–272.
5. Webster AC, Nagler EV, Morton RL, Masson P. Chronic kidney disease. *Lancet.* 2016;389(10075):1238–1252.
6. Grundy SM, Cleeman JI, Daniels SR, et al. Diagnosis and management of the metabolic syndrome: an American Heart Association/National Heart, Lung, and Blood Institute scientific statement. *Circulation.* 2005;112:2735–2752.
7. Thomas G, Sehgal AR, Kashyap SR, Srinivas TR, Kirwan JP, Navaneethan SD. Metabolic syndrome and kidney disease: a systematic review and meta-analysis. *Clin J Am Soc Nephrol.* 2011;6:2364–2373.
8. Hoehner CM, Greenlund KJ, Rith-Najarian S, Casper ML, McClellan WM. Association of the insulin resistance syndrome and microalbuminuria among nondiabetic native Americans: the Inter-Tribal Heart Project. *J Am Soc Nephrol.* 2002;13:1626–1634.
9. Locatelli F, Pozzoni P, Del VL. Renal manifestations in the metabolic syndrome. *J Am Soc Nephrol.* 2006;17:S81–S85.
10. Chen J, Muntner P, Hamm LL, et al. The metabolic syndrome and chronic kidney disease in U.S. adults. *Ann Intern Med.* 2004;140:167–174.
11. Huh JH, Yadav D, Kim JS, et al. An association of metabolic syndrome and chronic kidney disease from a 10-year prospective cohort study. *Metabolism.* 2017;67:54–61.
12. Porrini E, Delgado P, Bigo C, et al. Impact of metabolic syndrome on graft function and survival after cadaveric renal transplantation. *Am J Kidney Dis.* 2006;48:134–142.
13. de Vries AP, Bakker SJ, van Son WJ, et al. Metabolic syndrome is associated with impaired long-term renal allograft function; not all component criteria contribute equally. *Am J Transplant.* 2004;4:1675–1683.

14. Nashar K, Egan BM. Relationship between chronic kidney disease and metabolic syndrome: current perspectives. *Diabetes Metab Syndr Obes.* 2014;7:421–435.

15. Zhang X, Lerman LO. The metabolic syndrome and chronic kidney disease. *Transl Res.* 2016;83:14–25.

16. Kovesdy CP, Furth SL, Zoccali C. Obesity and kidney disease: hidden consequences of the epidemic. *Kidney Int.* 2017;91:260–262.

17. Hall ME, do Carmo JM, da Silva AA, Juncos LA, Wang Z, Hall JE. Obesity, hypertension, and chronic kidney disease. *Int J Nephrol Renovasc Dis.* 2014;7:75–88.

18. D'Agati VD, Chagnac A, de Vries AP, et al. Obesity-related glomerulopathy: clinical and pathologic characteristics and pathogenesis. *Nat Rev Nephrol.* 2016;12:453–471.

19. Fox CS, Yang Q, Cupples LA, et al. Genomewide linkage analysis to serum creatinine, GFR, and creatinine clearance in a community-based population: the Framingham Heart Study. *J Am Soc Nephrol.* 2004;15:2457–2461.

20. Pattaro C, Teumer A, Gorski M, et al. Genetic associations at 53 loci highlight cell types and biological pathways relevant for kidney function. *Nat Commun.* 2016;7:10023.

21. Ma J, Yang Q, Hwang SJ, Fox CS, Chu AY. Genetic risk score and risk of stage 3 chronic kidney disease. *BMC Nephrol.* 2017;18:32.

22. United States Renal Data System. *U S Renal Data System, USRDS 2016 Annual Data Report: Atlas of Chronic Kidney Disease and End-Stage Renal Disease in the United States.* Ann Arbor, MI: USRDS; 2016.

23. Inker LA, Shafi T, Okparavero A, et al. Effects of race and sex on measured GFR: the multiethnic study of atherosclerosis. *Am J Kidney Dis.* 2016;68:743–751.

24. Grace BS, Clayton P, Cass A, McDonald SP. Socio-economic status and incidence of renal replacement therapy: a registry study of Australian patients. *Nephrol Dial Transplant* 2012;11:4173–4180.

25. Ward MM. Socioeconomic status and the incidence of ESRD. *Am J Kidney Dis.* 2008;51:563–572.

26. Gray NA, Dent H, McDonald SP. Renal replacement therapy in rural and urban Australia. *Nephrol Dial Transplant.* 2012;27:2069–2076.

27. Fan ZJ, Lackland DT, Lipsitz SR, et al. Geographical patterns of end-stage renal disease incidence and risk factors in rural and urban areas of South Carolina. *Health Place.* 2007;13:179–187.

28. Luyckx VA, Bertram JF, Brenner BM, et al. Effect of fetal and child health on kidney development

and long-term risk of hypertension and kidney disease. *Lancet.* 2013;382:273–283.

29. Gansevoort RT, Matsushita K, van der Velde M, et al. Lower estimated GFR and higher albuminuria are associated with adverse kidney outcomes: a collaborative meta-analysis of general and high-risk population cohorts. *Kidney Int.* 2011;80:93–104.

30. Grams ME, Chow EK, Segev DL, Coresh J. Lifetime incidence of CKD stages 3–5 in the United States. *Am J Kidney Dis.* 2013;62:245–252.

31. Hoerger TJ, Simpson SA, Yarnoff BO, et al. The future burden of CKD in the United States: a simulation model for the CDC CKD Initiative. *Am J Kidney Dis.* 2015;65:403–411.

32. McMahon GM, Hwang SJ, Fox CS. Residual lifetime risk of chronic kidney disease. *Nephrol Dial Transplant* 2016;32(10):1705–1709.

33. Mills KT, Xu Y, Zhang W, et al. A systematic analysis of worldwide population-based data on the global burden of chronic kidney disease in 2010. *Kidney Int.* 2015;88:950–957.

34. Bruck K, Stel VS, Gambaro G, et al. CKD prevalence varies across the European general population. *J Am Soc Nephrol.* 2016;27:2135–2147.

35. De Broe ME, Gharbi MB, Elseviers M. Maremar, prevalence of chronic kidney disease, how to avoid over-diagnosis and under-diagnosis. *Nephrol Ther.* 2016;12(Suppl 1):S57–S63.

36. Ji E, Kim YS. Prevalence of chronic kidney disease defined by using CKD-EPI equation and albumin-to-creatinine ratio in the Korean adult population. *Korean J Intern Med.* 2016;31:1120–1130.

37. Xu R, Zhang L, Zhang P, Wang F, Zuo L, Wang H. Comparison of the prevalence of chronic kidney disease among different ethnicities: Beijing CKD survey and American NHANES. *Nephrol Dial Transplant.* 2009;24:1220–1226.

38. Coresh J, Selvin E, Stevens LA, et al. Prevalence of chronic kidney disease in the United States. *J Am Med Assoc.* 2007;298:2038–2047.

39. Stanifer JW, Jing B, Tolan S, et al. The epidemiology of chronic kidney disease in sub-Saharan Africa: a systematic review and meta-analysis. *Lancet Glob Health.* 2014;2:e174–e181.

40. Glassock RJ, Warnock DG, Delanaye P. The global burden of chronic kidney disease: estimates, variability and pitfalls. *Nat Rev Nephrol.* 2017;13:104–114.

41. NCD Risk Factor Collaboration. Worldwide trends in blood pressure from 1975 to 2015: a pooled analysis of 1479 population-based measurement studies with 19.1 million participants. *Lancet.* 2017;389:37–55.

42. NCD Risk Factor Collaboration. Worldwide trends in diabetes since 1980: a pooled analysis

of 751 population-based studies with 4.4 million participants. *Lancet.* 2016;387:1513–1530.

43. Ng M, Fleming T, Robinson M, et al. Global, regional, and national prevalence of overweight and obesity in children and adults during 1980–2013: a systematic analysis for the Global Burden of Disease Study 2013. *Lancet.* 2014;384:766–781.

44. Davids MR, Eastwood JB, Selwood NH, et al. A renal registry for Africa: first steps. *Clin Kidney J.* 2016;9:162–167.

45. Robinson BM, Akizawa T, Jager KJ, Kerr PG, Saran R, Pisoni RL. Factors affecting outcomes in patients reaching end-stage kidney disease worldwide: differences in access to renal replacement therapy, modality use, and haemodialysis practices. *Lancet.* 2016;388:294–306.

46. Couchoud C, Guihenneuc C, Bayer F, Lemaitre V, Brunet P, Stengel B. Medical practice patterns and socio-economic factors may explain geographical variation of end-stage renal disease incidence. *Nephrol Dial Transplant.* 2012;27:2312–2322.

47. Couchoud C, Guihenneuc C, Bayer F, Stengel B. The timing of dialysis initiation affects the incidence of renal replacement therapy. *Nephrol Dial Transplant.* 2010;25:1576–1578.

48. Caskey FJ, Kramer A, Elliott RF, et al. Global variation in renal replacement therapy for end-stage renal disease. *Nephrol Dial Transplant.* 2011;26:2604–2610.

49. Castledine CI, Gilg JA, Rogers C, Ben-Shlomo Y, Caskey FJ. How much of the regional variation in RRT incidence rates within the UK is explained by the health needs of the general population? *Nephrol Dial Transplant.* 2012;27:3943–3950.

50. Sparke C, Moon L, Green F, et al. Estimating the total incidence of kidney failure in Australia including individuals who are not treated by dialysis or transplantation. *Am J Kidney Dis.* 2013;61:413–419.

51. van de Luijtgaarden MW, Noordzij M, Van BW, et al. Conservative care in Europe:nephrologists' experience with the decision not to start renal replacement therapy. *Nephrol Dial Transplant.* 2013;28:2604–2612.

52. Susantitaphong P, Cruz DN, Cerda J, et al. World incidence of AKI: a meta-analysis. *Clin J Am Soc Nephrol.* 2013;8:1482–1493.

53. Lameire NH, Bagga A, Cruz D, et al. Acute kidney injury: an increasing global concern. *Lancet.* 2013;382:170–179.

54. Kolhe NV, Muirhead AW, Wilkes SR, Fluck RJ, Taal MW. National trends in acute kidney injury requiring dialysis in England between 1998 and 2013. *Kidney Int.* 2015;88:1161–1169.

55. Bouchard J, Mehta RL. Acute kidney injury in western countries. *Kidney Dis (Basel).* 2016;2:103–110.

56. Yang L. Acute kidney injury in Asia. *Kidney Dis (Basel).* 2016;2:95–102.

57. Coca SG, Singanamala S, Parikh CR. Chronic kidney disease after acute kidney injury: a systematic review and meta-analysis. *Kidney Int.* 2012;81:442–448.

58. Grams ME, Astor BC, Bash LD, Matsushita K, Wang Y, Coresh J. Albuminuria and estimated glomerular filtration rate independently associate with acute kidney injury. *J Am Soc Nephrol.* 2010;21:1757–1764.

59. James MT, Grams ME, Woodward M, et al. A meta-analysis of the association of estimated GFR, albuminuria, diabetes mellitus, and hypertension with acute kidney injury. *Am J Kidney Dis.* 2015;66:602–612.

60. Pannu N. Bidirectional relationships between acute kidney injury and chronic kidney disease. *Curr Opin Nephrol Hypertens.* 2013;22:351–356.

61. Hsu RK, Hsu CY. The role of acute kidney injury in chronic kidney disease. *Semin Nephrol.* 2016;36:283–292.

62. Tangri N, Stevens LA, Griffith J, et al. A predictive model for progression of chronic kidney disease to kidney failure. *J Am Med Assoc,* 2011;305:1553–1559.

63. Tangri N, Grams ME, Levey AS, et al. Multinational assessment of accuracy of equations for predicting risk of kidney failure: a meta-analysis. *J Am Med Assoc.* 2016;315:164–174.

64. Astor BC, Matsushita K, Gansevoort RT, et al. Lower estimated glomerular filtration rate and higher albuminuria are associated with mortality and end-stage renal disease: a collaborative meta-analysis of kidney disease population cohorts. *Kidney Int.* 2011;79:1331–1340.

65. Matsushita K, van d, V, Astor BC, et al. Association of estimated glomerular filtration rate and albuminuria with all-cause and cardiovascular mortality in general population cohorts: a collaborative meta-analysis. *Lancet.* 2010;375:2073–2081.

66. van der Velde M, Matsushita K, Coresh J, et al. Lower estimated glomerular filtration rate and higher albuminuria are associated with all-cause and cardiovascular mortality. A collaborative meta-analysis of high-risk population cohorts. *Kidney Int.* 2011;79:1341–1352.

67. Nitsch D, Grams M, Sang Y, et al. Associations of estimated glomerular filtration rate and albuminuria with mortality and renal failure by sex: a meta-analysis. *Brit Med J.* 2013;346:f324.

68. Fox CS, Matsushita K, Woodward M, et al. Associations of kidney disease measures

with mortality and end-stage renal disease in individuals with and without diabetes: a meta-analysis. *Lancet,* 2012;380:1662–1673.

69. Mahmoodi BK, Matsushita K, Woodward M, et al. Associations of kidney disease measures with mortality and end-stage renal disease in individuals with and without hypertension: a meta-analysis. *Lancet.* 2012;380:1649–1661.

70. Hallan SI, Matsushita K, Sang Y, et al. Age and association of kidney measures with mortality and end-stage renal disease. *J Am Med Assoc.* 2012;308:2349–2360.

71. Gansevoort RT, Correa-Rotter R, Hemmelgarn BR, et al. Chronic kidney disease and cardiovascular risk: epidemiology, mechanisms, and prevention. *Lancet.* 2013;382:339–352.

72. Denker M, Boyle S, Anderson AH, et al. Chronic Renal Insufficiency Cohort Study (CRIC): overview and summary of selected findings. *Clin J Am Soc Nephrol.* 2015;10:2073–2083.

73. White SL, Hirth R, Mahillo B, et al. The global diffusion of organ transplantation: trends, drivers and policy implications. *Bull World Health Organ.* 2014;92:826–835.

74. Bayat S, Macher MA, Couchoud C, et al. Individual and regional factors of access to the renal transplant waiting list in france in a cohort of dialyzed patients. *Am J Transplant.* 2015;15:1050–1060.

75. Nordio M, Limido A, Maggiore U, Nichelatti M, Postorino M, Quintaliani G. Survival in patients treated by long-term dialysis compared with the general population. *Am J Kidney Dis.* 2012;59:819–828.

76. European Renal Association–European Dialysis and Transplant Association. *ERA-EDTA Registry Annual Report 2013.* Amsterdam, The Netherlands: Academic Medical Center, Department of Medical Informatics; 2015.

77. Ashuntantang G, Osafo C, Olowu WA, et al. Outcomes in adults and children with end-stage kidney disease requiring dialysis in sub-Saharan Africa: a systematic review. *Lancet Glob Health.* 2017;5(4):e408–e417.

78. Global Burden of Disease Study 2013 Collaborators. Global, regional, and national incidence, prevalence, and years lived with disability for 301 acute and chronic diseases and injuries in 188 countries, 1990-2013: a systematic analysis for the Global Burden of Disease Study 2013. *Lancet.* 2015;386:743–800.

79. GBD 2013 Mortality and Causes of Death Collaborators. Global, regional, and national age-sex specific all-cause and cause-specific mortality for 240 causes of death, 1990-2013: a systematic analysis for the Global Burden of Disease Study 2013. *Lancet.* 2015;385: 117–171.

2

Pathogenesis of Acute Kidney Injury

DAVID P. BASILE AND BABU J. PADANILAM

OVERVIEW

Acute kidney injury (AKI) represents a major clinical concern that effects up to 5% of all hospitalized patients and is associated with significant mortality rates. Typically AKI is defined as an abrupt loss of kidney function associated with a decrease in glomerular filtration rate (GFR) resulting in increased nitrogenous waste. The term "AKI" has been provided as alternative to the term acute renal failure, which historically had not been uniformly defined in the literature. Several strategies for defining and classifying AKI have been adopted in recent years based on changes in serum creatinine levels and reductions in urine output.[1]

Causes of renal injury include ischemia, resulting from severe or protracted decreases in renal perfusion or nephrotoxins including aminoglycosides, cisplatinum, and radiocontrast agents, which have the potential to damage renal parenchymal cells.[2] Tubular epithelial cell injury and death are hallmark features of AKI. When damaged, this highly metabolic tissue may further compromise renal perfusion by influencing vascular tone, inflammation, or congestion associated with secondary cellular damage. Thus, an understanding of the pathophysiology of AKI requires an appreciation for the potential interplay between epithelial, vascular, and inflammatory activities leading to impaired function and also the repair processes necessary for successful recovery.

It is important to note that much of what is known regarding the pathophysiology of AKI derives from experimental models, primarily in rodents. How faithfully such models reflect the processes underlying AKI in human patients is unclear.[2] Species differences, perhaps due to anatomical differences, may alter sensitivity to insults such as ischemia reperfusion.

For example, prominent injuries with loss of GFR and epithelial cell necrosis are observed in mice with shorter ischemic times relative to rats. Dogs and pigs require much longer ischemic times with less prominent necrosis, while frank necrosis is a rare finding in human biopsies. These controversies are hampered by the relative lack of medullary tissue routinely obtained in human biopsies. In addition, human biopsies also identify alterations in distal tubule and thick ascending limb structures, which are not prominent in routinely used rodent models of ischemia/reperfusion injury.[3] Studies in animal models routinely use young healthy animals of a single sex, which fails to recapitulate all of the complications usually observed in patients at risk of AKI. Nevertheless, similarities in injury exist between human and animal models such as findings of increased vulnerability of S_3 segments of the proximal tubule regarding loss of brush border, cell detachment, sloughing of cells into the lumen, cast formation, and sublethal tubular injury as well as evidence of regenerating cells adjacent to areas of injury.[2] At the functional level, reduced GFR and a reversibility of tubular injury and renal function, based on the severity of the initial insult, are observed in both models and human patients. Animal models also manifest a prominent inflammatory response in the kidney, which does not appear to be prominent in human biopsies. Alterations in renal hemodynamics, in particular, related to vascular congestion are well described in animal models but have not been definitively assessed in human AKI.

HEMODYNAMICS

In animal models of AKI such as ischemia-reperfusion, there is typically an impairment in renal blood flow associated with lost renal function and tissue damage.[4] In models of sepsis, AKI may or may not occur in the presence of reduced total renal blood flow. Regardless, microvascular imaging studies have shown heterogeneous disturbances in microvascular perfusion in the early stages of both ischemic or sepsis models of AKI.[5] Laser Doppler flowmetry studies have been used to measure reductions in renal medullary blood flow following reperfusion injury and have shown that immediate vasodilator treatments can mitigate reductions in medullary flow and attenuate AKI severity.[6] Relative reductions in flow in the renal medulla may further enhance hypoxia in this region, following ischemia/reperfusion injury (IRI) or induction of sepsis, as demonstrated using the hypoxia-sensitive compound, pimonadizole, or the use of blood oxygen level-dependent magnetic resonance imaging.[7-9] The reduction in renal pO_2 may represent a significant challenge for the renal tubules to meet metabolic demands and the increased hypoxia is consistent with the greater degree of cellular injury and death that develops in the renal outer medulla.

Reductions in renal blood flow has been thought to be due, in part, to vasoconstriction, perhaps secondary to tubular glomerular feedback triggered by impaired sodium reabsorption[2] and the activity of adenosine on A1 receptors. However, if GFR is reduced, sustained tubular glomerular feedback is not likely to represent a continued contributor toward vasoconstriction.[5] Many other factors may affect vasoconstriction such as sympathetic nervous system activity, norepinephrine, angiotensin II, and endothelin, since pharmacological blockade of these factors are associated with reduced severity of injury.[2,10] Nitric oxide from nitric oxide synthase-2 and prostacyclin (prostaglandin E2) generated by cyclooxygenase (COX-1 or COX-2) help to maintain renal perfusion. COX-2 or NO synthase-2 inhibitors reduce the influence of these vasodilatory factors and can augment the severity of AKI, while infusion of the synthetic prostacyclin analog iloprost or NO donors can protect against the development of AKI.[10] However, as illustrated by the lack of effect of low-dose dopamine, vasodilator treatments have no effect in mitigating AKI. Therefore, enhanced vascular tone may play a role in the development of AKI, but it is not clear that vasoconstriction contributes significantly to sustained reductions in perfusion during the extension and maintenance phase of AKI.[10]

Significant attention has been directed toward the postglomerular peritubular capillaries and

venules contributing toward the development of AKI. Capillary damage has been observed in cadaveric grafts following transplant and the degree of vascular damage correlated with the immediate function of the graft.[11] Endothelial dysfunction can manifest as both an impairment in endothelial cell-dependent vasodilation as well as the activation of enhanced leukocyte adhesion molecules such as P-selectin, ICAM-1, or co-stimulatory factors.[4,10] Leukocyte adhesion not only promotes the liberation of injurious cytokines but can also contribute to rouleaux formation and impair perfusion. These events have been suggested as critical factors leading from the initiation phase to the extension phase of AKI as described by Molitoris and Sutton[12] (Fig. 2.1). Resistance to vasodilator therapy may therefore be due to a lack of effect on alleviating established microvascular congestion.[10] Interestingly, retrograde delivery of saline through the renal vein was shown to alleviate leukocyte adhesion, vascular congestion, and accelerate recovery of GFR in rats with established AKI.[13]

METABOLISM

Bioenergetics deficit is the major determinant of the pathophysiological consequences manifested in the kidney after an ischemic episode.[2] Following IRI, medullary pO_2 is restored to only 10% of its normal levels for at least 24 hours. Therefore, the outer medullary nephron segments may partially switch from respiration to glycolysis as a last resort to generate adenosine triphosphate (ATP). However, proximal tubule glycolysis and fatty acid oxidation (FAO) are inhibited, especially in the medullary proximal straight tubules (PST), resulting in sustained ATP depletion for a period up to 48 hour post-reperfusion.[12]

Glycolysis is the sequence of reactions that metabolizes 1 molecule of glucose to 2 molecules of pyruvate with the concomitant net production of 2 molecules of ATP. This process is anaerobic. Glyceraldehyde-3-phosphate dehydrogenase (GAPDH) plays a key role in glycolysis and gluconeogenesis by reversibly catalyzing the oxidation and phosphorylation of D-glyceraldehyde-3-phosphate to 1,3-diphospho-glycerate. The DNA repair enzyme, poly (adenosine diphosphate [ADP]-ribose) polymerase-1 (PARP-1), inhibits GAPDH during IRI (Fig. 2.2). PARP-1 transfers the ADP-ribose moiety of nicotinamide adenine dinucleotide (NAD^+) to nuclear proteins and to itself. PARP-1 is selectively induced and activated in PST following renal ischemia.[14] PARP-1

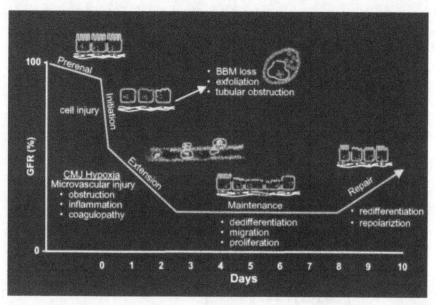

FIGURE 2.1 Relationship between the clinical phases and the cellular phases of ischemic acute renal failure and the temporal impact on organ function as represented by the glomerular filtration rate (GFR). Prerenal azotemia exists when a reduction in renal blood flow causes a reduction in GFR. A variety of cellular and vascular adaptations maintain renal epithelial cell integrity during this phase. The initiation phase occurs when a further reduction in renal blood flow results in cellular injury, particularly the renal tubular epithelial cells, and a continued decline in GFR. Vascular and inflammatory processes that contribute to further cell injury and a further decline in GFR usher in the proposed extension phase. During the maintenance phase, GFR reaches a stable nadir as cellular repair processes are initiated to maintain and reestablish organ integrity. The recovery phase is marked by a return of normal cell and organ function that results in an improvement in GFR. BBM = Brush border membrane. CMJ = corticomedullary junction. From Sutton TA, Fisher CJ, Molitoris BA. Microvascular endothelial injury and dysfunction during ischemic acute renal failure. *Kidney Int.* 2002;62:1539–1549, with permission from Kidney International.

activation inhibited GAPDH enzyme activity via poly (ADP-ribosyl)ation and thus inhibits glycolytic ATP synthesis after renal IRI. However, PARP-1 inhibition only partially preserved ATP levels and prevented necrotic cell death by only 33%, suggesting this pathway only partially accounts for the bioenergetic deficit observed after IRI.

Phosphofructokinase (PFK) is the most important control element in the mammalian glycolytic pathway. The activity of PFK increases when the ATP/AMP ratio is lowered while a fall in pH (acidosis) inhibits its activity. Another potent activator of PFK is fructose 2,6-bisphosphate (F-2,6-BP), which activates it by increasing its affinity for fructose 6-phosphate and diminishing the inhibitory effect of ATP. The p53 target gene, TIGAR (TP53-induced glycolysis and apoptosis regulator), plays a direct role in glucose metabolism by altering the concentration of fructose 2,6-bisphosphate (Fig. 2.2).[15] TIGAR

shares functional sequence similarities with the bisphosphatase domain (FBPase-2) of the bifunctional enzyme PFK-2/FBPase-2, which degrades fructose-2,6-bisphosphate (Fru-2,6-P_2). Fru-2,6-P_2 stimulates 6-phospho-1-kinase to convert fructose-6-phosphate to fructose-1,6-bisphosphate at the third rate limiting step in glycolysis; when Fru-2,6-P_2 decreases, the formation of fructose-6-phosphate is favored. TIGAR activation causes a decline in Fru-2,6-P_2 levels (by degrading Fru-2,6-P_2) and thereby blocks PFK activity and glycolysis at the third step resulting in inhibition of ATP synthesis. TIGAR is selectively induced and activated in PST during the early time periods following IRI and its expression persists up to 48 hours postinjury. TIGAR upregulation inhibited PFK-1 activity and glucose 6-phosphate dehydrogenase (G6PD) activity and induced ATP depletion, oxidative stress, autophagy, and apoptosis. Small interfering RNA-mediated TIGAR inhibition prevented the

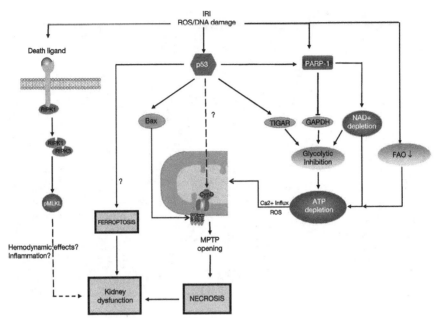

FIGURE 2.2 Scheme of regulation of bioenergetics and cell death in ischemic renal injury. In the ischemic renal injury model, necrosis in proximal tubular cells is a common type of cell death. Initial injury results in ROS-mediated DNA damage and rapid activation of p53 and PARP-1. p53 induces the expression of Bax, which will facilitate the MOMP for necrosis. Activated PARP-1 will rapidly deplete intracellular NAD+ and ATP and simultaneously inhibit glyceraldehyde-3-phosphate dehydrogenase, which reduces glycolytic capacity in proximal tubules. p53-induced TP53-induced glycolysis and apoptosis regulator expression inhibits the rate-limiting phosphofructokinase and the glycolytic pathway. Further, IRI leads to inhibition of proliferator-activated receptor alpha activity and decreased FAO and ATP synthesis. The severe ATP depletion resulting from decreased glycolysis and FAO shuts down ion homeostasis resulting in Ca2+ influx and uptake into mitochondria. PARP-1 as a transcriptional cofactor induces several cytokines and promotes infiltration of inflammatory cells to the injured renal parenchyma, all leading to increased ROS production. ROS and Ca2+, the most prominent mediators of permeability transition, increase the probability of mitochondrial permeability transition pore opening via activation of cyclophilin D and the ATP synthasome complex. Osmotic influx of water and solutes into the mitochondrial matrix leads to mitochondrial swelling and rupture of outer membrane to elicit mitochondrial dysfunction and necrosis. The contribution of necroptosis in proximal tubule cell death has recently been challenged and the mechanism by which RIP1K blockade prevents renal injury remains to be elucidated. Although, recent evidences suggest p53 translocation to mitochondrial matrix and activation of cyclophilin D, such a role for p53 is not established in kidney injury. ROS = reactive oxygen species. ATP = adenosine triphosphate. IRI = ischemia reperfusion injury. FAO = fatty acid oxidation. Modified with permission from Ying Y, Padanilam BJ. Regulation of necrotic cell death p53, PARP1 and Cyclophilin D-overlapping pathways of regulated necrosis. *Cell Mol Life Sci.* 2016;73:2309–2324.

aforementioned malevolent effects and protected the kidneys from functional and histological damage and reduced oxidative stress and apoptosis. Collectively, these results demonstrate that both PARP-1 and TIGAR impair glycolysis contributing to renal damage in the setting of severe renal ischemia reperfusion injury.[16]

However, FAO constitutes the major source of energy for the renal tissue and is inhibited during reperfusion. Reduced FAO and persistent increases of tubule cell nonessential fatty acid levels occur during ischemia and post-reperfusion

in vivo in association with downregulation of mitochondrial and peroxisomal enzymes of β-oxidation.[17] Feldkamp et al.[18] has demonstrated that proximal tubules subjected to hypoxia/reoxygenation exhibit decreased ATP. This energetic deficit was not due to loss of mitochondrial membrane integrity, decreased electron transport, or compromised F_1F_0-ATPase.[19] Rather, it was demonstrated that nonessential fatty acid overload is the primary cause of energetic failure of reoxygenated proximal tubules and impaired recovery of mitochondrial membrane potential

($\Delta\Psi_m$) during reoxygenation. Portilla et al.[20] demonstrated disturbances of mitochondrial and peroxisomal β-oxidation of fatty acids during both ischemic and cisplatin-induced AKI, which are driven by downregulation of gene transcription resulting from decreased DNA binding activity of the transcription factor peroxisome proliferator-activated receptor alpha (PPAR*a*) and decreased expression of its coactivator, peroxisome proliferator activated receptor-gamma coactivator-1 (PGC-1). Fibrates and other PPAR*a* ligands were shown to alleviate disturbances in FAO, improve renal function, and prevent cell death in cisplatin AKI. Importantly, the PPAR*a* agonist effects were not seen in PPAR*a* null mice, supporting specific mediation by this pathway in cisplatin nephrotoxicity.

INFLAMMATION

Renal injury may result in a dramatic increase in inflammation, including macrophages, dendritic cells, T and B lymphocytes, and natural killer cells, and the reader is referred to excellent review articles for a more comprehensive handling of the subject.[21,22] The liberation of signals driving inflammation may derive from either the activated endothelium, damaged tubular epithelial cells, or tissue resident macrophages activated by injury (Fig. 2.3). Such factors likely include cytokines such as tumor necrosis factor alpha (TNF-α), interleukin (IL) 1, IL-6, monocyte chemoattractant protein-1, and RANTES (and many others) damage-associated molecules or complement.

These pathways have been investigated primarily in mice using strategies such as immune depletion of specific cells, transgenic knockouts, and adoptive transfer approaches. A significant literature exists illustrating an important role for many leukocytes in the genesis of AKI in animal models such as IRI, cisplatin, or sepsis, although the potential contribution of inflammation in human AKI is not firmly established. Of particular interest, CD4+ T cells differentiate into T-helper cells that liberate cytokines, promoting either injury or repair. Evidence suggests that Th-1 cells, which liberate IFN-γ, as well as T helper-17 cells, which secrete the cytokine IL-17, may enhance kidney injury in response to ischemia or cisplatin. In contrast, T-regulatory cells have inhibitory activity and have been implicated in tissue repair following injury.[22]

Similarly, macrophages and dendritic cells have also been shown to mediate renal injury.

Classic studies using the liposomal clodronate showed that depletion of macrophages attenuated the degree of injury following ischemia.[22] Interestingly, the delayed administration of liposomal clodronate (2–3 days) resulted in worse injury and less efficient repair.[23] These different results are thought to be attributable to activities of different macrophage populations. Generally speaking, M1-type macrophages are activated early during the development of kidney injury and secrete factors such as IL12, which exacerbate inflammation and damage. In contrast, M2-type macrophages infiltrate the kidney at a later time, secrete anti-inflammatory IL-10, and promote repair.[23]

CELL INJURY AND DEATH

The bioenergetic deficit in models of renal injury, the sustained impairment in perfusion, and the liberation of damaging cytokines result in a variety of physiological processes that lead to cellular injury or death by processes such as necrosis, apoptosis, necroptosis, ferroptosis, and autophagy. Both the severity and duration of ATP depletion have been implicated as key determinants of cell fate,[2] while other extrinsic and intrinsic variables will influence the mode by which cell death is actuated.

Mitochondrial Permeability Transition Pore-Dependent Necrosis

Mitochondrial permeability transition pore (MPTP)-dependent necrosis is characterized by cell swelling with subsequent rupture of surface membranes and is a frequent consequence of IRI. ATP depletion leads to the inhibition of the membrane-bound Na+-K+-ATPase activity and causes a large intracellular increase of Na+ ions and water, with consequent edema. Increased Na+ in the cell causes a decrease in transmembrane sodium concentration gradient and potentiates Ca^{2+} entry via Na^+/Ca^{2+} exchanger.[2] The calcium overload is thought to increase reactive oxygen species at the mitochondrial level during the ischemia. Reactive oxygen species and Ca^{2+} are 2 of the major inducers of MPTP-mediated necrosis via activation of cyclophilin D (CypD). CypD belongs to the polypeptidyl-prolyl cis-trans isomerase family. CypD is located in the mitochondrial matrix and can interact with mitochondrial inner membrane proteins to induce the opening of the MPTP (Fig. 2.2). Accordingly, genetic deletion of CypD in mice led to significant protection against renal IRI as demonstrated

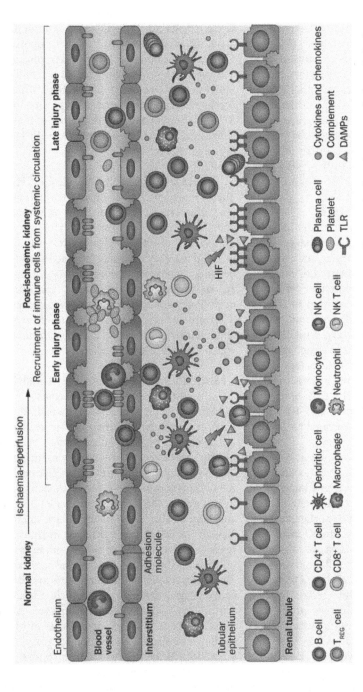

FIGURE 2.3 An immune response is initiated in postischemic kidneys by resident immune cells through the disrupted endothelium. TLRs, adhesion molecules, and DAMPs released from dying cells facilitate the recruitment and activation of various immune cells including neutrophils, macrophages, dendritic cells, NK cells, T cells, and B cells during the early injury phase. Activation of the complement system and increased production of proinflammatory cytokines and chemokines are important promoters of leucocyte infiltration into the postischemic kidney. Major effector cells of the innate immune system, such as macrophages, dendritic cells, and NK cells, are involved in the pathogenesis of renal injury after IRI. T cells, the major effector cells of the adaptive immune system, also substantially contribute to the development of renal injury from the early to late injury phase. Plasma cells seem to participate in the tubular damage process during the late injury phase. AKI = acute kidney injury. DAMPs = damage-associated molecular patterns. HIF = hypoxia-inducible factor. IRI = ischemiareperfusion injury. NK = natural killer. TLR = toll-like receptor. T_{REG} cell = regulatory T cell. Modified with permission from Jang HR and Rabb H. Immune cells in experimental acute kidney injury. *Nat Rev Nephrol.* 2015;11:88–101.

by increased renal function and morphological protection.[24]

PARP1-Dependent Necrosis

Excessive activation of poly(ADP-ribose) polymerase 1 (PARP1), such as in the setting of IRI, can lead to glycolytic inhibition,[25] depletion of NAD+, and consequent depletion of ATP. Pharmacological inhibition of PARP1 protects rats and mice kidneys from ischemic injury. PARP1 inhibition protected against IRI by improving renal function and tissue morphology, attenuated ATP depletion, leukocyte infiltration, and activation of inflammatory molecules but had no effect on apoptosis. Although clinical trials have not been attempted using PARP1 or CypD inhibitors in AKI, PARP1 inhibitors are currently in clinical trials for treatment of cancer (ClinicalTrials.gov identifier: NCT01215643, NCT01318694, and NCT01183169) and inhibitors for CypD are in development for clinical use.

p53-Dependent Necrosis

We reported that, after IRI, proximal tubule-specific p53-KO mice showed significantly reduced levels of plasma creatinine and blood urea nitrogen and improved renal morphology compared to wild-type control mice.[26] Quantitative studies indicated that necrosis is significantly reduced in the proximal tubules after IRI. Although the mechanism by which p53 deletion results in decreased necrosis is not defined, our data suggest that p53 depletion may attenuate the increased expression of PARP1. In addition, p53 depletion in postischemic proximal tubules results in reduced expression of Bax and Bid, important regulators of mitochondrial outer membrane permeability (Fig. 2.2). These data suggest that proximal tubule p53 may influence both apoptosis and necrosis pathways after IRI.

Apoptosis

Unlike necrosis, apoptosis confers advantages to the injured organ. During apoptosis, cellular components are packaged into apoptotic bodies and phagocytosed by macrophages and neighboring epithelial cells, which limits inflammatory cell recruitment. Mitochondrial outer membrane permeabilization permits proapoptotic proteins (cytochrome *c*, apoptosis inducing factor, and others, including Omi/HtrA2) to activate caspase-dependent and independent pathways.[27] In renal epithelial cells, Bax and Bak are the primary BCL2 family members

that increase membrane permeability, whereas Bcl-2 and Bcl-XL (B-cell lymphoma–extra large) antagonize "membrane attack" by Bax and Bak. Despite the current absence of human trials, several therapeutic interventions targeting the apoptotic pathway, including the use of caspase inhibitors such as zVAD, decrease apoptosis and improve organ function in diverse AKI models and warrants further investigation.[28]

Necroptosis, MPTP-Mediated Necrosis, and Ferroptosis

Necroptosis is a regulated form of necrosis, initiated through a wide range of triggers, including tumor necrosis factor-alpha (TNFα), first apoptotic signal ligand (FasL), and virus-activated pathways. Necroptosis leads to plasma membrane damage and the release of multiple damage (or danger)-associated molecular pattern molecules, such as interleukin-1α (IL-1α), high-mobility group box 1 (HMGB1), ATP, leading to activation of inflammation. The signaling pathway of necroptosis has been reviewed in detail recently.[29] Necroptosis generally occurs only if prosurvival transcriptional and/or apoptotic pathways are compromised. A potential contribution of necroptosis to ischemic injury in the kidney was suggested by the protective effect of necrostatin-1 (Nec-1), considered as an inhibitor of RIPK1 (see Fig. 2.2). However, Nec-1 might have off-target effects on ferroptosis, while other studies suggest that protection by Nec-1 in models of cyclosporine or contrast mediated injury was independent of an effect on cell death. These observations have raised doubt that the effect of genetic loss of RIPK3, FADD, or caspase-8 or Nec-1 inhibition on reducing kidney IRI are due to primary effects on necroptosis, but the effect rather may be due to extratubular effects including vascular diameter changes and hemodynamic alterations.[30]

In contrast, studies investigating Gpx4 (glutathione peroxidase-4) suggest an important role for ferroptosis, a nonapoptotic form of cell death, in AKI. Gpx4 catalyzes the reduction of hydrogen peroxide, organic hydroperoxides, and lipid peroxides utilizing reduced glutathione and protects against oxidative stress. Gpx4 knockdown renders human proximal tubule cells more susceptible to ferroptosis inducing agents, indicating Gpx4 regulates ferroptotic machinery in these cells. In a recent study, Linkermann et al.[30] reported a significant role for iron-dependent ferroptosis in necrosis of renal tubules in models of severe IRI and oxalate crystal-induced AKI. In addition, an inducible Gpx4-/- mutation results in lipid oxidation, tubular cell death, and AKI.[19]

Linkermann's group[30] also reported that double knockout of cyclophilin D and RIPK3 provides stronger protection against prolonged ischemic injury than the respective single knockout mice, suggesting an additive protective effect by blocking both necrosis and necroptosis. The use of the ferroptosis inhibitor ferrostatin (termed 16-86) to protect from renal IRI is superior to Nec-1 and to that of the cypD inhibitor, sanglifehrin A (SfA). A combination therapy with 16-86 and (Nec-1 + SfA) in a model of ultrasevere IRI (bilateral renal pedicle clamping for 50 minutes) reduced plasma levels of serum urea and serum creatinine, suggesting that a triple combination therapy with (Nec-1 + SfA) plus 16-86 is superior to double-combination therapy (Nec-1 + SfA) on the development of AKI. These data suggest that at least 3 independent pathways of regulated necrosis may be involved in ischemia/reperfusion-mediated organ damage.[30]

Autophagy

The role of autophagy in AKI if protective or deleterious remains controversial as several studies provided evidence for a renoprotective role, while others demonstrated autophagy as another form of cell death. Kimura et al.[31] demonstrated heightened renal ischemia–reperfusion injury in proximal tubule-specific Atg5-knockout mice, providing the first in vivo genetic evidence for a renoprotective role in this AKI model. Dong et al.[32] used both pharmacologic and genetic approaches to determine the role of autophagy in ischemic, as well as cisplatin nephrotoxic, AKI. Their results show that inhibition of autophagy by chloroquine or conditional Atg7 ablation from proximal tubules aggravates AKI, whereas activation of autophagy by rapamycin protects against AKI.

RECOVERY, MALADAPTIVE REPAIR, AND PROGRESSION

Following renal injury, resolution of renal function is typically observed in surviving patients. Importantly, repair processes are invoked immediately following renal injury and include the upregulation of cytoprotective compounds such as heat shock proteins, heme oxygenase, and/or other antioxidants, which may help in survival of sublethally damaged cells. An important component of tissue repair is the proliferation of proximal tubule epithelial cells following renal injury. It is widely accepted that the source of regenerating cells in the proximal tubule is from adjacent surviving proximal tubule cells, which dedifferentiate and undergo cell division and redifferentiation and are not derived from a population of stem cells.[2] Importantly, exogenous compounds such as growth factors or progenitor cell extracts appear to enhance the proliferative activity of these cells and result in better outcomes in rats and mice.

In contrast, it has become apparent in recent years that some patients experience progression to chronic kidney disease (CKD) following the initial episode. This AKI to CKD transition has been suggested to be the result of a balance between adaptive and maladaptive repair responses.[33] Interestingly, there is a less robust proximal tubule proliferation in aging mice that is associated with incomplete regeneration following injury and a predisposition toward CKD.[34] Moreover, it is becoming widely appreciated that some cells may become arrested in the G2 phase of the cell cycle or fail to completely redifferentiate. This state is associated with the liberation of pro-fibrotic cytokines such as transforming growth factor beta and may contribute to the development of CKD.[2] It is possible that these repair processes are further impaired in the setting of pre-existing renal insufficiency or with other risk factors such as diabetes.

Other elements of tissue repair following injury have also been identified that may be associated with the AKI to CKD progression. For example, there is a permanent reduction in peritubular capillaries, which is indicative of a lack of repair potential within the vascular compartment. The loss of capillaries exacerbates renal hypoxia and promotes the development of interstitial fibrosis following the initial recovery from AKI (Fig. 2.4). In addition, there are other alterations in the renal interstitium.[2] Following renal injury, pericytes detach from the endothelial cells, destabilizing the vasculature and differentiating into profibrotic myofibroblasts. In addition, persistent activation of innate and adaptive immune cells participate in the promotion of interstitial fibrosis and the development of hypertension. Thus, a complex milieu exists between incomplete tubular regeneration and an altered interstitial state, which influences the AKI to CKD transition.[2]

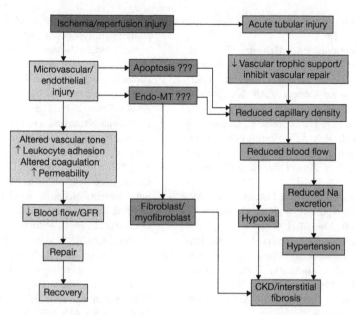

FIGURE 2.4 Putative model for the influence of vascular injury in the setting of renal IRI. The illustration suggests that IRI results in damage to both tubular epithelial and vascular cells. Alteration in vascular function results from damage to endothelial and smooth muscle cells that affect early blood flow and contribute to reduced GFR and continued injury to the tubular epithelium. Reduction in peritubular capillary density is associated with loss of endothelial cells through undetermined mechanisms. Loss of trophic support or production of inhibitory factors from the epithelium has been proposed. Alteration in capillary structure increases hypoxia-mediated fibrosis and alters proper hemodynamics that contribute to hypertension. IRI = ischemia reperfusion injury. GFR = glomerular filtration rate. Endo-MT = endothelial-mesenchymal transition. CKD = chronic kidney disease. With permission from Basile DP. The endothelial cell in ischemic acute kidney injury: implications for acute and chronic function. Kidney Int. 2007;72:151–156.

REFERENCES

1. Kidney Disease: Improving Global Outcomes (KDIGO) Acute Kidney Injury Work Group. KDIGO clinical practice guideline for acute kidney injury. *Kidney Int Suppl.* 2012;2(3):1–138.
2. Basile DP, Anderson M, Sutton TA. Pathophysiology of acute kidney injury. *Compr Physiol* 2012;2:1303–1353.
3. Heyman SN, Rosenberger C, Rosen S. Experimental ischemia–reperfusion: biases and myths—the proximal vs. distal hypoxic tubular injury debate revisited. *Kidney Int.* 2010;77:9–16.
4. Basile DP. The endothelial cell in ischemic acute kidney injury: implications for acute and chronic function. *Kidney Int.* 2007;72:151–156.
5. Matejovic M, Ince C, Chawla LS, et al. Renal hemodynamics in AKI: in search of new treatment targets. *J Am Soc Nephrol.* 2016;27:49–58.
6. Regner K, Roman R. Role of medullary blood flow in the pathogenesis of renal ischemia-reperfusion injury. *Curr Opin Nephrol Hy.* 2012;21:33–38.
7. Muroya Y, Fan F, Regner KR, et al. Deficiency in the formation of 20-hydroxyeicosatetraenoic acid

enhances renal ischemia-reperfusion injury. *J Am Soc Nephrol.* 2015;26:2460–2469.
8. Pohlmann A, Hentschel J, Fechner M, et al. High temporal resolution parametric MRI monitoring of the initial ischemia/reperfusion phase in experimental acute kidney injury. *PLoS One.* 2013;8:e57411.
9. Wang Z, Holthoff JH, Seely KA, et al. Development of oxidative stress in the peritubular capillary microenvironment mediates sepsis-induced renal microcirculatory failure and acute kidney injury. *Am J Pathol.* 2012;180:505–516.
10. Basile D, Yoder M. Renal endothelial dysfunction in acute kidney ischemia reperfusion. *Cardiovasc Hematol Disord Drug Targets.* 2014;14:3–14.
11. Kwon O, Hong S-M, Sutton TA, Temm CJ. Preservation of peritubular capillary endothelial integrity and increasing pericytes may be critical to recovery from postischemic acute kidney injury. *Am J Physiol Renal.* 2008;295:F351–F359.
12. Sutton TA, Fisher CJ, Molitoris BA. Microvascular endothelial injury and dysfunction during

ischemic acute renal failure. *Kidney Int.* 2002;62:1539–1549.

13. Collett J, Corridon PR, Mehrotra P, et al. Hydrodynamic isotonic fluid delivery ameliorates moderate to severe ischemia/reperfusion injury in rat kidneys. *J Am Soc Nephrol.* 2017;28(7):2081–2092.

14. Zheng J, Devalaraja-Narashimha K, Singaravelu K, Padanilam BJ. Poly(ADP-ribose) polymerase-1 gene ablation protects mice from ischemic renal injury. *Am J Physiol Renal.* 2005;288(2):F387–F398.

15. Bensaad K, Tsuruta A, Selak MA, et al. TIGAR, a p53-inducible regulator of glycolysis and apoptosis. *Cell 1.* 2006;126:107–120.

16. Kim J, Devalaraja-Narashimha K, Padanilam BJ. TIGAR regulates glycolysis in ischemic kidney proximal tubules. *Am J Physiol-Renal.* 2015;308:F298–F308.

17. Weinberg JM. Lipotoxicity. *Kidney Int.* 2006;70:1560–1566.

18. Feldkamp T, Park JS, Pasapulati R, Amora D, et al. Regulation of the mitochondrial membrane permeability transition in kidney proximal tubules and its alteration during hypoxia-reoxygenation. *Am J Physiol Renal Physiol.* 2009;297:F1632–F1646.

19. Friedmann Angeli JP, Schneider M, Proneth B, et al. Inactivation of the ferroptosis regulator Gpx4 triggers acute renal failure in mice. *Nat Cell Biol.* 2014;16:1180–1191.

20. Portilla D, Dai G, McClure T, et al. Alterations of PPARalpha and its coactivator PGC-1 in cisplatin-induced acute renal failure. *Kidney Int.* 2003;62:1208–1218.

21. Jang HR, Rabb H. Immune cells in experimental acute kidney injury. *Nat Rev Nephrol.* 2015;11:88–101.

22. Kinsey GR, Li L, Okusa MD. Inflammation in acute kidney injury. *Nephron Exp Nephrol.* 2008;109:e102–e107.

23. Lee S, Huen S, Nishio H, et al. Distinct macrophage phenotypes contribute to kidney injury and repair. *J Am Soc Nephrol.* 2010;22: 317–326.

24. Devalaraja-Narashimha K, Diener AM, and Padanilam BJ. Cyclophilin D gene ablation protects mice from ischemic renal injury. *Am J Physiol-Renal.* 2009;297:F749–F759.

25. Devalaraja-Narashimha K, Padanilam BJ. PARP-1 inhibits glycolysis in ischemic kidneys. *J Am Soc Nephrol.* 2009;20:95–103.

26. Ying Y, Kim J, Westphal SN, Long KE, Padanilam BJ. Targeted deletion of p53 in the proximal tubule prevents ischemic renal injury. *J Am Soc Nephrol.* 2014;25:2707–2716.

27. Green DR, Reed JC. Mitochondria and apoptosis. *Science.* 1998;281(5381):1309–1312.

28. Yang Y, Song M, Liu Y, et al. Renoprotective approaches and strategies in acute kidney injury. *Pharmacol Therapeut.* 206;163:58–73.

29. Linkermann A, Green DR. Necroptosis. *N Engl J Med.* 2014;370:455–465.

30. Linkermann A, Skouta R, Himmerkus N, et al. Synchronized renal tubular cell death involves ferroptosis. *P Natl Acad Sci USA.* 2014;111:16836–16841.

31. Kimura T, Takabatake Y, Takahashi A, et al. Autophagy protects the proximal tubule from degeneration and acute ischemic injury. *J Am Soc Nephrol.* 2011;22(5):902–913.

32. Jiang M, Wei Q-q, Dong G, Komatsu M, Su Y, and Dong Z. Autophagy in proximal tubules protects against acute kidney injury. *Kidney international.* 2012;82:1271–1283.

33. Basile DP, Bonventre JV, Mehta R, et al.; Group tAXW. Progression after AKI: understanding maladaptive repair processes to predict and identify therapeutic treatments. *J Am Soc Nephrol.* 2016;27:687–697.

34. Schmitt R, Marlier A, and Cantley LG. Zag expression during aging suppresses proliferation after kidney injury. *J Am Soc Nephrol.* 2008;19:2375–2383.

3

Adaptation in Acute Kidney Injury

Progression to Chronic Kidney Disease

NAVIN JAIPAUL

REPAIR AFTER AKI

Acute kidney injury (AKI) is typically the result of hemodynamic and nephrotoxic insults, occurring in isolation or combination and causing damage to the renal parenchyma. After injury develops, the kidney possesses the ability to repair itself (Fig. 3.1). Until recently, complete structural and functional recovery from AKI was traditionally considered the likely outcome if the clinical factors mediating the process could be reversed early and fully. It is now understood, however, that the biologic response to AKI depends on a variety of environmental and host factors predicated on the ability of the kidney to adapt in response to an insult.[1] Whether and the extent to which that adaptation is adequate or inadequate to restore structure and function to the organ ultimately determines the outcome of AKI. On one end of the spectrum is return to a condition indistinguishable from the uninjured kidney and on the other end is irreversible damage associated with increased risk of progression to chronic kidney disease (CKD) and the eventual development of end stage renal disease.[2] An admixture of appropriate and inappropriate adaptations, and the balance between them, in response to injury may be associated with partial (incomplete) renal recovery and CKD progression.

Structural damage and functional impairment often persist after development of AKI. Defining the resolution or progression of AKI in this context requires precise terminology of the processes implicated in the response to renal damage. To this effect, a working group of the 13th Acute Dialysis Quality Initiative[3] proposed new terms to describe the various phases and potential sequelae of renal response to injury: repair, adaptive repair, maladaptive repair, recovery, and progression. Repair refers to a biologic process conditioned on environmental and host factors. Adaptive repair is a desired response to injury where structural and functional abnormalities are fully reversed. Maladaptive repair is a misaligned response which results in persistence of structural changes and renal dysfunction over time. Recovery may be partial or complete, depending on the nature of the original injury and type of reparative response. Progression implies chronicity resulting from irreversible injury.

PROGRESSION TO CKD AFTER AKI

When a renal insult first occurs, injury and repair begin almost simultaneously. The immediate impact of this injury on the kidney may not be clinically evident by traditional serum markers such as creatinine or estimated glomerular filtration rate (eGFR), because residual renal reserve compensates for the presence of early damage. At this subclinical stage, however, specific biomarkers may be produced in response to the injury and be detected and measured via nontraditional methods.[4] As the injury evolves to overwhelm the compensatory mechanisms in the kidney, the structural and functional clinical manifestations of the process eventually become apparent. The balance between ongoing injury and the nature of the repair during these stages determine the degree to which resolution from the original insult is possible. For example, patients with mild renal injury will often benefit from adaptive repair processes where complete restoration of normal kidney function is achieved without long-term effects, whereas patients with more severe renal injury or injury superimposed

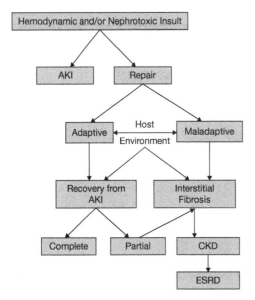

FIGURE 3.1 Repair after AKI. In response to an insult, onset of AKI and repair begin almost simultaneously. Depending on host and environmental factors, the balance between adaptive and maladaptive repair processes determines the outcome of AKI, ranging from complete to partial renal recovery or progression to CKD including ESRD. The hallmark of CKD progression is development of interstitial fibrosis, which may be the direct result of maladaptive repair or sequelae after partial renal recovery. AKI = acute kidney injury; CKD = chronic kidney disease; ESRD = end-stage renal disease.

and secretion of factors, which mediate paracrine fibrotic effects in the renal interstitium.[8] For example, tubular epithelial cells may produce cytokines such as transforming growth factor beta and extracellular matrix proteins like connective tissue growth factor, which accelerate proliferation of interstitial fibroblasts and expansion of interstitial matrix.[9] Progression is ultimately conditioned on the necessary presence of these maladaptive processes because the resulting interstitial fibrosis reduces functional renal reserve and predisposes to the additive effects of repeated renal injury over time. Maladaptation to AKI and the resulting fibrosis, however, are not by themselves sufficient to promote progression to CKD because renal fibrosis is not inherently progressive; it requires additional injury.[5] Fibrosis surrounds atrophic tubules and partially serves the purpose of protecting uninjured parenchyma from damage. It does not extend to intact portions of the tubulointerstitium unless additional nephrons are recruited by way of repetitive or severe injury.[5] Therefore, propagation of fibrosis is essentially the cumulative result of recurrent episodes of maladaptive responses in response to continued clinical or subclinical injury. The process may be slow and deliberate or rapidly progressive depending on the severity of the insult and the nature of the repair response that ensues.

on CKD may suffer the consequences of maladaptive repair resulting in fibrotic changes to the structure of the kidney that contribute to long-term functional impairment and further deterioration in renal reserve over time.[3]

The transition from AKI to CKD involves maladaptive repair processes that culminate in the development of interstitial fibrosis. This maladaptation occurs at multiple intrinsic kidney levels and through various mechanistic pathways elucidated by various animal models. For example, hemodynamic alterations in the kidney may predispose to capillary dropout causing sustained renal hypoxia, which prevents recovery of the affected segment and promotes tubular atrophy and interstitial fibrosis.[5,6] In addition to rarefaction at the vascular level, endothelial cells may exhibit a phenotypic transformation in favor of fibroblast production and enhanced interstitial fibrosis.[7] At the tubular level, cell division may arrest in the G2 phase of the cell cycle, and this prolongation may lead to the synthesis

BIOCHEMICAL PATHWAYS INVOLVED IN REPAIR RESPONSE TO AKI

Understanding that maladaptive repair is invoked in the transition of AKI to CKD, the natural question that arises is, what cellular processes are targetable to interfere with the progression of renal disease? Proposed pathways at the cellular level have included hypoxia and oxidative injury, cell cycle arrest, phenotypic changes in gene expression, and mitochondrial dysfunction (Table 3.1).[3]

As previously mentioned, the renal parenchyma, particularly the S3 segment of the proximal tubule, is especially sensitive to persistence of hypoxia and oxidative damage. To defend against these stressors, cells contain transcriptional factors like hypoxia-inducible factor (HIF) that, upon activation, upregulates various gene products that promote cell survival via angiogenesis and restored capillary density.[10] Animal models have demonstrated that HIF activation before induction of AKI both mitigates

TABLE 3.1. BIOCHEMICAL PATHWAYS AND POTENTIAL TARGETS FOR THERAPEUTIC INTERVENTION AFTER ACUTE KIDNEY INJURY

Pathway	Potential Targets	Target Response to Activation
Oxidation injury	Hypoxia-inducible factor	Before AKI: angiogenesis and restored capillary density
		After AKI: antiangiogenesis and increased capillary rarefaction
	Vascular endothelial growth factor	Early AKI: angiogenesis and restored capillary density
		Late AKI: antiangiogenesis and increased capillary rarefaction
	Nuclear factor (erythroid-derived 2)-like 2	Expression of antioxidant gene products
Cell cycle arrest	DNA damage response	Phase-specific checkpoints monitor, signal, and direct repair of DNA
Phenotypic alterations in gene expression	Vascular and tubular cell-specific elements	Profibrotic senescent secretory cell phenotype
Mitochondrial dysfunction	Mitochondria-specific elements	Decreased cellular ATP generation and increased mitochondrial reactive oxygen species

AKI = acute kidney injury. ATP = adenosine triphosphate.

the severity of renal injury and mediates an antifibrotic effect by preventing inflammatory sequelae and encouraging adaptive repair.[11] Activation of HIF after induction of AKI, however, may have the opposite effect to exaggerate a maladaptive response to injury. This may be the result of other antiangiogenic factors that blunt the normal response to HIF.[10] Therefore, HIF represents 1 possible therapeutic target to attenuate AKI to CKD progression, though its potential may be limited by a relatively early and short period of opportunity after injury. This same limitation applies to vascular endothelial growth factor (VEGF), which is stimulated by HIF and is protective when invoked in response to hypoxia in the early postinjury period but not in the later phases of kidney damage.[12] This may be related to the observation that VEGF expression is decreased in CKD, likely resulting from diminished production by damaged tubular epithelial cells, partly in response to reduced HIF activity, and suppression by the inflammatory milieu associated with the disease state.[10] Nuclear factor (erythroid-derived 2)-like 2 (Nrf2) is a third transcription factor and potential therapeutic target that is expressed throughout the body but is present in highest concentration in the kidney.[13] It is activated in response to hypoxia and upregulates

expression of antioxidant gene products that may blunt the effects of ischemic AKI.[14]

Ischemic or nephrotoxic kidney injury may also induce DNA damage at the cellular level. In response to DNA damage, cells activate a complex network of pathways that monitor, signal, and direct the repair of DNA to prevent potentially serious mutations from arising. This is referred to as the DNA damage response.[15] However, this process may also result in cell cycle arrest or cell death.[15] During the normal process of cell division, the cell cycle is divided into 4 distinct phases: G0-G1, S, G2, and M (Fig. 3.2). G0 is a resting phase during which the cell is not engaged in the cell cycle or division process. The G1 phase is defined by cell growth and synthesis of components required for DNA duplication, which occurs during the S phase. This is followed by a rapid phase of cell growth (G2) and finally the mitosis (M) phase, which is characterized by cessation of cell growth and progression to cell division. Each phase in the cell cycle also represents a checkpoint where problems that arise during cell division can be corrected before proceeding through the remainder of the cycle.[8] Disruptions in the safeguards that form the basis for this process may lead to

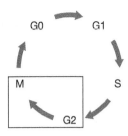

FIGURE 3.2 The cell cycle. During the normal process of cell division, cells proceed from a resting phase (G0) through a period of initial cell growth (G1), DNA synthesis (S), rapid cell growth (G2), and mitosis (M). Arrest of cell growth in the G2/M phase (boxed area) occurs during maladaptive repair, predisposing to a profibrotic senescent secretory phenotype.

undesirable outcomes. For example, during maladaptive repair, the cell cycle arrests in the G2/M phase of the cell cycle.[16] This pathologic growth arrest inhibits recovery from AKI by preventing dedifferentiated tubular cells from redifferentiating into a normal phenotype.[5] Instead, the cells assume the function of a profibrotic senescent secretory phenotype as previously mentioned.[8] This phenotypic alteration leads to expansion of interstitial matrix and progression to CKD. Therefore, the G2/M checkpoint in the cell cycle represents another potential target for therapeutic intervention.

Oxidative stress to the kidney has also been implicated in the development of mitochondrial dysfunction, which may further promote renal fibrosis.[17] The regulation of cellular metabolism is largely dependent on the intact function of mitochondria. Though the primary role of mitochondria is to generate adenosine triphosphate (ATP), the organelles also produce and detoxify reactive oxygen species. In an animal model treated with hypochlorite-modified albumin (HOCl-alb) to replicate oxidative stress, animals given HOCl-alb exhibited multiple manifestations of mitochondrial dysfunction culminating in increased interstitial fibrosis associated with deterioration in kidney function.[18] These effects ranged from decrease in mitochondrial membrane potential and ATP generation to increased production of mitochondrial reactive oxygen species in renal parenchyma. Administration of a mitochondrial-specific antioxidant peptide prevented these complications. This suggests that the mitochondrial pathway may represent another novel therapeutic target in the progression of AKI to CKD.

EMERGING METHODS TO DETECT EARLY OR SUBCLINICAL AKI

Despite the promising advances that have been made in understanding the physiologic basis for AKI to CKD progression and in identifying potential therapeutic targets for intervention, challenges remain for translating this knowledge into practical clinical applications and patient management tools. Currently, we lack effective interventions for attenuating or reversing the course of AKI. This difficulty is largely related to the challenge of identifying patients at highest risk for progression to CKD, because of limited diagnostic markers to detect early nephron injury in the kidney. Traditional serum markers like creatinine detect late kidney injury and are ineffective for recognizing subclinical AKI. Additionally, serum creatinine level may be influenced by other patient factors like age, gender, muscle mass, and nutritional supplement intake. In response to this, development of nontraditional serum biomarkers capable of detecting and quantifying early tubular injury has been an active field of investigation. Examples of proposed tubular biomarkers with predictive potential for CKD include kidney injury molecule-1 (KIM-1), neutrophil gelatinase-associated lipocalin (NGAL), liver-type fatty acid-binding protein (L-FABP), and interleukin-18 (1L-18).[19] KIM-1 is a 38.7-kD transmembrane protein minimally expressed in the normal kidney but upregulated in response to ischemia/reperfusion injury. It appears to promote regeneration and regulate apoptosis of proximal tubular epithelial cells, with a peak in activity approximately 48 hours after injury.[18] NGAL is a 25-kD protein expressed in various human tissues including the kidney. Expressed primarily in the thick ascending limb and renal collecting ducts, NGAL is markedly upregulated in response to ischemic or nephrotoxic kidney injury, with urinary levels detectable as early as 3 hours following the insult.[20] L-FABP is a 14-kD proximal tubule protein expressed soon after kidney injury with a urinary peak typically within 6 hours of the insult.[21] IL-18 is a 22-kD cytokine located in proximal tubular cells; it mediates an inflammatory renal response and is detectable in the urine as early as 4 hours after ischemic injury with peak levels around 12 hours.[22]

Despite the plausibility of utilizing these tubular biomarkers to detect subclinical AKI, they do not distinguish adaptive from maladaptive repair and therefore do not differentiate progression attributable to AKI from that due to underlying CKD. Urinary biomarker levels may also be influenced by the presence of other urinary findings like hematuria and pyuria.[23] Therefore, reliance on tubular biomarkers alone in detecting onset of AKI poses practical challenges. Alternative epigenetic biomarker approaches, such as analyzing DNA methylation patterns, may represent an emerging field of investigation to quantify the risk of progression in patients with already established CKD but not necessarily the transition from AKI to CKD.[24,25] Another area of emerging interest that shows promise for individualizing susceptibility risk for CKD after AKI is related to various magnetic resonance (MR) and positron emission tomography (PET) imaging techniques that target and detect collagen as a quantifiable marker of fibrosis. For example, stiffness of medullary renal parenchyma measured by magnetic resonance elastography (MRE) in a swine model correlated significantly with the histological degree of fibrosis.[26] Other animal models have also demonstrated utility of novel MR imaging contrast agents and Cu-labeled peptides in PET targeting collagen to detect liver or cardiac fibrosis,[27,28] so it is plausible that these techniques may offer potential to evaluate renal fibrosis as well.

FUTURE DIRECTIONS IN RISK IDENTIFICATION AND QUANTIFICATION FOR CKD PROGRESSION AFTER AKI

Due to the inherent limitations of single biomarker methods in predicting and quantifying the risk of progression to CKD after AKI, it is likely that some combination of biomarkers and traditional methods to evaluate renal function will be necessary to identify the patients with the highest likelihood of progression.[29] For example, elevation in injury-specific biomarkers concurrent with rise in serum creatinine may indicate a higher risk of progression than either occurrence in isolation.[29] By extension of that logic, the advances in the previously mentioned imaging techniques may offer potential in the future for further quantifying or modifying that risk.

Severity of initial AKI presentation, incomplete recovery after AKI, recurrent AKI, and AKI superimposed on CKD are all well-recognized clinical risk factors for progression to CKD.[30] Recently, AKI has also been identified as a risk factor for development of incident or worsening proteinuria,[31] consistent with maladaptive repair

physiology and the associated interstitial fibrosis contributing to CKD progression. In light of this, identification of patients at highest risk for CKD represents both an opportunity and a challenge to improve outcomes in patients who have suffered an AKI event. Researchers have sought to develop clinical risk prediction tools for CKD progression after AKI based predominantly on epidemiological data gathered from observational studies.[32] One such model derived from a cohort of hospitalized veterans included clinical variables such as age, AKI stage, albumin, baseline eGFR, time at risk, and need for renal replacement therapy to predict the risk for CKD development after recovery from AKI.[32] However, these risk prediction models have limited utility in their ability to capture or quantify risk associated with early AKI, when intervention to alter the course of disease progression may be most imperative. For example, we are not yet at the point where we can confidently assign or modify risk for CKD after subclinical onset of AKI. Because of this, the sequelae in patients with acute injury are managed similarly to patients with already established CKD and represents a lost opportunity to target potential therapeutic interventions implicated in the repair response to AKI. To refine the clinical approach to AKI management will require our ability to detect early AKI before it becomes clinically evident, differentiate adaptive from maladaptive repair processes, and define and quantify risk for progression to CKD based on a combination of clinical factors, biochemical and functional markers, and perhaps novel emerging imaging techniques (Table 3.2). To date, there are few human studies investigating the predictive value of kidney injury-specific or profibrotic biomarkers. Most research has been conducted in animal models, which lack disease states like hypertension or diabetes associated with the human condition and the potential to alter the risk for progression to CKD after an AKI insult. Nevertheless, the future holds much promise for continued investigation into the translational implications of animal-to-human research and the development of more precise and validated risk prediction models derived from incorporation of plausible combinations of clinical, functional, biochemical, and imaging factors. To achieve this desirable outcome will necessitate robust research studies that further refine and elucidate the complexities and adaptations involved in the AKI-induced progression to CKD.

TABLE 3.2 EMERGING METHODS FOR DETECTING AND QUANTIFYING CKD PROGRESSION AFTER ACUTE KIDNEY INJURY

Method	Examples	Implications
Injury-specific biomarkers	Kidney injury molecule-1 (KIM-1) Neutrophil gelatinase-associated Lipocalin Liver-type fatty acid-binding protein Interleukin 18	Detection of subclinical or early-onset AKI
DNA methylation patterns	Gene analysis of proinflammatory or profibrotic factors	Quantify risk of progression in patients with already established CKD
Radiologic imaging techniques	Magnetic resonance elastography Cu-labeled collagen-specific positron emission tomography	Individualize susceptibility risk for CKD after AKI based on detection and quantification of fibrosis

CKD = chronic kidney disease. AKI = acute kidney disease.

REFERENCES

1. Hsu CY. Yes, AKI truly leads to CKD. *J Am Soc Nephrol.* 2012;23:967–969.
2. Coca SG, Singanamala S, Parikh CR. Chronic kidney disease after acute kidney injury: a systematic review and meta-analysis. *Kidney Int.* 2012;81:442–448.
3. Basile DP, Bonventre JV, Mehta R, et al. Progression after AKI: Understanding maladaptive repair processes to predict and identify therapeutic treatments. *J Am Soc Nephrol* 2016;27:687–697.
4. Murray PT, Mehta RL, Shaw A, et al. ADQI 10 workgroup: Potential use of biomarkers in acute kidney injury: Report and summary recommendations from the 10th Acute Dialysis Quality Initiative Consensus Conference. *Kidney Intl* 2014;85:513–521.
5. Venkatachalam MA, Weinberg JM, Kriz W, Bidani AK. Failed tubule recovery, AKI-CKD transition, and kidney disease progression. *J Am Soc Nephrol* 2015;26:1765–1776.
6. Basile DP, Donohoe D, Roethe K, Osborn JL. Renal ischemic injury results in permanent damage to peritubular capillaries and influences long-term function. *Am J Physiol Renal Physiol* 2001;281:F887–F899.
7. Basile DP, Friedrich JL, Spahic J, et al. Impaired endothelial proliferation and mesenchymal transition contribute to vascular rarefaction following acute kidney injury. *Am J Physiol Renal Physiol* 2011;300:F721–F733.
8. Canaud G, Bonventre JV. Cell cycle arrest and the evolution of chronic kidney disease from acute kidney injury. *Nephrol Dial Transplant* 2015;30:575–583.
9. Venkatachalam MA, Griffin KA, Lan R, Geng H, Saikumar P, Bidani AK. Acute kidney injury: A springboard for progression to chronic kidney disease. *Am J Physiol Renal Physiol* 2010;298:F1078–F1094.
10. Tanaka S, Tanaka T, Nangaku M. Hypoxia and hypoxia-inducible factors in chronic kidney disease. *Renal Replacement Therapy* 2016;2:25.
11. Kapitsinou PP, Jaffe J, Michael M, et al. Pre-ischemic targeting of HIF prolyl hydroxylation inhibits fibrosis associated with acute kidney injury. *Am J Physiol Renal Physiol* 2012;302:F1172–F1179.
12. Leonard EC, Friedrich JL, Basile DP. VEGF-121 preserves renal microvessel structure and ameliorates secondary renal disease following acute kidney injury. *Am J Physiol Renal Physiol* 2008;295:F1648–1657.
13. Moi P, Chan K, Asunis I, Cao A, Kan YW. Isolation of NF-E2-related factor 2 (Nrf2), a NF-E2-like basic leucine zipper transcriptional activator that binds to the tandem NF-E2/AP1 repeat of the beta-globin locus control region. *Proc Natl Acad Sci USA* 1994;91:9926–9930.
14. Lui M, Reddy NM, Higbee EM, et al. The Nrf2 triterpenoid activator, CDDO-imidazolide, protects kidneys from ischemia-reperfusion injury in mice. *Kidney Int* 2014;85:134–141.

15. Jackson SP, Bartek J. The DNA-damage response in human biology and disease. *Nature* 2009;461:1071–1078.

16. Yang L, Besschetnova TY, Brooks CR, Shah JV, Bonventre JV. Epithelial cell cycle arrest in G2/M mediates kidney fibrosis after injury. *Nat Med* 2010;16:535–543.

17. Stallons LJ, Whitaker RM, Schnellmann RG. Suppressed mitochondrial biogenesis in folic acid-induced acute kidney injury and early fibrosis. *Toxicol Lett* 2014;224:326–332.

18. Zhao H, Liu YJ, Liu ZR, Tang DD, Chen XW, Chen YH, Zhou RN, et al. Role of mitochondrial dysfunction in renal fibrosis promoted by hypochlorite-modified albumin in a remnant kidney model and protective effects of antioxidant peptide SS-31. *Eur J Pharmacol* 2017;804:57–67.

19. Tan HL, Yap JQ, Qian Q. Acute kidney injury: Tubular markers and risk of chronic kidney disease and end-stage kidney failure. *Blood Purif* 2016;41:144–150.

20. Boligano D, Lacquaniti A, Coppolino G, et al. Neutrophil gelatinase-associated lipocalin (NGAL) and progression of chronic kidney disease. *Clin J Am Soc Nephrol* 2009;4:337–344.

21. Susantitaphong R, Siribamrungwong M, Doi K, Noiri E, Terrin N, Jaber BL. Performance of urinary liver-type fatty acid-binding protein in acute kidney injury: A meta-analysis. *Am J Kidney Dis* 2013;61:430–439.

22. Parikh CR, Jani A, Melnikov VY, Faubel S, Edelstein CL. Urinary interleukin-18 is a marker of human acute tubular necrosis. *Am J Kidney Dis* 2004;43:405–414.

23. Nadkarni GN, Coca SG, Meisner A, et al. Urinalysis findings and urinary kidney injury biomarker concentrations. *BMC Nephrol* 2017;18:218.

24. Wing MR, Devaney JM, Joffe MM, et al. Chronic Renal Insufficiency Cohort (CRIC) Study: DNA methylation profile associated with rapid decline in kidney function: findings from the CRIC study. *Nephrol Dial Transplant* 2014;29:864–872.

25. Wing MR, Ramezani A, Gill HS, Devaney JM, Raj DS. Epigenetics of progression of chronic kidney disease: Fact or fantasy? *Semin Nephrol* 2013;33:363–374.

26. Korsmo MJ, Ebrahimi B, Eirin A, et al. Magnetic resonance elastography noninvasively detects in vivo renal medullary fibrosis secondary to swine renal artery stenosis. *Invest Radiol* 2013;48:61–68.

27. Polasek M, Fuchs BC, Uppal R, et al. Molecular MR imaging of liver fibrosis: A feasibility study using rat and mouse models. *J Hepatol* 2012;57:549–555.

28. Kim JS, Kim I, Lee S-J, Kim H, Davies-Venn C, Won S, et al. Longitudinal analysis of PET imaging with Cu-64-labeled collagen specific peptides for detection of collagen in myocardial fibrosis in rats. *J Nucl Med* 2014;55:408.

29. McCullough PA, Shaw AD, Haase M, et al. Diagnosis of acute kidney injury using functional and injury biomarkers: Workgroup statements from the tenth Acute Dialysis Quality Initiative Consensus Conference. *Contrib Nephrol* 2013; 182:13–29.

30. Heung M, Chawla LS. Predicting progression to chronic kidney disease after recovery from acute kidney injury. *Curr Opin Nephrol Hypertens* 2012;21:628–634.

31. Parr SK, Matheny ME, Abdel-Kader K, et al. Acute kidney injury is a risk factor for subsequent proteinuria. *Kidney Int* 2017; [Epub ahead of print].

32. Chawla LS, Amdur RL, Amodeo S, et al. The severity of acute kidney injury predicts progression to chronic kidney disease. *Kidney Int* 2011;79:1361–1369.

4

Risk Factors for Chronic Kidney Disease

HANIA KASSEM AND BERNARD G. JAAR

Many risk factors for chronic kidney disease (CKD) have been identified and well described in the medical literature. Even though it might be difficult to prove causality in some cases, some associations are more convincing than others. In this chapter, known nonmodifiable and modifiable risk factors for CKD will be reviewed (Table 4.1). Some of those risk factors will be discussed in more detail in other chapters.

NONMODIFIABLE RISK FACTORS

Age

Data from the National Health and Nutrition Examination Surveys (NHANES) showed that all stages of CKD were more prevalent in older individuals. Some, but not all, of the increase in CKD prevalence was attributed to the increase in diabetes mellitus (DM) and hypertension (HTN) with age.[1] Age appears to be a risk factor for CKD; however, the rate of decline in renal function is variable in the elderly with different cohorts showing faster or slower decline with age.[2-5] On average, glomerular filtration rate (GFR) declines by 0.75 to 1 mL/min/year and by up to 2.7 mL/min/year in patients with diabetes.[3-5]

Many histologic changes take place in the aging kidney, including glomerular, vascular, and tubulointerstitial changes.[6] Based on renal biopsy findings in healthy kidney transplant donors, the prevalence of nephrosclerosis increased gradually with age, and was noted to be up to 73% in donors over 70 years of age compared to 2.7% in donors 18 to 29 years old.[7] Impaired autoregulation causing glomerular HTN as well as a variable response to vasodilators and vasoconstrictors in the renal vasculature might be responsible for some of the structural changes observed.[6]

It is, however, difficult to control for all the factors that affect kidney function and that are more prevalent with aging such as systemic illnesses or a longer exposure to a certain diet or toxins. It might also be inaccurate to assess kidney function based on serum creatinine alone in the elderly. Given those limitations, the variable rate of renal function decline with age, and the absence of CKD in a good proportion of the elderly population, age alone may be considered a controversial risk factor for CKD.

Gender

It is generally believed that men are at higher risk of CKD than women and according to data from the annual United States Renal Data System reports, the incidence of treated end stage renal disease (ESRD), examined periodically, is persistently higher in men.[8] The effect of gender on risk of CKD might be related to differences in renal structure and hemodynamics.[9] It might also be due to the antifibrotic properties of endogenous estrogens.[10] However, findings from different cohorts have not been consistent. In a cross-sectional study from Japan, low estimated GFR (eGFR) was more prevalent in men.[11] And the rate of decline of renal function was found to be lower in women based on a 10-year population-based study from Norway.[4] On the other hand, the CREDIT study from Turkey showed that CKD was more prevalent in women.[12] A meta-analysis, published in 2003, of randomized controlled trials evaluating the efficacy of angiotensin-converting enzyme inhibitors for slowing renal disease progression showed that women had a faster rate of decline in renal function.[13] Many possibilities could explain the discrepancy in those findings, including the proportion of postmenopausal women in each of those studies as well as the etiology of CKD in the participants, a factor that might not be easy

TABLE 4.1 MODIFIABLE AND NONMODIFIABLE RISK FACTORS FOR CHRONIC KIDNEY DISEASE

Nonmodifiable risk factors

Age

Gender

Ethnicity

Family history

Low birth weight

Modifiable risk factors

Acute kidney injury

Obstructive uropathies

Kidney stones

Obstructive sleep apnea

Smoking

Systemic illnesses	Diabetes mellitus
	Hypertension
	Hepatitis B and C
	HIV
	Systemic lupus, erythematosus, and other autoimmune diseases
	Sickle cell disease
	Cardiovascular disease
Drugs	Analgesics/NSAIDs
	Proton pump inhibitors
	Sodium phosphate
	Illicit drugs
Diet and the metabolic syndrome	Hyperuricemia
	Obesity
	Western-style diet

to delineate in population-based studies. The characteristics of each cohort are especially important when determining the effect of gender as it has been shown that there are significant gender differences in the established predictors of renal function decline.[14] Albuminuria, for instance, is a more important prognostic factor in men.[14] Furthermore, gender inequities in healthcare inevitably affect results reported from different geographic locations. The limitations of a creatinine-based eGFR will also have an impact on any comparison between genders. Those inaccuracies in estimating renal function are best illustrated by the discrepancy between the higher

prevalence of advanced stages of CKD in women and the significantly higher incidence of ESRD in men.[15]

Race

Race is a perfect example of a very complex risk factor for CKD, where other factors, not necessarily related to a certain genetic background, such as socioeconomic status and access to healthcare, may play a significant role.[16] Socioeconomic factors were linked to risk of CKD in whites as well as African Americans, with some analyses showing an even stronger correlation between a lower socioeconomic status and a higher risk of CKD in Whites than in African Americans.[17]

Furthermore, certain diseases that are directly linked to CKD, such as diabetes and HTN, may be more common in African Americans patients, which would also contribute to the increased risk of CKD seen in this group. However, when examining data from the NHANES, CKD was 2.7 times higher among African Americans compared with whites but only half of the increased risk could be attributed to modifiable factors such as sociodemographic, lifestyle, and clinical factors.[18]

In addition to the increase in the incidence of CKD, African Americans have a faster rate of progression of CKD compared to whites.[19]

Several years ago, missense mutations were identified in the apolipoprotein L-1 (APOL1) gene on chromosome 22 in people of West African descent. The product of this gene is a serum factor that lyses trypanosomes. APOL1 derived from risk alleles confers human resistance to *Trypanosoma brucei rhodesiense*, which is responsible for sleeping sickness. The gene variants were found to be strongly associated with focal segmental glomerulosclerosis, HTN-attributed ESRD, and HIV-associated nephropathy.[20] Those risk variants were later implicated in renal disease progression and the higher rates of ESRD in African Americans.[21]

Compared to whites, not only African Americans had higher rates of ESRD but also Hispanics, Asians, and Native Americans.[19,22–24] But unlike in African Americans, the reasons for the increased risk of CKD in other racial minorities are not fully understood and may not necessarily be related to any specific genetic predisposition.

Family History

A family history of kidney disease is a common finding in ESRD patients. Different reports showed that 20% to 23% of patients with ESRD reported having family members with the disease.[25,26] Race, of course, plays a major role in the association between family history and risk of CKD. Furthermore, the same factors that affect the relationship between race and CKD might also contribute to the familial clustering of CKD. Yet, multivariable analyses confirmed the relationship between family history and risk of ESRD independent of socioeconomic factors such as income, education, and living conditions.[26] On the other hand, family history of ESRD was found to be strongly associated with female gender, early age of onset of ESRD, etiology of the disease, and race of the patients with ESRD.[25,26]

Low Birth Weight

There is a strong association between low birth weight (LBW) and risk of CKD in childhood and adulthood. In one series, the odds ratio for CKD in patients with LBW was reported to be almost 3 times higher compared to normal controls.[27] A more recent meta-analysis confirmed this association and showed no association between high birth weight and risk of CKD.[28] To further analyze the association, and since both LBW and CKD tend to cluster in families, a recent study examined the data in siblings and determined that familial factors alone did not explain the association between LBW and risk of CKD.[29]

Nephrogenesis starts in the first trimester of pregnancy but the total number of nephrons is determined by 36 weeks gestation with more than half of nephrons forming in the last trimester.[30] Moreover, and based on autopsy findings in premature infants, postnatal nephrogenesis in infants born prematurely is impaired and is likely to stop completely 40 days after birth.[31] According to the Brenner's hypothesis, people with a low nephron number develop hyperfiltration in the remaining nephrons as a compensatory mechanism. Conversely, this compensation results eventually in glomerular HTN and glomerulosclerosis further reducing the number of nephrons.[32] Nevertheless, the risk of CKD in premature infants with LBW might not only be related to prenatal factors. Postnatal episodes of acute kidney injury (AKI) secondary to recurrent infections, hemodynamic instability, and nephrotoxic agents might also play a role in the increased risk of CKD in those patients.

MODIFIABLE RISK FACTORS

Other medical conditions that increase the risk of CKD are listed here under modifiable risk factors even though, in some of those conditions, the risk of CKD remains high compared to the general population despite available treatment and attempts at controlling the underlying disease. The role of the following modifiable risk factors will be discussed in detail elsewhere in this book: systemic illnesses, AKI, and obstructive uropathy.

Kidney Stones

Stone formers have been shown to be at increased risk of CKD.[33-35] The increased risk was noted even after a single episode of kidney stone.[34] However, surprisingly, when analyzing the data from the Atherosclerosis Risk in Communities (ARIC) study, nephrolithiasis was not found to be an independent risk factor for CKD except in participants with lower plasma uric acid levels.[36] On the other hand, a recent review confirmed the association between a history of kidney stones and an increased risk of CKD.[37] The risk of CKD is not affected by shock wave lithotripsy or ureteroscopy but is affected by certain stone characteristics such as type, size, and location.[38] Creatinine clearance is lower in cystine and struvite stone formers compared to other stone formers.[39] Kidney function also inversely correlates with cumulative stone size.[40] Furthermore, stone location affects the risk of kidney disease, with the highest risk noted in patients with a history of kidney stone followed by patients with a ureteral stone, and the lowest risk reported in patients with a bladder stone.[41]

Several mechanisms have been proposed to explain the etiology of CKD in stone formers, including acute or recurrent episodes of obstructive uropathy, recurrent pyelonephritis, obstruction of the ducts of Bellini (in brushite stone formers), and papillary necrosis (with staghorn calculi).[42]

Obstructive Sleep Apnea

Sleep apnea is a disorder where an individual experiences multiple episodes of apnea during sleep, frequently resulting in significant hypoxemia. Sleep apnea is further classified into central or obstructive with the latter being the most common and resulting from obstruction in the upper airway during sleep.[43] Both an increased prevalence of sleep apnea in patients with CKD and an increased prevalence of CKD in patients with sleep apnea have been reported.[43-45] This finding is to be expected since both diseases have similar risk factors including age, obesity, and smoking; it is also possible that each of those disorders increases the risk of developing the other.[46] However, establishing sleep apnea as independent risk factor for CKD remains a challenging task. One study in patients with no diabetes or HTN showed that the apnea-hypopnea index, which is the number of apneic and hypopneic episodes per hour of sleep time, was an independent predictor of urinary albumin to creatinine ratio and desaturation index independently predicted eGFR. Most confounding factors in this study were excluded or accounted for.[45] Another study showed an approximately 2-fold increase in the incidence of CKD and ESRD in patients with sleep apnea, independent of factors such as age, sex, and other common medical conditions. However, data on smoking and body mass index were not available in this study.[43] To further support the effect of sleep apnea on the risk of CKD, it has been shown that sleep apnea treatment with continuous positive airway pressure improved glomerular hyperfiltration.[47] On the other hand, a more recent study showed that sleep apnea was associated with an increased risk of CKD only in patients with metabolic syndrome, illustrating again the difficulty in proving an independent effect.[48]

Sleep apnea might correlate with CKD because of the high prevalence of comorbid conditions such as diabetes, HTN, and obesity in patients with sleep apnea. But sleep apnea may also directly affect the kidneys through multiple possible mechanisms. Intermittent hypoxia activates type I angiotensin II receptors causing an increase in blood pressure as well as inflammation and fibrosis, which are known consequences of activation of the renin–angiotensin–aldosterone system (RAAS) at the level of the kidneys.[49,50] The high sympathetic activity affecting renal hemodynamics, hypoxemia-induced reactive oxygen species, and endothelial dysfunction are additional mechanisms that have also been implicated in the increased risk of CKD in patients with sleep apnea.[51]

Smoking

Smoking remains one of the main modifiable risk factors in many diseases including CKD. Many of the large studies that examined different risk factors for CKD identified smoking as one of those risk factors. In a large prospective study of more than 20,000 participants from Maryland, smoking was found be associated with a 2.5-fold increase in the risk of CKD in both genders.[52] Another larger cohort from England showed

that smoking was one of the independent risk factors that determined development of moderate to severe CKD.[48] More recently, the ARIC study identified being a nonsmoker, among other 7 lifestyle factors, as a predictor of lower risk of CKD.[53]

Smoking may affect kidney function indirectly, through an increase in blood pressure, or directly, by affecting renal vasculature or causing cellular toxicity.[52]

Drugs

Nephrotoxicity is a frequently reported adverse reaction for numerous therapeutic agents. In this section, only drugs that have been associated with CKD will be discussed.

NSAIDS and Other Analgesics

Classic analgesic nephropathy will be discussed in this section. Nonsteroidal anti-inflammatory drugs (NSAIDs) will be discussed elsewhere in this book.

It was in 1953 when the association between intake of large amounts of analgesics and interstitial nephritis was first described.[54]

Subsequently, analgesic nephropathy was the entity used to describe kidney disease in patients who take large amounts of analgesics and was characterized by papillary necrosis and chronic interstitial nephritis.[55] Analgesic nephropathy usually results from the ingestion of a combination of analgesics including aspirin, acetaminophen, codeine, or caffeine, but it is also believed that it may result from the long-term intake of a single agent.[56] Nevertheless, some reports showed no association between the chronic use of aspirin or acetaminophen as single agents and an increased risk of kidney disease.[57,58] Overall, the data have been inconsistent, and early epidemiological studies had major limitations, making it difficult to draw any reliable conclusions.[59] Furthermore, with the decline in the rate of analgesic nephropathy after removal of phenacetin from the market, the risk of analgesic nephropathy in patients who chronically use non-phenacetin-based analgesics was questioned.[60] In another study, [61] that attempted to determine the sensitivity of noncontrast computerized tomography in detecting analgesic nephropathy, it was found that radiological findings of analgesic nephropathy were rare even in heavy analgesic users. Therefore, classic non-NSAIDS analgesic nephropathy remains a controversial entity that might not exist in users of non-phenacetin analgesics.

Proton Pump Inhibitors

Proton pump inhibitors (PPI) are very commonly used drugs that have been associated with significant side effects, including acute interstitial nephritis and chronic kidney disease and are sometimes being used without a good indication or beyond the time frame recommended for therapy.[62] Upon examining data from 11,656 participants in the ARIC study who were followed prospectively, the risk of CKD was found to be 20% to 50% higher in PPI users. The increased risk was observed after adjusting for multiple confounding variables including comorbidities and use of other medications.[62] More recently, another study from the Veterans Affairs[63] showed the increased risk of CKD among PPI users even after excluding patients who developed AKI. Chronic adverse effects on kidney function was confirmed in a recent review.[64] PPI's adverse effects on kidney function seem to be dose and duration dependent.[62,63] Even though, those results have been reproducible in very large cohorts, the association is based on findings from observational studies. Data from pharmacoepidemiologic studies might be confounded by the fact that patients who are given more drugs have more comorbidities making it difficult to determine whether the association with an adverse effect is related to the drug or to the underlying medical illness. Another limitation is that sicker patients seek medical attention more frequently and are more likely to get diagnosed with certain conditions including the outcome in question.[65] In this specific case, participants may have been started on PPI posthospitalization making the hospitalization itself or the illness that caused it possible causes for the negative effect on the kidneys.[66] However, the studies previously mentioned did attempt to control for all of those biases.

Undiagnosed acute interstitial nephritis may account for the association between the use of PPI and increased risk of CKD.[67] CKD has also been hypothesized to result from altered gastrointestinal flora and protein metabolism in PPI users.[68]

Given the extensive use of PPI for prolonged durations, a potential adverse kidney outcome has to be taken into account and monitored for.

Sodium Phosphate

Oral sodium phosphate (OSP) preparations are hyperosmolar solutions that contain high amounts of sodium and elemental phosphate and that, when ingested, result in increased water excretion into the intestinal lumen.[69] The relatively small volume of OSP required, compared to other bowel preparation agents, makes it ideal to use prior to colonoscopies and more effective as patients are more likely to take it compared to the other agents.[70] However, OSP may result in severe hyperphosphatemia, elevated calcium-phosphorous product, and hypocalcemia.[69] Acute phosphate nephropathy was first described in a patient who developed AKI and subsequent CKD after ingesting OSP for bowel preparation, with renal biopsy showing nephrocalcinosis as well as calcium phosphate crystals that caused tubular obstruction.[71] Since then, multiple biopsy-proven case reports and observational studies reported the same entity.[69,72,73] Nonetheless, and similarly to other CKD risk factors, some studies did not confirm the association between the use of OSP and worsening renal function.[74]

The pathogenesis of AKI and subsequent CKD in this setting is related to the combination of a high phosphate load in addition to potential diarrhea-induced hypovolemia, which lead to precipitation of calcium and phosphorous in the renal tubules.[73]

Illicit Drugs

The use of illicit drugs is another modifiable risk factor that has been linked to CKD with different possibilities of renal involvement including nephrotic syndrome, acute glomerulonephritis, amyloidosis, interstitial nephritis, and rhabdomyolysis.[75] Yet, many of the renal manifestations, previously attributed to illicit drug use and specifically to heroin nephropathy, were later found to be due to HIV and hepatitis B and C infections.[76] There was also the possibility of socioeconomic and genetic factors affecting the prevalence of specific pathologic entities in drug users such as focal segmental glomerulosclerosis, which was only described in patients of African descent.[75] However, a recent prospective study of adult participants residing in Baltimore, Maryland, showed that, even after adjusting for socioeconomic factors, HIV, and hepatitis, there was a statistically significant association between opioid and cocaine use and decreased eGFR and albuminuria, respectively.[77] Furthermore, in a postmortem study of illicit drug users in Germany, multiple renal pathologic changes were identified including interstitial inflammation, calcification of renal parenchyma, interstitial fibrosis, and tubular atrophy. Hypertensive and ischemic changes were mainly seen in cocaine users.[76]

It is speculated that renal damage might be the result of injury related to the pharmacologic properties of the drugs or the accompanying adulterants and diluents.[76] Cocaine, for instance, is a sympathomimetic; it activates the RAAS and may cause endothelial dysfunction. It may cause rhabdomyolysis, interstitial nephritis, thrombotic microangiopathy, renal infarction, and malignant HTN.[78] Mechanisms by which heroin independently causes renal damage are less clear, and there is not much evidence, overall, to currently support heroin nephropathy as an independent entity.[75]

Diet and the Metabolic Syndrome

The association between metabolic syndrome and CKD has been reported in multiple observational studies. The association, however, is very difficult to analyze given that HTN and hyperglycemia, which are common features of the metabolic syndrome, are both established risk factors for CKD. Based on the results of a meta-analysis that analyzed 11 studies with more than 30,000 participants, metabolic syndrome and its individual components were associated with an increased risk of CKD and proteinuria. In addition, the risk increased with the increase in the number of components of the metabolic syndrome (elevated blood pressure, elevated triglycerides, low HDL cholesterol, abdominal obesity, and impaired fasting glucose).[79] Moreover, another prospective study[80] from Japan, that examined a large cohort of participants and analyzed specifically nonobese participants, emphasized the association of the other components of the metabolic syndrome (high blood pressure, high triglycerides, low high-density lipoprotein cholesterol, and high fasting blood sugar) with CKD.

Obesity

Obesity itself, on the other hand, has also been described in multiple studies to be a risk factor for CKD and CKD progression, with risk of CKD being 2.5 times higher in obese individuals compared to the general population as described in one report.[81,82] More important, obesity has been shown to have renal effects without the presence of any other metabolic derangements. In a cohort study of more than 6,500 Chinese individuals followed over 5 years, hazard ratio for incident CKD was found to be almost 3 times higher in obese with metabolic syndrome compared to nonobese without

metabolic syndrome but was also found to be 2.4 times higher in obese without metabolic syndrome compared to nonobese without metabolic syndrome.[83] Another large study,[84] involving more than 60,000 participants, also showed that metabolically healthy overweight and obese participants had a higher incidence of CKD.

Hyperfiltration, glomerular hypertrophy, and increased single nephron GFR may explain the glomerulosclerosis seen in obese individuals. Based on animal models, as glomeruli hypertrophy, podocyte foot processes may detach from the basement membrane leading to proteinuria.[85] Activation of the RAAS and sympathetic stimulation may also contribute to further renal injury.[86] Furthermore, leptin as well as other adipose tissue-derived factors, such as tumor necrosis factor-α and interleukin-6 may also contribute to the development of CKD.[84]

Western-Style Diet

A Western diet, characterized by increased intake of red and processed meats as well as saturated fats and sweets, is associated with albuminuria and decline in renal function.[87] In addition, based on data from the ARIC study, increased intake of sugar sweetened sodas was associated with an increased prevalence of CKD.[88] High salt intake is also associated with increased risk of proteinuria and CKD.[89]

All the above dietary factors may affect renal function by affecting renal vasculature as well as hormonal regulation and by causing inflammation and oxidative stress.[89]

Hyperuricemia

The association between hyperuricemia and CKD is well established; however, hyperuricemia as an independent risk factor for CKD is a debatable topic. Numerous confounders may affect the association. Hyperuricemia is common in individuals with metabolic syndrome, which is, as previously described, a risk factor for CKD.[90] Hyperuricemia may also be a consequence of CKD rather than being a cause of CKD.[91]

Therefore, some of the more recent studies performed rigorous statistical analyses to control for many potential confounders. In a study analyzing pooled data from more than 13,000 participants from the ARIC and the Cardiovascular Health Study,[92] uric acid level at baseline was found to be an independent risk of incident CKD after adjusting for multiple variables including components of the metabolic syndrome, alcohol, smoking, and baseline kidney function. Another even larger study[93] from Austria confirmed those findings and showed that the higher the uric acid level, the higher the risk of incident CKD. To further support the independent role that hyperuricemia plays in increasing CKD risk, a randomized trial[94] showed that treatment with Allopurinol slowed down the progression of renal disease in patients with CKD. On the other hand, hyperuricemia was not found to be an independent risk factor for CKD progression in a recently published retrospective study from Brazil.[95]

Hyperuricemia may cause proteinuria, renal vascular changes, and renal fibrosis. It may also activate the RAAS and cyclooxygenase-2 system.[96] It may as well cause endothelial dysfunction and vascular smooth muscle cell proliferation.[97]

Other Risk Factors

Less commonly described risk factors for CKD, such as an increased heart risk and periodontal disease, have been reported, but there is paucity of evidence to support the association at this time.[98]

CONCLUSION

Nonmodifiable risk factors for CKD include age, gender, race, family history, and LBW whereas modifiable risk factors include systemic illnesses, AKI, obstructive uropathy, kidney stones, OSA, smoking, obesity, Western-style diet, and hyperuricemia. Drugs, such as NSAIDs and other analgesics, PPI, and sodium phosphate as well as illicit drugs, are also modifiable risk factors for CKD. Even though those factors have been associated with CKD, the association has not always been reproducible, and causality has not been fully established for most of those factors. However, given the increasing incidence of CKD, it is important to be aware of all the potential risk factors in case an intervention is warranted or even, in some cases, to determine the need for closer follow-up.

REFERENCES

1. Coresh J, Selvin E, Stevens LA, et al. Prevalence of chronic kidney disease in the United States. *J Am Med Assoc.* 2007;298(17):2038–2047.
2. Fox CS, Larson MG, Leip EP, Culleton B, Wilson PW, Levy D. Predictors of new-onset kidney disease in a community-based population. *J Am Med Assoc.* 2004;291(7):844–850.
3. Lindeman RD, Tobin J, Shock NW. Longitudinal studies on the rate of decline in renal function with age. *J Am Geriatr Soc.* 1985;33(4):278–285.
4. Eriksen BO, Ingebretsen OC. The progression of chronic kidney disease: a 10-year population-based study of the effects of gender and age. *Kidney Int.* 2006;69(2):375–382.
5. Hemmelgarn BR, Zhang J, Manns BJ, et al. Progression of kidney dysfunction in the community-dwelling elderly. *Kidney Int.* 2006;69(12):2155–2161.
6. Zhou XJ, Rakheja D, Yu X, Saxena R, Vaziri ND, Silva FG. The aging kidney. *Kidney Int.* 2008; 74:710–720.
7. Rule AD, Amer H, Cornell LD, et al. The association between age and nephrosclerosis on renal biopsy among healthy adults. *Ann Intern Med.* 2010;152(9):561.
8. Centers for Disease Control and Prevention. *Chronic Kidney Disease Surveillance System— United States.* http://www.cdc.gov/ckd
9. Silbiger S, Neugarten J. Gender and human chronic renal disease. *Gend Med.* 2008; 5(Suppl A):S3–S10.
10. Elliot SJ, Berho M, Korach K, et al. Gender-specific effects of endogenous testosterone: female alpha-estrogen receptor-deficient c57bl/6j mice develop glomerulosclerosis. *Kidney Int.* 2007;72: 464–472.
11. Takamatsu N, Abe H, Tominaga T, et al. Risk factors for chronic kidney disease in Japan: a community-based study. *BMC Nephrol.* 2009;10:34.
12. Süleymanlar G, Utaş C, Arinsoy T, et al. A population-based survey of Chronic REnal Disease In Turkey—the CREDIT study. *Nephrol Dial Transplant.* 2011;26(6):1862–1871.
13. Jafar TH, Schmid CH, Stark PC, et al. The rate of progression of renal disease may not be slower in women compared with men: a patient-level meta-analysis. *Nephrol Dial Transplant.* 2003;18(10):2047–2053.
14. Halbesma N, Brantsma AH, Bakker SJ, et al. Gender differences in predictors of the decline of renal function in the general population. *Kidney Int.* 2008;74(4):505–512.
15. Carrero JJ. Gender differences in chronic kidney disease: underpinnings and therapeutic implications. *Kidney Blood Press Res.* 2010;33:383–392.
16. McClellan WM, Flanders WD. Risk factors for progressive chronic kidney disease. *J Am Soc Nephrol.* 2003;14(7 Suppl 2):S65–S70.
17. Vart P, van Zon SKR, Gansevoort RT, Bültmann U, Reijneveld SA. SES, chronic kidney disease, and race in the U.S.: a systematic review and meta-analysis. *Am J Prev Med.* 2017;53(5):730–739.

18. Tarver-Carr ME, Powe NR, Eberhardt MS, et al. Excess risk of chronic kidney disease among African-American versus white subjects in the United States: a population-based study of potential explanatory factors. *J Am Soc Nephrol.* 2002;13(9):2363–2370.

19. Derose SF, Rutkowski MP, Crooks PW, et al. Racial differences in estimated GFR decline, ESRD, and mortality in an integrated health system. *Am J Kidney Dis.* 2013;62:236–244.

20. Genovese G, Friedman DJ, Ross MD, et al. Association of trypanolytic ApoL1 variants with kidney disease in African Americans. *Science.* 2010;329(5993):841–845.

21. Parsa A, Kao WH, Xie D, et al.; AASK Study Investigators; CRIC Study Investigators. APOL1 risk variants, race, and progression of chronic kidney disease. *N Engl J Med.* 2013;369(23):2183–2196.

22. Pugh JA, Stern MP, Haffner SM, Eifler CW, Zapata M. Excess incidence of treatment of end-stage renal disease in Mexican Americans. *Am J Epidemiol.* 1988;127:135–144.

23. Hoy WE, Megill DM. End-stage renal disease in southwestern Native Americans, with special focus on the Zuni and Navajo Indians. *Transplant Proc.* 1989;21:3906–3908.

24. Hall YN1, Hsu CY, Iribarren C, Darbinian J, McCulloch CE, Go AS. The conundrum of increased burden of end-stage renal disease in Asians. *Kidney Int.* 2005;68(5):2310–2316.

25. Freedman BI, Volkova NV, Satko SG, et al. Population-based screening for family history of end-stage renal disease among incident dialysis patients. *Am J Nephrol.* 2005;25(6):529–535.

26. Song EY, McClellan WM, McClellan A, et al. Effect of community characteristics on familial clustering of end-stage renal disease. *Am J Nephrol.* 2009;30(6):499–504.

27. Hsu CW, Yamamoto KT, Henry RK, De Roos AJ, Flynn JT. Prenatal risk factors for childhood CKD. *J Am Soc Nephrol.* 2014;25(9):2105–2111.

28. Das SK, Mannan M, Faruque AS, Ahmed T, McIntyre HD, Al Mamun A. Effect of birth weight on adulthood renal function: A bias-adjusted meta-analytic approach. *Nephrology (Carlton).* 2016;21(7):547–565.

29. Ruggajo P, Skrunes R, Svarstad E, Skjærven R, Reisæther AV, Vikse BE. Familial factors, low birth weight, and development of ESRD: a nationwide registry study. *Am J Kidney Dis.* 2016;67(4):601–608.

30. Carmody JB, Charlton JR. Short-term gestation, long-term risk: prematurity and chronic kidney disease. *Pediatrics.* 2013;131(6):1168–1179.

31. Rodríguez MM, Gómez AH, Abitbol CL, Chandar JJ, Duara S, Zilleruelo GE. Histomorphometric analysis of postnatal glomerulogenesis in extremely preterm infants. *Pediatr Dev Pathol.* 2004;7(1):17–25.

32. Luyckx VA, Brenner BM. Birth weight, malnutrition and kidney-associated outcomes—a global concern. *Nat Rev Nephrol.* 2015;11(3):135–149.

33. Hippisley-Cox J, Coupland C. Predicting the risk of chronic kidney disease in men and women in England and Wales: prospective derivation and external validation of the QKidney scores. *BMC Fam Pract.* 2010;11:49.

34. Alexander RT, Hemmelgarn BR, Wiebe N, et al.; Alberta Kidney Disease Network. Kidney stones and kidney function loss: a cohort study. *Brit Med J.* 2012;345:e5287.

35. Shoag J, Halpern J, Goldfarb DS, Eisner BH. Risk of chronic and end stage kidney disease in patients with nephrolithiasis. *J Urol.* 2014;192(5):1440–1445.

36. Kummer AE, Grams M, Lutsey P, et al. Nephrolithiasis as a risk factor for CKD: the Atherosclerosis Risk in Communities Study. *Clin J Am Soc Nephrol.* 2015;10(11):2023–2029.

37. Gambaro G, Croppi E, Bushinsky D, et al. The risk of chronic kidney disease associated with urolithiasis and its urological treatments: a review. *J Urol.* 2017;198:268–273.

38. Denburg MR, Jemielita TO, Tasian GE, et al. Assessing the risk of incident hypertension and chronic kidney disease after exposure to shock wave lithotripsy and ureteroscopy. *Kidney Int.* 2016;89(1):185–192.

39. Worcester EM, Parks JH, Evan AP, Coe FL. Renal function in patients with nephrolithiasis. *J Urol.* 2006;176(2):600–603.

40. Ahmadi F, Etemadi SM, Lessan-Pezeshki M, et al. Contribution of stone size to chronic kidney disease in kidney stone formers. *Int J Urol.* 2015;22(1):104–108.

41. Keller JJ, Chen YK, Lin HC. Association between chronic kidney disease and urinary calculus by stone location: a population-based study. *BJU Int.* 2012;110(11 Pt C):E1074–E1078.

42. Rule AD, Krambeck AE, Lieske JC. Chronic kidney disease in kidney stone formers. *Clin J Am Soc Nephrol.* 2011;6(8):2069–2075.

43. Han Lee YC, Hung SY, Wang HK, et al. Sleep apnea and the risk of chronic kidney disease: a nationwide population-based cohort study. *Sleep.* 2015;38(2):213–221.

44. Sakaguchi Y, Shoji T, Kawabata H, et al. High prevalence of obstructive sleep apnea and its association with renal function among nondialysis chronic kidney disease patients in Japan: a cross-sectional study. *Clin J Am Soc Nephrol.* 2011;6(5):995–1000.

45. Chou YT, Lee PH, Yang CT, et al. Obstructive sleep apnea: a stand-alone risk factor for chronic kidney disease. *Nephrol Dial Transplant.* 2011;26(7):2244–2250.

46. Mirrakhimov AE. Obstructive sleep apnea and kidney disease: is there any direct link? *Sleep Breath.* 2012;16(4):1009–1016.

47. Kinebuchi S, Kazama JJ, Satoh M, et al. Short-term use of continuous positive airway pressure ameliorates glomerular hyperfiltration in patients with obstructive sleep apnoea syndrome. *Clin Sci (Lond).* 2004;107(3):317–322.

48. Lee YJ, Jang HR, Huh W, et al. Independent contributions of obstructive sleep apnea and the metabolic syndrome to the risk of chronic kidney disease. *J Clin Sleep Med.* 2017;13(10):1145–1152.

49. Foster GE, Hanly PJ, Ahmed SB, Beaudin AE, Pialoux V, Poulin MJ. Intermittent hypoxia increases arterial blood pressure in humans through a renin-angiotensin system-dependent mechanism. *Hypertension.* 2010;56(3):369–377.

50. Ruiz-Ortega M, Rupérez M, Esteban V, et al. Angiotensin II: a key factor in the inflammatory and fibrotic response in kidney diseases. *Nephrol Dial Transplant.* 2006;21(1):16–20.

51. Adeseun GA, Rosas SE. The impact of obstructive sleep apnea on chronic kidney disease. *Nephrol Dial Transplant.* 2010;25(1):181–186.

52. Haroun MK, Jaar BG, Hoffman SC, Comstock GW, Klag MJ, Coresh J. Risk factors for chronic kidney disease: a prospective study of 23,534 men and women in Washington County, Maryland. *J Am Soc Nephrol.* 2003;14(11):2934–2941.

53. Rebholz CM, Anderson CA, Grams ME, et al. Relationship of the American Heart Association's impact goals (Life's Simple 7) with risk of chronic kidney disease: results from the Atherosclerosis Risk in Communities (ARIC) cohort study. *J Am Heart Assoc.* 2016;5(4):e003192.

54. V. Spühler, H. Zollinger. Die chronisch: interstitialle nephritis. *Z Klin Med.* 1953;151:1–50.

55. Murray TG, Goldberg M. Analgesic-associated nephropathy in the U.S.A.: epidemiologic, clinical and pathogenetic features. *Kidney Int.* 1978;13(1):64–71.

56. Henrich WL, Agodoa LE, Barrett B, et al. Analgesics and the kidney: summary and recommendations to the Scientific Advisory Board of the National Kidney Foundation from an ad hoc committee of the National Kidney Foundation. *Am J Kidney Dis.* 1996;27(1):162–165.

57. Perneger TV, Whelton PK, Klag MJ. Risk of kidney failure associated with the use of acetaminophen, aspirin, and nonsteroidal antiinflammatory drugs. *N Engl J Med.* 1994;331(25):1675–1679.

58. Kelkar M, Cleves M, Foster H, Hogan W, James L, Martin B. Acute and chronic acetaminophen use and renal disease: a case-control study using pharmacy and medical claims. *J Manag Care Pharm.* 2012;18(3):234–246.

59. Delzell E, Shapiro S. A review of epidemiologic studies of nonnarcotic analgesics and chronic renal disease. *Medicine (Baltimore).* 1998;77(2):102–121.

60. Feinstein A, Heinemann L, Curhan G, et al. Relationship between nonphenacetin combined analgesics and nephropathy: a review. Ad hoc committee of the International Study Group on Analgesics and Nephropathy. *Kidney Int.* 2000;58(6):2259–2264.

61. Henrich WL, Clark RL, Kelly JP, et al. Non-contrast-enhanced computerized tomography and analgesic-related kidney disease: report of the national analgesic nephropathy study. *J Am Soc Nephrol.* 2006;17(5):1472–1480.

62. Lazarus B, Chen Y, Wilson FP, et al. Proton pump inhibitor use and the risk of chronic kidney disease. *JAMA-Intern Med.* 2016;176(2):238–246.

63. Xie Y, Bowe B, Li T, Xian H, Yan Y, Al-Aly Z. Long-term kidney outcomes among users of proton pump inhibitors without intervening acute kidney injury. *Kidney Int.* 2017;91(6):1482–1494.

64. Nochaiwong S, Ruengorn C, Awiphan R, et al. The association between proton pump inhibitor use and the risk of adverse kidney outcomes: a systematic review and meta-analysis. *Nephrol Dial Transplant.* 2018;33(2):331–342.

65. Tomlinson LA, Fogarty DG, Douglas I, Nitsch D. Pharmacoepidemiology for nephrologists: do proton pump inhibitors cause chronic kidney disease? *Nephrol Dial Transplant.* 2017;32(Suppl 2):ii40–ii46.

66. Iannuzzella F, Corradini M, Pasquali S. Adverse effects of proton pump inhibitors in chronic kidney disease. *JAMA-Intern Med.* 2016;176(6):868–869.

67. Moledina DG, Perazella MA. Proton pump inhibitors and CKD. *J Am Soc Nephrol.* 2016;27(10):2926–2928.

68. Poesen R, Meijers B, Evenepoel P. Adverse effects of proton pump inhibitors in chronic kidney disease. *JAMA-Intern Med.* 2016;176(6):867–868.

69. Heher EC, Thier SO, Rennke H, Humphreys BD. Adverse renal and metabolic effects associated with oral sodium phosphate bowel preparation. *Clin J Am Soc Nephrol.* 2008;3(5):1494–1503.

70. Tan JJ, Tjandra JJ. Which is the optimal bowel preparation for colonoscopy: a meta-analysis. *Colorectal Dis.* 2006;8:247–258.

71. Desmeules S, Bergeron MJ, Isenring P: Acute phosphate nephropathy and renal failure. *N Engl J Med.* 2003;349:1006–1007.

72. Markowitz GS, Stokes MB, Radhakrishnan J, D'Agati VD: Acute phosphate nephropathy following oral sodium phosphate bowel purgative: an underrecognized cause of chronic renal failure. *J Am Soc Nephrol.* 2005;l16:3389–3396.

73. Markowitz GS, Perazella MA. Acute phosphate nephropathy. *Kidney Int.* 2009;76(10):1027–1034.

74. Layton JB, Klemmer PJ, Christiansen CF, et al. Sodium phosphate does not increase risk for acute kidney injury after routine colonoscopy, compared with polyethylene glycol. *Clin Gastroenterol Hepatol.* 2014;12(9):1514–1521.

75. Jaffe JA, Kimmel PL. Chronic nephropathies of cocaine and heroin abuse: a critical review. *Clin J Am Soc Nephrol.* 2006;1(4):655–667.

76. Buettner M, Toennes SW, Buettner S, Bickel M, Allwinn R, Geiger H, Bratzke H, Amann K, Jung O. Nephropathy in illicit drug abusers: a postmortem analysis. *Am J Kidney Dis.* 2014;63(6):945–953.

77. Novick T, Liu Y, Alvanzo A, Zonderman AB, Evans MK, Crews DC. Lifetime cocaine and opiate use and chronic kidney disease. *Am J Nephrol.* 2016;44(6):447–453.

78. Goel N, Pullman JM, Coco M. Cocaine and kidney injury: a kaleidoscope of pathology. *Clin Kidney J.* 2014;7(6):513–517.

79. Thomas G, Sehgal AR, Kashyap SR, Srinivas TR, Kirwan JP, Navaneethan SD. Metabolic syndrome and kidney disease: a systematic review and meta-analysis. *Clin J Am Soc Nephrol.* 2011;6(10):2364–2373.

80. Nishikawa K, Takahashi K, Okutani T, et al. Risk of chronic kidney disease in non-obese individuals with clustering of metabolic factors: a longitudinal study. *Intern Med.* 2015;54(4):375–382.

81. Chang A, Kramer H. CKD progression: a risky business. *Nephrol Dial Transplant.* 2012;27:2607–2609.

82. McMahon GM, Hwang SJ, Fox CS. Residual lifetime risk of chronic kidney disease. *Nephrol Dial Transplant.* 2017;32(10):1705–1709.

83. Cao X, Zhou J, Yuan H, Wu L, Chen Z. Chronic kidney disease among overweight and obesity with and without metabolic syndrome in an urban Chinese cohort. *BMC Nephrol.* 2015;16:85.

84. Chang Y, Ryu S, Choi Y, et al. Metabolically healthy obesity and development of chronic kidney disease: a cohort study. *Ann Intern Med.* 2016;164(5):305–312.

85. Wickman C, Kramer H. Obesity and kidney disease: potential mechanisms. *Semin Nephrol.* 2013;33(1):14–22.

86. Thethi T, Kamiyama M, Kobori H. The link between the renin-angiotensin-aldosterone system and renal injury in obesity and the metabolic syndrome. *Curr Hypertens Rep.* 2012;14:160–169.

87. Lin J, Fung TT, Hu FB, Curhan GC. Association of dietary patterns with albuminuria and kidney function decline in older white women: a subgroup analysis from the Nurses' Health Study. *Am J Kidney Dis.* 2011;57(2):245–254.

88. Bomback AS, Derebail VK, Shoham DA, et al. Sugar-sweetened soda consumption, hyperuricemia, and kidney disease. *Kidney Int.* 2010;77:609–616.

89. Odermatt A. The Western-style diet: a major risk factor for impaired kidney function and chronic kidney disease. *Am J Physiol Renal Physiol.* 2011;301(5):F919–F931.

90. Cirillo P, Sato W, Reungjui S, et al. Uric acid, the metabolic syndrome, and renal disease. *J Am Soc Nephrol.* 2006;17(Suppl 3):S165–S168.

91. Ishani A, Grandits GA, Grimm RH, et al. Association of single measurements of dipstick proteinuria, estimated glomerular filtration rate, and hematocrit with 25-year incidence of end-stage renal disease in the multiple risk factor intervention trial. *J Am Soc Nephrol.* 2006;17:1444–1452.

92. Weiner DE, Tighiouart H, Elsayed EF, Griffith JL, Salem DN, Levey AS. Uric acid and incident kidney disease in the community. *J Am Soc Nephrol.* 2008;19(6):1204–1211.

93. Obermayr RP, Temml C, Gutjahr G, Knechtelsdorfer M, Oberbauer R, Klauser-Braun R. Elevated uric acid increases the risk for kidney disease. *J Am Soc Nephrol.* 2008;19(12):2407–2413.

94. Goicoechea M, de Vinuesa SG, Verdalles U, et al. Effect of allopurinol in chronic kidney disease progression and cardiovascular risk. *Clin J Am Soc Nephrol.* 2010;5(8):1388–1393.

95. Chini LSN, Assis LIS, Lugon JR. Relationship between uric acid levels and risk of chronic kidney disease in a retrospective cohort of Brazilian workers. *Braz J Med Biol Res.* 2017;50(9):e6048.

96. Kang DH, Nakagawa T. Uric acid and chronic renal disease: possible implication of hyperuricemia on progression of renal disease. *Semin Nephrol.* 2005;25(1):43–49.

97. Johnson RJ, Kang DH, Feig D, et al. Is there a pathogenetic role for uric acid in hypertension and cardiovascular and renal disease? *Hypertension.* 2003;41(6):1183–1190.

98. Kazancioğlu R. Risk factors for chronic kidney disease: an update. *Kidney Int Suppl.* 2013;3(4):368–371.

5

Senescence of the Kidney

EOIN D. O'SULLIVAN AND DAVID A. FERENBACH

INTRODUCTION

Senescence derives from the Latin *senex* meaning "old" and was a term originally used by biologists interchangeably with the term "aging" to describe the decline in organism function with time. Since its seminal description by Hayflick as a phenomenon of prolonged cell culture in vitro over half a century ago, cellular senescence is now recognized to exist not only in vitro but as an important in vivo cellular response involved in successful embryogenesis and wound repair, but in other contexts it promotes inflammation, aging, and tissue fibrosis.

THE SENESCENT PHENOTYPE

Cellular senescence has been described as an irreversible process, induced in damaged cells by a variety of stressors, including critical telomere shortening, oncogenic stimuli, DNA damage, and mechanical stress (Fig. 5.1).[1]

Senescence is recognized to occur in mitotic cells including epithelial, endothelial, and stromal cells, as well as components of the haemopoietic system. One hallmark of a senescent cell is the loss of the ability to replicate. While a senescent cell may remain metabolically active, in vivo it will be unable to reenter the cell cycle. Senescent cells also demonstrate markedly altered gene expression and modified, condensed chromatin.[2] While postmitotic cells lack the ability to proliferate, and as such cannot "lose" this function and become senescent, it is now recognized that such cells can undergo heterochromatinization, synthesis of proinflammatory interleukins, and express high senescence-associated β-galactosidase activity levels, all features consistent with a "senescent" phenotype.[3]

A key characteristic of senescent cells is altered protein expression and secretion. This secretome can alter the local tissue microenvironment

affecting the function of neighboring cells. These cells have a tendency to express pathways that encourage growth arrest and repress pathways that encourage cell-cycle progression. This secretory function of senescence cells is described as the senescence associated secretory phenotype (SASP) and is of major interest to senescence researchers. SASP components include IL-6, IL-8, and WNT16B, which can act in both a paracrine and also autocrine fashion, leading to persistence and propagation of the senescent state.[3] The SASP may differ depending on the mode of senescence induction and cell type, although proinflammatory and immune cell attraction are common traits shared among most SASPs and appear a highly conserved characteristic. Other important effects of the SASP include modulating cell proliferation, angiogenesis, inflammation, wound healing, and an as yet partially understood role in postinjury fibrosis and effective tissue repair (Fig. 5.2).[4–7]

As our understanding of the underlying mechanisms and effects of senescence has changed, a broad classification of modes of senescence has become commonplace within the literature. Real biological systems rarely conform to simple classification, and it is likely that there is overlap between both the drivers and manifestations of each type of senescent cell.

REPLICATIVE SENESCENCE

In the classic senescence as described by Hayflick, cells remain viable in vivo but show altered morphology, altered surface marker expression, and accumulation of lipofuscin granules and lack any response to mitogenic stimuli. There is an association between replicative senescence and decreasing length of telomeres with age, and experimentally elongating telomeres can delay or arrest development of senescence entirely.[8]

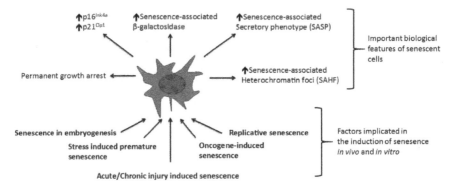

FIGURE 5.1 Cellular processes leading to the induction of senescence and the biological properties of the senescent cell. Emerging evidence shows that senescence is induced in normal embryogenesis (including formation of the kidney), after acute and chronic organ injury, and in response to cellular stress and oncogene activation (in vitro and in vivo) and after prolonged division in vitro. Senescent cells are permanently growth arrested, express one or both of p16^{Ink4a} and p21^{cip1}, senescence associated beta-galactosidase, and the senescence associated secretory phenotype (SASP). There is also nuclear reorganization with the formation of heterochromatin foci (senescence-associated heterochromatin foci). SASP = senescence-associated secretory phenotype.

Shortening telomeres are an important component of aging and replicative senescence, and as increasingly short telomeres become dysfunctional, this may lead to chromosomal instability and tumorigenesis. This can trigger a classical DNA damage response and subsequent senescence in the effected cell.

STRESS-INDUCED PREMATURE SENESCENCE

We understand that shortening telomeres are only one piece of the senescent puzzle. For example, mouse telomeres are much longer than human telomeres, and mouse cells express the protective telomerase enzyme, preventing genetic material from erosion through replication over time. Despite this, however, mouse cells still become senescent over time, like their human counterparts. An important driver here is thought to be accumulated cellular stress and injury. This is known as stress-induced premature senescence, which is a cellular response to insult and can be induced by oxidative stress, genotoxic damage, lack of nutrients, and

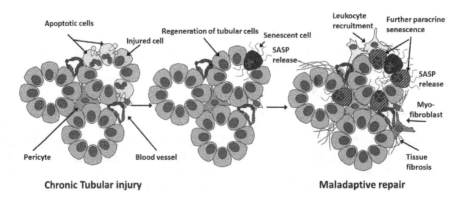

FIGURE 5.2 Mechanisms of senescent cell generation within the chronically injured kidney and the consequences of the senescence-associated secretory phenotype (SASP). Chronic tissue injury can include both lethal and sublethal cellular injury. Injured cells may become senescent and adopt the SASP, releasing factors promoting paracrine senescence of other cells and promote fibrosis, inflammation, and neoplasia in the affected tissue. The components of the SASP vary between cells and are not well characterized in the kidney. Emerging evidence suggests that heterogeneity exists between different senescent cells in the same tissue (e.g., DNA damaged vs. cytokine-induced senescence).

mitochondrial damage.[9] This occurs independently of telomere length and is characterized by activation of multiple intracellular pathways such as p38 and mitogen-activated protein kinase, which lead to p16-INK4a activation and ultimately to cellular senescence. This phenomenon of increased p16-INK4a expression is a key pathway for researchers in the field who use the presence of p16-INK4a as an important, if imperfect, experimental marker of senescence.

ONCOGENE-INDUCED SENESCENCE

Oncogenes are genes that have acquired mutations that alter their function and could potentially lead to cancer developing from the cell. The appearance of an oncogene in a cell can induce senescence, suggesting a protective, anticancer role of senescence. An alternative fate of cells that express oncogenes is apoptosis, although the factors that determine whether a cell undergoes senescence or apoptosis are poorly understood.

It is probable that within a given tissue there are simultaneous competing causes for cellular senescence, and there may be overlap between these cells groups, resulting in a "mosaic culture" of senescent cell types.[10] The significance and interaction of these different populations and resulting senescent phenotypes is still unclear to researchers.

ACUTE VERSUS CHRONIC SENESCENCE

An emerging paradigm is that of acute and chronic senescence and that the senescent phenotype displayed may be as a result of different modes of senescence induction and thus may have different impacts on tissue and organ physiology (Fig. 5.3). Acute senescence is thought to occur in settings such as renal embryogenesis, cutaneous wound healing, and normal tissue repair and potentially has a role in limiting fibrosis before senescent cells are subsequently removed by apoptotic or immune clearance.[11] This form of senescence seems a tightly controlled, scheduled process.

In contrast, chronic senescence is persistent and uncontrolled, probably because of multiple senescent-inducing stimuli (e.g., oxidative stress, activated oncogenes, etc.) acting simultaneously on a cell. A potentially impaired immune clearance may represent another key difference between acute and chronic senescence as chronically induced senescent cells seems resistant to apoptosis and immune clearance. It is speculated that these chronic senescent cells may then promote deleterious fibrosis, persistent inflammation, and alter the local tissue microenvironment.

WHAT ARE THE PHYSIOLOGICAL FUNCTIONS OF SENESCENCE?

Senescent cells are not unique to aging or disease states and have a role in normal development

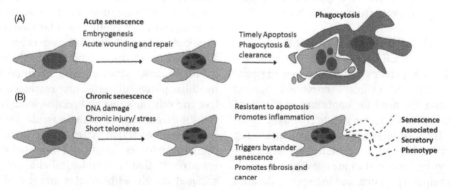

FIGURE 5.3 Differences in senescence-inducing stimuli and subsequent behavior of senescent cells in tissues. While further studies are needed, there is experimental evidence that cellular senescence is involved in normal embryogenesis of the kidney and that it forms an important part of successful cutaneous wound healing, with senescent cells undergoing timely apoptosis/phagocytosis (A). In contrast, senescence that occurs after DNA damage, through critically shortened telomeres or through chronic inflammation, injury, or stress is thought to produce senescent cells that are resistant to both apoptosis and phagocytosis (via poorly understood mechanisms) and contribute further senescence, vaculogenesis, immune recruitment, and inflammation and increase the chances of cancer formation (B). SASP = senescence-associated secretory phenotype.

and health. Senescence can be a defensive process that can "shut down" damaged cells, protect against malignant transformation, and may modulate fibrosis at both baseline and after injury.[12] The observation that oncogenes may induce senescence speak of its importance in opposition of malignancy. Animal models where senescence is blocked quickly succumb to accelerated cancerous growths.

Senescent cells are now understood to be important in embryonic development and in embryonic pattern signaling. These senescent cells are ultimately removed by apoptosis and by macrophage-mediated clearance.[13] This raises one potential question, as to whether senescence in disease states is a reactivation of embryonic pathways and whether the persistence of senescent cells is due to alterations in these clearance pathways with age.

Senescent cells also play a role in postinjury repair, but the specifics of that role are far from clear any may depend on the nature of the injury. For example, p16[INK4a] knockout mice exposed to experimental renal injury show improved recovery after ischemia reperfusion injury but worsened fibrosis after unilateral ureteric obstruction models.[14,15] Possibly related is the observation that senescent cells are required for healthy wound closure, and the presence of senescent cells can accelerate wound closure via increased myofibroblasts.[16] Thus, while many of the features of chronic senescence are now considered detrimental to health and lifespan, features of acute senescence appear to be important in early recovery from acute injury.

AN EVOLUTIONARY PERSPECTIVE

There is an apparent conflict between the protective effects of cellular senescence against cancer and the need for continued replications throughout life for repair and to maintain organ health. This can be recapitulated by considering senescence through an evolutionary lens. For a gene to be beneficial to an organism, it needs only to help it reproduce, and in the early decades of a human's life, the benefit of protecting from cellular injury and malignant transformation is large as it allows successful reproduction, and any bystander effect of organ "aging" has minimal impact on an organism. As decades pass and a human has successfully reproduced, the potential cumulative and deleterious effects of senescence grow, but the selective pressure has

now disappeared, and thus there will be no tendency to remove these genes from the broader gene pool. This hypothesis is known as antagonistic pleiotropthy.[17]

SENESCENCE IN RENAL AGING

An aged kidney is not a perfectly defined entity, but classically is characterized by structural changes such as increased nephrosclerosis, glomerular basement membrane changes, and decreased nephron size and number and by functional changes such as reduced glomerular filtration and impaired tubular function. Renal aging is a complex and multifactorial process with diverse drivers such as vascular and hemodynamic changes; altered histological structure; altered cell signaling; impaired response to oxidative stress and injury; genetic, telomeric, and transcriptomic hemodynamic changes; altered immunological function; and increased senescence.[18] It may be that senescence is both cause and consequence of some of these features of aging, but this remains unclear to researchers as yet. The specific mechanism through which senescent cells impact an aged kidney is still unclear, and it may be due to loss of replicative function, disordered repair and remodeling, or local inflammatory influence of the SASP.

There is evidence that some of the pathways implicated in cellular senescence, such as increased expression of pINK4a, are also implicated in issue aging.[19,20] With age, there is an increase in p16 and possibly related stem cell senescence, in association with tissue dysfunction, notably in the brain, bone marrow, and pancreas of aging mice.[21-23] While this is far from conclusive, it does suggest that this association is consistent across organs and increases with time.

In humans, senescence is maximal in the medulla, potentially reflecting increased oxidative and cellular stress and relative local hypoxia resulting from the age-related vascular changes.[24] It has been noted that increased age correlates to decreased telomere length and increased staining for p16[INK4a]. Similar histological changes are associated closely with tubular atrophy of native and transplanted kidneys, which were important determinants of clinical outcome. One could thus speculate that this increased senescence is responsible, at least in part, for the poor postinjury outcomes we see in our aged patients.

Senescence is present in the kidneys of children with renal disease and may play a role in their subsequent clinical course; however, the overall senescent burden is less than in adult kidneys, which may be a factor contributing to the superior repair in young kidneys following renal injury.[25]

While there may be increased production of senescent cells in aging due to increased formation secondary to cellular stress and telomeric shortening, it is unclear how senescent cell removal affects the overall senescent burden. Apoptosis is the programmed death of damaged cells and is an important anticancer process alongside senescence. Some populations of senescence cells have a decreased susceptibility to apoptosis. As alluded to earlier, the altered immune milieu in the elderly may result in less efficient senescent cell phagocytosis and removal.

SENESCENCE IN RENAL DISEASE
Given the increasing burden of renal disease with age and the parallels between the insults of disease and aging, there is likely much overlap between the mechanism of disease-related senescence. Indeed, increased senescent cell number can found in both aged and disease-affected human renal biopsies.[26-28]

Much of our early understanding of senescence was derived from observations made of senescent cells in vitro; however, recent decades have suggested that accumulation of senescent cells is associated with a number of chronic disease conditions including kidney disease.

Increased senescence is noted in patients with glomerular disease as compared to age-matched controls, indicated by increased p16-INK4a staining on biopsy specimins.[29] In immunoglobulin A (IgA) nephropathy, for example, shorter telomere lengths can be detected in the urine of patients with IgA nephropathy, suggesting that there is increased renal cell senescence in these patients, and there is a significant correlation between this telomere length and serum creatinine in these patients.[30] In patients with nephrotic syndrome due to minimal change disease, membranous nephropathy, and FSGS, increased markers of senescence could be detected in glomeruli, interstitial cells, and tubules.[31] This was more than was present in normal aging kidneys and interstitial nephritis, suggesting a role of senescent cells in glomerular disease.

Patients with diabetic nephropathy also exhibit increased senescence in tubular cells, podocytes, and glomerular mesangial cells as well as vascular endothelial cells.[32] There is murine and human in vivo data to suggest that hyperglycemia is an important driver of this senescence.[33]

Polycystic kidney disease provides an interesting alternative view of the role of senescence in disease, as cell cycle inhibitors and senescence were lower in patients with enlarging cysts and increasing the levels of senescent cells experimentally attenuated disease progression.[34] In vitro data support the protective role of senescence in such cystic disease and reminds us that not all senescent cells are harmful.[35] Commentators have noted that autosomal dominant polycystic kidney disease is associated with increased fibrosis, so a careful balance between the protective and detrimental effects of senescent cells would need to be struck if these cells were to be targeted for disease modulation[36]

Renal transplant biopsies have provided a unique insight into the role of senescent cells in renal disease. Access to pretransplant tissue samples allows identification of senescent cells and subsequent correlation to outcomes. Crucially, the presence of senescent cells in preimplantation biopsies predicts poorer long-term outcomes of renal transplants.[37,38] Studies in murine renal transplantation demonstrated transplanting genetically altered organs with reduced senescent cell load resulted in less pathological tubulointerstitial changes and interstitial fibrosis post-transplant.[39]

Further human studies have suggested senescence contributes to adverse long-term allograft outcomes. Posttransplant, renal biopsies demonstrate that the presence of senescent cells correlates significantly with chronic allograft nephropathy and are further increased locally in the vulnerable cortex.[26,40,41] Senescent cell markers such as p16[INK4a] and p27(Kip1) are present in both atrophic and nonatopic tubules in transplant biopsies with chronic allograft nephropathy, suggesting their association is not as specific tubular damage markers but rather a general marker of overall senescence.[29,42] Whether this senescence is simply a marker of a generally lower tolerance for cellular stress in the organ or rather responsible for the dysfunction is unclear.

MODULATING SENESCENCE
Senescent cells are potentially attractive therapeutic targets (Fig. 5.4). Work with progeroid mice with accelerated aging demonstrated that depletion of senescent cells attenuated age-related change in muscle and fat cells.[43] The use

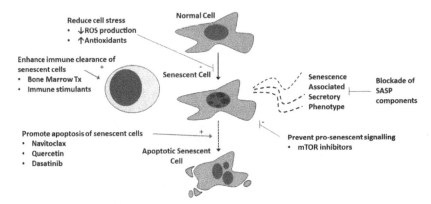

FIGURE 5.4 Potential approaches to therapeutic targeting of senescent cell generation and deletion. Efforts to alter the production and clearance of senescent cells are a focus of interest, with no treatments currently licensed for use in man. Interventions have been proposed to reduce oxidative stress and reduce senescent cell formation, or to enhance clearance using a transplanted young immune system. Interest has also focused on interventions to block proinflammatory components of the SASP. Exciting recent work has shown that clinically licensed mTor inhibitors inhibit pro-senescent signaling within cells, and that the licensed/clinically trialed agents navitoclax, quercetin and dastinib may trigger cell death in senescent cells. ROS = reactive oxygen species. SASP = senescence-associated secretory phenotype. Tx = transplantation. mTOR = mechanistic target of rapamycin.

of Bcl-2/xL inhibitors to deplete senescent cells in nontransgenic animals resulted in marrow rejuvenation.[44] Recent seminal studies used transgenic mice to allow depletion of p16^{INK4a}-expressing senescent cells with subsequent reduced markers of aging in multiple organs, including the kidney, which ultimately lead to increased organism lifespan.[45] Even in older age, transgenic removal of senescent cells has been demonstrated to delay aging phenotypes in muscles and eyes of mice.[46] Could a similar effect be demonstrated in a human kidney—a fountain of renal youth?

Senescent cell depletion is the most immediate method of cell removal and has the advantages of immediately removing senescent cells, halting the source of the SASP, and intermittent treatment regimens. This could take the form of directly senolytic or immune-mediated treatments.[47] Thus far, an elegant clinical solution to remove senescent cells does not exist in humans yet, but several suitable candidate drugs have emerged. Examples include dasatinib, a broad spectrum kinase inhibitor,[48] navitoclax, a BCL-2/xL inhibitor,[49] and quercetin, a flavanol.[50] No human data exist to support their use as senolytic agents in patients, but undoubtedly future research will explore this avenue.

Senescence can also be modulated in humans indirectly through effecting upstream pathways and protection from intracellular stress. One

such pathway is the mechanistic target of rapamycin (mTOR) which is considered a master growth regulator and modulates cell growth in response to environmental cues such as nutrient availability, cellular stress, and growth factors. As its name would suggested, rapamycin is an inhibitor of this pathway, and mice treated from birth with rapamycin had demonstrated greatly extended lifespans.[51] While these experiments did not measure senescent cells directly in these mice, we know that mTOR is an important upstream pathway in senescent cell induction, and a separate series of experiments demonstrate that rapamycin can suppress senescence in vitro.[52] Furthermore, rapamycin demonstrates an antifibrotic effect following ureteric obstruction injury models and in patients using rapamycin posttransplant. This raises the tantalizing questions of whether these observed life extending and antifibrotic effects of rapamycin could be due to senescent cell modulation.[53,54] Additional evidence is present as caloric restriction has long been noted to increased organism lifespan, and some authors suggest a common downstream pathway is responsible for this effect.[55]

Protection from reactive oxygen species (ROS) is a second potential indirect method of minimizing senescence. Both antioxidants and statins can delay the onset of replicative senescence by counteracting the increased ROS production and minimizing telomere shortening in an in vitro model of endothelial cell senescenese.[56,57] Atorvastatin and n-acetyl cysteine can reduce replicative senescence in an in vitro model via protecting from ROS-induced mitochondrial damage.[57] A further example of protection against mitochondrial damage and reduction of ROS species stress is the observation that long-term treatment with the peroxisome proliferator-activated receptor gamma (PPARγ) agonist pioglitazone ameliorates aging-related progressive renal injury and senescent cell burden in rats.[58]

Finally, more dramatic means of modulation exist such as marrow transplant. Reconstituting the bone marrow of old mice with young marrow had dramatic effects on reducing renal senescent cell populations and improved organ response to injury.[59] Given the effect young marrow will have on young circulating immune cells, this would lend some support to the notion that immune clearance is an important factor in senescent cell number in kidneys, and this may become impaired with age. In experiments where mice received either old or young marrow, the young marrow recipients did seem to suppress local senescent cell surface markers.

Such cell depletion studies hint at a potential therapeutic target to be used by clinicians in future, but much research still needs to be undertaken before fundamental questions surround cell depletion can be answered. Will depletion improve recovery postinjury and, if so, for specific injury types? Is there an optimal time or patient who should have their senescent cells depleted? What harmful side effects could we expose our patients to if we deplete their senescent cells? It is observed that senescent cells are important in wound healing for example. Impaired scar formation of a superficial skin wound is at best a nuisance, but impaired ventricular scar formation postmyocardial infarction could be catastrophic. For now, targeting senescent cells acutely remains a tantalizing but unproven prospect.

THE FUTURE OF RENAL SENESCENCE: GAPS IN OUR KNOWLEDGE

Senescence is an exciting area of research yet remains poorly understood as fundamental questions surround the role, regulation, and potential as a therapeutic target of senescent cells in both protecting and treating patients with kidney disease.

Why do senescent cells accumulate with age? Is the accumulation due to increased numbers of cells becoming senescent during aging or reduced immune clearance? And if increasing accumulation is a key factor, is it primarily replicative senescence or the accumulation of years of cellular injury leading to increased burden.

Is depletion safe or effective? Agents exist to deplete senescent cells, but their efficacy and safety are largely unknown. Minimizing development of senescent cells via modulating telomere length (caloric restriction, ibuprofen, angiotensin converting enzyme inhibitors) or minimizing genotoxic damage by reducing ROS burden (dietary changes, PPARγ) seems too proximal to have clinical relevance to elderly patients but perhaps have a role as preventative therapies in the young?

Are senescence cells important in recovery? It is entirely possible that optimal recovery postrenal injury requires the presence of adequate numbers of senescent cells at key timepoints, and a delicate balance is needed. The specific role of these cells in renal repair and development of fibrosis, however, is essentially unknown.

Senescent cell burden may possibly be a useful predictor of renal outcome postinjury or in the setting of progressive CKD. Current means of detection are not sufficiently specific and are largely impractical as they require stained tissue. Additionally, whether increased senescent cell number on renal biopsy predicts progression and functional decline better or additively to existing markers remains untested. Prospective studies following patients with differing numbers of senescent cells will be required to answer this question. Surrogate biomarkers would help researchers associate senescent burden with clinical phenotypes and outcomes, which helps inform basic science research and build a more complete understanding of their role.

Growing interest and research in senescent cells, will continue to shed light on these ubiquitous yet mysterious players in the aging and damaged kidney. With better understand of their role in damage and repair, it may become possible to target them therapeutically, without compromising their essential regulatory function in healing and cancer suppression.

REFERENCES

1. Sturmlechner I, Durik M, Sieben CJ, Baker DJ, van Deursen JM. Cellular senescence in renal ageing and disease. *Nat Rev Nephrol.* 2016;13(2):77–89.

2. Chandra T, Ewels PA, Schoenfelder S, et al. Global Reorganization of the Nuclear Landscape in Senescent Cells. *Cell Rep.* 2015;10(4):471–483.

3. van Deursen JM. The role of senescent cells in ageing. *Nature.* 2014;509(7501):439–446.

4. Jun J-I, Lau LF. The matricellular protein CCN1 induces fibroblast senescence and restricts fibrosis in cutaneous wound healing. *Nat Cell Biol.* 2010;12(7):676–685.

5. Krizhanovsky V, Yon M, Dickins RA, et al. Senescence of activated stellate cells limits liver fibrosis. *Cell.* 2008;134(4):657–667.

6. Freund A, Orjalo A V., Desprez P-Y, Campisi J. Inflammatory networks during cellular senescence: causes and consequences. *Trends Mol Med.* 2010;16(5):238–246.

7. Coppé J-P, Kauser K, Campisi J, Beauséjour CM. Secretion of vascular endothelial growth factor by primary human fibroblasts at senescence. *J Biol Chem.* 2006;281(40):29568–29574.

8. Blackburn EH. Switching and signaling at the telomere. *Cell.* 2001;106(6):661–673.

9. Yang H-C, Fogo AB. Fibrosis and renal aging. *Kidney Int Suppl.* 2014;4(1):75–78.

10. Ben-Porath I, Weinberg RA. The signals and pathways activating cellular senescence. *Int J Biochem Cell Biol.* 2005;37(5):961–976.

11. van Deursen JM. The role of senescent cells in ageing. *Nature.* 2014;509(7501):439–446.

12. Jun J-I, Lau LF. The matricellular protein CCN1 induces fibroblast senescence and restricts fibrosis in cutaneous wound healing. *Nat Cell Biol.* 2010;12(7):676–685.

13. Storer M, Mas A, Robert-Moreno A, et al. Senescence is a developmental mechanism that contributes to embryonic growth and patterning. *Cell.* 2013;155(5):1119–1130.

14. Lee DH, Wolstein JM, Pudasaini B, Plotkin M. INK4a deletion results in improved kidney regeneration and decreased capillary rarefaction after ischemia-reperfusion injury. *Am J Physiol Renal Physiol.* 2012;302(1):F183–F191.

15. Wolstein JM, Lee DH, Michaud J, Buot V, Stefanchik B, Plotkin MD. INK4a knockout mice exhibit increased fibrosis under normal conditions and in response to unilateral ureteral obstruction. *Am J Physiol Renal Physiol.* 2010;299(6):F1486–F1495.

16. Demaria M, Ohtani N, Youssef SA, et al. An essential role for senescent cells in optimal wound healing through secretion of PDGF-AA. *Dev Cell.* 2014;31(6):722–733.

17. Campisi J. Cancer and ageing: rival demons? *Nat Rev Cancer.* 2003;3(5):339–349.

18. O'Sullivan ED, Hughes J, Ferenbach DA. Renal aging: causes and consequences. *J Am Soc Nephrol.* 2017;28(2):407–420.

19. Kim WY, Sharpless NE. The regulation of INK4/ARF in cancer and aging. *Cell.* 2006;127(2):265–275.

20. Hornsby PJ. Cellular senescence and tissue aging in vivo. *J Gerontol A Biol Sci Med Sci.* 2002;57(7):B251–B256.

21. Molofsky A V., Slutsky SG, Joseph NM, et al. Increasing p16^{INK4a} expression decreases forebrain progenitors and neurogenesis during ageing. *Nature.* 2006;443(7110):448–452.

22. Janzen V, Forkert R, Fleming HE, et al. Stem-cell ageing modified by the cyclin-dependent kinase inhibitor p16^{INK4a}. *Nature.* 2006;443(7110):421–426.

23. Krishnamurthy J, Ramsey MR, Ligon KL, et al. p16^{INK4a} induces an age-dependent decline in islet regenerative potential. *Nature.* 2006;443(7110):453–457.

24. Melk A, Schmidt BMW, Takeuchi O, Sawitzki B, Rayner DC, Halloran PF. Expression of p16^{INK4a} and other cell cycle regulator and senescence associated genes in aging human kidney. *Kidney Int.* 2004;65(2):510–520.

25. Jacobi C, Hömme M, Melk A. Is cellular senescence important in pediatric kidney disease? *Pediatr Nephrol.* 2011;26(12):2121–2131.

26. Melk A, Schmidt BMW, Vongwiwatana A, Rayner DC, Halloran PF. Increased expression of senescence-associated cell cycle inhibitor p16/INK4a in deteriorating renal transplants and diseased native kidney. *Am J Transplant.* 2005;5:1375–1382.

27. Verzola D, Gandolfo MT, Gaetani G, et al. Accelerated senescence in the kidneys of patients with type 2 diabetic nephropathy. *Am J Physiol Renal Physiol.* 2008;295(5):F1563–F1573.

28. Sis B, Tasanarong A, Khoshjou F, Dadras F, Solez K, Halloran PF. Accelerated expression of senescence associated cell cycle inhibitor p16INK4A in kidneys with glomerular disease. *Kidney Int.* 2007;71(3):218–226.

29. Melk A, Schmidt BMW, Vongwiwatana A, Rayner DC, Halloran PF. Increased expression of senescence-associated cell cycle inhibitor p16^{INK4a} in deteriorating renal transplants and diseased native kidney. *Am J Transplant.* 2005;5(6):1375–1382.

30. Szeto CC, Poon PYK, Lai FMM, Chow KM, Szeto CYK, Li PKT. Chromosomal telomere shortening of kidney cells in IgA nephropathy by the measurement of DNA in urinary sediment. *Clin Nephrol.* 2005;64(5):337–342.

31. Sis B, Tasanarong A, Khoshjou F, Dadras F, Solez K, Halloran PF. Accelerated expression of senescence associated cell cycle inhibitor p16INK4A in kidneys with glomerular disease. *Kidney Int.* 2007;71(3):218–226.

32. Verzola D, Gandolfo MT, Gaetani G, et al. Accelerated senescence in the kidneys of patients with type 2 diabetic nephropathy. *AJP Ren Physiol.* 2008;295(5):F1563–F1573.

33. Kitada K, Nakano D, Ohsaki H, et al. Hyperglycemia causes cellular senescence via a SGLT2- and p21-dependent pathway in proximal tubules in the early stage of diabetic nephropathy. *J Diabetes Complications.* 2014;28(5):604–611.

34. Park J-Y, Schutzer WE, Lindsley JN, et al. p21 is decreased in polycystic kidney disease and leads to increased epithelial cell cycle progression: roscovitine augments p21 levels. *BMC Nephrol.* 2007;8(1):12.

35. Park J-Y, Park S-H, Weiss RH. Disparate effects of roscovitine on renal tubular epithelial cell apoptosis and senescence: implications for autosomal dominant polycystic kidney disease. *Am J Nephrol.* 2009;29(6):509–515.

36. Sturmlechner I, Durik M, Sieben CJ, Baker DJ, van Deursen JM. Cellular senescence in renal ageing and disease. *Nat Rev Nephrol.* 2017;13(2):77–89.

37. McGlynn LM, Stevenson K, Lamb K, et al. Cellular senescence in pretransplant renal biopsies predicts postoperative organ function. *Aging Cell.* 2009;8(1):45–51.

38. Koppelstaetter C, Schratzberger G, Perco P, et al. Markers of cellular senescence in zero hour biopsies predict outcome in renal transplantation. *Aging Cell.* 2008;7(4):491–497.

39. Braun H, Schmidt BMW, Raiss M, et al. Cellular senescence limits regenerative capacity and allograft survival. *J Am Soc Nephrol.* 2012;23(9):1467.

40. Ferlicot S, Durrbach A, Bâ N, Desvaux D, Bedossa P, Paradis V. The role of replicative senescence in chronic allograft nephropathy. *Hum Pathol.* 2003;34(9):924–928.

41. Halloran P, Melk A, Barth C. Rethinking chronic allograft nephropathy: the concept of accelerated senescence. *J Am Soc Nephrol.* 1999;10(1):167–181.

42. Chkhotua AB, Gabusi E, Altimari A, et al. Increased expression of p16(INK4a) and p27(Kip1) cyclin-dependent kinase inhibitor genes in aging human kidney and chronic allograft nephropathy. *Am J Kidney Dis.* 2003;41(6):1303–1313.

43. Baker DJ, Perez-Terzic C, Jin F, et al. Opposing roles for p16Ink4a and p19Arf in senescence and ageing caused by BubR1 insufficiency. *Nat Cell Biol.* 2008;10(7):825–836.

44. Chang J, Wang Y, Shao L, et al. Clearance of senescent cells by ABT263 rejuvenates aged hematopoietic stem cells in mice. *Nat Med.* 2016;22(1):78–83.

45. Baker DJ, Childs BG, Durik M, et al. Naturally occurring p16-positive cells shorten healthy lifespan. *Nature.* 2016;530(7589):184–189.

46. Baker DJ, Wijshake T, Tchkonia T, et al. Clearance of p16Ink4a-positive senescent cells delays ageing-associated disorders. *Nature.* 2011;479(7372):232–236.

47. Childs BG, Durik M, Baker DJ, van Deursen JM. Cellular senescence in aging and age-related disease: from mechanisms to therapy. *Nat Med.* 2015;21(12):1424–1435.

48. Zhu Y, Tchkonia T, Pirtskhalava T, et al. The Achilles' heel of senescent cells: from transcriptome to senolytic drugs. *Aging Cell.* 2015;14(4):644–658.

49. Chang J, Wang Y, Shao L, et al. Clearance of senescent cells by ABT263 rejuvenates aged hematopoietic stem cells in mice. *Nat Med.* 2015;22(1):78–83.

50. Malavolta M, Pierpaoli E, Giacconi R, et al. Pleiotropic effects of tocotrienols and quercetin on cellular senescence: introducing the perspective of senolytic effects of phytochemicals. *Curr Drug Targets.* 2016;17(4):447–459.

51. Harrison DE, Strong R, Sharp ZD, et al. Rapamycin fed late in life extends lifespan in genetically heterogeneous mice. *Nature.* 2009;460(7253):392–395.

52. Demidenko ZN, Zubova SG, Bukreeva EI, Pospelov VA, Pospelova T V., Blagosklonny M V. Rapamycin decelerates cellular senescence. *Cell Cycle.* 2009;8(12):1888–1895.

53. Wu M-J, Wen M-C, Chiu Y-T, Chiou Y-Y, Shu K-H, Tang M-J. Rapamycin attenuates unilateral ureteral obstruction-induced renal fibrosis. *Kidney Int.* 2006;69(11):2029–2036.

54. Özdemir BH, Özdemir AA, Erdal R, Özdemir FN, Haberal M. Rapamycin prevents interstitial fibrosis in renal allografts through decreasing angiogenesis and inflammation. *Transplant Proc.* 2011;43(2):524–526.

55. Cox LS, Mattison JA. Increasing longevity through caloric restriction or rapamycin feeding in mammals: common mechanisms for common outcomes? *Aging Cell.* 2009;8(5):607–613.

56. Assmus B, Urbich C, Aicher A, et al. HMG-CoA reductase inhibitors reduce senescence and increase proliferation of endothelial progenitor cells via regulation of cell cycle regulatory genes. *Circ Res.* 2003;92(9):1049–1055.

57. Haendeler J, Hoffmann J, Diehl JF, et al. Antioxidants inhibit nuclear export of telomerase reverse transcriptase and delay replicative senescence of Endothelial cells. *Circ Res.* 2004;94(6):768–775.

58. Yang H-C, Deleuze S, Zuo Y, Potthoff SA, Ma L-J, Fogo AB. The PPARgamma agonist pioglitazone ameliorates aging-related progressive renal injury. *J Am Soc Nephrol.* 2009;20(11):2380–2388.

59. Yang H-C, Rossini M, Ma L-J, Zuo Y, Ma J, Fogo AB. Cells derived from young bone marrow alleviate renal aging. *J Am Soc Nephrol.* 2011;22(11):2028–2036.

6

The Kidney in Pregnancy

SAMUEL MON-WEI YU AND ANJALI ACHARYA

PHYSIOLOGICAL CHANGES IN THE KIDNEYS DURING NORMAL PREGNANCY

Many physiologic changes that occur in the kidney within weeks of conception and continue through the middle of the third trimester[1,2–4] are attributed to the hormonal changes of pregnancy such as alterations in the renin–angiotensin–aldosterone system (RAAS), progesterone, and other hormones. Relaxin, a 6-kDa peptide produced by the corpus luteum, plays an important role as well.[5,6] As early as 6 weeks of gestation, the vasodilatory hormones reduce the vascular tone significantly, resulting in a decrease in blood pressure along with an increase in cardiac output. The nadir of blood pressure is seen between 18 and 24 weeks, with drop in blood pressure of approximately 10 mmHg. There is an increase in renal plasma flow by 60% to 80% and in glomerular filtration rate (GFR) by 40% to 60%.[7–9] In addition to the physiologic changes, there are anatomic changes taking place as well, such as increase in the size of kidney and dilatation of urinary collecting system. Up to 60% to 80% of pregnant women develop hydronephrosis, especially on the right side, with maximal incidence of hydronephrosis reported at 28 weeks.[10] In addition to hormonal changes, this physiologic dilatation in the collecting system is thought to be due to mechanical factors from ureteric compression between the iliopsoas muscle and gravid uterus at the level of the sacral promontory.[11] This dilatation may cause urinary stasis resulting in a higher susceptibility to urinary tract infections (UTIs), including pyelonephritis. These physiologic changes resolve by 4 to 6 weeks postpartum.

The glomerular hyperfiltration seen during pregnancy contributes to several metabolic changes, including a decrease of blood urea nitrogen, serum creatinine (SCr), and uric acid levels. The average SCr during pregnancy is 0.5 to 0.6 mg/dL, and a SCr of 1.0 mg/dL, despite being in the normal range, is indicative of kidney injury. Tubular function is affected as well with decreased tubular reabsorption of uric acid, amino acids, and β2-microglobulin, leading to lower serum levels compared with the nonpregnant state. Though the role of elevated uric acid level in predicting preeclampsia has been debated, it is suggested to be a biomarker to predict atherosclerotic complications later in life in the mother. Traditionally, glycosuria, despite normoglycemia seen during pregnancy, is attributed to excess amount of filtered glucose overwhelming the capacity of proximal tubular reabsorption; however, some studies have suggested altered maximal glucose reabsorption. The increase in proteinuria during pregnancy is attributed to the rise in GFR and selective alterations in glomerular charge. Mean levels of protein excretion are below 200 mg/24 hours.[12] Proteinuria greater than 300 mg on a 24-hour collection or >0.3 on a spot urine protein–creatinine ratio assessment is considered abnormal. Though proteinuria quantification on a spot urine sample is increasingly used in practice, 24-hour urine protein collection remains the gold standard.

Total body water increases by 6 to 8 L, the majority of which remains extracellular, and contributes to the edema in pregnancy. This volume expansion is dependent on activation of RAAS. Water and electrolyte balance are also affected during pregnancy. The antinatriuretic effects of aldosterone and deoxycorticosterone surpass the natriuretic hormones such as progesterone and atrial natriuretic peptide, consequently leading to water and sodium retention. Of note, despite the cumulative sodium retention of up to 900 to 1,000 mEq, plasma osmolality and serum sodium levels are lower than normal by 10 mOsm/L and 4 to 5 mEq/L, respectively. This is attributed to the lowering of threshold for secretion of antidiuretic hormone during pregnancy, mediated by β-human chorionic gonadotropin and relaxin among others. Polyuria (>3 L/day) is rare in pregnancy but can occur when there is overactivity of placental vasopressinase leading to transient diabetes insipidus due to increased degradation of the antidiuretic hormone.[13]

HYPERTENSIVE DISORDERS IN PREGNANCY

Hypertension defined as either a systolic blood pressure higher than 140 mmHg, diastolic blood pressure >90 mmHg, or both, taken on 2 occasions at least 4 hours apart occurs in about 10% of pregnancies. The hypertensive disorders during pregnancy are categorized into four groups: (i) chronic hypertension (CHT), (ii) gestational hypertension, (iii) preeclampsia–eclampsia, and (iv) CHT superimposed with preeclampsia.

It is important to rule out white coat hypertension with home blood pressure monitoring, preferably with ambulatory blood pressure monitoring to avoid overtreatment. In addition, though not a part of the classification, hypertension and preeclampsia as well as eclampsia can develop in the late postpartum period.

CHT is defined as hypertension antedating pregnancy, seen before 20 weeks of gestation or persisting longer than 12 weeks after delivery. It can be seen in 5% to 10% of pregnancies. The diagnosis is not in doubt in women on antihypertensive medication before pregnancy or those who are hypertensive during the first trimester. However, the diagnosis may be missed due to the physiologic drop in blood pressure soon after conception when there is no history of prior hypertension. If the woman seeks medical attention after the second trimester with elevated blood pressures, it may be misclassified as gestational hypertension and the diagnosis of CHT is made only after delivery. CHT is a recognized risk factor for preeclampsia, intrauterine growth retardation (IUGR), and placental abruption.

Gestational hypertension is defined as hypertension that develops after 20 weeks of gestation without proteinuria or other signs or symptoms of preeclampsia and is the most common cause of hypertension during pregnancy. A history of preeclampsia in a prior pregnancy, multifetal gestation, and obesity increase the risk of developing gestational hypertension. When systolic blood pressure is ≥160 mmHg and/or diastolic blood pressure is ≥110 mmHg on 2 consecutive readings at least 4 hours apart, it is classified as severe gestational hypertension.

Preeclampsia/Eclampsia

Preeclampsia a complex multisystem disease is defined as new onset of maternal blood pressure ≥140/90 mmHg on 2 occasions at least 4 hours apart after 20 weeks of gestation, with onset of proteinuria or with multisystem involvement in the absence of proteinuria. Proteinuria is defined as presence of >300 mg of protein in 24-hour urine collection or a spot urine protein–creatinine ratio >0.3. In the absence of proteinuria, presence of any of the following features is sufficient to make the diagnosis of preeclampsia:

- Thrombocytopenia (platelet count <100,000/μL)
- Abnormal liver function test (≥2 times upper normal limit), severe persistent right upper quadrant or epigastric pain
- Serum creatinine >1.1 mg/dL or ≥2 times baseline)
- Pulmonary edema
- New-onset cerebral or visual disturbances
- Women with preeclampsia are at an increased risk for life-threatening events, including placental abruption, acute kidney injury (AKI), cerebral hemorrhage, hepatic failure or rupture, pulmonary edema, disseminated intravascular coagulation, and progression to eclampsia.

Eclampsia refers to women with preeclampsia who develop new-onset, generalized, tonic–clonic seizure. HELLP (hemolysis, elevated liver enzymes, and low platelet count) syndrome is a severe form of preeclampsia.

Superimposed preeclampsia refers to development of preeclampsia in women with underlying CHT. Maternal factors such as severity and duration of prepregnancy hypertension, presence of secondary hypertension, diabetes mellitus, obesity, and history of chronic kidney disease (CKD) increase the risk of superimposed preeclampsia. Superimposed preeclampsia is considered severe when there is sudden worsening of blood pressure to greater than 160 mmHg systolic and 105 mmHg diastolic, and the identification of clinical symptoms (headache, vision changes, upper abdominal pain) or development of systemic manifestations of

HELLP syndrome, pulmonary congestion or development of doubling of SCr (SCr >1.1 mg/dL), or sudden increase in proteinuria.

Preeclampsia is a condition with widespread endothelial dysfunction, accompanying inflammation, vasoconstriction, and platelet activation. Normal placentation requires orchestration of several vascular processes including angiogenesis and adequate cytotrophoblast invasion and remodeling of the uterine spiral arteries. Abnormal placentation and uteroplacental malperfusion is thought to be the initial insult, leading to placental oxidative stress inflammatory response, endothelial dysfunction, and an imbalance between angiogenic and antiangiogenic factors. An abnormal angiogenic balance has shown to antedate the clinical manifestations of preeclampsia by at least 5 to 6 weeks and is useful in predicting development of preeclampsia.

A plethora of biomarkers have been explored to help predict preeclampsia in the past 2 decades. Soluble fms-like tyrosine kinase-1 (sFlt-1), placental growth factor (PlGF), vascular endothelial growth factor, and soluble endoglin have been extensively studied and sFlt-1–PlGF ratio has demonstrated a superior performance.[14–16] Multiparametric testing and addition of clinical parameters increase the sensitivity and specificity of these biomarkers. Newer candidate serum biomarkers,[17] urine and plasma metabolic profile, micro RNAs, and specific kidney injury markers including kidney injury molecule-1 and neutrophil gelatinase-associated lipocalin are undergoing further investigation.

PREGNANCY IN CKD

Both pregnancy and CKD can impact the outcome of the other. The conception rate in women with CKD has increased in the recent years, and pregnancy in women with CKD remains a challenge for nephrologists as well as obstetricians. Nephrologists caring for women of childbearing age with CKD must start conception counseling early to optimize care and to avoid any teratogenic effects of medications.

Pregnant Women with CKD

Older studies classified CKD during pregnancy by the level of SCr as mild (<1.5 mg/dL), moderate (1.5–2.5 mg/dL), and severe (>2.5 mg/dL). More recent studies instead used GFR to stage CKD though the most commonly used GFR estimation methods such as the Modification of Diet in Renal Disease[18] and the CKD Epidemiology Collaboration[19] underestimate GFR in pregnancy and result in misclassification of CKD stage. Cystatin-C-based determinations have been inconclusive, and furthermore these tests have not been validated in pregnant women.

Regardless of the CKD stage, women with hypertension or proteinuria are more likely to have worsening renal function during pregnancy. Even women with early CKD stage have a higher complication rate than the general population.[20] Therefore, clinicians are encouraged to be vigilant and monitor renal function carefully, particularly in women with risk factors such as prior hypertension or proteinuria. Adverse outcomes such as preterm delivery, small for gestational age, increased rates of caesarean section, and the need for neonatal intensive care unit use are more prevalent among women with advanced CKD.[20,21] Unfortunately, there are no clear guidelines or biomarkers to guide clinicians on the timing of delivery in such women.

Effect of Pregnancy on Kidney Disease

Pregnancy may have short-term or long-term consequences on GFR. Worsening of proteinuria, hypertension, and edema may occur during pregnancy that could resolve in the postpartum period. However, pregnancy can lead to permanent worsening of renal function in women with moderately decreased GFR. Most experts believe that the underlying etiology of CKD does not play a role on the course of the disease in pregnancy, except in women with lupus nephritis. The etiologies and workup of glomerular disease in pregnancy is similar to that in the nonpregnant population.

Lupus Nephritis and Antiphospholipid Antibody Syndrome

Systemic lupus erythematous (SLE) is a disease predominantly of women, with roughly 4,500 pregnancies reported in women with the diagnosis of SLE each year in the United States. Delaying pregnancy until the disease is inactive for at least 6 months is recommended to optimize maternal and fetal outcomes.[22] Preeclampsia and renal flare are the most common maternal complications, and preterm birth is the most common fetal complication in these women.

Most studies suggested that SLE patients have higher risks of developing disease flare during pregnancy due to altered immune modulation. Lupus nephritis can also occur for the first time during pregnancy, making it difficult to differentiate from preeclampsia unless there a high index of suspicion for the condition. PROMISSE (Predictors of Pregnancy Outcome: Biomarker in Antiphospholipid Antibody Syndrome and Systemic Lupus Erythematosus),[22] the largest multicenter, multiethnic and multiracial study to prospectively assess the frequency of adverse pregnancy outcomes showed that with inactive or stable mild/moderate activity at conception, maternal and fetal outcomes are good in over 80% of women. History of prior nephritis has been shown to be associated with IUGR, preterm delivery, and 2 to 3 times higher incidence of preeclampsia.[22,23]

Women with lupus nephritis should be followed closely by an interdisciplinary team including a nephrologist and a rheumatologist, in addition to maternal-fetal medicine experts. Testing for disease flare with complete blood count, comprehensive metabolic panel, complements C3 and C4, CH50 levels, autoimmune antibody profile (dsDNA, anti-Ro/La, lupus anticoagulant, anti-cardiolipin), urinalysis, and urine protein–creatinine ratio should be obtained during the first visit and at regular intervals thereafter. Conditions such as HELLP syndrome and preeclampsia could present with findings similar to lupus flare. Though establishing the correct diagnosis usually requires a renal biopsy, most clinicians have a conservative approach to renal biopsy during pregnancy, and biopsy after 32 weeks is not recommended. Kidney biopsy in pregnancy has the potential risk of major bleeding, severe obstetric complications, and early preterm deliveries, with the risk–benefit ratio varying according to gestational age. The pros and cons of empirical therapeutic approach versus kidney biopsy has to be individualized.

Pregnant Women with Renal Transplantation

Restoration of hypothalamic–pituitary–gonadal axis happens within a few weeks of transplantation and ovulation is restored soon after. Although the optimal timing of conception after transplant is still unclear, the American Society of Transplantation recommends that conception should be deferred for 1 year after a solid organ transplant and the following criteria should be met: (i) no rejection in the previous year, (ii) adequate and stable renal function (SCr <1.5 mg/dL), (iii) minimal or no proteinuria, (iv) no acute fetotoxic infections, and (v) stable function with nonteratogenic immunosuppression. European Best Practice Guidelines[24] recommend that conception be delayed until 2 years after transplant. A recent study showed the lowest allograft loss was seen in the third year after transplant. Prompt counseling and contraceptive use after renal transplantation are essential for optimal maternal and fetal outcomes.

Hypertension and preeclampsia are common after kidney transplant with a 6-fold higher risk compared to the general population.[25,26] Pregnancy has little or no effect on renal function in the transplant patient, provided there are no other risk factors[27] such as presence of hypertension, prepregnancy SCr >1.4 mg/dL, and proteinuria. Acute rejection may be difficult to diagnose based on rising SCr as this change may be subtle. A renal biopsy of the transplanted kidney may be required to establish the diagnosis. Preeclampsia is difficult to diagnose as protein excretion may be >500 mg after transplant during pregnancy. Ascending UTIs can occur in up to 40% of pregnant women after renal transplant.[28]

ACUTE KIDNEY INJURY DURING PREGNANCY

AKI, a term that has replaced acute renal failure, remains a frequent cause of poor maternal outcomes in many parts of the world. Lack of uniform defining criteria, physiologic changes in pregnancy that effect interpretation of laboratory tests, and regional differences in etiologic factors account for the variation in incidence across the globe. The recent increase reported in the United States and Canada could be due to higher maternal age, increased testing, and lowering of the threshold for diagnosing AKI possibly leading to an ascertainment bias.

According to gestational age, the etiologies of AKI can be divided into those seen in early, late, and postpartum periods, keeping in mind that some etiologies are unique to the pregnant state.

Due to advancing maternal age at conception, use of assisted fertility, and higher comorbidities in modern obstetric practice, women are at risk of developing AKI, and we encourage baseline assessment of renal function early in pregnancy. This will aid in making a timely diagnosis of AKI in pregnancy. The workup is no different than in the nonpregnant patients. Because of the heterogeneity of the etiology of AKI, during pregnancy, therapy must be tailored to the underlying condition and supportive care plays an important role.

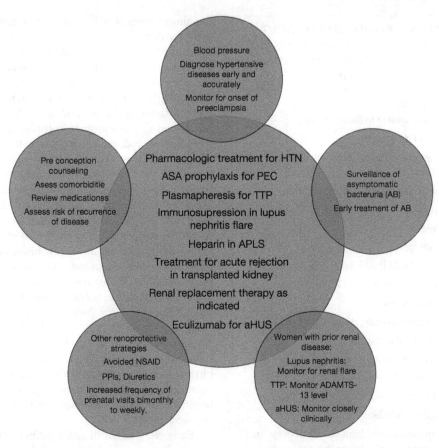

FIGURE 6.1 Multifaceted approach for renal protection in high-risk women. aHUS = atypical hemolytic uremic syndrome. APLS = antiphospholipid antibody syndrome. HTN = hypertension. NSAIDs = nonsteroidal anti-inflammatory drugs. PEC = preeclampsia. PPI = proton pump inhibitor. TTP = thrombotic thrombocytopenic purpura.

RENO-PROTECTIVE STRATEGIES AND MANAGEMENT OF WOMEN WITH KIDNEY DISEASE DURING PREGNANCY

Preconception counseling is important for women with CHT or known CKD to optimize maternal and fetal outcomes. Some of the antihypertensive medications such as angiotensin-converting enzyme inhibitors, angiotensin receptor blockers, and mineralocorticoid antagonists are known to cause adverse fetal effects and are contraindicated during pregnancy. Physicians are advised to switch to another class of antihypertensive medication before conception. Investigating for possible end-organ damage is recommended during the first visit, such as checking the SCr, electrolytes, liver enzymes, platelet count, and urine protein. Screening of secondary hypertension is essential if the patient is on multiple medications, since women with secondary

hypertension have higher risks of adverse maternal and fetal outcomes. Pheochromocytoma, hyperaldosteronism, Cushing disease, and CKD are common causes of secondary hypertension, and if features of secondary hypertension such as resistant hypertension or hypokalemia are present, referral to a specialist in this field should be considered. Nonpharmacological intervention such as aerobic exercise, weight loss, and low-salt diet are suggested for nonpregnant patients. However, these approaches are either not appropriate to pregnant women or have not proven to be beneficial. Due to potential maternal and fetal complications, mainly from volume contraction and decreased placental perfusion, diuretic use in pregnancy is not recommended except for symptomatic relief of pulmonary congestion in women with heart failure.

Gestational hypertension has been reported to recur in subsequent pregnancies and

TABLE 6.1 ETIOLOGIES OF ACUTE
KIDNEY INJURY DURING PREGNANCY
DURING VARIOUS GESTATIONAL
PERIODS

A. Early pregnancy

Prerenal states leading to kidney injury:

Hyperemesis Gravidarum

Hemorrhage due to missed abortion, uterine
  perforation

Sepsis from ascending UTI, septic abortion

Placenta previa

B. Late pregnancy

Placental abruption

Preeclampsia, HELLP, AFLP

TTP (ADAMTS13-deficient TMA), aHUS

Pulmonary embolism

Worsening of pre-existing glomerular disease

De novo glomerular disease

C. Postpartum period

Postpartum preeclampsia

Puerperal sepsis

Amniotic fluid embolism

Postpartum hemorrhage from uterine perforation,
  uterine atony, vascular injury during surgery

Bilateral ureteral injury during cesarean section

aHUS

NSAID use

D. At any gestational age

Gastroenteritis (common in some parts of the world),
  use of diuretics,

Exacerbation of CHF, or valvular heart disease,
  ascending UTI

Kidney injury in renal allograft
Recurrent disease CNI toxicity, acute rejection,
  infections such as CMV, BK virus

UTI = uninary tract infection. HELLP = hemolysis, elevated liver
enzymes, and low platelet. AFLP = acute fatty liver of pregnancy.
TTP = thrombotic thrombocytopenic purpura. TMA = thrombotic
microangiopathy. aHUS = atypical hemolytic uremic syndrome.
NSAID = nonsteroidal anti inflammatory drug. CHF = chronic
heart failure. CNI = calcineurin inhibitor. CMV = cytomegalo virus.

is associated with development of hypertension
later in life and, like CHT, is possibly associated with development of cardiovascular disease
and CKD. Therefore, close clinical monitoring
with an eye to early intervention should be

the aim in women with a history of gestational
hypertension.

As aspirin has been shown to have a modest
yet significant effect in decreasing preeclampsia,
the American College of Obstetricians and
Gynecologists[29] recommends prophylaxis with
aspirin starting in late first trimester, for primary
prevention in those women considered to be at
high baseline risk such as women with a history
of preterm delivery earlier than 34 weeks' gestation due to preeclampsia or preeclampsia in more
than 1 prior pregnancy, history of preeclampsia,
multifetal gestation, CHT, type 1 or 2 diabetes,
renal disease, or autoimmune disease. Aspirin
should be considered in women with severe risk
factors nulliparity, obesity, family history of preeclampsia, certain socioeconomic characteristics/
personal histories, and age >35 years. As per the
2014 US Preventive Services Task Force statement,[30] the use of low-dose aspirin (81–150 mg)
is recommended in those at high risk for preeclampsia between 12 and 28 weeks of gestation to
reduce the occurrence of preeclampsia, preterm
birth, and intrauterine growth restriction. It has
been demonstrated that there is no role for vitamin C, calcium, or antioxidants in prevention
of preeclampsia.

Early recognition of and treatment of hypovolemia in cases with volume depletion is crucial.
In women with hemorrhage, timely and adequate
resuscitation in an attempt to avoid cortical necrosis is prudent. This scenario, though self-
evident, remains a challenge in many remote
parts of the world.

All pregnant women should be given low-dose
aspirin post-transplantation for preeclampsia
prevention. Changes to immunosuppression
preconception may be warranted to avoid
fetotoxicity. For long-term immunosuppressive
agents, calcineurin inhibitors (tacrolimus, cyclosporine), azathioprine, and low-dose prednisone
are considered safe to use. Mycophenolate mofetil
and sirolimus should be stopped 6 weeks before
conception. Generally, pregnancy is considered
as "immunotolerant" state. However, antigens of
fetal origin may lead to acute rejection. Due to the
glomerular hyperfiltration during pregnancy, the
rise of SCr could be very subtle and unhelpful to
detect acute rejection necessitating an ultrasound
guided allograft biopsy. Gancyclovir prophylaxis
for cytomegalo virus is not recommended due to
possible teratogenicity.

The Infectious Disease Society of North
America[31]   recommends   screening   for

asymptomatic bacteriuria which is the presence of >10^5 bacterial colony forming units per milliliter (CFU/mL) of urine on urine culture with no local or systemic symptoms of UTI to be performed early in pregnancy. It is recommended to repeat urine culture in those with risk factors such as a history of prior UTI and women with diabetes mellitus and increased parity. Asymptomatic bacteria should be treated with antibiotics tailored to the susceptibility of the isolated organism, as 30% to 40% of women will develop ascending infections if untreated. A short course of 4 to 7 days is usually sufficient with a follow-up urine culture a week afterwards to confirm cure. In those women with a renal allograft, closer surveillance with monthly urine culture and longer duration of treatment (for 2 weeks) if positive, is recommended, and then prophylaxis should be continued throughout pregnancy. Antibiotics used to treat UTI include nitrofurantoin and cephalexin. Untreated UTI can precipitate acute rejection in the allograft.[32,33]

Since pregnancy can cause multiple maternal and fetal complications in SLE patients, timely prenatal counseling and contraception prescription to prevent unplanned pregnancy is essential. Switching immunosuppression therapy may be necessary in women who plan to conceive. Low-dose aspirin should be started to prevent preeclampsia in all pregnant women with SLE. Anticoagulation therapy is indicated for women with antiphospholipid syndrome or considered for patients with heavy proteinuria in nephrotic range, usually greater than 3 g in 24 hours. Unfractionated heparin or low molecular-weight heparin is the drug of choice, as warfarin is teratogenic when used in the first trimester, while exposure later in pregnancy can cause fetal bleeding including intracranial hemorrhage.[34] Cyclophosphamide and mycophenolate mofetil are teratogenic and are contraindicated in pregnancy. Corticosteroid, hydroxychloroquine, azathioprine, and calcineurin inhibitors are relatively safe for use. Newer biological agents use such as rituximab have not yet been well studied.

Which women with hypertension to treat is an important consideration so as to avoid fetal adverse effects due to low blood pressure. The target to initiate pharmacological treatment varies between different guidelines, with the American College of Obstetricians and Gynecologists[29] guideline recommending to start treatment if systolic blood pressure is 160 mmHg or higher or diastolic blood pressure is 105 mmHg or higher. The target blood pressure goal should be between 120 mmHg and 160 mmHg systolic and 80 and 105 mmHg diastolic. The National Institute of Health and Clinical Excellence[35] recommends treatment at blood pressure over 150 mmHg systolic, 100 mmHg diastolic, or both. Pharmacological treatment can be divided into chronic control or urgent blood pressure lowering in acute exacerbations of blood pressure. Labetalol, extended release form of nifedipine, and methyldopa are the recommended and commonly used agents. Diuretics are not recommended due to the concern of volume contraction contributing to further activation of RAAS and IUGR. Physicians could consider continuing diuretics (except for mineralocorticoid antagonists) if the patient is on diuretics before, or if they have evidence of pulmonary edema. Intravenous agents such as labetalol or hydralazine are used for control of severe acute elevation in blood pressure, with the objective of preventing maternal cardiovascular, renal, or cerebrovascular complications.

The management of preeclampsia requires a multidisciplinary approach, with the definitive treatment being delivery of the fetus. In addition to recommended obstetrical tests, such as fetal nonstress testing, twice-weekly blood pressure monitoring and weekly laboratory tests (complete blood count, SCr, liver function tests) are required to monitor preeclamptic women without severe features. Magnesium sulfate ($MgSO_4$) is used for women with severe features of preeclampsia in order to prevent eclampsia. In women with renal dysfunction, serum magnesium level should be tested every 6 hours to monitor for magnesium toxicity. Overdose of $MgSO_4$ should be reversed by intravenous calcium gluconate. Antihypertensive medication should not be initiated until blood pressure is >160/ 110 mmHg to prevent possible utero-placental insufficiency from hypotension.

General principles of management for those with CKD include increased frequency of prenatal visits, early detection and treatment of asymptomatic bacteriuria, serial monitoring of maternal renal function and for the treatment of hypertension, monitoring for the development of preeclampsia, and fetal surveillance with ultrasound and fetal heart rate. Preterm intervention including delivery may be necessitated by deteriorating renal function, severe preeclampsia, fetal growth restriction, or non-reassuring fetal testing as determined by continuous electronic

TABLE 6.2 SUGGESTED STRATEGIES AIMED AT RENAL PROTECTION

Preconception counseling in the high-risk group

Review of medications/switch of medications to avoid teratogenicity

Assess risk of recurrence of disease in pregnancy

Increased frequency of prenatal visits; every two to four weeks initially, until the third trimester and then weekly

Home BP monitoring (to rule out white coat hypertension, chronic hypertension with poor control, to diagnose onset of PE/SPEC)

Monitor for onset of PEC in those with CKD

Surveillance for asymptomatic bacteriuria and early treatment

Serial monitoring of maternal renal and liver function /Consider PRES in those with PE/SPEC

ASA prophylaxis

Pharmacologic therapy for hypertension

Evaluate for secondary HTN if BP is difficult to control or other features of secondary HTN are present

Avoid use of diuretics/OTC meds such as NSAID/PPIs

Monitor level of maternal ADAMTS13 activity in women with inherited TTP

Monitor for renal flare in women with SLE

BP = blood pressure. PE/SPEC = PEC = preeclampsia. CKD = chronic kidney disease. PRES = posterior reversible encephalopathy syndrome. ASA = acetylsalicylic acid. HTN = hypertension. OTC = over the counter. NSAID = nonsteroidal anti inflammatory drug. PPI = proton pump inhibitors. TTP = thrombotic thrombocytopenic purpura. SLE = systemic lupus erythematous.

fetal heart rate monitoring, via cardiotocography. If the patient requires renal replacement therapy for either AKI or CKD, intensive hemodialysis with a goal of maintaining the blood urea nitrogen under 50 mg/dL is recommended. Other supportive measures such as higher doses of erythropoietin, correction of metabolic acidosis, and management of electrolyte abnormalities are important.

Plasma exchange (PE) is the most effective therapy in thrombotic thrombocytopenic purpura (TTP). PE is also recommended if it is not possible to differentiate between preeclampsia, HELLP, and AFLP (acute fatty liver of pregnancy), and TTP/atypical hemolytic uremic syndrome (aHUS). For TTP presenting in the first trimester, regular PE with close monitoring may allow for continuation of pregnancy. In postpartum thrombotic microangiopathies (TMAs), PE is recommended if thrombocytopenia, hemolysis, or kidney failure continue to worsen 48 to 72 hours after delivery of the fetus. Eculizumab, a monoclonal humanized immunoglobulin G that inhibits complement activation, is available for use in aHUS or complement dysregulation TMAs. The risk of relapse of TTP in subsequent pregnancies varies between 20% for acquired defects and 100% in inherited disorders.[36,37] Close monitoring of maternal ADAMTS13 (a disintegrin and metalloprotease with thrombospondin type 1 motif 13 repeats) activity and evidence of ongoing hemolysis is required in these women. Prophylactic plasmapheresis may be indicated. In women with aHUS, genetic testing for mutations in the complement pathway proteins may help in risk stratification (Table 6.2).

CONCLUSION

In summary, since women with hypertension, preeclampsia, or CKD are a high-risk group, the general recommendations as described in this chapter should guide management. Diagnosis of superimposed preeclampsia is difficult in this population. In addition to the impact of the kidney disease on pregnancy, and vice versa, the possible effects of drugs on the fetus is a concern. Care of these women requires a multidisciplinary approach to minimize mishaps and improve renal maternal and fetal outcomes. Prevention of AKI is a priority due to the possible long-term sequelae of CKD and its associated comorbidities.

REFERENCES

1. Odutayo A, Hladunewich M. Obstetric nephrology: renal hemodynamic and metabolic physiology in normal pregnancy. *Clin J Am Soc Nephrol* .2012;7:2073–2080.
2. Hussein W, Lafayette RA. Renal function in normal and disordered pregnancy. *Curr Opin Nephrol Hypertens.* 2014;23:46–53.
3. Cheung KL, Lafayette RA. Renal physiology of pregnancy. *Adv. Chronic Kidney Dis.* 2013;20:209–214.
4. Acharya A. Management of acute kidney injury in pregnancy for the obstetrician. *Obstet Gynecol Clin N Am.* 2016;43:747–765.
5. Conrad KP. Maternal vasodilation in pregnancy: the emerging role of relaxin. *Am J Physiol Regul Integr Comp Physiol.* 2011;301:R267–R275.

6. Lafayette RA, Hladunewich MA, Derby G, Blouch K, Druzin ML, Myers BD. Serum relaxin levels and kidney function in late pregnancy with or without preeclampsia. *Clin Nephrol.* 2011;75:226–232.

7. Chapman AB, Abraham WT, Zamudio S, et al. Temporal relationships between hormonal and hemodynamic changes in early human pregnancy. *Kidney Int.* 1998;54:2056–2063.

8. Davison JM, Dunlop W. Renal hemodynamics and tubular function normal human pregnancy. *Kidney Int.* 1980;18:152–161.

9. Krutzen E, Olofsson P, Back SE, Nilsson-Ehle P. Glomerular filtration rate in pregnancy: a study in normal subjects and in patients with hypertension, preeclampsia and diabetes. *Scand J Clin Lab Invest.* 1992;52:387–392.

10. Cietak KA, Newton JR. Serial quantitative maternal nephrosonography in pregnancy. *Br J Radiol.* 1985;58:405–413.

11. Lin YJ, Ou YC, Tsang LC, Lin H. Diagnostic value of magnetic resonance imaging for successful management of a giant hydronephrosis during pregnancy. *J Obstet Gynaecol.* 2013;33:91–93.

12. Higby K, Suiter CR, Phelps JY, Siler-Khodr T, Langer O. Normal values of urinary albumin and total protein excretion during pregnancy. *Am J Obstet Gynecol.* 1994;171:984–989.

13. Schrier RW. Systemic arterial vasodilation, vasopressin, and vasopressinase in pregnancy. *J Am Soc Nephrol.* 2010;21:570–572.

14. Maynard SE, Min JY, Merchan J, et al. Excess placental soluble fms-like tyrosine kinase 1 (sFlt1) may contribute to endothelial dysfunction, hypertension, and proteinuria in preeclampsia. *J Clin Invest* 2003;111:649–658.

15. Thadhani R, Mutter WP, Wolf M, et al. First trimester placental growth factor and soluble fms-like tyrosine kinase 1 and risk for preeclampsia. *J Clin Endocrinol Metab.* 2004;89:770–775.

16. Bramham K, Seed PT, Lightstone L, et al. Diagnostic and predictive biomarkers for preeclampsia in patients with established hypertension and chronic kidney disease. *Kidney Int.* 2016;89:874–885.

17. Acharya A, Brima W, Burugu S, Rege T. Prediction of preeclampsia-bench to bedside. *Curr Hypertens Rep.* 2014;16:491.

18. Smith MC, Moran, P., Ward, M. K. & Davison, J. M. Assessment of glomerular filtration rate during pregnancy using the MDRD formula. *BJOG* 2008;115:109–112.

19. Alper AB, Yi Y, Rahman M, et al. Performance of estimated glomerular filtration rate prediction equations in preeclamptic patients. *Am J Perinatol.* 2011;28:425–430.

20. Zhang JJ, Ma XX, Hao L, Liu LJ, Lv JC, Zhang H. A systematic review and meta-analysis of outcomes of pregnancy in CKD and CKD outcomes in pregnancy. *Clin J Am Soc Nephrol.* 2015;10:1964-1978.

21. Hou S. Pregnancy in women with chronic renal disease. *N Engl J Med.* 1985;312:836–839.

22. Buyon JP, Kim MY, Guerra MM, et al. Predictors of pregnancy outcomes in patients with lupus: a cohort study. *Ann Intern Med.* 2015;163:153–163.

23. Smyth A, Radovic M, Garovic VD. Women, kidney disease, and pregnancy. *Adv Chronic Kidney Dis.* 2013;20:402–410.

24. Rose C, Gill J, Zalunardo N, Johnston O, Mehrotra A, Gill JS. Timing of pregnancy after kidney transplantation and risk of allograft failure. *Am J Transplant.* 2016;16:2360–2367.

25. Coscia LA, Constantinescu S, Moritz MJ, et al. Report from the National Transplantation Pregnancy Registry (NTPR): outcomes of pregnancy after transplantation. *Clin Transpl.* 2010;65–85.

26. Bramham K, Nelson-Piercy C, Gao H, et al. Pregnancy in renal transplant recipients: a UK national cohort study. *Clin J Am Soc Nephrol.* 2013;8:290–298.

27. Kim HW, Seok HJ, Kim TH, Han DJ, Yang WS, Park SK. The experience of pregnancy after renal transplantation: pregnancies even within postoperative 1 year may be tolerable. *Transplantation.* 2008;85:1412–1419.

28. Chuang P, Parikh CR, Langone A. Urinary tract infections after renal transplantation: a retrospective review at two US transplant centers. *Clin Transplant.* 2005;19:230–235.

29. American College of Obstetricians and Gynecologists. Hypertension in pregnancy: executive summary. *Obstet & Gynecol.* 2013; 122(5):1122–1131.

30. US Preventive Services Task Force. *Final Update Summary: Low-Dose Aspirin Use for the Prevention of Morbidity and Mortality From Preeclampsia: Preventive Medication.* September 2016. https://www.uspreventiveservicestaskforce. org/Page/Document/UpdateSummaryFinal/ low-dose-aspirin-use-for-the-prevention-of- morbidity-and-mortality-from-preeclampsia- preventive-medication

31. Nicolle LE, Bradley S, Colgan R, et al. Infectious Diseases Society of America guidelines for the diagnosis and treatment of asymptomatic bacteriuria in adults. *Clin Infect Dis.* 2005;40: 643–654.

32. Pelle G, Vimont S, Levy PP, et al. Acute pyelonephritis represents a risk factor impairing

long-term kidney graft function. *Am J Transplant.* 2007;7:899–907.

33. Lee JR, Bang H, Dadhania D, et al. Independent risk factors for urinary tract infection and for subsequent bacteremia or acute cellular rejection: a single-center report of 1166 kidney allograft recipients. *Transplantation.* 2013;96: 732–738.

34. Barbour LA. Current concepts of anticoagulant therapy in pregnancy. *Obstet Gynecol Clin North Am.* 1997;24:499–521.

35. Hypertension in pregnancy: diagnosis and management. https://www.nice.org.uk/guidance/cg107/chapter/1reference. Published date August 2010

36. Moatti-Cohen M, Garrec C, Wolf M, et al. Unexpected frequency of Upshaw-Schulman syndrome in pregnancy-onset thrombotic thrombocytopenic purpura. *Blood.* 2012;119: 5888–5897.

37. Vesely SK, Li X, McMinn JR, Terrell DR, George JN. Pregnancy outcomes after recovery from thrombotic thrombocytopenic purpura-hemolytic uremic syndrome. *Transfusion (Paris).* 2004;44:1149–1158.

SECTION II

Assessment of Kidney Disease

7

Laboratory Investigation of the Kidney

TIMOTHY S. LARSON

INTRODUCTION

Kidney disease and injury is largely silent with few overt clinical manifestations until disease or injury is quite advanced. For this reason, laboratory testing is the mainstay of the assessment and monitoring of kidney injury or disease. This chapter will review laboratory testing used in the assessment of kidney function and impairment.

URINALYSIS

Assessment of the urine, urinalysis, has been a cornerstone of the clinical assessment of patients suspected of having kidney disease, for monitoring of patients with kidney disease or for screening purposes. Most urinalysis is semiquantitative and can be divided into 2 components, urine chemistry analysis and urine microscopic analysis. The urine chemistry portion is often assessed by dipstick, but wet chemistry assessment has also been utilized.

Visual inspection of urine can provide useful information for the clinician. For example, although causes of red urine are most often due to blood or hemoglobin, other causes include myoglobin, ingestion of beets, and drugs such as pyridium. Other conditions that can cause changes in urine color include bilirubinuria, marked uric acid crystalluria, chyluria, porphyria, and alkaptonuria. Cloudy urine is usually a manifestation of urinary tract infection. Additionally, several drugs can result in coloration of the urine including rifampin (red/orange), methylene blue (blue), propofol (green), and phenazopyridine (red/orange). Cloudy or turbid urine may also occur as a nonspecific finding of a concentrated urine specimen that has cooled to room temperature or refrigerated.

Urine pH can be measured either by reagent strip or by ion electrode. The normal range is 4.5 to 7.8, and it can be of use for the assessment of patients with suspected metabolic acidosis. For example, patients with distal renal tubular acidosis are unable to acidify their urine (pH remains >5.5). It is also useful in the management of conditions that require the alkalization or acidification of urine. The urine pH is also important in the interpretation of urine microscopy.

Urine reagent strip testing includes testing for bilirubin and urobilinogen. Only conjugated bilirubin passes into the urine. Although the presence of bilirubin in the urine is indicative of liver disease, it is little clinical utility due to the poor sensitivity for detecting disease. False positives are also common.

Leukocyte esterase on urine reagent dipsticks detects the presence of leukocytes as a result of esterases released from lysed leukocytes. If urine is allowed to stand for prolonged periods of time, leukocytes may be lysed resulting in absence of leukocytes by microscopy but with positive esterase on reagent dipstick testing. False negative results can occur in the presence of high urine glucose or protein, or when the antibiotics cephalothin, tetracycline, and cephalexin are administered.[1] Urine nitrites indicate the presence of bacteria capable of reducing nitrate to nitrite. Many urinary pathogens have this capability though notably *Pseudomonas, Enterococcus,* and *Staphylococcus* albus cannot. Several hours of incubation are needed for the conversion; therefore, short urine retention time can result in false negatives. Additionally, false positives occur with diets rich in vegetables (high nitrate content). Specificity of urine nitrite testing is relatively high, but sensitivity is low.

The presence of glucose by dipstick occurs usually when blood glucose levels exceed 180 mg/dL. Glycosuria in the absence of hyperglycemia is a relatively common manifestation of proximal tubule injury, either in isolation such as with

Fanconi's syndrome or in conjunction with more widespread kidney injury. Dipstick methods detect glucose concentrations as low as 50 mg/dL; for more sensitive detection, the hexokinase method is required. False positive results occur in the presence of oxidizing detergents, and false negative results in the presence of large quantities of ascorbic acid and ketones. Proteinuria is addressed in the following discussion.

URINE MICROSCOPY

Urine microscopy is an essential component of urine assessment. Some advocate using the first morning void since it tends to be acidic (alkaline urine tends to favor lysis of red blood cells [RBC] and white blood cells [WBC]) and is more concentrated. Others recommend using the second morning void to avoid excessive lysis of cells that might occur with prolonged dwell of the urine in the bladder during the night. Ideally, it should be performed on as fresh of a specimen as possible (<2 hrs after voiding) to avoid the lysis of cellular components that occurs with prolonged standing, especially if the specimen did not have a urine stabilizer added. Refrigeration is discouraged, since although it may help to reduce the lysis of cellular components, it also tends to promote the precipitation of crystals.

Processing of the urine includes centrifugation, followed by decanting of the supernatant, leaving a sediment volume of approximately 0.50 mL. The sediment should then be resuspended by vigorous mixing. Approximately 25 μL of the mixed sediment should be pipetted to a microscopy slide to which a cover slip is applied. Alternatively, if an automated urine microscopy system is used, noncentrifuged urine is typically analyzed.[2,3]

Casts present in the urinary sediment should be identified by scanning the entire slide using low power (10× objective). Both brightfield and phase contrast microscopy are preferably used to properly identify casts due to their low refractive index. High power (40× objective) should be used to properly identify any elements contained within a cast. The identification of all other elements (RBCs, RBC morphology [e.g., dysmorphia], WBCs, bacteria, yeast, fat, crystals, etc.) is conducted by evaluating a minimum of 10 to 12 high power fields (40× objective). Ideally brightfield, phase contrast, and polarized microscopy should all be used to properly identify all elements present. (Fig. 7.1)

The addition of 25% acetic acid can aid in the identification of cells with difficult morphology, yeast, and monohydrate calcium oxalate and to clear samples with interfering amorphous phosphates or large numbers of RBCs. It is important to remember that 25% acetic acid will lyse the RBCs and occasionally casts present in the sample. Therefore, RBC numbers and morphology as well as cast identification needs to be evaluated prior to using acetic acid.

RBCs, WBCs, renal tubular epithelial cells, transitional epithelial cells, casts, parasites, sperm, fat, bacteria, and crystals are reported

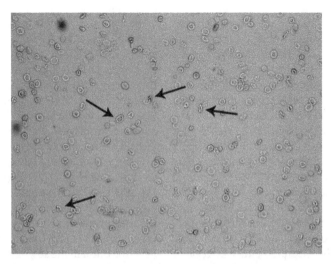

FIGURE 7.1 Waxy cast. Waxy cast by phase contrast microscopy at 40× magnification in a patient with advanced chronic kidney disease.

with urine microscopy. RBCs can be assessed for the presence of dysmorphic features (Fig. 7.2). The presence of dysmorphic cells is suggestive of glomerular origin, with the dysmorphia thought due to the passage of the RBC through the glomerular basement membrane and together with osmolality and pH changes as the cells traverse the tubules.[4-7] The amount of dysmorphic RBCs needed in the urine to indicate glomerular pathology, however, has not been definitively established. In our laboratory we use >25% dysmorphic RBCs as having clinical significance when there are >3 RBC/high power fields. Although dysmorphic RBCs are highly suggestive of glomerular pathology, false positives can occur.

RBC casts are almost always indicative of glomerulonephritis. WBC casts are typically an indication of acute interstitial nephritis or pyelonephritis but can also be seen in glomerulonephritides because there is often a component of accompanying interstitial nephritis. Fatty casts and free fat are often seen in patients with nephrotic syndrome or other glomerular diseases associated with significant proteinuria. Granular casts are observed in a number of disorders and are thought to be formed from partially degraded cellular casts or are protein-derived casts. Hyaline casts are not thought to be indicative of any disease process, but increased numbers may be seen in concentrated urine samples. Waxy casts and broad casts are most often observed in advanced kidney injury. Increased numbers of renal tubular cells are indicators of renal tubular injury and may be caused by a variety of drugs may that are known to be associated with renal tubular toxicity (e.g., calcineurin inhibitors, aminoglycosides, cisplatin, radio-contrast media, and acetaminophen overdose), in addition to interstitial nephritis, hypotension (surgical, sepsis, obstetric complications), heme pigments from hemoglobinuria or myoglobinuria from rhabdomyolysis. Newborns often shed renal tubular cells in their urine. The presence of squamous cells suggests that the sample may not have been an optimal clean-catch specimen and could be contaminated with skin flora.

Automated urine microscopy systems have utilized either flow cytometry or specialized imaging to characterize elements within the urine.[2,3] In our experience, we have found automated imaging systems useful in identifying and quantifying RBCs, dysmorphic RBCs, squamous cells, epithelial cells, and WBCs but less so with identification of urine casts. As such, we utilize an automated image system as an adjunct to manual microscopy, particularly in the analysis of urine that visually is clear and has low protein concentration.

Identification of crystals within the urine is also a required aspect of a thorough urinalysis, particularly in patients with known renal stone disease. Many crystals can develop upon cooling to room temperature or refrigeration in normal individuals. The presence of crystals should also be taken in the context of the urine pH and urine

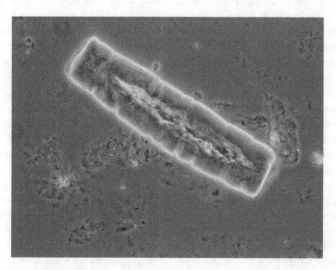

FIGURE 7.2 Dysmorphic red blood cells. Dysmorphic red blood cells (arrows) by brightfield microscopy at 40× magnification in a patient with acute glomerulonephritis.

concentration. Uric acid crystals and amorphous crystals are common, particularly in an acidic urine (pH <5.8). Calcium oxalate crystals are also common seen, particularly in urine with pH >5.4. Similarly, calcium phosphate crystals (brushite) are also relatively common in alkaline urine (pH >7.0). The presence of cystine crystals (characteristic hexagonal morphology) is indicative of the pathologic condition of cystinuria. These crystals form in acidic urine.

PROTEINURIA

Proteinuria is a common finding in clinical practice and may be due to a renal pathologic condition, such as a glomerulopathy, tubulointerstitial nephritis, dysproteinemia, or vasculitis. Clinicians should be aware that the causes of proteinuria are diverse; some cases are benign and are associated with a favorable prognosis (e.g., orthostatic or postural proteinuria, and benign persistent proteinuria), whereas others have more ominous implications.

Proteinuria is usually detected by dipstick analysis as a semiquantitative method of the protein concentration in urine. The degree of proteinuria is determined from a colorimetric reaction of an indicator dye (usually bromphenol blue in a citric acid buffer). The results are graded as negative, trace (10–20 mg/dL), 1+ (30 mg/dL), 2+ (100 mg/dL), 3+ (300 mg/dL), and 4+ (1,000 mg/dL). This method is more sensitive to albumin than globulins and other proteins. False positive results can occur in highly alkaline urine, in highly concentrated urine, in patients with gross hematuria, and in urine contaminated with certain antiseptics (such as chlorhexidine or benzalkonium chloride). False negative results can occur in dilute urine or in states in which the primary protein constituent is not albumin (e.g., immunoglobulin in the urine of patients with multiple myeloma).

Qualitative urine protein measurements, such as with dipstick analysis, are only crude estimates of the urine protein concentration. They are affected by the amount of urine produced and the degree to which the urine is diluted or concentrated in the random urine sample provided by the patient. As such, qualitative urine protein measurements correlate poorly with quantitative 24-hour urine protein determinations. Better correlation between the quantitative protein concentration in a random urine specimen and a 24-hour protein measurement is when the protein concentration in the sample is corrected for the

urine creatinine (protein-to-creatinine ratio) or urine osmolality (protein-to-osmolality ratio).[8,9] The protein-to-creatinine ratio or protein-to-osmolality ratio eliminates the effects of dilution of the urine and, therefore, aids in the assessment of proteinuria in a random urine collection. Furthermore, a reasonable correlation between these ratios and the 24-hour urine protein value has been found. Limitations of both of these methods are that they are based on the assumption of inter- and intraindividual comparable amounts of creatinine or osmole excretion.

Other methods exist for detecting protein in the urine, including precipitation methods (sulfosalicylic acid, or heat and acetic acid), dye-binding methods (Coomassie brilliant blue), chemical methods (biuret or Folin-Lowry assays), and immunologic methods (radial immunodiffusion, immunoelectrophoresis, immunoturbidimetry, nephelometry, and immunoassays for specific proteins). Precipitation methods with use of sulfosalicylic acid result in the denaturation and precipitation of the protein in the urine sample. With this method, the amount of protein present is estimated by the degree of turbidity; proteins other than albumin will be detected. The other methods are used primarily for quantifying total protein in 24-hour urine collections or for identifying and quantifying specific proteins in the urine.

If proteinuria is found to be persistent, a 24-hour urine collection for protein should be obtained. A normal value in healthy adults is less than 150 mg/day. Low-grade proteinuria (mild protein excretion) is less than 1 to 2 g/24 h. Nephrotic-range proteinuria is defined as 3.5 g/24 h or more and almost always is a reflection of significant glomerular disease. Usually, lipiduria (oval fat bodies, fatty casts, or free fat) accompanies nephrotic-range proteinuria, and additional testing should be directed toward further characterizing the probable glomerular disease. Several primary glomerular diseases and multisystem diseases are associated with nephrotic-range proteinuria.

When the degree of proteinuria is assessed on the basis of a 24-hour urine specimen, the results are directly dependent on an accurate collection by the patient. If an appreciable discrepancy exists between the expected 24-hour urine output of the patient and the amount of urine reported as collected for the urine protein determination (typical 24-hour urine output = 1 to 2.5 L), the patient should be questioned about the actual duration of collection and asked to provide another sample to ensure appropriate evaluation. A concomitant measurement of the creatinine clearance from the collected urine specimen can also be used to judge the completeness of collection. If a substantial discrepancy is noted between the expected clearance as predicted from the serum creatinine concentration and the measured creatinine clearance, an inaccurate collection of urine should be suspected.

Low-grade or mild proteinuria should be investigated further by obtaining overnight supine and daytime upright urine collections to determine whether orthostatic proteinuria is present. Normally, urinary protein excretion is slightly increased in the upright position as compared with the recumbent position. With orthostatic proteinuria, this difference is accentuated. In this condition, the proteinuria is usually less than 1 g/24 h; however, values of 2 to 3 g/24 h occasionally are noted. Long-term follow-up studies of patients with orthostatic proteinuria have indicated that the proteinuria often disappears with time and that a normal glomerular filtration rate (GFR) is maintained in these patients.

Further identification of the type of protein (or proteins) excreted should be considered in patients with persistent proteinuria. Protein electrophoresis of the urine can be done to determine the relative amounts of the protein components in the urine, and the results may provide clues about the cause of the proteinuria. For example, patients with nephrotic syndrome due to minimal change disease have mainly albumin in the urine, whereas patients with diseases of the renal tubules or interstitium fail to absorb low-molecular-weight proteins in the glomerular filtrate and thus will not have a preponderance of albumin. The presence of immunoglobulin light chains in the urine should be suspected when dipstick analysis for protein yields much lower results than those obtained by turbidimetric assay (e.g., the sulfosalicylic acid test). If this situation occurs, the protein can be characterized further by heating the urine specimen to assess for Bence Jones protein. If Bence Jones protein is present, the presence of light chains is suggested; however, false positive results can occur, and low-grade Bence Jones proteinuria will be found in many cases of heavy proteinuria because of the presence of polyclonal immunoglobulin light chains as a component of the proteinuria. Immunoelectrophoresis of the urine (and serum) is the definitive test for detection of monoclonal protein and should be performed in middle-aged and elderly patients with proteinuria or when the diagnosis of a paraprotein disorder is considered.

ALBUMINURIA

For the past several years, considerable attention has been given to the measurement of urine albumin in "micro" amounts, or microalbuminuria; that is, urine albumin excretion in patients who have negative results of protein determination on dipstick analysis. It has been recommended recently that the term "microalbuminuria" be abandoned and "albuminuria" be used instead, due to confusion about the meaning of the former term. Urine albumin determinations have been primarily used for monitoring the development of diabetic nephropathy. Albuminuria in patients with insulin-dependent diabetes mellitus has been demonstrated to predict the development of more advanced diabetic kidney disease. Enzyme-linked immunosorbent assay techniques, radioimmunoassays, or nephelometry is used for these determinations on overnight or 24-hour urine collections.[10] The normal 24-hour excretion of urine albumin is less than 30 mg. Usually, early albuminuria is defined as greater than 20 µg/min (or 30 mg/24 h) and less than 200 µg/min (or 300 mg/24 h).

Albumin excretion increases in patients with diabetes who are destined to develop diabetic nephropathy. More important, at this phase of increased albumin excretion before overt proteinuria develops, therapeutic maneuvers can be expected to significantly delay, or possibly prevent, development of nephropathy. Thus, there is a need for addressing small amounts of urinary albumin excretion (in the range of 30–300 mg/day; i.e., early albuminuria). The National Kidney Foundation convened an expert panel to recommend guidelines for the management of patients with diabetes and albuminuria. These guidelines recommend that all type 1 diabetic patients older than 12 years and all type 2 diabetic patients younger than 70 years should have their urine tested for albuminuria yearly when they are under stable glucose control.[11] Acceptable urine specimens can be from a 24-hour collection, a 10-hour overnight collection (9 PM to 7 AM) or a random collection, though KDIGO guidelines recommend obtaining a spot urine albumin-to-creatinine determination as initial screening, to be confirmed if positive by 2 additional samples.[11]

Several studies have addressed the optimal conditions for urine albumin collections (e.g., from a fasting urine, an exercised urine, or an overnight urine specimen). From these studies, it is clear that the first-morning urine specimen is less sensitive but more specific. A positive result should be confirmed by another first-morning random or 24-hour timed urine specimen.[12–14]

OTHER MARKERS OF KIDNEY INJURY

A large number of potential kidney injury biomarkers have been studied, and while several have potential utility for the diagnosis of kidney injury prior to a rise in serum creatinine, almost all are still considered investigational. The list includes markers of tubular injury, glomerular injury, acute kidney injury, renal fibrosis, and so on. Potential biomarkers of tubular injury include enzymes released from renal tubules (e.g., N-acetyl-beta-glucosaminidase, alkaline phosphatase, lactate dehydrogenase, gamma-glutamyltranspeptidase, alanine aminopeptidase, pi-glutathione S-transferase, alpha-glutathione S-transferase). Neutrophil gelatinase-associated lipocalin and kidney injury molecule-1 have been proposed as an early marker of acute tubular necrosis. Neutrophil gelatinase-associated lipocalin production by the kidney is increased with renal ischemia and kidney injury molecule-1 production by proximal tubular cells is similarly increased in settings of acute kidney injury. These, as well as several others, show promise for the diagnosis of acute kidney injury; however, their clinical validity and utility have yet to be clearly established.

Low molecular weight (LMWt) proteins (i.e., proteins 10–50 daltons) have been utilized as markers for tubular injury. Notably, the most commonly used LMWt proteins used for this purpose have been retinol binding protein, alpha-1 microglobulin and beta-2 microglobulin. These proteins are freely filtered at the glomerulus and then avidly reabsorbed by the proximal tubule such that under normal conditions little if any of these proteins are present in the final urine. In states of renal tubular injury, however, particularly those involving the proximal tubule, the urinary excretion of these LMWt proteins increase. Beta-2-microglobulin's stability in urine is influenced significantly by pH; it is degraded rapidly in acidic urine (both with urine residing in the bladder as well as after collection) resulting in unreliable measurements if the urine is not maintained in an alkaline state.

Markers for various glomerular diseases have been studied. Recent studies have shown that in approximately 70% of patients with primary membranous nephropathy (MN), the immune complexes consist of autoantibodies against the podocyte protein M-type phospholipase A2 receptor (PLA2R). There is also evidence that levels of anti-PLA2R autoantibodies correlate well with disease activity and progression.[15] The presence of anti-PLA2R antibodies could also potentially be used to differentiate primary MN from secondary MN (e.g., lupus membranous, etc.) or other causes of nephrotic syndrome if a biopsy is not possible. Among patients with chronic kidney disease (CKD) awaiting kidney transplantation, higher levels of anti-PLA2R could predict those more likely to recur after transplantation.[16]

There is extensive evidence to indicate that renal injury in primary focal glomerulosclerosis is due to a circulating factor that alters the permeability of glomerular basement membrane to proteins. This circulating permeability factor however has evaded precise identification despite extensive investigations though recent studies have implicated soluble urokinase plasminogen-activating receptor as a possible candidate.[17]

ASSESSMENT OF GFR

GFR is the aggregate of the filtration rate of individual nephrons. In normal individuals it is approximately 100 to 140 mL/min/1.73m^2 but is affected by a host of variables including age, gender, diet, body size, as well as a several other physiologic and pathophysiologic states and pharmacologic agents. It is often considered the best overall index of kidney function. Its decline correlates with other physiologic and clinical consequences and is a criterion in the definition and staging of AKI and CKD. It is essential but not sufficient for clinical assessment of kidney disease.

True GFR (tGFR) is the actual GFR. It, however, can never be known precisely because there is not a means to directly determine the GFR. As such, we rely on the laboratory assessment of either measured GFR (mGFR) or estimates of GFR (eGFR). Measured GFR is largely based on the clearance concept. The clearance of a substance can be defined as the amount of a given substance that is completely cleared from plasma per unit of time. For a substance that is cleared solely by the kidney and is (i) freely filtered; (ii) not protein bound; (iii) not reabsorbed, secreted, or metabolized by renal tubules; and (iv) stable in urine and is produced or infused at a steady state, then the amount of that substance (x) that is excreted in urine is equal to the product of the amount cleared by the kidney and its concentration in blood. This can be expressed in the following equations:

$$U_x \cdot V = Cl_x \cdot P_x$$

or

$$Cl_x = (U_x \cdot V) \div P_x$$

where U_x and P_x are the concentration of x in urine and plasma, respectively, Cl_x is the clearance of x and V is the urine flow. Given the properties of the substance as previously outlined, the clearance of x is equal to the GFR.

Several substances have been utilized as markers for the measurement of GFR (mGFR). Inulin historically has been considered the gold standard for mGFR. It is a fructose polymer derived from various plant products including the Jerusalem artichoke and chicory, among others. Many of the early seminal GFR measurement studies, both in humans and in animals, utilized inulin; however, it is rarely utilized recently due to lack of availability in the United States for human testing, as well as due to its cumbersome preparation and assay. Radiocontrast agents have largely replaced inulin for precise mGFR determinations. Iothalamate, either radiolabeled or non-radiolabeled is commonly used. Typically iothalamate is administered either as a continuous infusion or as a subcutaneous injection to achieve a steady plasma concentration followed by 1 or more timed urine collections. Its concentration in urine and plasma samples have utilized a variety of methods including, high-pressure liquid chromatography, mass spectrometry, and capillary electrophoresis (non-radiolabeled) as well as use of a scintillation counter for ^{125}I-iothalamate.

Plasma disappearance of a marker has been utilized in place of urinary clearance for the determination of mGFR. This method is based on the assumption that following a bolus injection the marker will first distribute relatively quickly into the extracellular fluid compartments (distribution phase) followed by a more prolonged elimination phase. The latter is directly proportional to the GFR. This method employs a bolus intravenous injection of the marker followed by a series of blood collections. The mGFR is then calculated based on formula derived from initial distribution phase and subsequent elimination phase, typically utilizing a 2 compartment model for the distribution of the marker. Iohexol is commonly used for plasma disappearance measurements. The primary advantage of plasma disappearance mGFR is that it does not require a timed urine collection.

Other methods for mGFR include the use of radionuclides diethylenetriaminepentaacetic acid (^{99m}Tc-DTPA) or ethylenediaminetetraacetic acid (^{51}Cr-EDTA). EDTA is used in Europe but not in the United States. A component of tubular reabsorption of EDTA and a degree of protein binding of DTPA can lead to an underestimation of GFR when using either of these agents.

The use of creatinine clearance has been widely used as an approximation of mGFR. Typically creatinine clearance measurements utilize a 24-hour urine collection and a single plasma sample. Although use of an endogenous marker has the advantage of not requiring the administration of an exogenous substance, it is well known that due to a component of tubular secretion of creatinine, the creatinine clearance tends to exceed other measures of GFR (e.g., inulin, iothalamate, iohexol) by 10% to 35%. Moreover, 24-hour urine collections are known to be prone to frequent and significant inaccuracies.

Creatinine is a product of muscle metabolism through the hydrolysis of phosphocreatine. Creatinine is largely eliminated through the kidneys. Creatinine is not protein bound, is freely filtered, and not reabsorbed or metabolized, but a component is reabsorbed by proximal renal tubules. Because creatinine elimination is largely dependent on glomerular filtration, its blood levels are inversely related to the GFR. However, nonglomerular factors affect serum creatinine concentrations, notably factors that affect muscle mass such as age, gender, race, physical activity, nutritional status, and so on. Additionally, dietary protein intake and drugs that compete with the tubular reabsorption of creatinine also can affect creatinine plasma levels independent of GFR.

A number of empirically derived equations utilizing serum creatinine have been developed as a way to provide eGFR.[18-22] Table 7.1 lists a few of the more commonly used eGFR equations. Most equations have been derived from populations of patients with stable chronic kidney disease. As such, the equations may not apply to all patient

TABLE 7.1 ESTIMATED GFR EQUATIONS

Cockcroft-Gault Equation[a]

$$C_{Cr} = \frac{(140 - Age) \times Weight\ (kg)}{72 \times S_{Cr}\ (mg/dL)} \times (0.85\ if\ female)$$

Schwartz Equation (for pediatric patients age 1–18 years)[b]

$$GFR = \frac{0.413 \times Height\ (cm)}{S_{Cr}}$$

MDRD Study Equation[c]

$$GFR = 175 \times Scr\ (mg/dL)^{-1.154} \times Age^{-0.203}$$
$$\times 0.742\ (if\ female) \times 1.21\ (if\ black)$$

CKD-EPI Equation for creatinine[d]

$$GFR = 141 \times \min(Scr/\kappa,1)^{-\alpha} \times \max(Scr/\kappa,1)^{-1.209}$$
$$\times 0.993^{Age} \times 1.018\ (if\ female) \times 1.157\ (if\ black)$$

where κ is 0.7 for females and 0.9 for males, α is −0.329 for females and −0.411 for males, min indicates the minimum of Scr/κ or 1, and max indicates the maximum of Scr/κ or 1.

CKD-EPI Equation for creatinine and cystatin C[e]

$$GFR = 135 \times \min(Scr/\kappa,1)^{-\alpha} \times \max(Scr/\kappa,1)^{-0.601}$$
$$\times \min(Scyst/0.8,1)^{-0.375} \times \max(Scyst/0.8,1)^{-0.711}$$
$$0.995^{Age} \times 0.969\ (if\ female) \times 1.08\ (if\ black)$$

where κ is 0.7 for females and 0.9 for males, α is −0.248 for females and −0.207 for males, min indicates the minimum of Scr/κ or 1, of Scyst/0.8 or 1; and max indicates the maximum of Scr/κ or 1, or Scys/0.8 or 1.

[a]Cockcroft DW, Gault MH. Prediction of creatinine clearance from serum creatinine. *Nephron.* 1976;16:31–41.
[b]Schwartz GJ, Munoz A, Schneider MF, et al. New equations to estimate GFR in children with CKD. *J Am Soc Nephrol.* 2009;20:629–637.
[c]Levey AS, Coresh J, Greene T, et al. Using standardized serum creainine values in the Modification of Diet in Renal Disease study equation for estimating glomerular filtration rate. *Ann Intern Med.* 2006;145:247–254.
[d]Levey AS, Stevens LA, Schmid CH, et al. A new equation to estimate glomerular filtration rate. *Ann Intern Med.* 2009;150:604–612.
[e]Inker LA, Schmid CH, Tighiouart H, et al. Estimating glomerular filtration rate from serum creatinine and cystatin C. *N Engl J Med.* 2012;367:20–29.

groups. Moreover, the degree of accuracy is limited. For example, the Chronic Kidney Disease Epidemiology Collaboration equation is based on 81% of eGFR values that are within 30% of the measured GFR. Additionally, eGFR equations are dependent on serum creatinine, which is affected by age, gender, race, physical activity, nutritional status, and so on. Dietary protein intake and drugs that compete with the tubular reabsorption of creatinine also can affect creatinine plasma levels independent of GFR.

Cystatin C is an endogenous low molecular weight protein that is constitutively produced by most cells, is freely filtered by the glomerulus, and is not protein bound. Its elimination appears to be solely the kidney. Unlike creatinine, however, filtered cystatin C is actively reabsorbed and metabolized by proximal tubule cells. Similar to creatinine its blood level is inversely related to GFR, but, unlike creatinine, it is not affected by muscle mass or diet. As such, it has inherent advantages over serum creatinine, particularly in situations with extremes of muscle mass (e.g., cachectic patients, children). Empiric equations for eGFR determinations have been derived utilizing cystatin C, either alone, or with serum creatinine (Table 7.1). Although cystatin C is not directly affected by muscle mass or diet there appear to be other yet to be clearly defined nonglomerular factors that can affect its levels.[23]

Beta-trace protein, another low molecular weight protein that is freely filtered by the kidneys, has been proposed as a marker of GFR. Beta-trace protein, also known as prostaglandin D2 synthase, is primarily expressed in the central nervous system but also expressed in the human heart. In addition to being freely filtered, similar to cystatin C, it is avidly taken up and degraded by renal proximal tubule cells. Several studies have indicated that as a marker of GFR it may compare similarly to cystatin, though its clinical utility has yet to be established.[24]

REFERENCES

1. Beer JH, Vogt A, Neftel K, et al. False positive results for lucocytes in urine dipstick test with common antibiotics. *Brit Med J.* 1996;313:25.
2. Linko S, Kouri TT, Toivonen E, et al. Analytical performance of the Iris iQ200 automated urine microscopy analyzer. *Clin Chim Acta.* 2006;372:54–64.
3. Delanghe JR, Kouri TT, Huber AR, et al. The role of automated urine particles: flow cytometry in clinical practice. *Clin Chim Acta.* 2000;301:1–18.
4. Fairley K, Birch DF. Hematuria: a simple method for identifying glomerular bleeding. *Kidney Int.* 1982;21:105–108.

5. Rath B, Turner C, Hartley B, Chantler C. What makes red cells dysmorphic in glomerular hematuria? *Paediatr Nephrol.* 1992;6:424–427.

6. Birch DF, Fairley KF. Haematuria: glomerular or non-glomerular? *Lancet.* 1979;2:845–846.

7. Pollock C, Liu PL, Györy AZ, et al. Dysmorphism of urinary red blood cells—value in diagnosis. *Kidney Int.* 1989;36:1045–1049.

8. Price CP, Newall R, Boyd JC. Use of protein/creatinine ratio measurements on random urine samples for prediction of significant proteinuria: A systematic review. *Clin Chem.* 2005;51:1577–1586.

9. Wilson DM, Anderson RL. Protein-osmolaltiy ratio for the quatntitative assessment of proteinuria from a random urinalysis sample. *Am J Clin Pathol.* 1993;100:419–424.

10. Sacks DB, Arnold M, Bakris GL, et al. Executive summary: guidelines and recommendations for laboratory analysis in the diagnosis and management of diabetes mellitus. *Clin Chem.* 2011;57:793–798.

11. Kidney Disease: Improving Global Outcomes (KDIGO) CKD Work Group. KDIGO 2012 clinical practice guideline for the evaluation and management of chronic kidney disease. *Kidney Int Suppl.* 2013;3:1.

12. Mogensen CE, Vestbo E, Poulsen PL, et al. Microalbuminuria and potential confounders. A review and some observations on variability of urinary albumin excretion. *Diabetes Care.* 1995;18:573–581.

13. Schwab SJ, Dunn FL, Feinglos MN. Screening for microalbuminuria: a comparison of single sample methods of collection and techniques of albumin analysis. *Diabetes Care.* 1992;15:1581–1584.

14. Witte EC, Lambers Heerspink HJ, de Zeeuw D, et al. First morning voids are more reliable than spot urine samples to assess microalbuminuria. *J Am Soc Nephrol.* 2009; 20:436–443.

15. Beck LH Jr, Bonegio RG, Lambeau G, et al. M-type phospholipase A2 receptor as target antigen in idiopathic membranous nephropathy. *N Engl J Med.* 2009;361:11–21.

16. Seitz-Polski B, Payré C, Ambrosetti D, et al. Prediction of membranous nephropathy recurrence after transplantation by monitoring of anti-PLA2R1 (M-type phospholipase A2 receptor) autoantibodies: a case series of 15 patients. *Nephrol Dial Transplant.* 2014;29:2334–2342.

17. Wei C, El Hindi S, Li J, et al. Circulating urokinase receptor as a cause of focal segmental glomerulosclerosis. *Nat Med.* 2011;17:952–960.

18. Schwartz GJ, Munoz A, Schneider MF, et al. New equations to estimate GFR in children with CKD. *J Am Soc Nephrol.* 2009;20:629–637.

19. Cockcroft DW, Gault MH. Prediction of creatinine clearance from serum creatinine. *Nephron.* 1976;16:31–41.

20. Levey AS, Coresh J, Greene T, et al. Using standardized serum creainine values in the Modification of Diet in Renal Disease study equation for estimating glomerular filtration rate. *Ann Intern Med.* 2006;145:247–254.

21. Levey AS, Stevens LA, Schmid CH, et al. A new equation to estimate glomerular filtration rate. *Ann Intern Med.* 2009;150:604–612.

22. Inker LA, Schmid CH, Tighiouart H, et al. Estimating glomerular filtration rate from serum creatinine and cystatin C. *N Engl J Med.* 2012;367:20–29.

23. Stevens LA, Schmid CH, Greene T, et al. Factors other than glomerular filtration rate affect serum cystatin C levels. *Kidney Int.* 2009;75:652–660.

24. Inker LA; Tighiouart H; Coresh J; et al. GFR estimation using beta-trace protein and beta2-microglobulin in CKD. *Am J Kid Dis.* 201;67:40–48.

8

Imaging of the Kidney

DAVID C. WYMER AND DAVID T. G. WYMER

INTRODUCTION

Imaging is an integral part in the evaluation of the renal patient. Radiology has a mandate to help provide a diagnosis while balancing the benefits of imaging against the potential adverse effect encountered in the imaging process. Major considerations in deciding on how to best image a given patient include radiation exposure, contrast allergies, potential contrast toxicity (including systemic effects such as nephrogenic systemic fibrosis [NSF]), psychological effects (such as claustrophobia), and renal trauma secondary to interventional procedures. The imaging toolbox includes ultrasound, computer tomography (CT) scan, magnetic resonance imaging (MRI) scan, and nuclear imaging. The choice of the best imaging in any given patient should include dialogue with the radiologist and online reference to the American College of Radiology[1] appropriate use criteria.

The focus of this chapter will be the use of imaging in providing the information necessary to protect the kidney from insults (metabolic and physical) and when needed to evaluate effects of age-related renal changes, drugs, treatments, and trauma on renal function. In-depth image evaluation and discussions on how to interpret images is left to other textbooks.

ULTRASOUND

Ultrasound is relatively inexpensive and non-invasive and can quickly assess renal location, contour, size, and obstructive uropathy without radiation exposure. Portable ultrasound is increasingly used and very useful in the pediatric or emergency setting. In cases of hematuria, evaluation for obstructing renal calculi can be readily performed, and renal masses can be identified as cystic or solid. The progression or regression of hydronephrosis in cases of obstructive uropathy is readily undertaken. Color Doppler imaging permits assessment of renal vascularity and perfusion. Limitations of ultrasound include lack of an acoustic window due to bowel gas or body habitus and poor patient cooperation.

The kidney is imaged in transverse and sagittal planes and is normally 9 to 12 cm in length in adults. The normal renal cortex is hypoechoic compared with the fat-containing echogenic renal sinus, and the cortical echotexture is defined as isoechoic or hypoechoic compared with the liver or spleen. The cortex is characteristically hyperechoic compared with the liver and the spleen. In adults, an increase in cortical echogenicity is a sensitive marker for parenchymal renal disease but is nonspecific. Decreased cortical echogenicity can be found in acute pyelonephritis and acute renal vein thrombosis. The renal pelvis and proximal ureter are anechoic. An extrarenal pelvis refers to the renal pelvis location outside the renal hilum. Due to its small size, the ureter is not identified beyond the pelvis in nonobstructed patients.

Obstruction can be identified by the presence of hydronephrosis. Parenchymal and pelvicalyceal nonobstructing renal calculi, as well as ureteral obstructing calculi, can be readily detected. False negative ultrasound examination findings with no hydronephrosis occasionally occur in early obstruction. Obstruction without ureteral dilation may also occur in retroperitoneal fibrosis and in transplanted kidneys as a result of periureteral fibrosis.

Cysts can be identified as anechoic lesions and are a frequent coincidental finding during renal imaging. Ultrasound usually readily identifies renal masses as cystic or solid. However, proteinaceous and hemorrhagic cysts may be mistakenly called solid because of increased echogenicity. Differentiation of cysts as simple or complex is required to plan intervention.

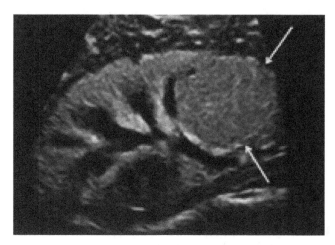

FIGURE 8.1 Contrast-enhanced ultrasound showing vascularity of renal tumor.

The Bosniak classification of cystic renal masses is widely used. Complex cysts identified by ultrasound require further evaluation by contrast-enhanced CT (or MRI) to identify abnormal contrast enhancement of the cyst wall, mural nodule, or septum, which may indicate malignancy.

Contrast-enhanced ultrasound using microbubbles is a new technique that shows vascularity of lesions (Fig. 8.1), while color Doppler investigation of the kidneys provides a detailed evaluation of the renal vascular anatomy. The main renal arteries can be identified in most patients. Power Doppler imaging is a more sensitive indicator of flow but provides no information about flow direction and cannot be used to assess vascular waveforms. Color Doppler sonography is used to evaluate renal artery stenosis. The narrowing in the artery causes a velocity change commensurate with the degree of stenosis as well as a change in the normal renal artery waveform downstream from the lesion. It also results in a decrease in the resistive index, defined as the end-diastolic velocity (EDV) subtracted from the peak systolic velocity (PSV) divided by PSV: (PSV − EDV)/PSV. The normal resistive index is 0.70 to 0.72.

When it is technically successful, Doppler ultrasound has a negative predictive value of more than 90%.[2] Doppler studies have several advantages such as being noninvasive, inexpensive, and widely available and do not expose the patient to radiation or contrast material.

Ultrasound is also used to guide renal biopsies. This will be discussed later.

PLAIN RADIOGRAPHY AND INTRAVENOUS UROGRAPHY

The simple plain film (or KUB—kidneys, ureters, and urinary bladder) provides a quick overview of the abdomen and with regards to the kidneys can identify large stones of the urinary tract but is otherwise an insensitive tool for complete renal evaluation. Intravenous urography (or intravenous pyelogram) historically was a useful exam to evaluate renal function and renal masses, but due to its lack of sensitivity and specificity, it has been completely replaced in most places by ultrasound, CT and MRI.

COMPUTED TOMOGRAPHY

While a downside of CT imaging is that it usually comes at a price of radiation exposure to the patient, new reconstruction software with what is called iterative reconstruction significantly reduces radiation exposure such that, unless multiple scans are required over short intervals of follow-up, the radiation risks to the patient are minimal. The CT data can be reconstructed in multiple planes and even 3D for improved anatomic visualization and localization (Fig. 8.2). CT examination of the kidneys is performed to evaluate suspect renal masses, locate ectopic kidneys, investigate calculi, assess retroperitoneal masses, and evaluate the extent of parenchymal involvement in patients with acute pyelonephritis. Noncontrast CT scans give the most robust evaluation of the patient in cases of urinary calculi and are considered the first line of imaging in those cases.[3,4] A primary drawback of CT is the patient radiation exposure.

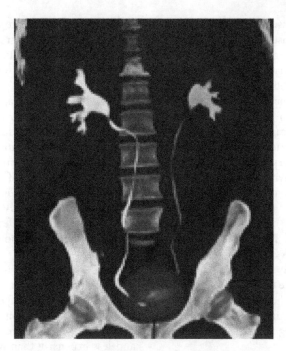

FIGURE 8.2 Coronal reconstruction from computed tomography intravenous pyelogram nicely demonstrating collecting system.

Contrast-Enhanced Computed Tomography

For additional renal evaluation, the kidneys are imaged after contrast administration (CT urography). The kidneys are imaged in the corticomedullary phase for evaluation of the renal vasculature as well as in the nephrographic phase for evaluation of the renal parenchyma. The degree of enhancement can be assessed in both solid masses and complex cysts. Delayed images through the kidneys and bladder are performed for evaluation of the opacified and distended collecting system, ureters, and bladder (Fig. 8.3). The CT study can be tailored to the individual clinical scenario. For example, the corticomedullary phase can be eliminated to decrease the radiation dose if there is no concern about a vascular abnormality or no need for presurgical planning. A diuretic or saline bolus can be administered after contrast to better distend the collecting system and ureters during the excretory phase.

Computed Tomographic Angiography

Computed tomographic angiography (CTA) produces images similar to conventional angiograms but requires no invasive catheterization. A bolus of contrast material is administered, and the images are reconstructed at narrow intervals. The contrast bolus is timed for optimal

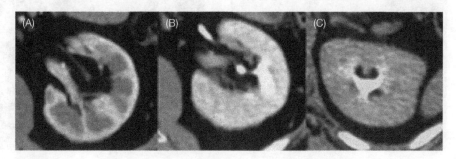

FIGURE 8.3 Images from a computed tomography intravenous pyelogram showing 3 different time points of scanning: (A) early arterial, (B) venous, and (C) excretory phases.

enhancement of the vessels. The aorta and branch vessels are well demonstrated. This technique is now widely used in living transplant donor evaluation, providing information not only on arterial and venous anatomy but also on size, number, and location of the kidneys as well as any ureteral anomalies of number or position.

In addition, CTA can be used to screen for atheromatous renal artery stenosis and helps in planning renal artery revascularization. The renal CTA has a sensitivity of 96% and specificity of 99% for the detection of hemodynamically significant stenosis.

MAGNETIC RESONANCE IMAGING

Although it should only rarely be the first examination used to evaluate the kidneys, MRI is typically an adjunct to other imaging. MRI allows direct multiplanar imaging and involves no radiation exposure, making it especially desirable in children.

There are multiple MRI imaging sequences that can be used, some of which allow very rapid image acquisition and, therefore, less chance of patient motion. The most common sequences are known as T1 and T2 (commonly a fast spin echo [FSE] sequence) with additional sequences that can suppress fat allowing differentiation of fat-containing masses. Fluid, such as urine, is dark or low in signal on T1-weighted sequences and bright or high in signal on T2 FSE sequences. The T2 image set is particularly useful in evaluating the renal pelvis, ureters, and bladder. Fat is bright on T1 and not as bright on T2 FSE sequences. Contrast material, gadolinium-based chelates, which are paramagnetic, can be intravenously administered to evaluate enhancement patterns of tissues. Notably, nephrotoxicity to gadolinium agents appears to be very uncommon, although in rare cases patients with renal insufficiency have been reported to develop NSF, which is discussed in another chapter. The sequences and imaging planes used for any given patient must be tailored to the individual MRI study.

A relatively new technique gaining popularity is diffusion-weighted imaging (DWI), which evaluates the freedom of water molecules to diffuse in tissues. Restriction of diffusion is imaged as bright areas on the DWI image set. The DWI data can be used to differentiate normal or benign tissues from infection, cancer, and ischemia (Fig. 8.4).

MRI is superior to CT in identifying noncalculous causes of renal obstruction, whereas CT is superior in identifying calculi as a cause of obstruction. Calcific stones are poorly visualized on MRI. CT is also more widely available, faster, and less expensive than MRI. However, MRI is better suited in patients with allergy to iodinated contrast agents and in children when radiation is an issue.

The disadvantages of MRI include the fact that the table and gantry are confining, so claustrophobic patients may be unable to cooperate. Patients with some types of internal metallic hardware cannot undergo MRI. MRI safety guidelines have been developed with an extensive list of devices that are or are not MRI approved, and any devices in the patient need to be checked against this list. Even with the new, fast-imaging techniques, patients need to be able to cooperate with breath-holding instructions to minimize motion-related artifacts. Patients

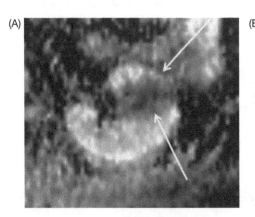
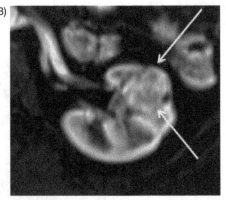

FIGURE 8.4 (A) Diffusion weighted imaging showing restricted diffusion (dark area) in renal cell carcinoma. (B) Contrast-enhanced magnetic resonance in same patient showing vascularity in tumor.

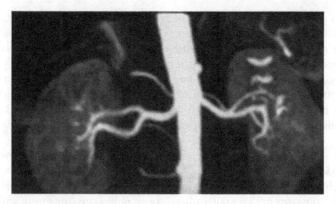

FIGURE 8.5 Magnetic resonance angiogram showing renal arteries.

in the intensive care unit and other critically ill patients can only be scanned if they are stable enough to be transported to the MRI suite and have no implanted metallic devices. Ventilated patients can undergo MRI; however, specific MRI-compatible, nonferromagnetic ventilators and other life support devices must be used. And finally, MRI with gadolinium has until recently been contraindicated in patients with glomerular filtration rate (GFR) below 30 mL/min/1.73m² because of the risk of nephrogenic systemic fibrosis.

Magnetic Resonance Angiography

Although MRA can be performed with or without intravenous contrast, contrast typically provides better images. The aorta and branch vessels are beautifully demonstrated (Fig. 8.5). By adjustment of timing and type of sequences, either the abdominal arterial or venous structures can be visualized (Fig. 8.6). MRA is performed to evaluate the renal arteries for stenosis and is less invasive than catheter angiography. Where MRA is unavailable, Doppler ultrasound can be used to evaluate renal artery stenosis.

Dual Energy CT

Dual energy CT (DECT) is a developing technology wherein two CT data sets are acquired using different tube potentials, usually 140 and 80 kV, which have different X-ray spectra. The density values at both acquired spectra differentiate

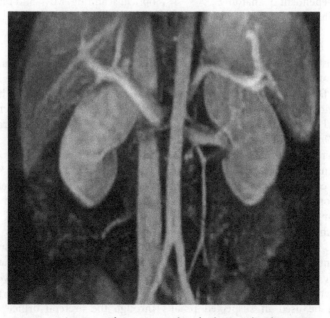

FIGURE 8.6 Magnetic resonance angiogram with imaging to show both arterial and venous structures.

materials (such as administered iodine or renal stones) on the basis of the photoelectric effect. One primary use of DECT is to allow kidney stone differentiation (i.e., differentiation of uric acid from magnesium or calcium), allowing tailored treatment strategies.[5,6] Additionally, uric acid deposits can be identified, and research is ongoing to use DECT to help characterize renal masses.

Nuclear Medicine

Nuclear scintigraphy primarily evaluates function and, to some extent, the anatomy seen with other diagnostic imaging modalities. Radiotracers are designed to accumulate in the renal parenchyma or collecting systems based on renal physiology. The gamma camera captures the photons from a radiotracer within the patient and generates an image. Three categories of radiotracers that differ in mode of renal clearance are used in renal imaging: glomerular filtration, tubular secretion, and tubular retention agents.

Nuclear scintigraphy provides an accurate assessment of renal function, used, for example, in estimating the expected reduction in renal function after nephron-sparing surgery and in the evaluation of the renal transplant patient. Both CTA and MRA have replaced nuclear scintigraphy in the evaluation of renal artery stenosis and in evaluation of benign renal masses, such as a column of Bertin. Nuclear medicine is still used to assess the functional significance of renal artery stenosis independent of anatomy.

Glomerular filtration agents can be used to measure GFR. Technetium Tc-99m–labeled diethylenetriaminepentaacetic acid (^{99m}Tc-DTPA) is the most common glomerular agent used for imaging and can also be used for GFR calculation. ^{99m}Tc-DTPA is also used along with lasix administration to evaluate obstructive uropathy and renal transplant follow-up.

Technetium-99m MAG3 is handled primarily by tubular secretion and can be used to estimate effective renal plasma flow. ^{99m}Tc-MAG3, like ^{99m}Tc-DTPA can be used to evaluate the renal transplant for rejection, cyclosporine toxicity, acute tubular necrosis, and posttransplant complications such as renal vascular issues or urine leaks.

The most commonly used tubular retention agent is ^{99m}Tc-labeled dimercaptosuccinate (DMSA). This agent provides excellent cortical imaging and can be used in suspected renal scarring or infarction, in pyelonephritis, and

for clarification of renal pseudotumors. DMSA binds with high affinity to sulfhydryl groups on the surface of proximal tubular cells. The cortical study is used most frequently for evaluation of renal scarring, particularly in children with reflux or chronic infections. Cortical imaging may be better than ultrasound in the evaluation of the young patient with urinary tract infection.

Positron Emission Tomography and Molecular Imaging

Positron emission tomography (PET) scanning uses radioactive positron emitters, most often ^{18}F-labeled fluorodeoxyglucose (FDG). FDG is intravenously injected and distributes in the body according to metabolic activity. Any process, such as a tumor or infection, that causes increased metabolic activity will result in an area of increased uptake on the scan. Because FDG is cleared through the kidneys and excreted in the urine, which can obscure renal masses or infection, PET scanning has a limited role in renal imaging but is useful in the staging and follow-up of metastatic renal cancer.

The term "molecular imaging" refers to the assessment of specific molecular differences in tissues and disease processes. Molecular imaging studies dynamic processes such as metabolic activity, cell proliferation, apoptosis, receptor status, and antigen modulation. Typically, this involves imaging of biochemical and physiologic processes. Techniques are being developed with optical scanning, MRI, and ultrasound as well as with radionuclides.

Applications are established in clinical practice, particularly in oncology (e.g., CD20 imaging in lymphoma), and work is under way for renal-specific molecular imaging. For example, MR renal cell imaging may soon be available to help differentiate acute tubular necrosis from renal rejection and renal cell cancer from benign tumors.

RETROGRADE AND ANTEGRADE PYELOGRAPHY

Retrograde pyelography is performed when the ureters are poorly visualized on other imaging studies or when samples of urine need to be obtained from the kidney for cytology or culture. Patients who have severe allergies to contrast agents or impaired renal function can be evaluated with retrograde pyelography. The examination is performed by placing a catheter through the ureteral orifice under cystoscopic guidance and advancing it into the renal pelvis.

With use of fluoroscopy, the catheter is slowly withdrawn while radiocontrast is injected. This technique provides excellent visualization of the renal pelvis and ureters.

Antegrade pyelography is performed through a percutaneous renal puncture and is used when retrograde pyelography is not possible. Ureteral pressures can be measured, hydronephrosis evaluated, and ureteral lesions identified.

Imaging Contrast Issues

Contrast administration continues to be a key part of diagnostic imaging. Although recent advances have allowed for imaging without contrast to characterize anatomy and pathology in ways that used to require contrast, many disease processes still require the use of intravenous contrast to be accurately and definitively characterized. Historically, medical dogma has stated that contrast agents (both for CT and MRI) carried risks in patients with impaired renal function that outweighed the benefits to the imaging. However, new data as well as newer contrast agents suggest that this may not be entirely accurate.

CT Contrast

CT utilizes iodinated intravenous contrast agents for imaging. A tri-iodinated benzene ring is the chemical basis of these agents. Older "conventional" agents had high osmolality up to 5 times greater than plasma. These were largely replaced by low-osmolar agents (which are still hyperosmolar to plasma), and more recently there are iso-osmolar nonionic agents. Iodinated contrast agents are renally excreted (by as much as 99%), with a biologic half-life of 1 to 2 hours in patients with normal renal function. If renal function is compromised, half-life can increase to 2 to 4 hours in dialysis patients, and extrarenal excretion predominantly through the gastrointestinal tract plays a larger role.

Reactions to contrast can be classified as anaphylactoid or chemotoxic. Anaphylactoid reactions are on the spectrum of allergic responses and will not be discussed in detail. Chemotoxic reactions are those thought to be a direct toxic effect of the material itself. It is in this category that the so-called contrast-induced nephropathy (CIN) belongs.

The threat of CIN is one of the largest factors preventing the use of contrast to obtain diagnostically more useful studies. The original studies and case reports that led to where we are today came from observations in patients who had received cardiac catheterization, and most of these studies did not have adequate control groups. These cases also used older generation (ionic high-osmolar) contrast agents, which are generally believed to be more nephrotoxic. More recent studies have shown that patients with normal renal function have no increased risk of renal impairment after the administration of intravenous contrast than those of the general population.[7] Furthermore, studies have shown that even in patients with impaired renal function, the overall risk of progressing to dialysis dependence or death is negligible.[7]

Over the years, there have been several theories on the pathogenesis of CIN including renal vasoconstriction, direct nephrotoxicity, and uricosuria (induced by the contrast agent). Damage from renal vasoconstriction was thought to be attributable to derangements in nitric oxide, which were thought to account for the reported increased incidence of CIN in patients with diabetes and heart failure, as these patients have altered nitric oxide metabolism at baseline.

Although the risk of CIN has likely been markedly overestimated, it is still reasonable to question the use of iodinated contrast in nondialysis-dependent renally impaired patients. In patients with a GFR of less than 45 mL/min, the clinical utility of a contrasted study should be questioned before proceeding. If it is necessary for the care of the patient and there is significant risk in delay in diagnosis by obtaining a noncontrasted study (such as possible stroke, dissection, or hemodynamically unstable bleeding), there should be no hesitation to administer intravenous contrast. In those patients who can afford to wait for a diagnosis, seeking alternative imaging such as MRI or ultrasound (depending on the clinical situation) is not unreasonable.[8]

For those patients receiving contrast who have decreased renal function, simple hydration with intravenous saline likely has the most benefit. Administration of sodium bicarbonate has not been shown to be superior to saline. Oral N-acetylcysteine, which has also been used, has shown no evidence of utility. This topic is discussed in greater detail in Chapter 25 of this book.

MR Contrast

MRI utilizes gadolinium-based contrast agents. These agents consist of a gadolinium atom that is tightly chelated to another organic molecule, as free gadolinium is highly toxic. These agents are classified by the type (shape) of molecule that the gadolinium is bound to (linear or macrocyclic) and the type of chemical bond that is made to the gadolinium (nonionic or ionic). In general, ionic binds the gadolinium tighter than nonionic, and macrocyclic binds the gadolinium tighter than linear. As with CT-iodinated contrast agents, the primary method of excretion for these agents is renal excretion (up to 99%) with the exception of gadoxetic acid (which is 50% renal, 50% hepatobiliary).

The main risk that physicians fear in using MR contrast is the risk of NSF. This entity is a rare fibrosing dermopathy that can cause severe morbidity or mortality. Initial studies showed that administration of gadolinium-based agents to patients with impaired renal function (GFR <30 mL/min) was the primary risk factor to developing NSF.[9] These cases were reported with the earlier agents that were linear nonionic (gadodiamide and gadoversetamide). Since that time, new agents have been developed that appear to have a much lower risk of NSF. The only linear ionic agent to have reported cases of NSF is gadopentetate dimeglumine, and all other linear ionic as well as macrocyclic ionic and nonionic formulations have, to date, demonstrated no cases of NSF. More recent studies have even shown that some of these agents (gadobenate dimeglumine and gadoterate meglumine) may not cause NSF even in patients on dialysis.[9]

As with iodinated contrast agents, it is still reasonable to question the use of gadolinium-based contrast in patients with severely impaired renal function. In patients with a GFR of less than 30 mL/min, the diagnostic utility of contrast should be called into question. If alternative imaging means are available to answer the clinical question, then these methods should be pursued. However, if MR contrast is deemed necessary to establish the diagnosis or direct further care for a patient, it is reasonable to administer contrast in these situations. These patients should receive contrast that has a very good risk profile, preferably gadobenate dimeglumine or gadoterate meglumine (if available) as these have the best evidence of their safety to date. Agents that have documented cases of NSF should always be avoided in patients with impaired renal function.

Recent evidence has also shown that gadolinium from these contrast agents has a degree of long-term retention and deposition in tissues. The brain has been identified as one of the main sites of deposition, especially after multiple administrations of contrast. There are no known adverse events associated with this, and it is unclear if this has any relation to renal function.

Renal Biopsy

Protecting the kidney from adverse effects of biopsy is paramount. Percutaneous renal biopsy is usually performed under ultrasonic guidance so the exact site of biopsy can be observed in real time. Ultrasonography can localize the desired lower pole site (at which the risk of puncturing a major vessel is minimized), determine renal size, and detect the unexpected presence of cysts that might necessitate using the contralateral kidney.

The usual approach is to try to obtain 2 cores of renal tissue, and adequacy of tissue sampling can be confirmed with microscopy immediately during the procedure. Bleeding is the primary complication of renal biopsy.

After a percutaneous renal biopsy, observing the patients for at least 12 hours is prudent to assure clinical stability.

Percutaneous renal biopsy for the detection of primary renal disease is generally not pursued in the following settings (relative contraindications):

- Small hyperechoic kidneys (less than 9 cm), which are generally indicative of chronic irreversible disease
- Solitary native kidney
- Multiple, bilateral cysts or a renal tumor
- Severe hypertension that cannot be controlled with antihypertensive medications
- Hydronephrosis
- Active renal or perirenal infection
- Skin infection over the biopsy site

Absolute contraindications for the performance of a percutaneous native kidney renal biopsy were defined in a position paper by the Health and Public Policy Committee of the American College of Physicians in 1988.[10] These include uncontrolled severe hypertension, uncontrollable bleeding diathesis, uncooperative patient, and a solitary native kidney.

SUMMARY

Renal ultrasound is often the first test in evaluating the kidneys since it is relatively inexpensive and noninvasive and can quickly assess renal location, contour, size, obstructive uropathy and renal vasculature without radiation exposure.

Noncontrast CT is the modality of choice for workup of calculi of the urinary tract, and with new iterative reconstruction software, the radiation dose is minimal. Contrast-enhanced CT is useful in evaluating renal masses, complex cysts, and the renal vasculature.

MRI has significant advantages is evaluating renal cysts and masses as well as obstructive uropathy in that it allows direct multiplanar acquisition with no radiation.

Nuclear medicine has strengths in evaluating obstructive uropathy and renal transplant functional analysis.

REFERENCES

1. American College of Radiology. ACR Appropriateness Criteria˙. https://www.acr.org/Clinical-Resources/ACR-Appropriateness-Criteria

2. Radermacher J, Chavan A, Schaffer J, et al. Detection of significant renal artery stenosis with color Doppler sonography: combining extrarenal and intrarenal approaches to minimize technical failure. *Clin Nephrol.* 2000;53:333–343.

3. Sommer FG, Jeffrey RB Jr, Rubin GD, et al. Detection of ureteral calculi in patients with suspected renal colic: value of reformatted non-contrast helical CT. *Am J Radiol.* 1995;165:509–513.

4. Lanoue MZ, Mindell HJ. The use of unenhanced helical CT to evaluate suspected renal colic. *Am J Radiol.* 1997;169:1579–1584.

5. Yeh BM, Shepherd JA, Wang ZJ, Teh HS, Hartman RP, Prevrhal S. Dual-energy and low-kVp CT in the abdomen. *Am J Roentgenol.* 2009;193:47–54.

6. Thorsten R. C. Johnson dual-energy CT: general principles *Am J Roentgenol.* 2012;199(5 Suppl):S3–S8.

7. Wilhelm-Leen E, Montez-Rath ME, Chertow GJ. Estimating the risk of radiocontrast-associated nephropathy. *Am Soc Nephrol.* 2017;28(2):653–659.

8. Merten GJ, Burgess WP, Gray LV, et al. Prevention of contrast-induced nephropathy with sodium bicarbonate. *J Am Med Assoc.* 2004;291:2328–2334.

9. Thomsen HS, Morcos SK, Almén T, et al. Nephrogenic systemic fibrosis and gadolinium-based contrast media: updated ESUR Contrast Medium Safety Committee guidelines. *Eur Radiol.* 2013;23:307–318.

10. Anon. Clinical competence in percutaneous renal biopsy. Health and Public Policy Committee. American College of Physicians. *Ann Intern Med.* 1988;108:301–303.

9

Fundamental of Kidney Pathology

SERENA M. BAGNASCO

PATHOLOGICAL EVALUATION OF THE RENAL BIOPSY

Percutaneous renal biopsy is the most common sampling technique for the pathological examination of native and transplanted kidney parenchyma.

Adequacy

The biopsy should contain both cortex and medulla, ideally with at least 2 separate cores including 10 or more glomeruli and 2 or more arteries. A minimum of 7 glomeruli and 1 artery has been proposed for transplanted kidneys.[1]

Light Microscopy

Light microscopy (LM) evaluation should be conducted on multiple, 2- to 4-μm thick serial sections of formalin-fixed, paraffin-embedded renal tissue, stained with hematoxylin and eosin, periodic acid Schiff (PAS) stain, methenamine silver-periodic acid stain (Jones, MS-PAS), and Masson trichrome stain. Additional special stains may be needed for identification of amyloid (Congo red, thioflavin T) or microorganisms.

Immunohistological Stains

Immunohistological stains are performed using antibodies conjugated with fluorescent dyes for immunofluorescence (IF) or enzyme-labeled for immunohistochemistry (IHC) to detect presence of specific protein antigens in the renal tissue. IF-based staining of frozen sections is used routinely for identification of pathologic immunoglobulins (IgG, IgA, IgM, and kappa and lambda light chains) and complement in glomeruli, tubules and interstitium, and vessels, and stain for albumin is used as a convenient way to highlight the glomerular and tubular basement membranes by virtue of its low-level, nonspecific stain of these structures. Additional immunostains for evaluation of glomerular pathology include IgG subclasses for identification of monoclonal IgG heavy chains and phospholipase A2 receptor antibodies (PLA2R); for evaluation of idiopathic membranous nephropathy. Other instances requiring immunohistochemical stains include identification of cell types and their distribution in renal inflammatory infiltrates to differentiate from lymphoproliferative disorders and identification of viral infections, myoglobin, amyloid.

Electron Microscopy

For electron microscopy (EM) examination, the tissue is fixed in gluteraldehyde, postfixed in osmium, embedded in resin or plastic, and cut in very thin sections. Sections stained with uranyl acetate and lead citrate are then placed on copper grid and examined. EM is valuable for identifying abnormal ultrastructural characteristic of glomerular and, to a lesser degree, tubular and vascular compartments. In the glomeruli, EM can identify abnormal thickness and structure of the glomerular basement membrane (GBM) relative to the age of the patient with estimated normal range of 230 to 430 nm for adult males and 215 to 395 nm for adult females.[2] Electron microscopy can show the distribution of glomerular immune deposits and the type of substructure in glomerular organized deposits and can reveal morphologic abnormality and injury of epithelial, mesangial, or endothelial glomerular cells such as podocyte foot process effacement, endothelial swelling, or abnormal cytoplasmic inclusions.

General Considerations

Several classic studies have correlated renal histology and renal function,[3-5] and the main purpose of existing histopathological classifications of renal diseases is to identify sets of features with predictive value for response to treatment that can ultimately arrest disease progression to end stage renal disease. Glomerular and tubulointerstitial scarring represent the end result of different pathological processes: primary glomerulopathies, systemic diseases, and tubulointerstitial and vascular diseases. Global glomerulosclerosis indicates complete obliteration by scarring of the glomerular tuft. It occurs with normal aging and various estimates generally place the number of globally sclerosed glomeruli in normal individuals from 1% to 10% up to middle age and even higher in older individuals.[6] A schema with the upper 95th percentile reference limit for the number of globally sclerosed glomeruli in normal individuals based on age and number of glomeruli per biopsy section has recently been published.[7] There is no generally accepted higher limit for tubular atrophy and interstitial fibrosis in the cortex, although up to 5% of interstitial fibrotic expansion can be considered normal.

PATHOLOGIC FEATURES OF MAJOR GLOMERULOPATHIES

Minimal Change Disease

Minimal change disease (MCD) is characterized by absence of pathologic glomerular changes by light microscopy, but ultrastructural evidence of podocyte injury is detectable by EM. MCD can be idiopathic but can also be secondary with use of certain drugs or in the presence of neoplasia, such as lymphoproliferative malignancies.

Light Microscopy

The glomeruli show normal appearance. Focal global glomerulosclerosis can be present but should not be exceeding the number of sclerosed glomeruli appropriate for the age of the patient. Tubular cytoplasmic protein droplets may be prominent with heavy proteinuria. Focal tubular atrophy and interstitial fibrosis may be present in older patients.

Immunofluorescence

IF staining should be negative for immune complex deposition.

Electron Microscopy

EM should reveal extensive effacement (also termed "fusion") of the podocyte foot processes, at least involving more than 50% of the capillary surface. Other evidence of podocyte injury include enlargement, microvillous transformation, vacuolization, and cytoplasmic protein or lipid droplets. Response to treatment, partial or complete, results in variable decrease or disappearance of foot process effacement.

Glomerular Tip Lesion

Light Microscopy

One or more glomeruli show a small area of the glomerular tuft located at the origin of the proximal convoluted tubule showing adhesion to the Bowman's capsule sometimes with foamy cells, with otherwise normal glomeruli by light microscopy.

Immunofluorescence

No immune deposits should be present.

Electron Microscopy

Diffuse effacement of the podocyte foot processes is usually present.[8] The glomerular tip lesion was originally described in 1984. The relation of glomerular tip lesion (GTL) with focal segmental glomerulosclerosis (FSGS) and clinical course has been the subject of several studies. The incidence of GTL varies in different studies ranging from 2% up to 13.5% and even 66%.[8,9] GTL appears to include cases that can behave like MCD and cases that behave like FSGS, without specific histologic features that can reliably predict the outcome.[9]

Focal Segmental Glomerulosclerosis

FSGS is defined as partial scarring of the glomerular tuft (segmental) affecting some but not all of the glomeruli (focal). FSGS can be encountered in renal diseases of different etiology involving the glomerulus. FSGS is a significant cause of nephrotic syndrome in 20% of children and 40% of adults.[10] Based on etiology, FSGS is classified as primary or idiopathic in the absence of a specific cause and secondary when associations can be established with genetic mutation in podocyte genes, certain viral infections, certain drugs, and adaptation to progressive reduction of renal mass in various conditions (postadaptive FSGS).

Light Microscopy

The glomeruli may be enlarged. Involved glomeruli typically show segmental solidification with obliteration of the capillaries by acellular matrix, which is highlighted by positive PAS and silver stain, variably extended areas of adhesion of the scarred glomerular capillaries to the Bowman's capsule, eosinophilic material (hyalinosis) resulting from plasma protein entrapment, and occasional foamy cells can be seen. Other features include enlarged visceral epithelial cells (podocytes) overlying sclerosed areas (capping), protein droplets in the podocyte cytoplasm, and enlargement and contact of the podocytes with parietal epithelial cells lining the Bowman's capsule. Tubular cytoplasmic protein droplets may be prominent with heavy proteinuria. Tubulointerstitial changes are often seen in FSGS, with variable degree of interstitial inflammation, tubular atrophy, and interstitial fibrosis.

Immunofluorescence
No immune complex deposits should be present.

Electron Microscopy
Variable degree of podocyte foot process effacement is present, typically mild, involving less than 50% of the capillary surface in secondary forms of FSGS such as postadaptive forms and more pronounced in primary forms.

A histopathological classification of FSGS based on light microscopy features has been proposed,[11] and includes five variants: FSGS not otherwise specified, perihilar, cellular, tip, and collapsing. This classification has not been robustly validated and is based solely on histological features that not infrequently can be found all together in the same biopsy. The form of FSGS that is generically defined by segmental consolidation, scarring, and obliteration of the glomerular capillaries by acellular matrix (not otherwise specified in the previously listed classification) is the most common lesion in primary and secondary forms of FSGS: 32% to 73% in different studies.[12] Glomerular collapsing changes, also referred to as collapsing glomerulopathy when not associated with obvious segmental lesion of FSGS, is characterized by severe narrowing of the capillary lumen with wrinkled glomerular capillary walls and apparent expansion of the urinary space, with marked hypertrophic changes in the podocytes (Fig. 9.1A). By EM, the podocytes

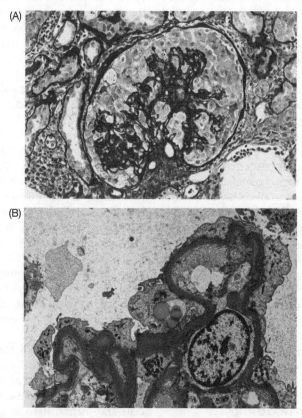

FIGURE 9.1 Collapsing glomerulopathy. (A) Light microscopy periodic acid Schiff- methenamine silver stain shows collapse of the glomerular capillary tuft with marked podocyte hypertrophy and hyperplasia. (B) Electron microscopy image showing wrinkling of the glomerular basement membrane and diffuse effacement of the podocyte foot processes.

show diffuse foot process effacement and detachment from the capillary wall surface (Fig. 9.1B), sometimes with intervening electrolucent material. Collapsing features are associated with severe nephrotic syndrome and rapid progression. Collapsing glomerulopathy is a characteristic pathologic glomerular injury associated with HIV infection and HIV-associated nephropathy (HIVAN).[13]

Membranous Nephropathy

Membranous glomerulopathy is characterized by the presence of immune complex deposits in the subepithelial aspect of the GBM. Based on etiology, membranous nephropathy (MN) can be classified on primary or idiopathic or secondary when associated with treatment with certain drugs, malignancies, infections, or autoimmune diseases.

Light Microscopy

The glomeruli are generally enlarged and show variable thickening of the glomerular capillary walls. The presence of deposits is best appreciated on silver-stained sections, where the glomerular capillary walls show vacuoles, or "spikes," representing projection of GBM matrix protruding on the subepithelial side of the capillary wall surface. There may be variable focal global or segmental glomerular scarring, and variable interstitial fibrosis and tubular atrophy (IFTA). Interstitial clusters of foamy cells are often seen.

Immunofluorescence

IF typically shows positive granular staining in the glomerular capillary walls, with or without mesangial staining, for IgG, kappa and lambda light chains, and C3; positive staining for IgM, and less frequently for IgA and C1q can also be present. Immunostain (IF or IHC) for PLA2R showing positive granular staining in the glomerular capillary walls can be used to differentiate primary from secondary forms of MN, with good sensitivity and specificity for primary MN.[14,15] Immunostain for thrombospondin type I domain-containing 7A (THSD7A) has also been used successfully to identify a small subset of primary MN.[16]

Electron Microscopy

EM shows electron dense deposits in the GBM and, in some cases, in the mesangium. Reactive podocyte changes with foot process effacement are usually present. The size and distribution of the deposits varies depending on the age and severity of the glomerular lesion, and includes 5 progressive stages according to a classification originally proposed by Ehrenreich and Churg[17] in 1968:

Stage I: small sparse deposits on the subepithelial aspect of the GBM, without intervening projection of GBM matrix

Stage II: subepithelial deposits generally larger and more closely spaced, with intervening projection of GBM matrix

Stage III: electron dense deposits are encircled by GBM matrix and appear intramembranous

Stage IV: deposits show evidence of reabsorption leaving behind electrolucent spaces

Stage V: sclerosing changes of the capillary walls.

These stages may be overlapping and do not correlate with proteinuria or clinical progression of the disease. In general, the degree of tubular atrophy and interstitial fibrosis have been found to be strong predictors of outcome in proteinuric glomerulopathies.[18]

Membranoproliferative Glomerulonephritis

Membranoproliferative glomerulonephritis (MPGN) refers to a glomerular lesion, with characteristic pathologic features. Historically, MPGN used to be classified in 3 morphological types (types I, II, and III). This is no longer appropriate since dense deposit disease (formerly MPGN II) has now be included among a group of diseases caused by abnormalities in the complement cascade also referred to as C3 glomerulopathies.[19,20] Regarding etiology, MPGN with immune complex deposits can be idiopathic but is most often associated with a variety of conditions including infections, autoimmune diseases, neoplasms, dysproteinemia, and paraproteins.

Light Microscopy

The glomeruli are usually enlarged with lobular appearance. There is hypercellularity with influx of inflammatory cells and an increase in mesangial cells and matrix, narrowing or obliterating the capillary lumen; typically all glomeruli are globally involved. The capillary walls are thickened and show a characteristic "double contours" due to new deposition of GBM-like material secreted by mesangial or endothelial cells, as well as by immune deposits accumulation on the subendothelial aspect of the glomerular capillary walls. These changes are best highlighted by PAS and silver stains. Crescents can be seen but are infrequent. The tubules may show protein reabsorption droplets and red blood cells in the lumen forming focal casts. Variable degree of interstitial inflammation, glomerular, and tubulointerstitial scarring may be present.

Immunofluorescence
IF shows positive granular staining for IgG (can have IgA and IgM), characteristically most evident in the peripheral glomerular capillary walls, accompanied by positive staining for C3, kappa, and lambda. Absence of immunoglobulin staining in the presence of positive C3 could indicate C3 glomerulopathy or dense deposits disease (defined by positive staining for C3 along the capillary walls, in the absence of staining for immunoglobulins, and by presence of electron dense continuous, ribbon-like deposits within the GBM, with or without mesangial deposits).

Electron Microscopy
EM shows subendothelial electron dense deposits as well as mesangial deposits, with scattered subepithelial/intramembranous deposits (MPGN with a large number of subepithelial deposits has been referred to as MPGN type III or Burkholder type). Of note, some cases of MPGN associated with cryoglobulinemia can show microtubular substructure of the subendothelial electron dense deposits.

IgA Nephropathy
IgA nephropathy is defined by the presence of IgA-dominant immune deposits in the glomerular mesangium. Most instances of IgAN can be considered primary or idiopathic, including the glomerular lesions of Henoch-Schoenlein purpura. Familial forms of IgAN have been described. Secondary forms of IgAN occur in association with a variety of conditions including hepatobiliary and intestinal diseases, infections such as HIV, some neoplasias, and some dermatologic diseases.

Light Microscopy
IgAN manifestations can vary, including normal glomerular appearance, FSGS, variable degree of mesangial expansion and mesangial hypercellularity, focal or diffuse endocapillary proliferation, and segmental or diffuse crescentic glomerular lesions. Red blood cell in the tubular lumen and red blood cell casts are usual. Variable degree of global glomerulosclerosis, interstitial inflammation, and tubulointerstitial scarring can be present.

Immunofluorescence
IF shows granular mesangial staining with strongest intensity for IgA with a positive stain for kappa and lambda, with or without IgG, IgM, or C3.

Electron Microscopy
Electron dense deposits should be evident in the mesangium, some extending into the subendothelial aspect of immediately adjacent capillary walls (paramesangium). Scattered subepithelial deposits can be present. Podocyte injury in the form of foot process effacement can also be present.

Several histopathological classifications have been proposed for IgAN. The most recent Oxford classification[21] and its recent update,[22] includes 5 parameters: absence (M0) or presence (M1) of mesangial hypercellularity; absence (E0) or presence (E1) of glomerular endocapillary hypercellularity; absence (S0) or presence (S1) of segmental glomerular sclerosis; percent of cortex showing IFTA asT0 if 0% to ≤25%, T1 if 26% to 50%, and T2 if >50%; and absence (C0) or presence of crescents in <25% (C1) or >25% (C2) of the glomeruli. Of these parameters, presence of mesangial hypercellularity (M1), segmental sclerosis (S1), IFTA >25% (T1), and crescents (C1, C2) have negative prognostic implications.

In general, the degree of tubular atrophy and interstitial fibrosis have been found to be strong predictors of outcome in different types of proteinuric glomerulopathies.[5,18,23]

Glomerulopathies Associated with Infections
Immune complex mediated glomerulonephritis can occur with active ongoing infection, or after the infection has subsided (postinfectious). Symptoms of infection can be absent, and the infection can be undetected or subclinical at the time when the glomerulonephritis is diagnosed. Glomerulonephritis can be associated with several types of bacterial infections and other infectious agents, including viral infections such as

hepatitis and HIV. The histologic manifestations can vary, depending on the type of infectious agent, the site of infection and amenability to treatment, and the time of diagnosis relative to the course of the infection, resulting in several patterns.

Light Microscopy

The classic features of poststreptococcal glomerulonephritis include diffuse, global glomerular hypercellularity with numerous intracapillary neutrophils (Fig. 9.2A) and red blood cell casts. However, the degree of endocapillary inflammatory cells may be subtle or focal. The glomeruli may show mesangial expansion and mesangial hypercellularity membranoproliferative features, and crescents may be present. Variable degree of global glomerulosclerosis, interstitial

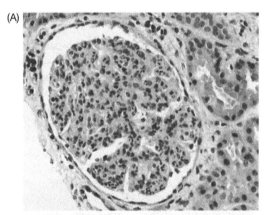

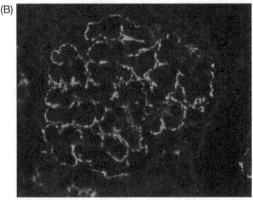

FIGURE 9.2 Postinfectious glomerulonephritis. (A) Light microscopy hematoxylin and eosin stain shows a hypercellular glomerulus with numerous neutrophils in the capillary lumen. (B) Immunofluorescence stain for immunoglobin G shows diffuse granular staining in the glomerular capillary walls indicating the presence of immune deposits.

inflammation, and tubulointerstitial scarring can be present.

Immunofluorescence

IF shows coarse granular staining in the capillary walls for IgG and C3 (Fig. 9.2B), which can be also seen in the mesangium, particularly in the resolving phase of glomerulonephritis. IgA can be present, showing dominance or codominance with IgG, particularly with staphylococcal infections.[24] A "full-house" immunostain positivity for IgG, IgA, IgM, C3, and C1q, typically seen in lupus nephritis, can be seen in some cases, particularly in association with HIV infection.[25]

Electron Microscopy

EM shows characteristically large, discrete, "hump-like" subepithelial electron dense deposits, irregularly distributed on the capillary walls. Mesangial deposits are usually present, and rare subendothelial deposits can be seen.

RENAL PATHOLOGIC CHANGES IN SYSTEMIC DISEASE

Diabetes

Diabetic nephropathy comprises several histologic changes reflecting progressive stages of the disease, best studied in type I diabetes and most evident in the glomeruli.

Light Microscopy

Initially there is glomerular enlargement, followed by diffuse thickening of the GBM and mesangial matrix accumulation in the absence of significant hypercellularity, best highlighted by PAS stain, and resulting in reduced patency of the glomerular capillaries. The mesangial expansion eventually assumes a nodular configuration detectable as at least 1 time and a half the size of the normal mesangial space. Loss of anchoring of the glomerular capillary walls to the mesangium may produce microaneurisms of the peripheral capillaries. As the lesion progresses, segmental adhesion to the Bowman's capsule, hyaline material accumulation may become visible in sclerosing segments of the glomerulus, and in the Bowman's capsule. Foam cells may be present. Progressive reduction of the number of podocytes occurs in diabetic nephropathy. Worsening glomerulosclerosis is usually accompanied by increased tubular atrophy and interstitial fibrosis often with marked thickening of the tubular basement membrane and variable degrees of mixed interstitial inflammation. Arteries manifest intimal thickening with or without duplication of the internal elastic lamina, and accumulation of hyaline material is typically seen in the arteriolar wall with narrowing of the lumen.

Immunofluorescence

There is increased intensity of albumin staining in the glomerular capillary loops but no immune deposits.

Electron Microscopy

EM often shows thickening of the GBM but no electron dense immune deposits.

Other renal lesions (e.g., immune-complex–mediated glomerulonephritis or podocyte injury with foot process effacement) may be superimposed on the diabetic lesion, in the not-infrequent scenario when biopsies are obtained from patients who present with unusually high proteinuria or hematuria.

A histopathologic classification of diabetic glomerulopathy was proposed in 2010,[26] featuring 4 classes with increased severity of glomerular abnormalities: class I: thickened GBM only (>395 nm in females and >430 nm in males); class II: mesangial expansion (IIa mild; IIb severe); class III: at least 1 convincing mesangial nodule; and Class IV: global glomerulosclerosis in >50% glomeruli. This classification has not been fully validated, and it has been suggested that the degree of IFTA may be a more effective predictor of renal survival than the glomerular lesions.[27]

Hypertension

The pathologic changes induced by chronic hypertension in the renal parenchyma affect primarily the arterial tree but result in chronic ischemic damage to glomeruli, tubule, and interstitium.

Light Microscopy

Small subcapsular scars may be evident in the renal superficial cortex. The glomeruli may show shrinking of the glomerular tuft and wrinkled glomerular capillary walls, with reduced lumen space in the glomerular capillaries, relative expansion of the urinary space, and mild fibrotic thickening of the glomerular capsule. These changes progress to glomerular scarring with solidification and replacement by collagen leading to global glomerulosclerosis; atrophic changes

develop in the tubules, and fibrotic expansion of the interstitium occurs. The arcuate and interlobular size arteries show fibrotic thickening of the intimal layer and splitting of the internal elastic lamina, all resulting in reduction in the caliber of the lumen. The arterioles commonly show subendothelial accumulation of hyaline material also reducing their lumen caliber. These changes are commonly observed as part of the chronic evolution of other renal diseases, when hypertension may accompany progressive renal deterioration. Acute, severe injury, described later for thrombotic microangiopathy (TMA), develops in the arteries and may involve the glomeruli in severe hypertension and may be superimposed on chronic hypertensive changes.

Immunofluorescence and Electron Microscopy

IF and EM do not show specific diagnostic findings.

Thrombotic Microangiopathy

TMA is a lesion in the microvasculature, which can be observed in different conditions including infections, genetic or acquired abnormalities of coagulation or of the complement system, exposure to certain drugs, eclampsia and pre-eclampsia, autoimmune diseases, malignancies, severe hypertension and scleroderma, hematopoietic stem cells transplantation, and antibody-mediated rejection in transplanted solid organs. Histologically, the renal involvement may vary from very focal to diffuse, localized in glomeruli or in small arteries and arterioles, or both.

Light Microscopy

Early glomerular lesion may manifest with congestion, swelling of the endothelial cells with occlusion of the capillary lumen conferring a bloodless appearance, fragmented red blood cells, fibrin, and platelet thrombi, with glomerular necrosis in the most severe instances. At a later stage, glomerular capillary walls are thickened, and by silver stain there may be double contours of the capillary walls, which, if very subtle, may be detectable only by EM. The arterial wall acutely shows endothelial cell swelling, intimal edema, fragmented red blood cells, and fibrinoid necrosis; at later stages, the vascular wall undergoes circumferential, multi-layered fibrotic thickening with onion skin-like appearance and severe narrowing of the lumen.

Immunofluorescence

No immune complex deposits are present but IF can show positive stain for fibrinogen in involved glomeruli and arteries.

Electron Microscopy

No electron dense deposits are present. Fibrin appears as bundles of very electron dense fibrillary material with some periodicity. EM may show chronic glomerular changes of TMA with thickening of the capillary walls, subendothelial space widening, cytoplasmic interposition, and new deposition of GBM material.

Lupus Nephritis

Involvement of the kidney in systemic lupus erythematosus (SLE) may manifest itself with different histomorphological patterns of injury, reflecting multiple pathogenetic mechanisms contributing to the disease. The histopathological classification of lupus nephritis has been periodically updated since its first publication in 1982, endorsed by the World Health Organization. The latest version in 2004[28] includes 6 classes with features summarized in Table 9.1.

Some ultrastructural features that can be detected by EM in any class of lupus nephritis

---

TABLE 9.1 CLASSES OF LUPUS NEPHRITIS

Class I	**Minimal mesangial lupus nephritis**
	LM: normal glomeruli;
	IF: "full house" deposits in the mesangium;
	EM: mesangial electron dense deposits
Class II	**Mesangial proliferative lupus nephritis**
	LM: mesangial enlargement and hypercellularity;
	IF: "full house" mesangial deposits with a few isolated subepithelial or subendothelial deposits; EM: mesangial electron dense deposits, with a few isolated subepithelial or subendothelial deposits
Class III	**Focal lupus nephritis[a]**
	LM: <50% of all glomeruli showing endocapillary proliferation/crescents;
	IF: "full house," mesangial deposits, focal subendothelial and subepithelial deposits;
	EM: electron dense mesangial deposits, focal subendothelial and subepithelial deposits
Class IV	**Diffuse lupus nephritis[a]**
	LM: ≥ 50% of all glomeruli showing endocapillary proliferation/crescents;
	IF: "full house" mesangial deposits and deposits in the glomerular capillary walls;
	EM: diffuse electron dense subendothelial deposits (wire loop) can have mesangial and subepithelial deposits
Class V	**Membranous lupus nephritis**
	LM: variable thickening of the glomerular capillary walls, with or without mesangial expansion, and generally little or no proliferative changes;
	IF: "full house" deposits in the glomerular capillary walls;
	EM: diffuse membranous deposits, mesangial deposits usually present
Class VI	**Advanced sclerosis lupus nephritis**: ≥90% globally sclerosed glomeruli, without residual active lesions

[a]Glomerular and tubulointerstitial scarring can be present with lesions in class III and IV.
LM = light microscopy. IF = immunofluorescence. EM = electron microscopy. "Full house" IF pattern describes positive staining for immune deposits containing IgG, IgA, IgM, C3, C1q, and kappa and lambda light chains.

include tubuloreticular inclusions and substructure of electron dense deposits such as tubulofibrillary arrays with parallel or curvilinear (fingerprint-like) orientation.

Specific pathologic features have been shown to have prognostic value for outcome. The NIH index of activity and chronicity proposed in 1983[29] was based on semiquantitative scores (from 0 to 3) of endocapillary hypercellularity, glomerular cellular crescents, glomerular necrosis/karyorrhexis, glomerular leukocyte infiltration, "wire loops," and interstitial inflammation for activity and on semiquantitative scores of glomerular sclerosis, fibrous crescents, tubular atrophy, and interstitial fibrosis for chronicity. More recent studies suggest that scoring fibrinoid necrosis and tubulointerstitial scarring may be of value for outcome prediction.[30,31] Although not included in the previously discussed schema, TMA may occur in patient with antiphospholipid antibodies as part of SLE, with or without concurrent lupus glomerulonephritis. Another infrequent pathological lesion, lupus podocytopathy has been described in patients with SLE and nephrotic range proteinuria, characterized by diffuse podocyte injury and foot process effacement in the absence of or with minimal immune complex deposits or proliferative changes.[32,33]

Renal Manifestation of Systemic Vasculitis

The kidney can be involved in different types of vasculitis defined by the Chapel Hill classification,[34] most often in small vessel vasculitis, including IgA vasculitis (Henoch-Schoenlein), cryoglobulinemic vasculitis, antineutrophil cytoplasmic antibody (ANCA) associated vasculitis (microscopic polyangiitis, granulomatosis with polyangiitis or Wegener's, eosinophilic granulomatosis with polyangiitis or Churg-Strauss's syndrome, and anti-GBM diseases. ANCA-associated vasculitides represent the largest group and comprises renal-limited and systemic forms of the disease.

Light Microscopy

The hallmark lesion is a crescentic and necrotizing glomerulonephritis. In the acute phase, the glomeruli show cellular crescents and fibrinoid necrosis resulting from breaks of the GBM, which can involve a variable number of glomeruli in global or segmental fashion (Fig. 9.3). Eventually the glomeruli undergo scarring with development of fibrocellular/fibrous crescents and partial or global glomerulosclerosis. Noninvolved glomeruli are typically normal without proliferative changes. Light microscopy can also reveal fibrinoid necrosis and inflammation in the walls of small arteries, and in rare cases lesions are evident only in the medullary capillaries. The tubulointerstitial compartment can show tubular red blood cell casts and variable degree of inflammation; granulomatous inflammation is a feature of Wegener's disease. Eosinophils are prominent in the interstitial inflammatory infiltrate of eosinophilic granulomatosis with polyangiitis (Churg-Strauss).

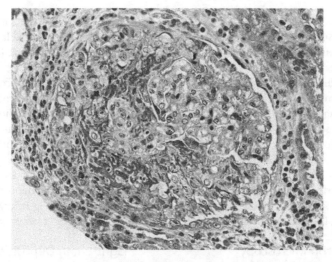

FIGURE 9.3 Light microscopy Masson trichrome stain shows glomerular fibrinoid necrosis and a cellular crescent in antineutrophil cytoplasmic antibody–associated crescentic, necrotizing paucimmune glomerulonephritis.

In term of differential diagnosis, ANCA-associated crescentic/necrotizing glomerular lesions do not show immune deposits by IF or EM and are defined as "paucimmune," a strongly positive, linear IF staining for IgG along the capillary walls in a crescentic/necrotizing glomerulonephritis is diagnostic of anti-GBM disease. A histopathological classification of ANCA-associated glomerulonephritis in 4 classes has been proposed in 2010[35] and is based on whether ≥50% of the glomeruli are normal (focal), show cellular crescents (crescentic), or are globally sclerotic (sclerotic), or none of these conditions are met (mixed). The sclerotic class seems to have the worst outcome.

Renal Disease Associated with Paraproteins and Plasma Cell Dyscrasias
Amyloidosis

Renal involvement can be seen with amyloid proteins of various natures, including light chains, as well as amyloid derived from other precursors. In the kidney, amyloid material can be found in the glomeruli, vascular walls, and the interstitium.

Light Microscopy

The histologic features of amyloid deposits are the same irrespective of the type of amyloid, and amyloid is recognizable as accumulation of amorphous material that is weakly eosinophilic, PAS negative, and silver negative. Amyloid is stained in orange-red by the Congo red stain, and when Congo red stain is examined under polarized light, the positive areas should show a green birefringence.

Immunofluorescence and Immunostains

Congo red-positive areas under fluorescence microscope appear orange with a fluorescein isothiocyanate filter and red with a tetramethylrhodamine isothiocyanate filter. Thioflavin stain examined with fluorescence microscopy can also detect amyloid deposits, which appear green with a fluorescein isothiocyanate filter. Amyloid typing with antibodies can be used for detection of kappa or lambda amyloid and amyloid A; further characterization of other types of amyloids can be achieved by mass spectroscopy analysis of Congo red positive tissue.[36]

Electron Microscopy

Ultrastructurally, amyloidosis is characterized by deposits of fibrillary material with nonbranching fibrils in random orientation measuring 8 to 12 nm in diameter.

Electron Microscopy in the Differential Diagnosis of Glomerulopathies with Organized Deposits

In the differential diagnosis of the EM findings in amyloid and other types of organized deposits, it is important to consider other glomerulopathies that may be associated with monoclonal immunoglobulins, may have variable light microscopy features, and are characterized by organized deposits with fibrillar-tubular ultrastructural appearance. They include fibrillary glomerulopathy, with fibrillary deposits of 16 to 24 nm in size containing IgG with polyclonal light chains; immunotactoid glomerulonephritis with parallel microtubules of 30 to 50 nm in diameters containing IgG or IgM with mostly monoclonal light chains; and cryoglobulinemic glomerulonephritis with parallel, often curved microtubules of 30 to 100 nm containing mostly IgM and IgG or IgM.[37]

Nonamyloid Renal Diseases Associated with Paraproteins and Plasma Cell Dyscrasias with Specific Pathologic Findings
Light Microscopy

The pathologic changes involve the tubules, particularly the medullary tubules, which typically show obstruction of the lumen by rigid, angulated casts, with fractures, occasionally surrounded by multinucleated cells. Unlike the usual tubular casts found in atrophic tubules, these casts are PAS negative.

Immunostains

When stained for kappa and lambda light chains the casts are typically positive for either kappa or lambda light chains (Fig. 9.4).

Rarely, renal biopsies from patients with plasma cell dyscrasias may show monoclonal light chain, detectable with immunostains and by EM as crystalline inclusions in the proximal tubules, without evidence of light chain tubular casts.

Other glomerulopathies associated with paraproteins include monoclonal IgG deposition diseases (MIDD) with deposits of monoclonal light chains (LCDD), Ig heavy chains (HCDD), or both monoclonal Ig heavy and light chains.[38]

Light Chain Deposition Disease

Light chain deposition disease is the most frequent of these manifestation and is associated

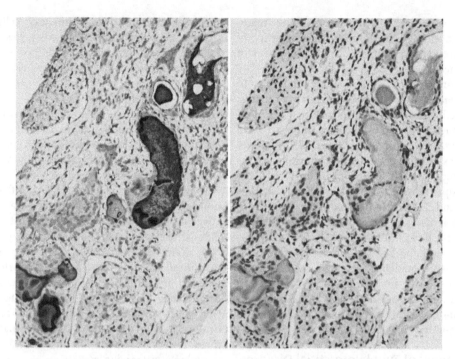

FIGURE 9.4 Light chain cast nephropathy in plasma cell dyscrasia. Immunostains for kappa light chain (left) and lambda light chain (right) show strongly positive tubular cast stain for kappa light chain with minimal weak staining for lambda light chain in a cases of multiple myeloma with monoclonal kappa light chain production.

with kappa light chain restriction in the majority of cases. In this lesion, monoclonal light chain deposits are found in the glomerular and tubular basement membrane. By light microscopy, the glomeruli may show increased mesangial matrix sometimes with a nodular configuration with variable hypercellularity, and the tubules may show thickening of the tubular basement membrane. The light chain deposits are detectable by immunostains for kappa and lambda light chains generally with a linear pattern and, by EM, appear as powdery electron dense deposits lining the subendothelial aspect of the GBM and the tubular basement membranes, and present in glomerular mesangium.

Renal Injury with HIV Infection and Its Treatment

HIV infection is associated with a variety of pathological changes in the kidney. HIVAN was described in the early phase of the HIV-AIDS epidemic between 1984 and 1988 as a characteristic combination of glomerular and tubular changes.

Light Microscopy

The glomerular lesion is described as collapsing glomerulopathy or collapsing FSGS. The glomeruli show visceral epithelial cell enlargement and hyperplasia, sometimes resembling crescents; vacuolization and protein droplets in the cytoplasm are also common. The glomerular capillaries show wrinkling and folding of the capillary walls with collapse of the lumen. There may be segmental consolidation with adhesion to the capsule; these areas of glomerular solidification may be covered by enlarged podocytes. The tubules are dilated focally forming microcysts, with scalloping clear spaces over the tubular cells and eosinophilic proteinaceous casts, associated with tubular cell injury. The interstitium is edematous and shows variable inflammatory infiltration mostly by lymphocytes which may be focally dense. Nonspecific vascular changes may be present.

Immunofluorescence

IF is typically negative for immune deposits.

Electron Microscopy

EM shows podocyte injury with vacuolization of the cytoplasm, microvillous changes of the cell membrane, and diffuse effacement of the foot processes that may appear detached from the folded surface of the GBM, with layers of electrolucent basement membrane material. Another typical feature is the presence of tubuloreticular inclusions in the cytoplasm of endothelial cells.

If untreated, HIVAN rapidly progresses to end stage renal disease in a matter of few months. With effective antiretroviral treatment, HIVAN is seen less commonly nowadays and other renal diseases, such as noncollapsing FSGS, immune-complex–mediated glomerulonephritis such as IgA and "lupus-like" nephropathies, diabetic nephropathy, and, to a lesser extent, amyloidosis and TMA have become more frequent in kidney biopsies of patients with well-controlled HIV infection. Antiretroviral drug toxicity has become an important cause in kidney disease in HIV-positive patients, who may develop interstitial nephritis, nonspecific tubular cell injury and, in some cases, intratubular crystal precipitation (indinavir) and ultrastructural alteration of mitochondria (tenofovir).

Pathology of Tubulointerstitial Diseases

Injury to tubules and interstitium can be primary or associated with glomerular disease.

Acute tubular injury due to ischemia or other noxious agent in its mildest form may be limited to loss of brush border in the proximal tubular cells. Histologic features of more severe tubular damage include loss of apical tubular cell cytoplasm in the lumen, cytoplasmic vacuolization, flattening of the tubular cells, cell detachment from the tubular basement membrane, cell necrosis, and formation of granular casts in the tubular lumen. Tubular injury caused by crystalline deposits most commonly is due to precipitation of calcium phosphate, oxalate, or uric acid.

Tubular atrophy histologically may appear as thickening of the tubular basement membrane with variable narrowing of the tubular lumen and dilatation with proteinaceous casts, which, if clustered, is often referred to as "thyroid-like."

Interstitial nephritis is usually associated with tubular injury, hence the term tubulointerstitial nephritis/nephropathy (TIN).

TIN is defined by infiltration of the interstitium by inflammatory cells. Tubulitis, defined by infiltration of inflammatory cells beyond the tubular basement membrane into the tubular epithelial lining, is often present.

Acute TIN

Interstitial edema is a prominent feature of acute TIN, in association with various types and combinations of inflammatory cells, including polymorphonuclear leukocytes such as neutrophils and eosinophils as well as lymphocytes, monocytes, and plasma cells.

Chronic TIN

Tubular atrophy and interstitial fibrosis with variable degree of mostly mononuclear interstitial inflammation are the hallmark of chronic interstitial nephritis. However, variable mix of acute and chronic lesion may be seen.

Neutrophil-rich interstitial inflammation and intratubular neutrophils are indicative of infection—bacterial in most cases. Tubular cells nuclear inclusions may indicate viral infection requiring immunostain for identification of the virus. Eosinophil-rich interstitial inflammation is a classic feature of drug-related TIN. Granulomatous inflammation with multinucleated cells may be seen in drug-related TIN, but the differential diagnosis includes sarcoidosis, Crohn's disease, Wegener's granulomatosis, and infections.

Immune-Complex–Mediated TIN

Immune-complex–mediated tubulointerstitial inflammation is rare. Lupus nephritis may show immune complex deposition in the tubular basement membrane detectable by IF and EM. IgG4-related TIN shows a characteristic combination of pathologic findings: numerous IgG4-positive plasma cells in the inflammatory infiltrate (>10 IgG4 positive plasma cells/high-power field is a diagnostic criteria), IgG4 immune complex deposits in the tubular basement membrane, and a characteristic "storiform" pattern of fibrosis of the interstitium.

Atherosclerosis and Atheroembolic Disease

Atherosclerosis can be a cause of renal artery stenosis and secondary hypertension and is more common when extrarenal vessels are affected. In the renal artery, atherosclerotic plaques tend to be located at the bifurcation from the aorta and consist of thickened intima by amorphous matrix containing lipid-laden macrophages and fibroblasts. Disruption of the plaques from any artery with embolization of plaque fragments in the circulation can result in atheroembolic disease.

Examination of renal biopsies by light microscopy can detect cholesterol emboli in the kidney as needle-like empty spaces or "cholesterol clefts" in the wall of small renal arteries often encircled by inflammatory and fibrotic re-action with variable obstruction of the lumen. Downstream glomeruli and tubules may show ischemic changes.

PATHOLOGY OF THE TRANSPLANTED KIDNEY

Renal allograft biopsies are usually performed when there is clinical evidence of decreased renal function or, less frequently, with stable renal function (protocol biopsies). Protocol biopsies are usually in the setting of clinical trials or in high-risk transplant recipients. The renal allograft biopsy may reveal many patterns of injury, reflecting different pathologic conditions besides rejection including acute tubular injury, calcineurin inhibitor nephrotoxicity, drug-induced interstitial nephritis, pyelonephritis, BK virus nephropathy, recurrent disease, de novo glomerulopathy, and posttransplant lymphoproliferative disorders.

Tubular injury due to calcineurin inhibitor nephrotoxicity may show characteristic Isometric vacuolization appearing as small vacuoles in tubular cells. Vacuolization of the arteriolar myocytes indicating vasoconstriction can also be seen as acute effect of these drugs, whereas nodular accumulation of hyaline material in the arteriolar wall may take longer to develop.

Rejection

The pathologic diagnosis of rejection in the kidney is based on a complex set of features defined in the Banff schema for classification of transplant rejection.[39] This schema relies on the semi-quantitative score (from 0 to 3) of several histologic features in glomeruli, tubules, interstitium, and vessels (abbreviation for each feature score is shown in parenthesis below) indicating the degrees of acute inflammation and chronic changes, including interstitial inflammation (i), tubulitis (t), intimal arteritis (v), glomerulitis or presence of inflammatory cells in the glomerular capillaries (g), peritubular capillaritis or presence of inflammatory cells in the peritubular capillaries (ptc)(Fig. 9.5A), total inflammation (ti), staining for the complement

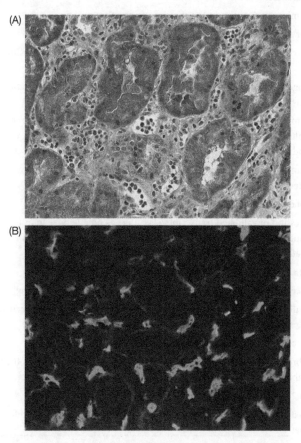

FIGURE 9.5 Allograft biopsy showing features of active antibody mediated rejection. (A) Severe peritubular capillaritis (ptc3), Masson trichrome stain. (B) Diffuse linear C4d staining in peritubular capillaries by immunofluorescence (C4d3).

fraction C4d in the peritubular capillary wall (C4d) (Fig. 9.5B), double contours of the glomerular capillary walls (cg), mesangial expansion (mm), arteriolar hyalinosis (ah), arterial intimal thickening (cv), interstitial fibrosis (ci), and tubular atrophy (ct).

The most recent Banff diagnostic schema, at the time of this writing, was formulated at the 2017 Banff meeting, and is reported in Table 9.2.[39]

BK nephropathy by light microscopy is characterized by tubular injury with basophilic ground-glass intranuclear inclusions in the tubular cells, mostly involving the medullary tubules. These inclusions are stained by immunostain for the large T antigen of the SV40 virus. There can be variable interstitial inflammation, usually containing several plasma cells.

TABLE 9.2 CLASSIFICATION OF RENAL ALLOGRAFT REJECTION

Banff 2017 classification of ABMR and TCMR in renal allografts

Category 1: Normal biopsy or nonspecific changes

Category 2: Antibody-mediated changes

Active ABMR; all 3 criteria must be met for diagnosis

1. Histologic evidence of acute tissue injury, including 1 or more of the following:

   - Microvascular inflammation (g > 0 and/or ptc > 0), in the absence of recurrent or de novo glomerulonephritis, although in the presence of acute TCMR, borderline infiltrate or infection, ptc ≥1 alone is not sufficient and g must be ≥1

   - Intimal or transmural arteritis (v > 0)1

   - Acute thrombotic microangiopathy, in the absence of any other cause

   - Acute tubular injury, in the absence of any other apparent cause

2. Evidence of current/recent antibody interaction with vascular endothelium, including 1 or more of the following:

   - Linear C4d staining in peritubular capillaries (C4d2 or C4d3 by IF on frozen sections, or C4d > 0 by IHC on paraffin sections)

   - At least moderate microvascular inflammation ([g + ptc] ≥2) in the absence of recurrent or de novo glomerulonephritis, although in the presence of acute TCMR, borderline infiltrate, or infection, ptc ≥ 2 alone is not sufficient and g must be ≥1

   - Increased expression of gene transcripts/classifiers in the biopsy tissue strongly associated with ABMR, if thoroughly validated

3. Serologic evidence of donor-specific antibodies (DSA to HLA or other antigens).

   C4d staining or expression of validated transcripts/classifiers as noted above in criterion 2 may substitute for DSA; however thorough DSA testing, including testing for non-HLA antibodies if HLA antibody testing is negative, is strongly advised whenever criteria 1 and 2 are met

Chronic active ABMR; all 3 criteria must be met for diagnosis

1. Morphologic evidence of chronic tissue injury, including 1 or more of the following:

   - Transplant glomerulopathy (cg >0) if no evidence of chronic TMA or chronic recurrent/de novo glomerulonephritis; includes changes evident by electron microscopy (EM) alone (cg1a)

   - Severe peritubular capillary basement membrane multilayering (requires EM)

   - Arterial intimal fibrosis of new onset, excluding other causes; leukocytes within the sclerotic intima favor chronic ABMR if there is no prior history of TCMR, but are not required

2. Identical to criterion 2 for active ABMR, above

3. Identical to criterion 3 for active ABMR, above, including strong recommendation for DSA testing whenever criteria 1 and 2 are met

TABLE 9.2 CONTINUED

C4d Staining without Evidence of Rejection; all 4 features must be present for diagnosis

1. Linear C4d staining in peritubular capillaries (C4d2 or C4d3 by IF on frozen sections, or C4d>0 by IHC on paraffin sections)

2. Criterion 1 for active or chronic, active ABMR not met

3. No molecular evidence for ABMR as in criterion 2 for active and chronic, active ABMR

4. No acute or chronic active TCMR, or borderline changes

Category 3: Borderline changes; Suspicious (Borderline) for acute TCMR

Foci of tubulitis (t > 0) with minor interstitial inflammation (i0 or i1), or moderate-severe interstitial inflammation (i2 or i3) with mild (t1) tubulitis

No intimal or transmural arteritis (v = 0)

Category 4: TCMR

Acute TCMR

- Grade IA   Interstitial inflammation involving >25% of nonsclerotic cortical parenchyma (i2 or i3) with moderate tubulitis (t2) involving 1 or more tubules, not including tubules that are severely atrophic

- Grade IB   Interstitial inflammation involving >25% of nonsclerotic cortical parenchyma (i2 or i3) with severe tubulitis (t3) involving 1 or more tubules, not including tubules that are severely atrophic

- Grade IIA   Mild to moderate intimal arteritis (v1), with or without interstitial inflammation and/or tubulitis

- Grade IIB   Severe intimal arteritis (v2), with or without interstitial inflammation and/or tubulitis

- Grade III   Transmural arteritis and/or arterial fibrinoid necrosis of medial smooth muscle with accompanying mononuclear cell intimal arteritis (v3), with or without interstitial inflammation and/or tubulitis

Chronic Active TCMR

Grade IA   Interstitial inflammation involving >25% of the total cortex (ti score 2 or 3) and >25% of the sclerotic cortical parenchyma (i-IFTA score 2 or 3) with moderate tubulitis (t2) involving 1 or more tubules, not including severely atrophic tubules; other known causes of i-IFTA should be ruled out

Grade IB   Interstitial inflammation involving >25% of the total cortex (ti score 2 or 3) and >25% of the sclerotic cortical parenchyma (i-IFTA score 2 or 3) with severe tubulitis (t3) involving 1 or more tubules, not including severely atrophic tubules; other known causes of i-IFTA should be ruled out

Grade II   Chronic allograft arteriopathy (arterial intimal fibrosis with mononuclear cell inflammation in fibrosis and formation of neointima)

ABMR = antibody-mediated rejection. TCMR = T cell-mediated rejection. IHC = immunohistochemistry.
Source: Haas M, Loupy A, Lefaucheur C, et al. The Banff 2017 Kidney Meeting Report: revised diagnostic criteria for chronic active T cell-mediated rejection, antibody-mediated rejection, and prospects for integrative endpoints for next-generation clinical trials. *Am J Transpl.* 2018; 18:293–307.

Posttransplant Lymphoproliferative Disorder

Posttransplant lymphoproliferative disorder (PTLD) may involve the kidney allograft, and its pathological features may be difficult to differentiate from rejection, which may require immunophenotyping for B and T cell, stains for kappa and lambda light chains, and in situ hybridization for small nuclear RNAs of Epstein-Barr virus. Histologically, PTLD includes 4 major types[40]:

Plasmacytic hyperplasia and infectious mononucleosis-like PTLD
Polymorphic PTLD
Monomorphic PTLD
Classical Hodgkin lymphoma-like PTLD

Plasmacytic hyperplasia and infectious mononucleosis-like PTLD are generally polyclonal B cell lesion with preserved architecture of the involved tissue.

Polymorphic PTLD consists of variably differentiated B cells with destructive infiltrative pattern, may have kappa or lambda restriction, and may show positive in situ hybridization for Epstein-Barr virus small nuclear RNAs.

Monomorphic PTLD has 4 subtypes: diffuse large B cell lymphoma, Burkitt lymphoma, plasma cell neoplasm, and peripheral T cell lymphoma not otherwise specified.

REFERENCES

1. Racusen LC, Solez K, Colvin RB, et al. The Banff 97 working classification of renal allograft pathology. *Kidney Int.* 1999;55(2):713–723.

2. Haas M. Alport syndrome and thin glomerular basement membrane nephropathy: a practical approach to diagnosis. *Arch Pathol Lab Med.* 2009;133(2):224–232.

3. Striker GE, Schainuck LI, Cutler RE, et al. Structural-functional correlations in renal disease. I. A method for assaying and classifying histopathologic changes in renal disease. *Hum Pathol.* 1970;1:615–630.

4. Schainuck LI, Striker GE, Luther RE, et al. Structural-functional correlations in renal disease. II. The correlations. *Hum Pathol.* 1970;1:631–641.

5. Bohle A, Mackensen-Haen S, von Giese H, et al. The consequences of tubulo-interstitial changes for renal function in glomerulopathies. A morphometric and cytological analysis. *Pathol Res Pract.* 1990;186:135–144.

6. Olson J. The nephrotic syndrome and minimal change disease. In: Jennetter CJ OJ, Silva FG, D'Agati VD, eds. *Heptinstall's Pathology of the Kidney.* 7th ed. Philadelphia, PA: Wolters Kluwer; 2015: 173–205.

7. Kremers WK, Denic A, Lieske JC, et al. Distinguishing age-related from disease-related glomerulosclerosis on kidney biopsy: the Aging Kidney Anatomy study. *Nephrol Dial Transpl.* 2015;30(12):2034–2039.

8. Howie AJ, Brewer DB. The glomerular tip lesion: A previously undescribed type of segmental glomerular abnormality. *J Pathol.* 1984;142(3):205–220.

9. Howie A, Pankhurst T, Sarioglu S, et al. Evolution of nephrotic-associated focal segmental glomerulosclerosis and relation to the glomerular tip lesion. *Kidney Int.* 2005;67:987–1001.

10. D'Agati VD, Kaskel FJ, Falk RJ. Focal segmental glomerulosclerosis. *N Engl J Med.* 2011;365(25):2398–2411.

11. D'Agati VD, Fogo AB, Bruijn JA, et al. Pathologic classification of focal segmental glomerulosclerosis: a working proposal. *Am J Kidney Dis.* 2004;43(2):368–382.

12. D'Agati VD. Focal segmental glomerulosclerosis. In: Jennetter CJ O, JL, Silva FG, D'Agati VD, ed. *Heptinstall's Pathology of the Kidney.* Philadelphia, PA: Wolters Kluwer; 2015: 207–254.

13. Cohen AH, Nast CC. HIV-associated nephropathy: a unique combined glomerular, tubular, and interstitial lesion. *Mod Pathol.* 1988;1:87–97.

14. Debiec H, Ronco P. PLA2R autoantibodies and PLA2R glomerular deposits in membranous nephropathy. *N Engl J Med.* 2011;364(7):689–690.

15. Larsen CP, Messias NC, Silva FG, et al. Determination of primary versus secondary membranous glomerulopathy utilizing phospholipase A2 receptor staining in renal biopsies. *Mod Pathol.* 2013;26(5):709–715.

16. Larsen CP, Cossey LN, Beck LH. THSD7A staining of membranous glomerulopathy in clinical practice reveals cases with dual autoantibody positivity. *Mod Pathol.* 2016;29(4):421–426.

17. Churg J, Ehrenreich T. Membranous nephropathy. *Perspect Nephrol Hypertens.* 1973;1 Pt 1:443–448.

18. Mariani L, Martini S, Barisoni L, et al. Interstitial fibrosis scored on whole-slide digital imaging of kidney biopsies is a predictor of outcome in proteinuric glomerulopathies. *Nephrol Dial Transpl.* 2018;33(2):310–318.

19. Bomback AS, Appel GB. Pathogenesis of the C3 glomerulopathies and reclassification of MPGN. *Nat Rev Nephrol.* 2012;8(11):634–642.

20. Cook HT, Pickering MC. Histopathology of MPGN and C3 glomerulopathies. *Nat Rev Nephrol.* 2015;11(1):14–22.

21. Cattran D, Coppo R, Cook H, et al. The Oxford classification of IgA nephropathy: rationale, clinicopathological correlations, and classification. *Kidney Int.* 2009;76(5):534–545.

22. Haas M, Verhave JC, Liu Z-H, et al. A multicenter study of the predictive value of crescents in IgA nephropathy. *J Am Soc Nephrol.* 2017;28:691–701.

23. D'Amico G. Natural history of idiopathic IgA nephropathy: role of clinical and histological prognostic factors. *Am J Kidney Dis.* 2000;36(2):227–237.

24. Haas M, Racusen LC, Bagnasco SM. IgA-dominant postinfectious glomerulonephritis: a report of 13 cases with common ultrastructural features. *Hum Pathol.* 2008;39(9):1309–1316.

25. Haas M, Kaul S, Eustace J. HIV-associated immune complex glomerulonephritis with "lupus-like" features: a clinicopathologic study of 14 cases. *Kidney Int.* 2005;67:1381–1390.

26. Tervaert TWC, Mooyaart AL, Amann K, et al. Pathologic classification of diabetic nephropathy. *J Am Soc Nephrol.* 2010;21(4):556–563.

27. Okada T, Nagao T, Matsumoto H, et al. Histological predictors for renal prognosis in diabetic nephropathy in diabetes mellitus type 2 patients with overt proteinuria. *Nephrology.* 2012;17(1):68–75.

28. Weening JJ, D'Agati VD, Schwartz MM, et al. The classification of glomerulonephritis in systemic

lupus erythematosus revisited. *J Am Soc Nephrol.* 2004;15(2):241–250.

29. Austin III HA, Muenz LR, Joyce KM, et al. Prognostic factors in lupus nephritis: Contribution of renal histologic data. *Am J Med.* 1983;75(3):382–391.

30. Rijnink EC, Teng YKO, Wilhelmus S, et al. Clinical and histopathologic characteristics associated with renal outcomes in lupus nephritis. *Clin J Am Soc Nephrol.* 2017;12(5):734–743.

31. Yu F, Wu L-h, Tan Y, et al. Tubulointerstitial lesions of patients with lupus nephritis classified by the 2003 International Society of Nephrology and Renal Pathology Society system. *Kidney Int.* 2010;77(9):820–829.

32. Kraft SW, Schwartz MM, Korbet SM, et al. Glomerular podocytopathy in patients with systemic lupus erythematosus. *J Am Soc Nephrol.* 2005;16(1):175–179

33. Hertig A, Droz D, Lesavre P, et al. SLE and idiopathic nephrotic syndrome: Coincidence or not? *Am J Kidney Dis.* 2002;40(6):1179–1184.

34. Jennette JC, Falk RJ, Bacon PA, et al. 2012 revised International Chapel Hill Consensus Conference Nomenclature of Vasculitides. *Arthritis Rheum.* 2013;65(1):1–11.

35. Berden AE, Ferrario F, Hagen EC, et al. Histopathologic classification of ANCA-associated glomerulonephritis. *J Am Soc Nephrol.* 2010;21(10):1628–1636.

36. Herrera G, Picken M. Renal diseases associated with plasma cell dyscrasias, amyloidoses, and Wladenstrom macroglobulinemia. In: Jennette JC, Olson J, Silva FG, et al., eds. *Heptinstall's Pathology of the Kidney.* Philadelphia, PA: Wolters Kluwer; 2015: 951–1014.

37. Motwani SS, Herlitz L, Monga D, et al. Paraprotein-related kidney disease: glomerular diseases associated with paraproteinemias. *Clin J Am Soc Nephrol.* 2016;11(12):2260–2272.

38. Doshi M, Lahoti A, Danesh FR, et al. Paraprotein-related kidney disease: kidney injury from paraproteins—what determines the site of injury? *Clin J Am Soc Nephrol.* 2016;11(12):2288–2294.

39. Haas M, Loupy A, Lefaucheur C, et al. The Banff 2017 Kidney Meeting Report: revised diagnostic criteria for chronic active T cell-mediated rejection, antibody-mediated rejection, and prospects for integrative endpoints for next-generation clinical trials. *Am J Transpl.* 2018; 18:293–307.

40. Swerdlow S, Campo E, Harris N, et al. *World Health Organization Classification of Tumours of Haematopoietic and Lymphoid Tissues.* Lyon, France: IARC Press; 2008.

SECTION III

General Concepts in Protecting Kidney Function

10

Pharmacologic Renal Protection

WAEL F. HUSSEIN AND AUSTIN G. STACK

INTRODUCTION

Chronic kidney disease (CKD) is a major chronic noncommunicable disease that affects between 7% and 20% of adults globally[1,2] and is associated with substantial morbidity and mortality. The complications of CKD are frequent and complex, and for many patients, the risk of progression to end-stage kidney disease (ESKD) is high. Current risk reduction strategies are broad and multifaceted with a major goal of preventing the risk of CKD progression, treatment of CKD-associated metabolic complications, and mitigating the risk of lethal cardiovascular events. Clinical studies have elucidated a broad array of complex pathophysiological mechanisms responsible for the development and progression of CKD. These serve as the target for existing and novel pharmacological interventions. While substantial progress has been made in the identification and testing of agents that block the renin–angiotensin–aldosterone system, intervention strategies to target other systems are still at early phases of development. In this chapter, we describe the expanding list of pharmacological interventions that are designed to prevent CKD progression and its attendant complications.

ANTI-HYPERTENSIVE THERAPY

Hypertension is common among patients with CKD and affects approximately one-third of this population.[3] It ranks second after diabetes as a cause of ESKD in the United States.[3] Hypertension may also develop in the course of CKD and contribute to increased risk of ESKD.[4–6] Salt and water retention, dysregulation of the renin–angiotensin system (RAS) and the sympathetic nervous systems, and increased vascular resistance are all mechanisms that contribute to the development or worsening of hypertension in CKD patients.[7] Effective management of hypertension in CKD patients and those at risk of CKD serves to reduce the risk of kidney disease progression, as well as the huge cardiovascular risk present in this population. Anti-hypertensive agents are effective in reducing CKD progression either directly by reducing systemic blood pressure or indirectly by several blood pressure independent mechanisms.

Renin-Angiotensin System Blockade

Downregulation of RAS is an integral part in the management of proteinuric CKD. Renin, secreted by the juxta-glomerular apparatus, cleaves angiotensinogen to angiotensin I, which in turn is hydrolyzed by angiotensin converting enzymes (ACE) to angiotensin II (Ang II). Stimulation of angiotensin-1 (AT-1) receptors induces vasoconstriction, tubular sodium reabsorption, activation of aldosterone synthesis and secretion, stimulation of vasopressin secretion, and modulation of the sympathetic nervous system among other effects.[8] AT-1 receptors are also involved in tubulo-interstitial fibrosis. Moreover, Ang II has proinflammatory and profibrotic effects through other receptors. RAS inhibitors are indicated in the treatment of heart failure[9] and postmyocardial infarction,[10] as well as in the treatment of proteinuric CKD, which we address in the following discussion. ACE inhibitor (ACEI) monotherapy produces a blood pressure-lowering effect that is similar to other first-line antihypertensive drugs.[11]

RAS Inhibitors in Nondiabetic Proteinuric CKD Patients

The benefits of RAS inhibitors on renal outcomes are independent of their blood pressure lowering effect.[12–14] RAS blockers also reduce proteinuria more than other agents. In one meta-analysis, ACEI reduced proteinuria by 40%, as compared to a reduction of 17% achieved by other agents.[15] Similar effects were noted with angiotensin receptor blockers (ARBs).[14] This important effect is mediated through the preferential vasodilatory effect of RAS blockers on the efferent more than the afferent glomerular arterioles, reducing the intraglomerular pressure. This, in turn, leads to greater reduction in proteinuria than is observed by other agents.[15,16] A reduction in proteinuria is associated with lower rates of CKD progression.[16,17]

This additional benefit of RAS blockers on progression of CKD has been observed in several clinical trials. Among 583 CKD patients with different etiologies, benazepril almost halved the risk of the combined outcome of doubling of serum creatinine (SCr) or need for dialysis over a 3-year follow-up. Risk reduction was greater in patients with baseline proteinuria of more than 1 g/24 h.[18] Patients randomized to ramipril who had proteinuria ≥3 g/day in the Ramipril Efficacy in Nephropathy (REIN) trial[19] experienced significantly slower rates of decline in glomerular filtration rate (GFR) compared to placebo (monthly decline of GFR 0.53 ml/min and 0.88 ml/min, respectively). Doubling of SCr or ESKD occurred in 18 and 40 patients randomized to ramipril and the placebo arms, respectively. The African American Study of Kidney Disease and Hypertension (AASK) trial[20] included more than 1,000 African American patients with hypertensive renal disease with a follow up of 3 to 6.4 years after randomization. Patients treated with ramipril had significant reduction in the clinical composite outcome (50% reduction in GFR [≥25 ml/min/1.73m2], ESKD, or death) compared to metoprolol (22% reduction; 95% confidence interval [CI]: 1%–38%) or amlodipine (38% reduction; 95% CI: 14%–56%).

In a meta-analysis of 11 randomized trials that included 1,860 nondiabetic CKD patients with a mean follow-up of 2.2 years, patients treated with ACEI had a relative risk of 0.69 (CI: 051–0.94) for ESKD and 0.70 (CI :0.55–0.88) for a combined outcome of doubling SCr or ESKD,[21] compared to patients not on ACEI. In a recent systematic review of randomized trials, the relative benefits of ACEI and ARB therapy over other agents were further demonstrated. Treatment with ACEI or ARB had relative risks of 0.67 (95% CI: 0.54–0.84) and 0.78 (95% CI: 0.66–0.90) for ESKD and 0.62 (95% CI: 0.46–0.84) and 0.78 (95% CI 0.68–0.90) for doubling of SCr, respectively.[22]

RAS Inhibition in Diabetic Nephropathy

Effects of RAS inhibition on progression of diabetic kidney disease were similar to effects in nondiabetic proteinuric CKD.

Type 1 Diabetes Mellitus

Reduction of blood pressure reduces risk of diabetic complications. In a follow-up of participants of the UK Prospective Diabetes Study (UKPDS),[23] each 10 mmHg reduction in systolic blood pressure was associated with a 12% reduction overall in diabetic complications and a 13% reduction in microvascular complications.[24]

In patients with type 1 diabetes and microalbuminuria, captopril decreased albuminuria and progression to overt diabetic nephropathy.[12,25] In patients with proteinuria ≤500 mg per day, captopril treatment was associated with slower increases in SCr and less progression to ESKD or death.[26] Patients with nephrotic range proteinuria were more likely to have regression of proteinuria with captopril than with placebo.[27]

Type 2 Diabetes Mellitus

In the Irbesartan Diabetic Nephropathy Trial (IDNT),[13] 1,715 patients with nephropathy secondary to type 2 diabetes were randomized to irbesartan, amlodipine, or placebo. The combined endpoint (doubling of SCr, ESKD, or death) was 23% and 20% lower with irbesartan than amlodipine or placebo, respectively. Similarly, among 1,513 patients with type 2 diabetes and nephropathy in the Reduction of Endpoints in NIDDM with the Angiotensin II Antagonist Losartan (RENAAL) study,[14] patients treated with losartan experienced a 25% reduction in doubling of SCr and 28% lower incidence of ESKD.

Nonproteinuric CKD

A meta-analysis of 1,860 nondiabetic CKD patients from 11 randomized clinical trials found no benefit of ACEI therapy on renal outcomes for patients with proteinuria <500 mg/day.[28]

Effect on Serum Creatinine and Potassium

Initiation of RAS inhibitor therapy is associated with an acute rise in SCr. This results from their effect on intraglomerular pressure and does not usually represent kidney injury. RAS inhibitors should only be stopped if SCr increases by more than 30% within the first 2 months after initiation of therapy.[29] Hyperkalemia is another concern, particularly in patients with diabetes and type 4 renal tubular acidosis, and requires monitoring patients after initiation of therapy.

Dual Blockade of the RAS System

Studies that have combined an ACEI with an ARB (or a direct renin inhibitor in conjunction with an ACEI or an ARB) have found a greater reduction in proteinuria than either agent alone. This, however, has not translated into improved renal outcomes. Evidence from the Ongoing Telmisartan Alone or in Combination with Ramipril Global Endpoint Trial (ONTARGET; ramipril and telmisartan),[30] the Veterans Affairs Nephropathy in Diabetes (VA NEPHRON-D; losartan and lisinopril),[31] and the Aliskerin Trial in Type 2 Diabetes Using Cardiorenal Endpoints (ALTITUDE; aliskiren with ACEI or ARB) study[32] have failed to show a positive impact on short term and longer term renal outcomes. In these clinical trials, combination therapy elevated the risks of hypotension, acute kidney injury (AKI), and hyperkalemia.

Mineralocorticoid Receptor Antagonists

Aldosterone levels are inappropriately high for patients with CKD.[33] This may be secondary to elevated renin levels due to renal hypoperfusion or due to direct stimulation by hyperkalemia among other factors.[33] Elevated aldosterone levels may also occur in patients on optimal treatment with RAS blockers, a phenomena called "aldosterone breakthrough."[33] Besides its role in sodium and water retention, mineralocorticoid receptor antagonists (MCR) activation contributes to renal injury through oxidative stress, vascular and renal inflammation, podocyte injury, mesangial expansion, and renal fibrosis.[34-37]

A recent meta-analysis of 19 clinical trials including 1,646 CKD patients found that the addition of MCR antagonists to RAS inhibition resulted in further significant reductions in proteinuria over and above that of RAS blockers.[38] Sample size limitations, however, did not allow for testing of hard renal outcomes such as cardiovascular events or death.

Hyperkalemia is a serious risk associated with use of MCR antagonist therapy especially in combination with RAS inhibitors. The recent availability of potassium binders (patiromer and sodium zirconium cyclosilicate) offer new opportunities to expand the use of MCR antagonist therapy in patients with advanced CKD.[39] Diuretic therapy may also help in controlling

hyperkalemia but requires careful monitoring to avoid volume depletion and AKI.

Calcium Channel Blockers

Dihydropyridine calcium channel blockers (dpCCB; e.g., nifedipine) have minimal effects on proteinuria. On the other hand, nondihydropyridine CCB (ndpCCB; e.g., diltiazem and verapamil), despite having a smaller effect on blood pressure, significantly reduce proteinuria by 20% to 30%.[15,40] This was also observed in patients on RAS inhibitor therapy.[40] This antiproteinuric effect results from preferential glomerular efferent arteriolar dilatation, a process that is similar to the effect of RAS inhibitors on renal hemodynamics. Additional factors including an effect on permeability of the glomerular basement membrane may be involved.[40]

Despite the effect of ndpCCB on proteinuria, no long-term studies are available to demonstrate an association with hard renal outcomes. ndpCCBs can be considered as an add-on therapy for patients on maximum RAS inhibitor therapy or as an alternative to RAS inhibitors in patients with contraindications or intolerance to these agents.[7]

Agents such as amlodipine exert their effects through L-type receptors, which are predominantly distributed on vascular smooth muscles. In addition to affecting L-type receptors, cilnidipine, a new calcium channel blocker, also blocks receptors on sympathetic nerve endings (N-type receptors). Use of cilnidipine showed promising effects on heart rate and uric acid production.[41,42] In proteinuric hypertensive patients, switching from amlodipine to cilnidipine resulted in modest reductions in proteinuria for similar blood pressure effects and suppressed uric acid production.[43] To our knowledge, there are no ongoing trials currently investigating the effect of cilnidipine on long-term renal outcomes.

Diuretics

Diuretics contribute to the management of hypertension in patients with CKD due to better control of salt and water excretion. They are also effective in preventing and, indeed, treating hyperkalemia especially in high-risk patients on RAS therapy or MCR. Use of diuretics in combination with RAS inhibitors can further reduce proteinuria especially when combined with salt restriction.[44-46] Caution is required with this approach, however, as dehydration in the setting of RAS inhibitor therapy may precipitate AKI. In addition, long-term clinical trials with hard outcomes to support this approach are not available.

HYPOGLYCEMIC AGENTS

Approximately 40% of patients with CKD have diabetes, and it remains the leading primary cause of ESKD.[3] Treatment of hypertension, particularly with RAS inhibitors, is a major component in the management of patients with diabetic nephropathy (as previously discussed) to prevent progression of CKD. Tight glycemic control on the other hand delays onset and progression of proteinuria, but not hard renal outcomes.[47,48] Below, we highlight the potential importance of two newer oral hypoglycemic agents that have demonstrated clinical benefit.

Emergence of the SGLT-2 Inhibitors

Sodium-glucose co-transporter 2 (SGLT-2) is expressed almost exclusively in cells of the proximal tubule. By blocking sodium and glucose absorption, SGLT-2 inhibitors improve glycemic control and reduce weight and blood pressure.[49,50] Increased sodium delivery to the distal tubule stimulates afferent glomerular vasoconstriction through tubuloglomerular feedback, reducing the intraglomerular pressure. This, in turn, reduces proteinuria.[49,50] GFR initially declines secondary to reduced intraglomerular pressure, an effect similar to that seen with use of RAS inhibitors.[51,52] Reducing energy demands of proximal tubular cells by blocking SGLT-2 may contribute to the beneficial effects of these agents.[53]

Empagliflozin, a selective SGLT-2 inhibitor, reduced major adverse cardiovascular events in patients with type 2 diabetes at high risk of cardiovascular events in the Empagliflozin, Cardiovascular Outcomes, and Mortality in Type 2 Diabetes (EMPA-REG OUTCOME) trial.[54] Patients were randomized to one of two doses of empagliflozin or placebo. The threshold GFR for inclusion was 30 mL/min/1.73 m². The effects of empagliflozin on prespecified renal outcomes were subsequently reported.[51] Patients randomized to empagliflozin experienced lower incidence of worsening nephropathy (39% relative risk reduction): doubling of SCr (44% relative risk reduction), and initiation of renal replacement therapy (55% relative risk reduction). Importantly, the benefits were observed even among patients on RAS inhibitors. Moreover,

progression to macroalbuminuria was lower in the empagliflozin group (38% relative risk reduction).

Similarly, in a secondary analysis of the CANATA-SU study, type 2 diabetics treated with canagliflozin experienced better renal outcomes.[52] In this study, patients were randomized to one of two doses of canagliflozin or to glimepiride as active control. The rate of GFR decline was lower in the canagliflozin groups (0.5 and 0.9 mL/min/1.73 m²/year) compared to the glimepiride group (3.3 mL/min per 1.73 m²/year). Patients with macroalbuminuria experienced reductions of 32% and 49% in albumin excretion and these results were consistent regardless of RAS inhibitor use. This trial excluded patients with GFR <55 ml/min/1.73m².

There is concern that these agents may increase the risk of AKI. This may be secondary to their diuretic action, in addition to an effect on increasing medullary hypoxia.[55] To reduce the risk of AKI, it is suggested that these agents be stopped prior to contrast exposure.[55] Despite the hugely promising results, no trials have directly investigated the impact of SGLT-2 inhibitors on renal outcomes. Several trials are currently underway to address this gap in our knowledge (Clinicaltrials.gov identifiers: NCT02065791, NCT01989754, and NCT02547935).

Dipeptidyl Peptidase IV Inhibitors

Dipeptidyl peptidase IV inhibitors prevent degradation of glucagon-like peptide 1, thereby stimulating insulin secretion and reducing glucagon secretion. Of particular interest is linagliptin, an agent with nonrenal clearance, enabling its use in all stages of CKD without need for adjustment.[56]

Among patients with type 2 diabetes and renal impairment receiving RAS inhibitor therapy, addition of linagliptin significantly reduced albuminuria in 24 weeks by 28%, an effect that was independent of glycemic or blood pressure control.[57] It is still not clear how linagliptin affects albuminuria, but suggested mechanisms include prevention of podocyte damage and antiinflammatory and antioxidative effects.[57]

A meta-analysis of 5,466 patients from 13 randomized clinical trials found that patients treated with linagliptin had a 16% lower hazard of composite renal events compared to placebo.[58] The primary composite outcome consisted of new onset of moderate elevation of albuminuria, new onset of severe elevation of albuminuria, reduction in kidney function, halving of estimated

GFR (eGFR), AKI, or death from any cause. A clinical trial is currently underway to investigate the long-term effects of linagliptin on cardiovascular and renal outcomes (ClinicalTrials.gov identifier: NCT01897532).

STATINS

Statins are used in CKD patients to reduce cardiovascular risk and mortality.[59,60] In the latest recommendations by Kidney Disease: Improving Global Outcomes (KDIGO)[61] guidelines, statins are recommended for patients who are 50 years of age or older and those with high cardiovascular risk.

Dyslipidemia is associated with glomerular injury in animal models through inflammation, glomerular hypertension, and altered production of matrix proteins.[62,63] In humans, statin therapy was associated with lower inflammation, improved vascular stiffness,[64–66] and reduction of albuminuria.[67,68]

Large human studies have, however, failed to show a beneficial effect of statins on hard renal outcomes. In the SHARP trial,[59] patients with CKD were randomized to simvastatin plus ezetimibe or placebo. A secondary analysis[69] investigated renal outcomes in 6,245 nondialysis CKD patients. There was no difference in the outcome of ESKD, ESKD or death, or composite risk of ESKD or doubling of SCr. There was also no significant effect on the rate of change in eGFR between the two groups. This lack of effect on renal outcomes was further corroborated in a Cochrane meta-analysis[60] that included 38 studies with more than 37,000 nondialysis CKD patients. Whereas statin use compared to placebo reduced the risk of cardiovascular events and mortality, effects on progression of CKD were uncertain.

URATE LOWERING THERAPY

In rats, hyperuricemia is associated with afferent arteriolopathy, glomerular hypertension, cortical vasoconstriction, tubulointerstitial inflammation and fibrosis. Treatment with an oxidase inhibitor, such as allopurinol, was found to ameliorate some of these effects.[70–72] In humans, most (but not all) observational studies in large population cohorts have shown a strong independent association between high serum uric acid with progression of CKD[73] and with the risk of incident kidney disease.[74–76]

The effect of lowering uric acid levels with xanthine oxidase inhibitors on renal outcomes has been studied in a few small randomized trials. In the largest of these trials (and the one with the longest follow-up), 113 CKD patients were randomized to allopurinol or placebo, with a follow up of 24 months. eGFR decline was slower in the allopurinol arm (−1.3 +/− 1.3 vs. 3.3 +/− 1.2 mL/min/1.73 m^2).[77] Similarly, CKD stage 3 patients randomized to febuxostat had a significantly higher GFR than those on placebo (difference of 6.5 mL/min/1.73 m^2 after 6 months follow-up).[78]

Several meta-analyses[79–81] have linked uric acid-lowering agents with renal protection. Despite the increasing body of evidence linking hyperuricaemia to CKD, it remains unclear as to whether treatment with urate-lowering therapies will reduce the risk of disease progression and ESKD. While recent randomized controlled trials have suggested a protective effect of urate-lowering therapy in preventing the progression of CKD, large randomized clinical trials of sufficient size, diversity, and follow-up have yet to prove conclusively that lowering serum uric acid levels leads to a reduction in major metabolic and cardiovascular outcomes. The latest KDIGO[57] guidelines document, while acknowledging the growing evidence to support the association between hyperuricemia and renal outcomes, does not recommend use of uric acid lowering agents to delay progression of CKD because of insufficient evidence.

ALKALI REPLACEMENT THERAPY

Metabolic acidosis is common in patients with CKD,[82,83] with a prevalence of 7%, 13%, and 37% in stage 2, 3, and 4 respectively.[83] Metabolic acidosis causes complement activation leading to tubulointerstitial fibrosis.[84] In humans, alkali therapy in patients with metabolic acidosis reduced urinary albumin,[85,86] endothelin,[85,87] N-acetyl-β-D-glucosaminidase,[85–87] and angiotensinogen[86] levels. Observational studies and post hoc analysis of clinical trials have reported worsening of renal outcomes and mortality with metabolic acidosis in most[88–92] but not all[93,94] studies. Prospective trials, however, are encouraging as we discuss below.

In a prospective open-label trial of 134 patients with stage 4 CKD and metabolic acidosis, treatment with oral sodium bicarbonate slowed the rate of CKD progression over 2 years compared to routine care (rate of GFR decline was 1.88 versus 5.93 mL/min/1.73m^2 in the treatment versus control arms respectively).

Treatment with oral sodium bicarbonate also reduced the rate of progression to ESKD (6.5% vs. 33% in the treatment vs. control arms, respectively).[95] A second study of 59 patients with hypertensive nephropathy patients followed for 2 years found that treatment with sodium citrate reduced the rate of CKD progression by 4.8 mL/min/1.73m² (27.8 vs. 23.0 for treatment vs. control, $p = 0.008$).[87] Similarly, correction of metabolic acidosis with fruits and vegetables or sodium bicarbonate resulted in greater stabilization of renal function after 3 years follow-up.[86] The protective benefits of sodium bicarbonate therapy also extend to patients with mild CKD with slower rates of GFR decline.[85]

A particular concern about use of sodium bicarbonate or sodium citrate is the development of hypervolemia and worsening of hypertension. These complications were not observed in the reported trials. Larger studies with longer follow-up are underway to examine the effects of alkali therapy on outcomes. The latest KDIGO[57] guidelines suggest treating CKD patients with bicarbonate level lower than 22 meq/L by oral sodium bicarbonate unless contraindicated (grade 2B).

ENDOTHELIN RECEPTOR ANTAGONISTS

Endothelin may promote renal damage by several mechanisms, including vasoconstriction, proteinuria, inflammation, and fibrosis.[96] Use of atrasentan, a selective endothelin A receptor antagonist, was associated with reduced levels of proteinuria in patients with type 2 diabetic nephropathy.[97] Average reduction in albumin-to-creatinine ratio after 12 weeks follow-up was 35% and 38% for atrasentan 0.75 mg and 1.25 mg daily, respectively, compared to placebo. All patients were on RAS inhibitors. A significant concern with use of endothelin receptor blockers is the risk of fluid retention. This is probably mediated through endothelin-B receptor blockade and is more likely to occur if high doses of endothelin receptor blockers are used.[96,97] The effect of atrasentan on a composite of doubling of SCr or the onset of ESKD is being assessed in the Study of Diabetic Nephropathy with Atrasentan (SONAR), which is currently recruiting (Clinicaltrials.gov identifier: NCT01858532).

BARDOXOLONE METHYL

Bardoxolone methyl, an agent with antioxidant and anti-inflammatory effects, was initially shown to have promising effects on GFR.[98] A subsequent trial examining the effect of bardoxolone methyl in patients with stage 4 CKD with diabetic nephropathy was terminated early, as there was a significantly increased risk of cardiovascular events with no effect on progression to ESKD.[99] This was likely mediated through modulation of the endothelin pathway, leading to salt and water retention.[100]

PENTOXYFILLINE

Pentoxyfilline (PTF) is a promising agent that may slow progression of CKD. It is a nonselective phosphodiesterase inhibitor used for the treatment of peripheral vascular occlusive disease and has anti-inflammatory, antiproliferative, and antifibrotic effects.[101,102] Goicoechea et al.[101] reported lower rates of CKD progression among 91 patients with established CKD randomized to PTF and followed for 1 year. Subsequently, a larger study by Navarro-Gonzalez et al.[102], found lower rates of decline among diabetic patients with stage 3 and 4 CKD when treated with PTF versus placebo. Moreover, there was also an associated significant decline in proteinuria. The effect of PTF on primary renal endpoints is currently being evaluated in a large multicenter randomized double-blind trial with follow-up for 3 years (Clinicaltrials.gov identifier: NCT01377285).

PIRFENIDONE

The antifibrotic agent pirfenidone, which inhibits transforming growth factor beta 1, may have a role in slowing progression of CKD. A recent trial by Sharma et al.[103] randomized 77 patients with diabetic nephropathy to placebo or one of two doses of pirfenidone. Improvements in GFR over time were observed in the low-dose pirfenidone group (+3.3 ± 8.5 mL/min/1.73 m²) but not in the high dose pirfenidone or placebo group (−2.2 ± 4.8 mL/min/1.73 m²). It should be noted, however, that this trial had several limitations including small sample size and large dropout rates. Most of the dropouts were because of fatigue and gastrointestinal symptoms. A second study addressing the potential benefit of pirfenidone is currently recruiting participants. (Clinicaltrials. gov identifier: NCT02689778).

CONCLUSION

In this chapter, we highlight the benefits of existing and newer pharmacological agents in reducing the progression of CKD. The past decade has witnessed the emergence of more selective therapeutic options targeting several pathways. The increasing number of clinical trials is a welcome boost. However, more robust evidence is required to support the clinical benefits of several new drugs on hard clinical outcomes and demonstrate that these benefits extend to diverse subgroups irrespective of demography, cause, and stage of kidney disease. Further research is also required to address interactions between these medications and the variation in therapeutic effect in the context of polypharmacy. In the interim, healthcare professionals caring for these patients should expect quite a challenging and hugely important task of balancing the clinical benefits demonstrated in large trials against potential complications in the individual patient.

REFERENCES

1. Coresh J, Selvin E, Stevens LA, et al. Prevalence of chronic kidney disease in the United States. *J Am Med Assoc.* 2007;298(17):2038–2047.
2. Bruck K, Stel VS, Gambaro G, et al. CKD prevalence varies across the European general population. *J Am Soc Nephrol.* 2016;27(7):2135–2147.
3. United States Renal Data System. *2016 USRDS annual data report: epidemiology of kidney disease in the United States.* Bethesda, MD: USRDS; 2016.
4. Ishani A, Grandits GA, Grimm RH, et al. Association of single measurements of dipstick proteinuria, estimated glomerular filtration rate, and hematocrit with 25-year incidence of end-stage renal disease in the multiple risk factor intervention trial. *J Am Soc Nephrol.* 2006;17(5):1444–1452.
5. Palit S, Chonchol M, Cheung AK, Kaufman J, Smits G, Kendrick J. Association of BP with death, cardiovascular events, and progression to chronic dialysis in patients with advanced kidney disease. *Clin J Am Soc Nephrol.* 2015;10(6):934–940.
6. Anderson AH, Yang W, Townsend RR, et al. Time-updated systolic blood pressure and the progression of chronic kidney disease: a cohort study. *Ann Intern Med.* 2015;162(4):258–265.
7. Sternlicht H, Bakris GL. The kidney in hypertension. *Med Clin N Am.* 2017;101(1):207–217.
8. Catt KJ, Mendelsohn FA, Millan MA, Aguilera G. The role of angiotensin II receptors in vascular regulation. *J Cardiovasc Pharmacol.* 1984;6(Suppl 4):S575–S586.
9. Mazurek JA, Jessup M. Understanding heart failure. *Heart Fail Clin.* 2017;13(1):1–19.
10. Pfeffer MA, Braunwald E, Moye LA, et al.; SAVE Investigators. Effect of captopril on mortality and morbidity in patients with left ventricular dysfunction after myocardial infarction: results of the survival and ventricular enlargement trial. *N Engl J Med.* 1992;327(10):669–677.
11. The Treatment of Mild Hypertension Research Group. The treatment of mild hypertension study: a randomized, placebo-controlled trial of a nutritional-hygienic regimen along with various drug monotherapies. *Arch Intern Med.* 1991;151(7):1413–1423.
12. The Microalbuminuria Captopril Study Group. Captopril reduces the risk of nephropathy in IDDM patients with microalbuminuria. *Diabetologia.* 1996;39(5):587–593.
13. Lewis EJ, Hunsicker LG, Clarke WR, et al. Renoprotective effect of the angiotensin-receptor antagonist irbesartan in patients with nephropathy due to type 2 diabetes. *N Engl J Med.* 2001;345(12):851–860.
14. Brenner BM, Cooper ME, de Zeeuw D, et al. Effects of losartan on renal and cardiovascular outcomes in patients with type 2 diabetes and nephropathy. *N Engl J Med.* 2001;345(12):861–869.
15. Gansevoort RT, Sluiter WJ, Hemmelder MH, de Zeeuw D, de Jong PE. Antiproteinuric effect of blood-pressure-lowering agents: a meta-analysis of comparative trials. *Nephrol Dial Transpl.* 1995;10(11):1963–1974.
16. Sarafidis PA, Khosla N, Bakris GL. Antihypertensive therapy in the presence of proteinuria. *Am J Kidney Dis.* 2007;49(1):12–26.
17. Gansevoort RT, Matsushita K, van der Velde M, et al. Lower estimated GFR and higher albuminuria are associated with adverse kidney outcomes: a collaborative meta-analysis of general and high-risk population cohorts. *Kidney Int.* 2011;80(1):93–104.
18. Maschio G, Alberti D, Janin G, et al.; The Angiotensin-Converting-Enzyme Inhibition in Progressive Renal Insufficiency Study Group. Effect of the angiotensin-converting-enzyme inhibitor benazepril on the progression of chronic renal insufficiency. *N Engl J Med.* 1996;334(15):939–945.
19. The GISEN Group (Gruppo Italiano di Studi Epidemiologici in Nefrologia).Randomised placebo-controlled trial of effect of ramipril on decline in glomerular filtration rate and risk of terminal renal failure in proteinuric, non-diabetic nephropathy. *Lancet.* 1997;349(9069):1857–1863.
20. Wright JT Jr, Bakris G, Greene T, et al. Effect of blood pressure lowering and antihypertensive drug class on progression of hypertensive kidney disease: results from the AASK trial. *J Am Med Assoc.* 2002;288(19):2421–2431.
21. Jafar TH, Schmid CH, Landa M, et al. Angiotensin-converting enzyme inhibitors and

progression of nondiabetic renal disease. A meta-analysis of patient-level data. *Ann Intern Med.* 2001;135(2):73–87.

22. Maione A, Navaneethan SD, Graziano G, et al. Angiotensin-converting enzyme inhibitors, angiotensin receptor blockers and combined therapy in patients with micro- and macroalbuminuria and other cardiovascular risk factors: a systematic review of randomized controlled trials. *Nephrol Dialy Transpl.* 2011;26(9):2827–2847.

23. UK Prospective Diabetes Study Group. Tight blood pressure control and risk of macrovascular and microvascular complications in type 2 diabetes: UKPDS 38. *BMJ-Clin Res.* 1998;317(7160):703–713.

24. Adler AI, Stratton IM, Neil HA, et al. Association of systolic blood pressure with macrovascular and microvascular complications of type 2 diabetes (UKPDS 36): prospective observational study. *BMJ-Clin Res.* 2000;321(7258):412–419.

25. Viberti G, Mogensen CE, Groop LC, Pauls JF; European Microalbuminuria Captopril Study Group. Effect of captopril on progression to clinical proteinuria in patients with insulin-dependent diabetes mellitus and microalbuminuria. *J Am Med Assoc.* 1994;271(4):275–279.

26. Lewis EJ, Hunsicker LG, Bain RP, Rohde RD; The Collaborative Study Group. The effect of angiotensin-converting-enzyme inhibition on diabetic nephropathy. *N Engl J Med.* 1993;329(20):1456–1462.

27. Hebert LA, Bain RP, Verme D, et al.; Collaborative Study Group. Remission of nephrotic range proteinuria in type I diabetes. *Kidney Int.* 1994;46(6):1688–1693.

28. Kent DM, Jafar TH, Hayward RA, et al. Progression risk, urinary protein excretion, and treatment effects of angiotensin-converting enzyme inhibitors in nondiabetic kidney disease. *J Am Soc Nephrol.* 2007;18(6):1959–1965.

29. Bakris GL, Weir MR. Angiotensin-converting enzyme inhibitor-associated elevations in serum creatinine: is this a cause for concern? *Arch Int Med.* 2000;160(5):685–693.

30. Yusuf S, Teo KK, Pogue J, et al. Telmisartan, ramipril, or both in patients at high risk for vascular events. *N Engl J Med.* 2008;358(15):1547–1559.

31. Fried LF, Emanuele N, Zhang JH, et al. Combined angiotensin inhibition for the treatment of diabetic nephropathy. *N Engl J Med.* 2013;369(20):1892–1903.

32. Parving HH, Brenner BM, McMurray JJ, et al. Cardiorenal end points in a trial of aliskiren for type 2 diabetes. *N Engl J Med.* 2012;367(23):2204–2213.

33. Bomback AS, Klemmer PJ. Mineralocorticoid receptor blockade in chronic kidney disease. *Blood Purificat.* 2012;33(1–3):119–124.

34. Bianchi S, Batini V, Bigazzi R. The renal effects of mineralocorticoid receptor antagonists. *Int J Cardiol.* 2015;200:20–24.

35. Brem AS, Gong R. Therapeutic targeting of aldosterone: a novel approach to the treatment of glomerular disease. *Clin Sci.* 2015;128(9):527–535.

36. Bernardi S, Toffoli B, Zennaro C, et al. Aldosterone effects on glomerular structure and function. *J Renin Angio Aldo S.* 2015;16(4):730–738.

37. Kadoya H, Satoh M, Sasaki T, Taniguchi S, Takahashi M, Kashihara N. Excess aldosterone is a critical danger signal for inflammasome activation in the development of renal fibrosis in mice. *FASEB J.* 2015;29(9):3899–3910.

38. Currie G, Taylor AH, Fujita T, et al. Effect of mineralocorticoid receptor antagonists on proteinuria and progression of chronic kidney disease: a systematic review and meta-analysis. *BMC Nephrol.* 2016;17(1):127.

39. Pitt B, Bakris GL. New potassium binders for the treatment of hyperkalemia: current data and opportunities for the future. *Hypertension.* 2015;66(4):731–738.

40. Bakris GL, Weir MR, Secic M, Campbell B, Weis-McNulty A. Differential effects of calcium antagonist subclasses on markers of nephropathy progression. *Kidney Int.* 2004;65(6):1991–2002.

41. Das A, Kumar P, Kumari A, et al. Effects of cilnidipine on heart rate and uric acid metabolism in patients with essential hypertension. *Cardiol Res.* 2016;7(5):167–172.

42. Masaki M, Mano T, Eguchi A, et al. Long-term effects of L- and N-type calcium channel blocker on uric acid levels and left atrial volume in hypertensive patients. *Heart Vessels.* 2016;31(11):1826–1833.

43. Uchida S, Takahashi M, Sugawara M, et al. Effects of the N/L-type calcium channel blocker cilnidipine on nephropathy and uric acid metabolism in hypertensive patients with chronic kidney disease (J-CIRCLE study). *J Clin Hypertens.* 2014;16(10):746–753.

44. Vogt L, Waanders F, Boomsma F, de Zeeuw D, Navis G. Effects of dietary sodium and hydrochlorothiazide on the antiproteinuric efficacy of losartan. *J Am Soc Nephrol.* 2008;19(5):999–1007.

45. Esnault VL, Ekhlas A, Delcroix C, Moutel MG, Nguyen JM. Diuretic and enhanced sodium restriction results in improved antiproteinuric response to RAS blocking agents. *J Am Soc Nephrol.* 2005;16(2):474–481.

46. Buter H, Hemmelder MH, Navis G, de Jong PE, de Zeeuw D. The blunting of the antiproteinuric efficacy of ACE inhibition by high sodium intake can be restored by hydrochlorothiazide. *Nephrol Dialy Transpl.* 1998;13(7):1682–1685.

47. Ismail-Beigi F, Craven T, Banerji MA, et al. Effect of intensive treatment of hyperglycaemia on microvascular outcomes in type 2 diabetes: an analysis of the ACCORD randomised trial. *Lancet.* 2010;376(9739):419–430.

48. Fullerton B, Jeitler K, Seitz M, Horvath K, Berghold A, Siebenhofer A. Intensive glucose control versus conventional glucose control for type 1 diabetes mellitus. *Cochrane Db Syst Rev.* 2014(2):Cd009122.

49. Cherney DZ, Perkins BA, Soleymanlou N, et al. Renal hemodynamic effect of sodium-glucose cotransporter 2 inhibition in patients with type 1 diabetes mellitus. *Circulation.* 2014;129(5):587–597.

50. Fioretto P, Stefansson BV, Johnsson E, Cain VA, Sjostrom CD. Dapagliflozin reduces albuminuria over 2 years in patients with type 2 diabetes mellitus and renal impairment. *Diabetologia.* 2016;59(9):2036–2039.

51. Wanner C, Inzucchi SE, Lachin JM, et al. Empagliflozin and progression of kidney disease in type 2 diabetes. *N Engl J Med.* 2016;375(4):323–334.

52. Heerspink HJ, Desai M, Jardine M, Balis D, Meininger G, Perkovic V. Canagliflozin slows progression of renal function decline independently of glycemic effects. *J Am Soc Nephrol.* 2017;28(1):368–375.

53. de Boer IH, Kahn SE. SGLT2 inhibitors-sweet success for diabetic kidney disease? *J Am Soc Nephrol.* 2017;28(1):7–10.

54. Zinman B, Wanner C, Lachin JM, et al. Empagliflozin, cardiovascular outcomes, and mortality in type 2 diabetes. *N Engl J Med.* 2015;373(22):2117–2128.

55. Heyman SN, Khamaisi M, Rosen S, Rosenberger C, Abassi Z. Potential hypoxic renal injury in patients with diabetes on sglt2 inhibitors: caution regarding concomitant use of NSAIDs and iodinated contrast media. *Diabetes Care.* 2017;40(4):e40–e41.

56. Graefe-Mody U, Friedrich C, Port A, et al. Effect of renal impairment on the pharmacokinetics of the dipeptidyl peptidase-4 inhibitor linagliptin(*). *Diabetes, Obes Metab.* 2011;13(10):939–946.

57. Groop PH, Cooper ME, Perkovic V, Emser A, Woerle HJ, von Eynatten M. Linagliptin lowers albuminuria on top of recommended standard treatment in patients with type 2 diabetes and renal dysfunction. *Diabetes Care.* 2013;36(11):3460–3468.

58. Cooper ME, Perkovic V, McGill JB, et al. Kidney disease end points in a pooled analysis of individual patient-level data from a large clinical trials program of the dipeptidyl peptidase 4 inhibitor linagliptin in type 2 diabetes. *Am J Kidney Dis.* 2015;66(3):441–449.

59. Baigent C, Landray MJ, Reith C, et al. The effects of lowering LDL cholesterol with simvastatin plus ezetimibe in patients with chronic kidney disease (Study of Heart and Renal Protection): a randomised placebo-controlled trial. *Lancet.* 2011;377(9784):2181–2192.

60. Palmer SC, Navaneethan SD, Craig JC, et al. HMG CoA reductase inhibitors (statins) for people with chronic kidney disease not requiring dialysis. *Cochrane Db Syst Rev.* 2014(5):Cd007784.

61. Wanner C, Tonelli M. KDIGO clinical practice guideline for lipid management in CKD: summary of recommendation statements and clinical approach to the patient. *Kidney Int.* 2014;85(6):1303–1309.

62. Keane WF, O'Donnell MP, Kasiske BL, Schmitz PG. Lipids and the progression of renal disease. *J Am Soc Nephrol.* 1990;1(5 Suppl 2):S69–S74.

63. Muhlfeld AS, Spencer MW, Hudkins KL, Kirk E, LeBoeuf RC, Alpers CE. Hyperlipidemia aggravates renal disease in B6.ROP Os/+ mice. *Kidney Int.* 2004;66(4):1393–1402.

64. Panichi V, Paoletti S, Mantuano E, et al. In vivo and in vitro effects of simvastatin on inflammatory markers in pre-dialysis patients. *Nephrol Dialy Transpl.* 2006;21(2):337–344.

65. Kosch M, Barenbrock M, Suwelack B, Schaefer RM, Rahn KH, Hausberg M. Effect of a 3-year therapy with the 3-hydroxy-3-methylglutaryl coenzyme a reductase-inhibitor fluvastatin on endothelial function and distensibility of large arteries in hypercholesterolemic renal transplant recipient. *Am J Kidney Dis.* 2003;41(5):1088–1096.

66. Ichihara A, Hayashi M, Ryuzaki M, Handa M, Furukawa T, Saruta T. Fluvastatin prevents development of arterial stiffness in haemodialysis patients with type 2 diabetes mellitus. *Nephrol Dialy Transpl.* 2002;17(8):1513–1517.

67. Nakamura T, Ushiyama C, Hirokawa K, Osada S, Shimada N, Koide H. Effect of cerivastatin on urinary albumin excretion and plasma endothelin-1 concentrations in type 2 diabetes patients with microalbuminuria and dyslipidemia. *Am J Nephrol.* 2001;21(6):449–454.

68. Nakamura T, Ushiyama C, Hirokawa K, et al. Effect of cerivastatin on proteinuria and urinary podocytes in patients with chronic

glomerulonephritis. *Nephrol Dialy Transpl.* 2002;17(5):798–802.

69. Haynes R, Lewis D, Emberson J, et al. Effects of lowering LDL cholesterol on progression of kidney disease. *J Am Soc Nephrol.* 2014;25(8):1825–1833.

70. Sanchez-Lozada LG, Tapia E, Santamaria J, et al. Mild hyperuricemia induces vasoconstriction and maintains glomerular hypertension in normal and remnant kidney rats. *Kidney Int.* 2005;67(1):237–247.

71. Sanchez-Lozada LG, Tapia E, Soto V, et al. Effect of febuxostat on the progression of renal disease in 5/6 nephrectomy rats with and without hyperuricemia. *Nephron Physiol.* 2008;108(4):69–78.

72. Kang DH, Nakagawa T, Feng L, et al. A role for uric acid in the progression of renal disease. *J Am Soc Nephrol.* 2002;13(12):2888–2897.

73. Chonchol M, Shlipak MG, Katz R, et al. Relationship of uric acid with progression of kidney disease. *Am J Kidney Dis.* 2007;50(2):239–247.

74. Weiner DE, Tighiouart H, Elsayed EF, Griffith JL, Salem DN, Levey AS. Uric acid and incident kidney disease in the community. *J Am Soc Nephrol.* 2008;19(6):1204–1211.

75. Obermayr RP, Temml C, Gutjahr G, Knechtelsdorfer M, Oberbauer R, Klauser-Braun R. Elevated uric acid increases the risk for kidney disease. *J Am Soc Nephrol.* 2008;19(12):2407–2413.

76. Madero M, Sarnak MJ, Wang X, et al. Uric acid and long-term outcomes in CKD. *Am J Kidney Dis.* 2009;53(5):796–803.

77. Goicoechea M, de Vinuesa SG, Verdalles U, et al. Effect of allopurinol in chronic kidney disease progression and cardiovascular risk. *Clin J Am Soc Nephrol.* 2010;5(8):1388–1393.

78. Sircar D, Chatterjee S, Waikhom R, et al. Efficacy of febuxostat for slowing the GFR decline in patients with CKD and asymptomatic hyperuricemia: a 6-month, double-blind, randomized, placebo-controlled trial. *Am J Kidney Dis.* 2015;66(6):945–950.

79. Kanji T, Gandhi M, Clase CM, Yang R. Urate lowering therapy to improve renal outcomes in patients with chronic kidney disease: systematic review and meta-analysis. *BMC Nephrol.* 2015;16:58.

80. Zhang YF, He F, Ding HH, et al. Effect of uric-acid-lowering therapy on progression of chronic kidney disease: a meta-analysis. *J Huazhong Univ Sci-Med.* 2014;34(4):476–481.

81. Bose B, Badve SV, Hiremath SS, et al. Effects of uric acid-lowering therapy on renal outcomes: a systematic review and meta-analysis. *Nephrol Dialy Transpl.* 2014;29(2):406–413.

82. Eustace JA, Astor B, Muntner PM, Ikizler TA, Coresh J. Prevalence of acidosis and inflammation and their association with low serum albumin in chronic kidney disease. *Kidney Int.* 2004;65(3):1031–1040.

83. Raphael KL, Zhang Y, Ying J, Greene T. Prevalence of and risk factors for reduced serum bicarbonate in chronic kidney disease. *Nephrology.* 2014;19(10):648–654.

84. Nath KA, Hostetter MK, Hostetter TH. Increased ammoniagenesis as a determinant of progressive renal injury. *Am J Kidney Dis.* 1991;17(6):654–657.

85. Mahajan A, Simoni J, Sheather SJ, Broglio KR, Rajab MH, Wesson DE. Daily oral sodium bicarbonate preserves glomerular filtration rate by slowing its decline in early hypertensive nephropathy. *Kidney Int.* 2010;78(3):303–309.

86. Goraya N, Simoni J, Jo CH, Wesson DE. Treatment of metabolic acidosis in patients with stage 3 chronic kidney disease with fruits and vegetables or oral bicarbonate reduces urine angiotensinogen and preserves glomerular filtration rate. *Kidney Int.* 2014;86(5):1031–1038.

87. Phisitkul S, Khanna A, Simoni J, et al. Amelioration of metabolic acidosis in patients with low GFR reduced kidney endothelin production and kidney injury, and better preserved GFR. *Kidney Int.* 2010;77(7):617–623.

88. Dobre M, Yang W, Chen J, et al. Association of serum bicarbonate with risk of renal and cardiovascular outcomes in CKD: a report from the Chronic Renal Insufficiency Cohort (CRIC) study. *Am J Kidney Dis.* 2013;62(4):670–678.

89. Shah SN, Abramowitz M, Hostetter TH, Melamed ML. Serum bicarbonate levels and the progression of kidney disease: a cohort study. *Am J Kidney Dis.* 2009;54(2):270–277.

90. Kovesdy CP, Anderson JE, Kalantar-Zadeh K. Association of serum bicarbonate levels with mortality in patients with non-dialysis-dependent CKD. *Nephrol Dialy Transpl.* 2009;24(4):1232–1237.

91. Navaneethan SD, Schold JD, Arrigain S, et al. Serum bicarbonate and mortality in stage 3 and stage 4 chronic kidney disease. *Clin J Am Soc Nephrol.* 2011;6(10):2395–2402.

92. Driver TH, Shlipak MG, Katz R, et al. Low serum bicarbonate and kidney function decline: the Multi-Ethnic Study of Atherosclerosis (MESA). *Am J Kidney Dis.* 2014;64(4):534–541.

93. Schutte E, Lambers Heerspink HJ, Lutgers HL, et al. Serum bicarbonate and kidney disease progression and cardiovascular outcome in patients with diabetic nephropathy: a post hoc analysis of the RENAAL (Reduction of End Points

in Non-Insulin-Dependent Diabetes With the Angiotensin II Antagonist Losartan) Study and IDNT (Irbesartan Diabetic Nephropathy Trial). *Am J Kidney Dis.* 2015;66(3):450–458.

94. Menon V, Tighiouart H, Vaughn NS, et al. Serum bicarbonate and long-term outcomes in CKD. *Am J Kidney Dis.* 2010;56(5):907–914.

95. de Brito-Ashurst I, Varagunam M, Raftery MJ, Yaqoob MM. Bicarbonate supplementation slows progression of CKD and improves nutritional status. *J Am Soc Nephrol.* 2009;20(9): 2075–2084.

96. Kohan DE, Pollock DM. Endothelin antagonists for diabetic and non-diabetic chronic kidney disease. *Brit J Clin Pharmacol.* 2013;76(4): 573–579.

97. de Zeeuw D, Coll B, Andress D, et al. The endothelin antagonist atrasentan lowers residual albuminuria in patients with type 2 diabetic nephropathy. *J Am Soc Nephrol.* 2014;25(5):1083–1093.

98. Pergola PE, Raskin P, Toto RD, et al. Bardoxolone methyl and kidney function in CKD with type 2 diabetes. *N Engl J Med.* 2011;365(4):327–336.

99. de Zeeuw D, Akizawa T, Audhya P, et al. Bardoxolone methyl in type 2 diabetes and stage 4 chronic kidney disease. *N Engl J Med.* 2013;369(26):2492–2503.

100. Chin MP, Reisman SA, Bakris GL, et al. Mechanisms contributing to adverse cardiovascular events in patients with type 2 diabetes mellitus and stage 4 chronic kidney disease treated with bardoxolone methyl. *Am J Nephrol.* 2014;39(6):499–508.

101. Goicoechea M, Garcia de Vinuesa S, Quiroga B, et al. Effects of pentoxifylline on inflammatory parameters in chronic kidney disease patients: a randomized trial. *Journal of nephrology.* 2012;25(6):969–975.

102. Navarro-Gonzalez JF, Mora-Fernandez C, Muros de Fuentes M, et al. Effect of pentoxifylline on renal function and urinary albumin excretion in patients with diabetic kidney disease: the PREDIAN trial. *J Am Soc Nephrol.* 2015;26(1):220–229.

103. Sharma K, Ix JH, Mathew AV, et al. Pirfenidone for diabetic nephropathy. *J Am Soc Nephrol.* 2011;22(6):1144–1151.

11

Evaluation and Management of Acute Kidney Injury

BHAGWAN DASS, WILLIAM HAHN, AND RAJESH MOHANDAS

INTRODUCTION

Acute kidney injury (AKI) is defined as a sudden or abrupt decrease in the glomerular filtration rate (GFR). The past decade has seen numerous attempts to standardize the diagnostic criteria for AKI. All of the criteria use a combination of changes in serum creatinine (SCr) and urine output to define and stage the severity of AKI. The Acute Kidney Injury Network (AKIN) criteria defines AKI as an increase in SCr greater than 0.3 mg/dl in 48 hours or a 50% increase in SCr from baseline, or a urine output less than 0.5 ml/kg/hour for greater than 6 hours.[1] KDIGO clinical practice guidelines extended the definition by specifying the decrease in GFR to occur within a week.[2] However, unlike SCr, the urine output criteria have not been prospectively validated in clinical trials and there is concern that a decreased urine output alone might overestimate those with AKI.[3]

ETIOPATHOGENESIS

An understanding of the etiopathogenesis of AKI is essential to develop effective preventive strategies for AKI. The majority of intrinsic AKI, at least in the hospital setting, occurs from acute tubular necrosis (ATN). Decreased renal blood flow commonly precedes ATN. When blood pressure falls below 80 mmHg systolic, autoregulation fails to maintain glomerular perfusion and ischemia results.[4] Autoregulatory mechanisms can be impaired by diabetes, chronic kidney disease (CKD), and drugs such as angiotensin converting enzyme inhibitors (ACEI) and contrast or nonsteroidal anti-inflammatory drugs. Lack of autoregulation can lead to disruption in renal blood flow even in the absence of overt hypotension particular with abrupt drops in blood pressure, called "normotensive ischemic AKI."[5] The decreased blood flow results in endothelial cell injury, disruption of the renal microvasculature, and tubular damage.[6] Although termed "acute tubular necrosis," the degree of cellular injury in ATN is usually mild. How this mild cellular dysfunction results in profound reductions in GFR is not well known. Several hypotheses have been proposed, of which the most widely accepted are (i) afferent arterial vasoconstriction, (ii) intraluminal tubular obstruction, and (iii) back leak of the filtrate. In established ATN, particularly in AKI due to nephrotoxins such as contrast and myoglobin, there is vasoconstriction of the afferent renal artery resulting in decreased GFR and worsening medullary hypoxia. The proximal tubular dysfunction accompanying ATN results in increased distal delivery of chloride to the macula densa, which activates the tubuloglomerular feedback loop and inhibits the GFR. Intraluminal tubular obstruction is caused by cells and cellular debris that forms casts with the Tamm-Horsfall proteins and is augmented in the presence of volume depletion. Tubular ischemia also results in loss of integrity of tubular cell junctions, causing filtrate to leak into the interstitium as well as bloodstream resulting in a decrease in GFR. The early initiation phase of AKI is followed by an extension phase characterized by intense inflammation. Hypoxia, acting directly on the proximal tubular cells or indirectly via the innate immune system composing of complements and toll-like receptors, induces several proinflammatory cytokines and chemokines. Neutrophils and mononuclear cells have been identified in peritubular capillaries in biopsy specimens, and depletion of neutrophils and T cells mitigates AKI in animal models. All of this suggests a prominent role for the immune system in AKI.

RISK STRATIFICATION

Preventing AKI requires accurately identifying those at risk to enable close monitoring of high-risk patients, timely institution of preventative therapy, and early diagnosis and treatment of established AKI to prevent complications. The risk of AKI depends on the extent and nature of injury as well as patient susceptibility factors. Exposures that can result in AKI in susceptible populations include sepsis, shock, surgery, burns, heart failure, and liver failure. Risk factors characterized by the clinical settings are summarized in Table 11.1. Of the patient susceptibility factors, age has consistently been shown to be a risk factor for AKI whereas the influence of gender and race seem to be modulated by the clinical setting in which AKI occurs. Other risk factors for developing AKI include comorbidities such as CKD, diabetes, mechanical ventilation, and exposure to nephrotoxic agents. Genetic studies using an unbiased approach or candidate genes regulating inflammation or vasomotor pathway have largely been unsuccessful in identifying and validating genes conferring risk for AKI. Injury-specific scoring systems have been devised to quantify the risk of AKI. However, most have modest predictive ability and have not been widely adapted into clinical practice.

CLINICAL ASSESSMENT

The clinical assessment targeted to prevent AKI must include a careful review of the chart to minimize or avoid nephrotoxic medications, as well as an assessment of volume status. Echocardiography, assessment of stroke volume variation or invasive hemodynamic monitoring might be required to accurately estimate intravascular volume in obese critically ill patients. A low fractional excretion of sodium might be helpful in identifying volume depletion in oliguric patients without cardiac or liver dysfunction. In patients with established AKI, attempts must be made to pinpoint a specific cause of AKI when possible. An accurate etiological diagnosis is helpful to streamline further diagnostic workup and institute appropriate and timely secondary prevention strategies. Timing and choice of preventive therapies in established AKI is predicated on the probability of spontaneous recovery. Identifying patients who are likely to recover is important to avoid unnecessary therapy. It is estimated that almost half the patients recover without need for dialysis, even with stage 3 AKI. The furosemide challenge test assesses the response of patients with AKI given 1 mg/kg of furosemide intravenously (1.5 mg/kg of furosemide if they have received diuretics in the past

TABLE 11.1 RISK FACTORS FOR ACUTE KIDNEY INJURY IN SELECTED CLINICAL ENTITIES

Setting	Specific
Burns	Severe burns >30%, multiple surgeries, cumulative positive fluid balance, multiple organ failure, sepsis, nephrotoxic medications
Cardiac surgery	(TAA>valves>CABG), redo surgery, CPB >200min, off-pump, LVEF <45%
Contrast-induced AKI	eGFR < 45 ml/min, IABP, dose of contrast agent, high-osmolar contrast, dehydration, hypotension, age >70 years
Heart failure	Older age, systolic dysfunction, CKD, low blood pressure
Liver failure	Spontaneous bacterial peritonitis, large volume paracentesis without albumin replacement, gastrointestinal bleeding, CKD
Rhabdomyolysis	High CK levels, ALT >259 IU/L, AST>95 IU/L, hypoalbuminemia, hypocalcemia, metabolic acidosis,
Sepsis	Bacteremia, cytopenias, advanced age, CKD, delay in administration of antibiotics
Tumor lysis syndrome	High tumor burden, LDH levels, hyperuricemia (> 6 mg/dL)

TAA = thoracic aortic aneurysm. CPB = cardio pulmonary bypass. CABG = coronary artery bypass grafting. IABP = intra-aortic balloon pump. CK = creatinine kinase. ALT = alanine amino transferase. AST = aspartate amino transferase. CKD = chronic kidney disease. LDH = lactate dehydrogenase.

7 days). To prevent hypovolemia an equivalent amount of saline is infused to match the urine output. A urine output greater than 200 mL in 2 hours had a sensitivity of 97% and specificity of 84% in predicting recovery from AKI.[7]

BIOMARKERS

SCr is not a sensitive marker for glomerular filtration, and serum levels of creatinine do not increase until substantial kidney function has been lost. Moreover, increases in creatinine can occur due to hemodynamic changes without any accompanying changes in GFR. Given the shortcomings of SCr, there has been an interest in developing novel biomarkers that can better predict AKI. Cystatin C is a 13kDa cysteine protease inhibitor that is produced by all nucleate cells, freely filtered at the glomerulus, and completely metabolized by the proximal tubular cells with no evident tubular secretion. Although cystatin production was thought to be constant, later studies have shown that it is influenced by age, gender, body mass index, smoking, inflammation, thyroid function, and immunosuppressive medication. Observational studies in diverse settings have shown area under the curve (AUC) ranging from 0.62 to 0.82. Biomarkers that reflect tubular injury as well as cellular and molecular events during different phases of AKI were proposed to overcome some of the shortcomings of functional biomarkers such as creatinine and cystatin. One of the earliest and most well-studied markers is neutrophil gelatinase-associated lipocalin, which was first isolated from neutrophil granules. Neutrophil gelatinase-associated lipocalin is also produced in renal epithelial cells and is upregulated as early as 3 hours following ischemia or nephrotoxic agents.[8] Although initial studies in children undergoing cardiac surgery suggested robust ability to predict AKI with AUCs of 0.998,[9] subsequent studies in more diverse patient cohorts have shown varying and more modest ability to identify patients at risk of AKI, with AUCs ranging from 0.50 to 0.93 after cardiac surgery and 0.54 to 0.99 in intensive care units (ICUs).[10] Kidney injury molecule (KIM-1) is a transmembrane phosphatidylserine receptor that is transiently upregulated in proximal tubular cells following AKI. The ectodomain of KIM-1 is shed in the urine after renal injury and can be detected using enzyme-linked immunosorbent assays. Prospective observational studies have shown widely varying sensitivity, ranging from 0.40 to 0.92 and specificities of 0.58 to 0.81, to detect AKI, depending on the patient population studied. Interleukin-18 and liver-type fatty acid–binding protein all have had modest success in predicting AKI. The predictive value of biomarkers varies depending on the clinical setting and the pretest probability of AKI. The pooled predictive values of selected biomarkers are summarized in Table 11.2. Further, tubular injury, which is identified by many biomarkers, might not be associated with reductions in GFR, particularly when the injury is mild. Recently tissue inhibitor of metalloproteinase-2 (TIMP-2) and insulin-like growth factor (IGF) binding protein 7 were shown to have much better predictive value in critically ill patients, with AUC of 0.79 and 0.76, respectively. NephroCheck™, an easy-to-use bedside test that incorporates TIMP and IGF-2 to predict an AKI risk score, has been approved by the Federal Drug Agency for clinical use in critically ill patients and is commercially

TABLE 11.2 PERFORMANCE OF SELECTED BIOMARKERS IN PREDICTING ACUTE KIDNEY INJURY

	AUC	Sensitivity	Specificity
Functional niomarkers			
Cystatin C	**0.89** (0.86, 0.91)	**0.89** (0.75, 0.87)	**0.82** (0.78, 0.86)
Tubular injury markers			
NGAL	**0.82** (0.73–0.89)	**0.76** (0.70–0.82)	**0.85** (0.77–0.91)
KIM-1	**0.86** (0.83–0.89)	**0.74** (0.61–0.84)	**0.86** (0.74–0.93)
TIMP-2 * IGFB-7	0.88	**0.84** (0.80–0.88)	**0.57** (0.55–0.60)

AUC = area under the curve. NGAL = neutrophil gelatinase-associated lipocalin. KIM-1 = kidney injury molecule. TIMP-2 = tissue inhibitor of metalloproteinase-2 (TIMP-2). IGFB-7 = insulin-like growth factor binding protein-7.

available. An AKI risk score greater than 0.3 predicts those who are likely to develop moderate or severe AKI within 12 hours. However, NephroCheck™ has not yet been widely adapted into clinical practice because the utility of biomarkers to improve resource utilization or clinical outcomes remains to be proven.

PREVENTION OF AKI

A proper risk assessment is essential for instituting timely preventive measures for AKI. It is termed "primary prevention" if therapy is instituted before tubular injury occurs and "secondary prevention" if therapy is initiated after AKI is established and with the goal of preventing complications of AKI. The distinction is often difficult and arbitrary since subclinical tubular damage might be present even if there is no overt AKI. Preventive measures for AKI include optimization of volume status, vasoactive agents, natriuretics, statin therapy, growth factors, remote ischemic preconditioning, prophylactic dialysis, and experimental therapies.

Selected randomized controlled trials are summarized in Table 11.3.

Preventive Measures for AKI
Optimization of Volume Status

Expanding intravascular volume has been shown to be beneficial in settings such as pigment related nephropathy, tumor lysis syndrome, and contrast-induced AKI. A meta-analysis of small randomized controlled trial (RCT) suggests that perioperative hemodynamic monitoring and optimizing volume might also prevent ischemic ATN associated with cardiac surgery.[11] Both crystalloids and colloids seem equally effective in expanding plasma volume and correcting hypotension.[12] Blood transfusion on the other hand has been associated with increased risk of AKI post cardiac surgery and angiogram. Although cause and effect cannot be established from these observational studies, minimizing blood transfusions seems prudent given that packed cell transfusions are associated with other complications, including transfusion reaction and acute lung injury. The benefits of volume expansion are less certain in patients with established AKI, in whom the benefits of volume repletion have to be balanced against the risks of volume overload. Several studies have clearly shown that volume overload is associated with excess mortality.[13] In patients with Acute Respiratory Distress Syndrome on mechanical ventilation, the Fluid and Catheter Treatment Trial (FACTT)[14] study showed that a conservative fluid management strategy resulted in decreased time on ventilator and in the ICU although there was no significant difference in the primary outcome of 60-day mortality or the use of dialysis.

Vasoactive Agents

The use of vasopressors is required if hypotension persists despite optimization of intravascular volume. Clinical decisions surrounding the use of vasopressors include the choice of vasopressor and target blood pressures. Theoretically, vasopressors such as dopamine that are associated with renal vasodilation might have an advantage over nonselective agents such as norepinephrine. However, data from observational studies and small RCTs suggest that the outcomes are similar and that norepinephrine might be more efficacious than dopamine.[15,16] The choice of vasopressors is thus dictated by the clinical scenario and possible side effects of therapy such as arrhythmias. There are no RCTs to guide target blood pressures. Many clinical guidelines, including Surviving Sepsis Campaign,[17] recommend a target mean arterial pressure (MAP) of at least 65 mmHg.[18] However, the optimal MAP required for restoring tissue perfusion is still unclear. In a recent study,[19] patients with sepsis randomized to a MAP of 80 to 85 mmHg, as compared to those who were randomized to a MAP of 65 to 70 mmHg, were less likely to require dialysis if they had a history of hypertension, although there were no differences in mortality. The kidney has a higher perfusion threshold and pressure flow curve than other vascular beds. So, particularly in patients with long-standing hypertension that is associated with vascular remodeling, a higher MAP might be needed to maintain adequate perfusion. This needs to be evaluated further in RCTs. Numerous clinical trials and subsequent meta-analyses have found that low dopamine is ineffective in preventing AKI. Fenoldopam, a selective D1 receptor agonist that lacks effects on the beta-adrenergic receptor, is thought to selectively dilate renal blood vessels. Although a meta-analysis of several small studies found that fenoldopam reduced risk of AKI and need for dialysis, a subsequent RCT of 667 cardiac surgery patients found evidence for neither.[20] The role of fenoldopam to prevent AKI thus remains unclear.

TABLE 11.3 SELECTED RANDOMIZED CONTROLLED TRIALS OF INTERVENTIONS IN ACUTE KIDNEY INJURY

Study	Setting	Intervention	Primary Outcome	Secondary Outcome	Important Findings
		Optimizing volume status			
Comparison of two fluid-management strategies in acute lung injury[a]	1,000 patients with acute lung injury	Liberal vs. conservative fluids	60-day mortality	Oxygenation Lung Injury score Ventilator-free days ICU length of stay Prevalence of shock Dialysis requirement	No difference in mortality. Conservative fluids improved oxygenation, lung injury score and ICU stay.
A comparison of albumin and saline for fluid resuscitation in the ICU[b]	6,997 patients in ICU	4% Albumin or Normal Saline	28-day death from any cause		No difference in mortality
Effect of a buffered crystalloid solution vs saline on acute kidney injury among patients in the ICU: the SPLIT randomized clinical trial[c]	2,278 patients in medical and surgical ICU not receiving dialysis	Saline or buffered crystalloid for alternating 7 week blocks	Proportion of patients with AKI (2-fold increase in serum creatinine level of ≥3.96 mg/dL with an increase of ≥0.5 mg/dL)	Incidence of RRT use and in-hospital mortality.	No difference in AKI
		Vasoactive agents			
Effect of fenoldopam on use of renal replacement therapy among patients with acute kidney injury after cardiac surgery[d]	667 patients post cardiac surgery	Fenoldopam or Placebo	Rate of RRT	30-day mortality Hypotension	No difference in RRT between fenoldopam (20%) or placebo (18%) $p = 0.47$. No difference in mortality. Hypotension more common in fenoldopam.

(continued)

TABLE 11.3 CONTINUED

Study	Setting	Intervention	Primary Outcome	Secondary Outcome	Important Findings
Natriuretics					
Recombinant human atrial natriuretic peptide in ischemic acute renal failure: a randomized placebo-controlled trial[e]	61 postsurgical patients with heart failure and normal renal function	Recombinant h-ANP (50 ng/kg/min) or placebo	Dialysis at 21 days	Dialysis free survival at 21-days Creatinine clearance	Enhances renal excretory function, decreases the probability of dialysis, and improves dialysis-free survival
Atrial natriuretic factor in oliguric acute renal failure. Anaritide Acute Renal Failure Study Group[f]	222 critically ill patients with oliguric AKI	Anaritide (0.2 microgram per kilogram of body weight per minute) or placebo	Dialysis-free survival for 21 days	60-day mortality Hypotension	No benefit of Anaritide in dialysis free survival or 60-day mortality but associated with increased hypotension
Statins					
Short-term rosuvastatin therapy for prevention of contrast-induced acute kidney injury in patients with diabetes and chronic kidney dsiease[g]	2,998 patients with DM and CKD undergoing angiography	Rosuvastain 10 mg/day for 5 days or standard of care	Contrast-induced AKI (increase in Cr >0.5 mg/dl or 0.25% above baseline at 72 hours)		Rosuvastatin lower CI-AKI (2.3% vs. 3.9%)
Ischemic preconditioning					
Effect of remote ischemic preconditioning on kidney injury among high-risk patients undergoing cardiac surgery[h]	329 patients undergoing CABG	Ischemic preconditioning or standard of care	Rate of AKI 72 hours after cardiac surgery.	Use of renal replacement therapy Duration of ICU stay Occurrence of myocardial infarction and stroke In-hospital and 30-day mortality Change in AKI biomarkers	Ischemic preconditioning significantly reduced AKI (37.5% vs. 52.5%) Need for renal replacement therapy 5.8% vs 15.8% ICU stay (3 vs 4 days No effect on myocardial infarction, stroke, or mortality.

Remote ischemic preconditioning and outcomes of cardiac surgery[i]	1,612 patients undergoing CABG	Ischemic preconditioning or sham	1-year death from cardiovascular causes, nonfatal myocardial infarction, coronary revascularization, or stroke,	Myocardial injury Use of vasopressors within 72 hours AKI ICU LOS Total LOS 6-minute walk test QOL	No difference in primary or secondary outcomes

Diuretics

High-dose furosemide for established ARF: a prospective, randomized, double-blind, placebo-controlled, multicenter trial[j]	338 patients with AKI requiring dialysis	Furosemide (25 mg/kg/d intravenously or 35 mg/kg/d orally) or matched placebo	Survival	Number of dialysis sessions	No difference in survival or dialysis requirements

[a]Wiedemann HP, Wheeler AP, Bernard GR,et al.; The National Heart, Lung, and Blood Institute Acute Respiratory Distress Syndrome (ARDS) Clinical Trials Network. Comparison of two fluid-management strategies in acute lung injury. *N Engl J Med.* 2006;354(24):2564–2575.

[b]Finfer S, Bellomo R, Boyce N, et al. A comparison of albumin and saline for fluid resuscitation in the intensive care unit. *N Engl J Med.* 2004;350(22):2247–2256.

[c]Young P, Bailey M, Beasley R, et al.; SPLIT investigators; ANZICS CTG. Effect of a buffered crystalloid solution vs saline on acute kidney injury among patients in the intensive care unit: the SPLIT randomized clinical trial. *J Am Med Assoc.* 2015;314(16):1701–1710.

[d]Bove T, Zangrillo A, Guarracino F, et al. Effect of fenoldopam on use of renal replacement therapy among patients with acute kidney injury after cardiac surgery a randomized clinical trial. *J Am Med Assoc.* 2014;312(21):2244–2253.

[e]Sward K, Valsson F, Odencrants P, Samuelson O, Ricksten SE. Recombinant human atrial natriuretic peptide in ischemic acute renal failure: a randomized placebo-controlled trial. *Crit Care Med.* 2004;32(6):1310–1315.

[f]Lewis J, Salem MM, Chertow GM, et al.; Anaritide Acute Renal Failure Study Group. Atrial natriuretic factor in oliguric acute renal failure. *Am J Kidney Dis.* 2000;36(4):767–774.

[g]Han Y, Zhu G, Han L, et al. Short-term rosuvastatin therapy for prevention of contrast-induced acute kidney injury in patients with diabetes and chronic kidney disease. *J Am Coll Cardiol.* 2014;63(1):62–70.

[h]Zarbock A, Schmidt C, Van Aken H, et al. Effect of remote ischemic preconditioning on kidney injury among high-risk patients undergoing cardiac surgery a randomized clinical trial. *J Am Med Assoc.* 2015;313(21):2133–2141.

[i]Hausenloy DJ, Candilio L, Evans R, et al. Remote ischemic preconditioning and outcomes of cardiac surgery. *N Engl J Med.* 2015;373(15):1408–1417.

[j]Cantarovich F, Rangoonwala B, Lorenz H, Verho M, Esnault VLM; High-Dose Flurosemide in Acute Renal Failure Study Group. High-dose furosemide for established ARF: a prospective, randomized, double-blind, placebo-controlled, multicenter trial. *Am J Kidney Dis.* 2004;44(3):402–409.

ICU = intensive care unit. AKI = acute kidney injury. RRT = renal replacement therapy. hANP = human atrial natriuretic peptide. DM = diabetes mellitus. CKD = chronic kidney disease. CI-AKI = contrast induced acute kidney injury. CABG = coronary artery bypass grafting. LOS = length of stay. QOL = quality of life.

Natriuretics

The atrial natriuretic peptide (ANP) and brain natriuretic peptide improve glomerular filtration by dilating the afferent arteriole and constricting the efferent arteriole. They also inhibit salt reabsorption in different segments of the tubules, block the renin–angiotensin–aldosterone system, and have anti-inflammatory as well antiapoptotic effects. All of these physiological effects of natriuretic peptides should be beneficial in AKI and have been shown to mitigate renal injury in animal models of ischemia reperfusion. However, a large multicenter trial of synthetic ANP showed no benefit in improving mortality or dialysis-free survival.[21,22] Although post hoc analysis suggested that ANP might improve dialysis free survival in oliguric patients, an RCT that enrolled 222 patients with oliguric renal failure failed to confirm these findings.[23] In another RCT, brain natriuretic peptide was associated with decreased incidence of AKI but did not decrease the incidence of 21-day mortality or need for dialysis.[24] Currently there are no data to substantiate the clinical use of natriuretics in AKI.

Loop Diuretics

Physiological studies have suggested that loop diuretics might decrease tubular reabsorption of sodium and decrease overall metabolic demand. However, a small randomized trial in 50 patients undergoing cardiac surgery randomized to saline or furosemide showed no difference in the incidence of AKI.[2] Observational studies suggest that diuretic therapy might be associated with detrimental effects. Increases in distal tubule sodium delivery induced by loop diuretics can increase the metabolic cost of sodium reabsorption and activate the renin–angiotensin–aldosterone system and sympathetic nervous system, which might negate the benefits of inhibiting salt reabsorption in the more proximal segments. Therefore, we recommend that the use of diuretics in AKI be restricted to patients with fluid overload, which is an important predictor of adverse events in critically ill patients.

Statins

Short-term statin treatment has antioxidant as well as anti-inflammatory effects and can improve endothelial dysfunction, all of which can potentially be beneficial in AKI. However, in clinical trials involving patients undergoing cardiac surgery, statins improved markers of inflammation but failed to improve incidence of or recovery from AKI.[25] RCTs have demonstrated that short-term statin therapy decreases the incidence of contrast-induced AKI.[26] However, it does not decrease mortality or the need for renal replacement therapy. This might be because most patients with contrast-induced AKI improve, and incidence of mortality and need for dialysis is low in contrast-induced AKI. On the other hand, long-term statin therapy has been associated with worsening renal function in retrospective studies. Larger RCTs are required before widespread adoption of statins to prevent AKI in clinical settings.

Growth Factors

Since recovery from AKI involves regeneration of tubular epithelial cells and studies have shown increased levels of growth factors during recovery, there has been interest in the use of growth factors to facilitate recovery from ATN. Rodent models of AKI have shown that insulin-like growth factor-1 and erythropoietin mitigate AKI in ischemia reperfusion models of AKI. However, there have been no adequately powered RCTs in humans. In a small study of 162 ICU patients considered high risk for AKI, erythropoietin did not decrease the incidence of AKI.[27] It is unclear whether animal models of ischemia recapitulate human pathology since the patterns of injury seem to be very different between rodents and humans. Moreover, the timing of drug administration in relation to injury might be important. The use of growth factors in clinical practice needs further validation.

Remote Ischemic Preconditioning

Ischemic preconditioning involves inducing short periods of hypoxia in a remote organ to make the kidneys more resistant to subsequent hypoxia. While initial single-center trials showed a clinical benefit by reducing AKI,[28,29] subsequent multicenter trials that included a sham procedure failed to show any benefit of preconditioning.[30,31]

Renal Replacement Therapy

Prophylactic dialysis has been evaluated in the setting of contrast nephropathy and certain toxins. Contrast is removed by hemodialysis or hemofiltration. A single session of dialysis removes about 60% to 90% of contrast media. However, meta-analysis of small studies in patients receiving contrast and at high risk for contrast-induced AKI have not demonstrated any improvements in incidence of AKI with dialysis.[32]

Whether hemofiltration, which removes contrast more effectively in combination with volume expansion, might have a role remains unproven.

Experimental Therapies

AKI is associated with oxidative stress and inflammation. So antioxidants such as alpha lipoid acid and selenium, as well as anti-inflammatory mediators such as sphingosine-1-phosphate analogues and dipeptidyl peptidase-4 inhibitors, are being studied for use in prevention and treatment of AKI. Small interfering RNA, which inhibits p53, is also being evaluated to affect cell cycle and tubular regeneration. However, these interventions need to be validated before therapeutic use in humans.

Prevention of Complications

The complications of AKI include volume overload, hyperkalemia, metabolic acidosis, and uremic encephalopathy.

Volume Overload

Although studies have not shown benefit from diuretics in the prevention of AKI, in the setting of volume overload, most clinicians would consider a trial of loop diuretics. In patients with AKI already on hemodialysis or hemofiltration, use of diuretics is not associated with freedom from dialysis.[33] The role of natriuretics and aquaretics remains to be proven.

Hyperkalemia

Hyperkalemia can be potentially life threatening due to its effects on the conducting system of the heart. If electrocardiogram changes are observed, telemetry and immediate administration of calcium gluconate to stabilize the membrane are essential. The onset of action is within minutes and lasts for 30 to 60 minutes. Calcium gluconate does not alter the serum potassium levels, and therapy to shift potassium intracellularly or enhance excretion must be instituted simultaneously. Insulin, in combination with glucose given to prevent hypoglycemia, will lower potassium within 20 to 30 minutes and lasts for 2 to 6 hours. In patients who are not oliguric, sodium chloride infusion along with a loop diuretic to promote kaliuresis is effective. Oligoanuric patients will likely need dialysis. Kayexalate should be avoided since it is generally ineffective and associated with potentially serious side effects. The newer ion exchange resins patiromer and sodium zirconium cyclosilicate have not yet been evaluated in AKI.

Metabolic Acidosis

AKI results in metabolic acidosis from accumulation of organic anions and impaired ammoniagenesis. Mild metabolic acidosis is of little or no consequence in the short term. Although clinical trials of sodium bicarbonate therapy in sepsis or lactic acidosis do not show any apparent benefit, these studies recruited relatively small number of participants and were underpowered. There is concern that sodium bicarbonate might worsen intracellular acidosis, hypernatremia, and volume overload. We recommend avoiding bicarbonate therapy unless the pH is below 7.2 or associated with compromised hemodynamic status or impending respiratory fatigue. In organic acidosis, particularly in younger individuals, it might be prudent to wait until the pH falls below 6.8. Severe acidosis, particularly in the setting of volume overload, often warrants dialysis.

RENAL REPLACEMENT THERAPY

Dialysis is often required to prevent or treat the secondary complications of AKI, including volume overload, acidosis, hyperkalemia and uremia. The therapeutic decisions involving renal replacement therapy include modality, timing, and dose of dialysis.[34] In the United States, the most widely used modalities for renal replacement therapy are intermittent hemodialysis and continuous renal replacement therapy (CRRT). Theoretically, CRRT is associated with improved hemodynamic stability as well as solute clearance and possibly has immunomodulatory effects due to enhanced removal of cytokines. However, RCTs comparing the efficacy of CRRT and daily or every other day hemodialysis have not found any difference in mortality or chances of renal recovery between the two.[34] The kidney is relatively resistant to ischemia, and it has been suggested that when renal injury is severe enough to result in AKI, the morbidity and mortality is unlikely to be affected by dialysis dose or modalities. Cross-over RCTs have suggested that perhaps hemodiafiltration, which is associated with better clearance of middle molecules, might be beneficial in AKI. However, this needs to be substantiated in larger RCTs, and, as such, hemodiafiltration is not yet available in the United States. In the absence of life-threatening complications such as hyperkalemia, severe acidosis, volume overload, or encephalopathy, the optimal timing for initiating renal replacement therapy remains unclear. Recently 2 large RCTs have examined the issue and come to very different conclusions. The Early Versus Late Initiation of Renal Replacement Therapy in Critically Ill Patients with Acute Kidney Injury (ELAIN) trial[35] was a single-center trial that compared early (renal replacement therapy started within 8 hours of established stage 2 AKI) with late dialysis (renal replacement therapy started soon after an absolute indication for dialysis or within 12 hours of stage 3 AKI) in predominantly surgical patients. Early dialysis was associated with a 15% reduction in 90-day mortality and recovery of renal function compared with delayed dialysis. However, the relatively large improvement in mortality observed because of modest 21-hour delay in initiation of dialysis between groups seemed rather remarkable. The Artificial Kidney Initiation in Kidney Injury (AKIKI) trial[36] was a multicenter trial that included 620 critically ill patients with stage 3 AKI who were receiving mechanical ventilation and/or vasopressors. The study found no difference in outcomes despite a difference of 57 hours between those assigned to early or late dialysis. Interestingly, half the patients in the delayed arm did not require dialysis and had a lower incidence of catheter-related bloodstream infection compared with the early strategy. These 2 studies had significant differences, including the patient population, the protocol for volume expansion, and the stage of AKI studied. The conclusions derived in one population might not be applicable to another. The dose of dialysis delivered in AKI is difficult to quantify because of the altered generation and volume of distribution of urea and creatinine. Intensified dialysis regimens targeting a Kt/V >3.9 have not shown differences in renal recovery or mortality.[37] While small single-center trials suggested a possible benefit of intensified hemofiltration, 2 large multicenter trials both showed effluent volumes of 20 to 25 mL/kg/hour gave no different results than volumes of 35 to 40 mL/kg/hour.[38] Given that CKD literature supports a Kt/V of 1.2 three times a week and that the delivered dose is often substantially less than the prescribed dose in acute settings, KDIGO[39] guidelines recommend targeting a Kt/V of 3.9 for intermittent hemodialysis and an effluent volume of 20 to 25 mL/kg/hour for CRRT.

CONCLUSION

Prevention of AKI requires risk stratification to identify individuals who are at high risk for AKI. The use of biomarkers to aid in risk stratification requires further study. Optimization of volume status and avoiding nephrotoxins are recommended for all patients. We do not recommend the routine use of dopamine, natriuretic peptides, statins, or growth factors. There is no role for prophylactic dialysis, and the optimal timing for initiation of renal replacement therapy remains controversial.

REFERENCES

1. Mehta RL, Kellum JA, Shah SV, et al. Acute Kidney Injury Network: report of an initiative to improve outcomes in acute kidney injury. *Crit Care*. 2007;11(2):R31.
2. Mahesh B, Yim B, Robson D, Pillai R, Ratnatunga C, Pigott D. Does furosemide prevent renal dysfunction in high-risk cardiac surgical patients? Results of a double-blinded prospective randomised trial. *Eur J Cardio-Thorac*. 2008;33(3):370–376.
3. Ralib AM, Pickering JW, Shaw GM, Endre ZH. The urine output definition of acute kidney injury is too liberal. *Crit Care*. 2013;17(3).
4. Shipley RE, Study RS. Changes in renal blood flow, extraction of inulin, glomerular filtration rate, tissue pressure and urine flow with acute alterations of renal artery blood pressure. *Am J Physiol*. 1951;167(3):676–688.
5. Abuelo JG. Normotensive ischemic acute renal failure. *N Engl J Med*. 2007;357(8):797–805.
6. Bonventre JV, Yang L. Cellular pathophysiology of ischemic acute kidney injury. *J Clin Invest*. 2011;121(11):4210–4221.
7. Chawla LS, Davison DL, Brasha-Mitchell E, et al. Development and standardization of a furosemide stress test to predict the severity of acute kidney injury. *Crit Care*. 2013;17(5):R207.
8. Mishra J, Ma Q, Prada A, et al. Identification of neutrophil gelatinase-associated lipocalin as a novel early urinary biomarker for ischemic renal injury. *J Am Soc Nephrol*. 2003;14(10):2534–2543.
9. Mishra J, Dent C, Tarabishi R, et al. Neutrophil gelatinase-associated lipocalin (NGAL) as a biomarker for acute renal injury after cardiac surgery. *Lancet*. 2005;365(9466):1231–1238.
10. Martensson J, Bellomo R. The rise and fall of NGAL in acute kidney injury. *Blood Purificat*. 2014;37(4):304–310.
11. Brienza N, Giglio MT, Marucci M, Fiore T. Does perioperative hemodynamic optimization protect

renal function in surgical patients? A meta-analytic study. *Crit Care Med*. 2009;37(6):2079–2090.

12. Finfer S, Bellomo R, Boyce N, et al. A comparison of albumin and saline for fluid resuscitation in the intensive care unit. *N Engl J Med*. 2004;350(22):2247–2256.

13. Bouchard J, Soroko SB, Chertow GM, et al. Fluid accumulation, survival and recovery of kidney function in critically ill patients with acute kidney injury. *Kidney Int*. 2009;76(4):422–427.

14. Wiedemann HP, Wheeler AP, Bernard GR,et al.; The National Heart, Lung, and Blood Institute Acute Respiratory Distress Syndrome (ARDS) Clinical Trials Network. Comparison of two fluid-management strategies in acute lung injury. *N Engl J Med*. 2006;354(24):2564–2575.

15. Martin C, Papazian L, Perrin G, Saux P, Gouin F. Norepinephrine or dopamine for the treatment of hyperdynamic septic shock? *Chest*. 1993;103(6):1826–1831.

16. Martin C, Viviand X, Leone M, Thirion X. Effect of norepinephrine on the outcome of septic shock. *Crit Care Med*. 2000;28(8):2758–2765.

17. Rhodes A, Evans LE, Alhazzani W, et al. Surviving sepsis campaign: international guidelines for management of sepsis and septic shock: 2016. *Intensive Care Med*. 2017;43(3):304–377.

18. De Backer D, Biston P, Devriendt J, et al. Comparison of dopamine and norepinephrine in the treatment of shock. *N Engl J Med*. 2010;362(9):779–789.

19. Asfar P, Meziani F, Hamel JF, et al. High versus low blood-pressure target in patients with septic shock. *N Engl J Med*. 2014;370(17):1583–1593.

20. Bove T, Zangrillo A, Guarracino F, et al. Effect of fenoldopam on use of renal replacement therapy among patients with acute kidney injury after cardiac surgery a randomized clinical trial. *J Am Med Assoc*. 2014;312(21):2244–2253.

21. Sward K, Valsson F, Odencrants P, Samuelsson O, Ricksten SE. Recombinant human atrial natriuretic peptide in ischemic acute renal failure: a randomized placebo-controlled trial. *Crit Care Med*. 2004;32(6):1310–1315.

22. Allgren RL, Marbury TC, Rahman SN, et al. Anaritide in acute tubular necrosis. Auriculin Anaritide Acute Renal Failure Study Group. *N Engl J Med*. 1997;336(12):828–834.

23. Lewis J, Salem MM, Chertow GM, et al.; Anaritide Acute Renal Failure Study Group. Atrial natriuretic factor in oliguric acute renal failure. *Am J Kidney Dis*. 2000;36(4):767–774.

24. Ejaz AA, Martin TD, Johnson RJ, et al. Prophylactic nesiritide does not prevent dialysis or all-cause mortality in patients undergoing high-risk cardiac surgery. *J Thorac Cardiov Sur*. 2009;138(4):959–964.

25. Chello M, Patti G, Candura D, et al. Effects of atorvastatin on systemic inflammatory response after coronary bypass surgery. *Crit Care Med*. 2006;34(3):660–667.

26. Han Y, Zhu G, Han L, et al. Short-term rosuvastatin therapy for prevention of contrast-induced acute kidney injury in patients with diabetes and chronic kidney disease. *J Am Coll Cardiol*. 2014;63(1):62–70.

27. Endre ZH, Walker RJ, Pickering JW, et al. Early intervention with erythropoietin does not affect the outcome of acute kidney injury (the EARLYARF trial). *Kidney Int*. 2010;77(11):1020–1030.

28. Thielmann M, Kottenberg E, Kleinbongard P, et al. Cardioprotective and prognostic effects of remote ischaemic preconditioning in patients undergoing coronary artery bypass surgery: a single-centre randomised, double-blind, controlled trial. *Lancet*. 2013;382(9892):597–604.

29. Zarbock A, Schmidt C, Van Aken H, et al. Effect of remote ischemic preconditioning on kidney injury among high-risk patients undergoing cardiac surgery a randomized clinical trial. *J Am Med Assoc*. 2015;313(21):2133–2141.

30. Meybohm P, Bein B, Brosteanu O, et al. A multicenter trial of remote ischemic preconditioning for heart surgery. *N Engl J Med*. 2015;373(15):1397–1407.

31. Hausenloy DJ, Candilio L, Evans R, et al. Remote ischemic preconditioning and outcomes of cardiac surgery. *N Engl J Med*. 2015;373(15):1408–1417.

32. Cruz DN, Goh CY, Marenzi G, Corradi V, Ronco C, Perazella MA. Renal replacement therapies for prevention of radiocontrast-induced nephropathy: a systematic review. *Am J Med*. 2012;125(1):66–78 e63.

33. Cantarovich F, Rangoonwala B, Lorenz H, Verho M, Esnault VLM; High-Dose Flurosemide in Acute Renal Failure Study Group. High-dose furosemide for established ARF: a prospective, randomized, double-blind, placebo-controlled, multicenter trial. *Am J Kidney Dis*. 2004;44(3):402–409.

34. Pannu N, Klarenbach S, Wiebe N, Manns B, Tonelli M; Alberta Kidney Disease Network. Renal replacement therapy in patients with acute renal failure: a systematic review. *J Am Med Assoc*. 2008;299(7):793–805.

35. Zarbock A, Kellum JA, Schmidt C, et al. Effect of early vs delayed initiation of renal replacement therapy on mortality in critically ill patients with acute kidney injury: The ELAIN randomized clinical trial. *J Am Med Assoc*. 2016;315(20):2190–2199.

36. Gaudry S, Hajage D, Schortgen F, et al. Initiation strategies for renal-replacement therapy in the intensive care unit. *N Engl J Med.* 2016;375(2):122–133.

37. Network VNARFT, Palevsky PM, Zhang JH, et al. Intensity of renal support in critically ill patients with acute kidney injury. *N Engl J Med.* 2008;359(1):7–20.

38. Bellomo R, Cass A, et al.; Investigators RRTS. Intensity of continuous renal-replacement therapy in critically ill patients. *N Engl J Med.* 2009;361(17):1627–1638.

39. National Kidney Foundation. KDOQI clinical practice guideline for hemodialysis adequacy: 2015 update. *Am J Kidney Dis.* 2015;66(5):884–930.

12

Slowing Progression of Chronic Kidney Disease

MARTINE POLLACK-ZOLLMAN AND JOSEPH A. VASSALOTTI

INTRODUCTION

The definition of chronic kidney disease (CKD) progression and related conceptual terms is shown in Table 12.1. In general, progression reflects loss of kidney function below the normal threshold of 60 mL/min/1.73m². Progression may also be assessed using other surrogate markers for specific CKD etiologies. Examples include increases in albuminuria/proteinuria, fibrosis or glomerulosclerosis on biopsy for glomerular diseases, and increase in kidney cyst or overall kidney volume for autosomal dominant polycystic kidney disease (ADPKD).

Progression of CKD is defined as a change in glomerular filtration rate (GFR) stage (i.e., G3b to G4) or albuminuria category with an accompanying 25% change in GFR from baseline. A sustained decline in GFR >5 mL/min/1.73m² per year is considered rapid progression and should be followed more closely. Fluctuations in GFR are observed as a result of biologic variability, bias in serum creatinine assays, or hemodynamic changes so that small changes may not indicate true progression.

By increasing frequency of serum creatinine testing and duration of follow-up, physicians can more confidently assess and confirm progression. Extrapolation of data for risk of end stage renal disease (ESRD) can be performed with >4 measurements over 3 years of data when decline is linear.[1] The cause of CKD should be determined since this may also help predict progression; for example, focal segmental glomerulosclerosis generally progresses more rapidly than ADPKD. Distinguishing rapid progression from acute kidney injury (AKI) may be challenging clinically for outpatients with infrequent serum creatinine monitoring. Patients with CKD should be monitored based on their CKD risk (Fig. 12.1).

PREDICTORS OF PROGRESSION

The following risk factors have been associated with CKD progression: cause of CKD, level of GFR, albuminuria, age, sex, race/ethnicity, elevated blood pressure (BP), hyperglycemia, dyslipidemia, smoking, obesity, cardiovascular disease (CVD), and ongoing exposure to nephrotoxic agents.

The individual course of CKD progression and complications are very heterogeneous and can be difficult to predict.[2] In an ongoing prospective trial of 1,741 patients with stage 3 CKD in the United Kingdom, Shardlow et al.[3] found a majority of patients with CKD stage G3a category A1 or no significant albuminuria were unlikely to progress to ESRD or death.

The 4-variable Kidney Failure Risk Equation by Tangri et al.[4] (http://kidneyfailurerisk.com/) is an externally validated publicly available tool that can help predict kidney failure in patients with CKD stages G3 to G5 at 2 and 5 years, using estimated GFR (eGFR), urine albumin–creatinine ratio (ACR), age, and gender. This relatively new prediction tool is not widely accepted in clinical practice. Some kidney failure risk thresholds have been proposed on the basis of physician surveys and decision analyses (>3 or 5% risk at 5 years for nephrology referral, >20 or 40% risk at 2 years for hemodialysis vascular access planning) and should be evaluated further in cluster randomized trials.

Currently, the best markers of progression are albuminuria and eGFR using the CKD-EPI creatinine equation, which is more accurate and less biased than the Modification of Diet in Renal Disease study creatinine-based equation compared to the gold-standard measured GFR.[5] The CKD-EPI equations, which were validated across a wider spectrum of kidney function than

TABLE 12.1 CKD PROGRESSION AND RELATED TERMS

Condition	Comment
Normal aging	Normal loss of GFR in the range of 0.5-1 mL/min/1.73 m² per year that begins at approximately age 50 years in epidemiologic studies.
CKD incidence	Onset of eGFR less than 60 mL/min/1.73 m²
CKD progression	A drop in GFR category accompanied by a >25% or greater drop in eGFR from baseline.
Rapid CKD progression	A sustained decline in GFR >5 mL/min/1.73 m² per year.
Acute kidney injury	Increase in serum creatinine by 0.3 mg/dL or more within 48 hours.

GFR = glomerular filtration rate. eGFR = estimated glomerular filtration rate. CKD = chronic kidney disease.

CKD is classified based on: • Cause (C) • GFR (G) • Albuminuria (A)				Albuminuria categories Description and range		
				A1	A2	A3
				Normal to mildly increased	Moderately increased	Severely increased
				<30 mg/g <3 mg/mmol	30–299 mg/g 3–29 mg/mmol	≥300 mg/g ≥30 mg/mmol
GFR categories (ml/min/1.73m²) Description and range	G1	Normal or high	≥90	1 if CKD	Treat 1	Refer* 2
	G2	Mildly decreased	60–89	1 if CKD	Treat 1	Refer* 2
	G3a	Mildly to moderately decreased	45–59	Treat 1	Treat 2	Refer 3
	G3b	Moderately to severely decreased	30–44	Treat 2	Treat 3	Refer 3
	G4	Severely decreased	15–29	Refer* 3	Refer* 3	Refer 4+
	G5	Kidney failure	<15	Refer 4+	Refer 4+	Refer 4+

FIGURE 12.1 Risk of chronic kidney disease progression, frequency of visits, and referral to nephrology according to estimated glomerular filtration rate (eGFR) and albuminuria. The glomerular filtration rate (GFR) and albuminuria grid depict the risk of progression, morbidity, and mortality by color, from best to worst (green, yellow, orange, red, deep red). The numbers in the boxes are a guide to the frequency of visits (number of times per year). Green can reflect CKD with normal eGFR and albumin-to-creatinine ratio (ACR) only in the presence of other markers of kidney damage, such as imaging showing polycystic kidney disease or kidney biopsy abnormalities, with follow-up measurements annually; yellow requires caution and measurements at least once per year; orange requires measurements twice per year; red and deep red require measurements at 3 and 4 times per year, respectively. These are general parameters only, based on expert opinion, and must take into account underlying comorbid conditions and disease state, as well as the likelihood of impacting a change in management for any individual patient. "Refer" indicates nephrology services are recommended.

'Referring clinicians may wish to discuss with their nephrology service, depending on local arrangements regarding treating or referring.

the older MDRD equation, also includes equations that use serum cystatin C alone or both serum cystatin C and creatinine. The identification of additional biomarkers of CKD progression is an area of vigorous investigation.

PATHOGENESIS

A final common pathway leads to significant nephron loss and damage for most proteinuric causes of CKD. Initially, there is adaptive or compensatory hyperfiltration. This leads to activation of renin–angiotensin–aldosterone system (RAAS) and increased glomerular permeability that causes proteinuria. These microinflammatory and nephrotoxic perturbations culminate in remodeling and scarring that cause secondary focal segmental glomerulosclerosis morphology, tubulointerstitial fibrosis, and progressive CKD. Unfortunately, no intervention has been shown to be safe and efficacious in reversing fibrosis.

TREATMENT—SLOWING CKD PROGRESSION

The main aims of treating CKD are to prevent progression and prevent CKD complications (see Fig. 12.2). There are often modifiable secondary factors of CKD that when treated can improve CVD risk, bone health, development of ESRD, morbidity, and mortality. The main areas of intervention are healthy lifestyle choices, BP and glycemic control, use of RAAS blockers, correction of metabolic acidosis, identifying potentially reversible causes, and preventing AKI. Determining the cause of CKD is also important to distinguish primary glomerular diseases in which reduction in progression may be achieved with immunosuppressive therapy that is beyond the scope of this chapter.

Proteinuria

Attenuating proteinuria slows CKD progression mainly by RAAS blockade with the use of angiotensin converting enzyme inhibitors (ACEI) or angiotensin receptor blockers (ARB). Patients with proteinuric CKD have slower loss of eGFR and improved albuminuria with RAAS blockade versus placebo when hypertension is present, independent of BP control in several trials.[6–8] There is limited evidence to support use of ACEI or ARB in the absence of hypertension for proteinuria attenuation.

Besides improving BP, attenuation of proteinuria occurs with the decrease in intraglomerular pressure that is achieved with RAAS blockade compared to other classes of antihypertensives. ACEI/ARB may also have antifibrotic effects[9] and increase nephrin, which improves glomerular selectivity.[10,11]

The decreased intraglomerular pressure results in an expected short-term decrease in GFR with the initiation of ACEI/ARB. Typically, a 30% decrease in GFR or less over 3 months is acceptable after initiating RAAS blockade. The risks of ACEI and/or ARB include AKI (especially with hypovolemia or bilateral renal artery stenosis) and hyperkalemia.

Theoretically, dual RAAS blockade with ACEI and ARB would more completely block RAAS

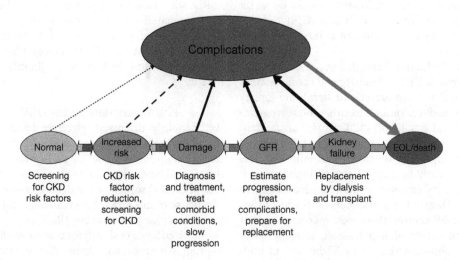

FIGURE 12.2 Conceptual model for chronic kidney disease development and progression with areas of intervention along the continuum of disease. GFR = glomerular filtration rate. EOL = end of life.

and decrease proteinuria more efficiently, leading to a slower decline in GFR. Unfortunately, the proteinuria attenuation with dual blockade is also associated with increased risk of AKI, and hyperkalemia as seen in the VA-NEPHRON-D[12], ALTITUDE[13] and ON-TARGET[14] trials.

Hypertension

Hypertension is an independent risk factor for progression to ESRD[15] and CVD. RAAS inhibition is both an anti-hypertensive and reno-protective class of drugs, as previously discussed. Diuretics are used concomitantly with ACEI/ARBs to decrease extracellular volume and further activate the RAAS.

The KDIGO hypertension guidelines[16] recommend a BP goal of <140/90 mmHg for nonproteinuric patients with CKD with or without diabetes (grade 1B) and goal BP <130/80 mmHg for patients with CKD and ACR >30 mg/g (grade 2). There is strong evidence to recommend use of an ACEI/ARB for A3 albuminuria (grade 1B) in all patients with hypertension. Based on the guidelines, use of ACEI/ARB is suggested to be beneficial for A3 albuminuria (grade 2D), though more controversial. The guidelines do not recommend specific first-line BP lowering medications for nonproteinuric patients with CKD and hypertension and should be at the discretion of the clinician based on other clinical factors.

Recently there has been a debate on the optimal BP target for patients with hypertension with and without CKD, proteinuria, and/or diabetes. The JNC-8 consensus panel[17] recommends patients with CKD and diabetes have a target BP <140/90 mmHg (grade E), and ACEI or ARB should be first-line treatment in those with CKD (grade B).

The Sprint trial[18] enrolled over 9,000 patients with systolic BP >130 mmHg and cardiovascular (CV) risk without diabetes or significant kidney disease and randomized to either intensive treatment (goal systolic BP <120 mmHg) or standard care (systolic BP <140 mmHg). The trial, focused on cardiovascular outcomes and mortality, was stopped early because of overall lower rates of the primary outcome in the intensive treatment group. Despite the overall beneficial effect of intensive BP control, there were increased serious adverse events of hypotension, syncope, electrolyte abnormalities, and AKI but not of injurious falls in the intensive treatment group. The overall number of renal events were small in both

groups and thus not well powered to assess renal outcomes. They found no significant difference in patients with CKD at baseline who progressed to ESRD and a higher proportion of patients in the intensive group without CKD at baseline experienced progression (eGFR <60 mL/min/1.73 m^2 and decrease in eGFR by 30%). Longer randomized controlled trials (RCTs) powered to determine renal outcomes are needed.

Hyperglycemia/Diabetes Mellitus
Treatment Targets

Diabetic kidney disease (DKD) is the leading cause of CKD and ESRD in the developed world and is a significant CVD risk factor. Genetic and environmental factors play a role in the development of DKD since only about one-third of patients with diabetes develop DKD. The mechanism of DKD involves hyperglycemia, activation of RAAS leading to glomerular hyperfiltration and hypertension (vasoconstriction of the efferent arteriole), inflammation from cytokines and oxidative stress, and fibrosis. Though the mainstay of treatment is glycemic control (hemoglobin A1c [HbA1c] target 7%) and use of RAAS blockade, significant renal outcomes (doubling of serum creatinine, ESRD, death) were not improved in the intensive glycemic control group compared to placebo in a 2012 meta-analysis of 7 different trials[19] and intensive glycemic control increased cardiac mortality in patients with high-risk CVD and type 2 diabetes mellitus, as seen in the ACCORD trial.[20] However, subsequently published kidney outcomes from the ADVANCE group[21] revealed a significant 65% reduction in ESRD with intensive glycemic control HbA1c 6.5% compared to standard control HbA1c 7.3%. The number of patients needed to treat over 5 years to prevent 1 ESRD event ranged from 410 in the overall study to 41 with A3 albuminuria at baseline.

Pharmacotherapy for DKD

As previously discussed, glycemic control and RAAS blockade for A3 proteinuria are the main treatment options for DKD. Based on large RCT, dual RAAS blockade is not recommended due to lack of clinical superiority with an increased risk of adverse events (AKI, hyperkalemia, and need for renal replacement therapy [RRT]).

Elevated levels of aldosterone have been linked to progressive renal and cardiac disease as well as inflammation and fibrosis. There is also a concept of "aldosterone escape," which occurs in 30% to

50% of patients within a year of RAAS blocker initiation. A systematic review in 2008 by Bomback et al.[22] suggests blocking the mineral corticoid receptor in addition to RAAS-inhibition therapy attenuates proteinuria in CKD. A 3-arm small RCT in 2009 randomized 81 patients with DM, hypertension, and ACR >300 mg/g already on Lisinopril 80 mg daily to spironolactone 25 mg daily versus losartan 100 mg daily versus placebo for 48 weeks. At the end of the trial, the spironolactone group had a significant 34% reduction in ACR (95% confidence interval [CI]: −51.0%, −11.2%, P = 0.007) compared to placebo. The reduction of proteinuria in the losartan versus placebo group was not significant, 16.8% (95% CI, −37.3%, +10.5%, p = 0.20). The BP and eGFR were not different across the groups, although there was more hyperkalemia in the spironolactone and losartan arms compared to placebo.[23] There is an ongoing larger Figaro-CKD RCT[24] investigating finerenone.

Sodium-glucose transport proteins 2 (SGLT2) are located exclusively in the proximal tubules where they increase sodium-glucose reabsorption, especially in hyperglycemic states in which they are upregulated. By inhibiting the SGLT2, glycosuria ensues with a proposed restoration of tubuloglomerular feedback as a result of increased sodium reaching the macula densa. This leads to afferent arteriole constriction, decreased intraglomerular pressures and improvement in albuminuria. Through these 2 putative mechanisms, these drugs confer both cardiac and renal protection. The EMPA-REG OUTCOME group[25] showed a significant reduction in the composite cardiovascular outcome and, in secondary prespecified analyses, significant renal protection for 7,020 patients with type 2 diabetes mellitus and established CVD treated with 10 or 25 mg empagliflozin compared to the standard of care. Another RCT, published in 2017 by Heerspink et al.,[26] found that 1,450 patients with type 2 diabetes mellitus on metformin randomized to 100 or 300 mg canagliflozin daily had a slower decline in eGFR decline and improved albuminuria compared to glimepiride daily. Importantly, these agents are not recommended by the US Food and Drug Administration (FDA) for low eGFR: canagliflozin <45, dapagliflozin <60, and empagliflozin <45 (all in mL/min/1.73m²). The FDA has a black box warning for this class of medications including risk of diabetic ketoacidosis and AKI and increased risk of urinary tract infections with urosepsis and genitourinary yeast infections. Increased risk of AKI and diabetic ketoacidosis was not seen in the EMPA-REG OUTCOME trials. See Table 12.2 for a chart of past and ongoing RCTs for DKD.

Polycystic Kidney Disease

ADPKD is the most commonly inherited form of kidney disease and the fourth leading cause of ESRD globally. Typically, patients with ADPKD progress to CKD, hypertension, ESRD, and death. Lower BP targets with RAAS blockade plus possibly use of vasopressin 2-receptor inhibitors and increased water intake to decrease ADH stimulation are all therapeutic targets to decrease progression.[27–30]

Managing CKD Metabolic Acidosis

Metabolic acidosis is a complication of CKD. Prior experimental models and observational studies have shown that decreased serum bicarbonate is a risk factor for CKD progression and current guidelines recommend serum bicarbonate levels between 24 and 26 meq/L and to begin treatment for levels <22 meq/L. In an interventional study, De Brito et al.[31] found that bicarbonate therapy compared to placebo in 134 patients from the United Kingdom with CKD stage 4 and serum bicarbonate 16 to 20 meq/L delayed the rate of progression to ESRD and improved nutritional status. The observational longitudinal Chronic Renal Insufficiency Cohort (CRIC) study[32] of 3,939 patients with CKD stages 2 to 4 showed the composite renal end point (ESRD or 50% decrease in GFR) was 3% lower per 1 mEq/L increase in serum bicarbonate, although the risk of heart failure increased by 14% by every 1 mEq/L increase in serum bicarbonate level over 24 mEq/L. The serum bicarbonate level was not associated independently with atherosclerotic events or death in the adjusted models, including diuretic use. The investigators excluded patients with New York Heart Association classes III and IV heart failure, which can both lead to metabolic alkalosis, primary and compensatory, respectively.

Hyperuricemia With or Without Gout

CKD is a risk factor for hyperuricemia and gout; hyperuricemia is a putative risk factor for incident CKD, yet interventional data are controversial and lacking. Many patients with gout have urate crystal nephropathy, which is crystal deposition in the interstitium or collecting tubules that can lead to nephrolithiasis, obstruction of

TABLE 12.2 PAST AND ONGOING CLINICAL TRIALS FOR DIABETIC KIDNEY DISEASE

Trial	Drug	Mechanism of Action	Outcome Measured
ASCEND[a] Terminated early due to adverse safety concerns n = 1,392	Avosentan	ET_A receptor antagonist	Composite of death, ESRD, or doubling of Cr NS; significantly increased risk of CHF compared to placebo (6.1% vs 2.2%, $p = 0.05$) and trend toward increased death.
Pirfenidone for Diabetic Nephropathy[b] n = 77	Pirfenidone	Inhibits TGFβ and TNF-α	Change in eGFR from baseline over 12 months; mean eGFR was improved in the 1,200 mg/d group compared to the placebo group (+3.3±8.5 mL/min per 1.73 m² vs. −2.2±4.8 mL/min per 1.73 m²; $p = 0.026$); higher dose was NS compared to placebo with higher drop-out rate.
ALTITUDE[c] n = 8,561 Terminated early due to adverse safety concerns	Aliskiren + ACEI or ARB	Direct renin inhibition + classic RAS blockade	Composite of CV death, MI, CVA, and unplanned hospitalization for heart failure; ESRD or doubling of the baseline serum Cr level NS. Increased risk of hyperkalemia (11.2% vs. 7.2%, $p < 0.001$) and reported hypotension (12.1% vs. 8.3%, $p < 0.001$).
BEACON[d] n = 2,185 Terminated early due to adverse safety concerns	Bardoxolone	Activates the nuclear factor-related factor2 (Nrf2) pathway	Composite of ESRD or cardiovascular death NS; HR 1.83; 95% CI, 1.32 to 2.55; $p < 0.001$ for hospitalization for heart failure or death from heart failure in intervention group compared to placebo.
VA-NEPHRON-D[e] n = 1,448 Terminated early due to adverse safety concerns	Losartan + Lisinopril	Dual RAS Blockade	Time to first occurrence of primary end points: change in eGFR, ESRD, or death, NS. Increased risk of hyperkalemia (6.3 events per 100 person-years vs. 2.6 events per 100 person-years with monotherapy; $p < 0.001$) and AKI (12.2 vs. 6.7 events per 100 person-years, $p < 0.001$).
EMPA-REG OUTCOME[f] n = 7,020	Empagliflozin	SGLT2 inhibitor	Incident or worsening nephropathy occurred in (12.7% vs.18.8%) in the SGLT2 arm and placebo group, respectively (HR empagliflozin group, 0.61; 95% CI, 0.53 to 0.70; $p < 0.001$). There were significant relative risk reductions for doubling of the serum creatinine level of 44% and RRT of 55% relative risk in the empagliflozin group. The adverse-event profile of empagliflozin in patients with impaired kidney function at baseline was similar to that reported in the overall trial population.

Trial	Drug	Class	End points
CANVAS[g] n = 1,0142	Canagliflozin	SGLT2 inhibitor	Composite of primary end points: CV death, nonfatal MI, nonfatal CVA (HR 0.86; 95% CI 0.75–0.97 favoring protection with canagliflozin with p = 0.02 for superiority). Secondary renal outcomes: >30% change in albuminuria or change in A class; >40% reduction in eGFR, need for RRT, death from renal cause (HR 0.6; 95% CI, 0.47–0.77 favoring protection with canagliflozin). There was a higher risk of amputations, genital infections, and volume depletion in intervention group.
FIGARO-DKD[h] NCT02545049 Phase III, recruiting	Finerenone	Aldosterone antagonist	Composite of cardiovascular death and nonfatal cardiovascular events (MI, stroke, or hospitalization for heart failure).
SONAR[i] NCT01858532 Phase III, recruiting	Atrasentan	ET$_A$ receptor antagonist	Composite of doubling of Cr or ESRD.
CREDENCE[j] NCT02065791 Phase III, recruiting	Canagliflozin	SGLT2 inhibitor	Composite of ESRD, doubling of Cr, renal or cardiovascular death.
Dapa-CKD[k] NCT03036150 Phase III, recruiting	Dapagliflozin	SGLT2 inhibitor	First occurrence of ≥50% sustained decline in eGFR or reaching ESRD or CV death or renal death.

[a]Mann JFE, Green D, Jamerson K, et al. Avosentan for overt diabetic nephropathy. *J Am Soc Nephrol.* 2010;21:527.
[b]Sharma K, Ix JH, Mathew AV, et al. Pirfenidone for diabetic nephropathy. *J Am Soc Nephrol.* 2011;22:1144–1151.
[c]Parving HH, Brenner BM, McMurray JJV, et al.; ALTITUDE Investigators. Cardiorenal end points in a trial of aliskiren for type 2 diabetes. *N Engl J Med.* 2012;367:2204–2213.
[d]de Zeeuw D, Akizawa T, Audhya P, et al.; BEACON Trial Investigators. Bardoxolone methyl in type 2 diabetes and stage 4 chronic kidney disease. *N Engl J Med.* 2013;369(26):2492–2503.e
[e]Fried LF, Emanuele N, Zhang JH, et al.; VA NEPHRON-D Investigators. Combined angiotensin inhibition for the treatment of diabetic nephropathy. *N Engl J Med.* 2013;369(20):1892–1903.
[f]Wanner C, Inzucchi SE, Lachin JM, et al. Empagliflozin and progression of kidney disease in type 2 diabetes. *N Engl J Med.* 2016;375:323–334.
[g]Neal B, Perkovic V, Mahaffey KW, et al.; CANVAS Program Collaborative Group. Canagliflozin and cardiovascular and renal events in type 2 diabetes. *N Engl J Med.* 2017 Aug 17;377(7):644–657.
[h]Efficacy and safety of finerenone in subjects with type 2 diabetes mellitus and the clinical diagnosis of diabetic kidney disease. ClinicalTrials.gov. 2015–. https://clinicaltrials.gov/ct2/show/study/NCT02545049?term=finerenone&rank=2&show_locs=Y#locn
[i]Study of diabetic nephropathy with atrasentan. ClinicalTrials.gov. 2018. https://clinicaltrials.gov/ct2/show/NCT01858532?term=sonar&rank=2
[j]Evaluation of the effects of canagliflozin on renal and cardiovascular outcomes in participants with diabetic nephropathy. ClinicalTrials.gov. 2014–. https://clinicaltrials.gov/ct2/show/NCT02065791?term=CREDENCE&rank=2
[k]A study to evaluate the effect of dapagliflozin on renal outcomes and cardiovascular mortality in patients with chronic kidney disease. ClinicalTrials.gov. 2017–. https://clinicaltrials.gov/ct2/show/NCT03036150?term=dapa-ckd&rank=1

ESRD = Cr = creatine. CHF = chronic heart failure. TGFβ = transforming growth factor beta. TNF-α = tumor necrosis factor α. eGFR = estimated glomerular filtration rate. RAS = renin-angiotensin system. CV = cardiovascular. MI = myocardial infarction. CVA = cerebrovascular accident. ESRD = end stage renal disease. AKI = acute kidney injury. SGLT2 = sodium glucose cotransporter 2. HR = hazard ratio. CI = confidence interval. RRT = renal replacement therapy urinary flow, inflammation, and/or fibrosis with CKD progression. Urate lowering therapy with allopurinol or febuxostat may attenuate CKD progression. In a meta-analysis by Kanji et al.[33] of 992 participants in 19 RCTs, there was insufficient evidence to support the use of allopurinol to prevent ESRD and CV events, although there was a significant difference in eGFR +3.2 mL/min/1.73 m^2 and improvement in the BP and uric acid levels in the treatment groups. Further larger adequately powered RCTs are needed before routine treatment of asymptomatic hyperuricemia can be recommended.

Folic Acid Supplementation

Epidemiologic studies have shown hyperhomocysteinemia is associated with the risk of developing CKD, although interventional studies of folic acid and vitamin B supplementation in populations with folic acid diet fortification showed no significant or even harmful effects on eGFR trajectory. The Renal Substudy of the China Stroke Primary Prevention trial[34] was an RCT of enalapril with or without folic acid supplementation in a Chinese population without dietary folic acid fortification. The baseline mean folic acid levels were low 7.6 to 7.7 ng/mL and increased significantly with supplementation (+15.4 ng/mL). A 56% reduction in risk of CKD progression and a 44% slower eGFR decline was shown in the folic intervention group compared to control. The investigators speculated that the previous negative studies were the result of nephrotoxic doses of cyanocobalamin, supported by the massively supratherapeutic levels of folate achieved in study populations that were not folic acid deficient. Folic acid supplementation is a promising simple way to prevent CKD progression in developing countries without folate dietary fortification, but the findings are probably not generalizable to developed countries like the United States.

Obstructive Sleep Apnea and CKD Progression

Like CKD, obstructive sleep apnea (OSA) carries a high risk of cardiovascular morbidity and mortality and is a common cause for secondary hypertension. Hypertension, DM, and obesity are risk factors for both CKD and OSA. Epidemiological and retrospective studies have shown a link between OSA and risk of progressive CKD but there have been limited prospective trials to establish the risk of incident and progressive CKD in patients with OSA. Nocturnal hypoxia in OSA causes a catecholamine storm that leads to tubulointerstitial stress, damage and eventual fibrosis. Further, hypoxia may exacerbate renal sympathetic nerve activation, which leads to afferent vasoconstriction and reduced eGFR. There is also evidence of systemic inflammation and endothelial dysfunction in OSA that may lead to decline in eGFR. A small nonrandomized trial of 38 men with diagnosed OSA from Japan treated with continuous positive airway pressure for 3 months showed a significant improvement in serum creatinine and eGFR from baseline (creatinine 0.87 to 0.82, $p = 0.013$; eGFR 72.9 to 79.3, $p = 0.014$).[35]

CKD Complications: Anemia and CKD Mineral and Bone Disorder

Recent animal studies have shown erythropoietin stimulating agents (ESA) may confer renal survival by increasing tissue perfusion of O_2, limiting red blood cell apoptosis, and promoting anti-inflammatory effects. In a meta-analysis, Elliot et al.[36] found no improvement in CKD progression between anemic patients who received erythropoietin stimulating agents versus those who did not (relative risk 0.99, 0.88–1.11), although there was a nonsignificant trend for improvement in the transplant subpopulation with AKI.

Observational longitudinal studies demonstrated correlation with higher phosphorus levels and CKD progression, but interventional studies are lacking. Currently, management of CKD mineral and bone disorder is recommended for their efficacy on bone health outcomes, though direct vascular and nephrotoxic effects of phosphorus is plausible.[37]

Lifestyle

As previously mentioned, lifestyle modifications and other modifiable risk factors are important in preventing CKD progression and often overlooked. As recommended by KDIGO,[38] exercise in encouraged to reduce CVD risk. There is no evidence it slows eGFR decline, though exercise improved quality of life, uremia symptoms scores, achieved better BP control, less arterial stiffness, weight loss, and improved exercise tolerance.

There is a direct association with obesity and glomerular hyperfiltration or secondary focal segmental glomerulosclerosis, and an indirect CKD association through the major risk factors, hypertension, and type 2 diabetes mellitus. Several meta-analyses that show improvement in BP and proteinuria with weight loss and stabilization of eGFR, though follow-up was short.

Smoking cessation has been well established to slow CKD progression and reduce CVD risk in all patients with CKD.

RCTs of fixed-dose statin-based therapies in CKD have shown a reduced risk of primary and secondary atherosclerotic events, but no benefit has been demonstrated for all-cause mortality or slower progression of CKD.[39]

The dietary needs of patients with CKD are complex and differ at various stages of CKD and ESRD. KDIGO CKD guidelines[1] recommend involvement with a dietician/nutritionist to assist in these patients' complex needs. Dietary management of sodium, potassium, phosphorous, and protein are all important in CKD care.

Protein restriction reduces BP and albuminuria in animal models and excessive protein intake can lead to accumulation of uremic toxins in patients with advanced CKD. Severe protein restriction can lead to malnutrition in a population already at risk. Data are controversial on optimal protein intake in CKD patients. The MDRD study[40] randomized low-protein diet (0.58 g/kg/day) to usual protein diet (1.3g/kg/day) in patients with moderate CKD (eGFR 25–55 mL/min/1.73 m^2) and very low-protein diet (0.28 g/kg/day supplemented by keto amino acids compared to 0.58) in patients with advanced CKD (3–24 mL/min/1.73 m^2) did not significantly slow CKD progression in either cohort. Furthermore, in a follow-up study, patients in the very low-protein diet had increased risk of mortality. The Nurses Health study,[41] an 11-year prospective cohort study of 1,624 women showed high (nonnimal) protein intake was associated with eGFR decline in patients with CKD at baseline but not observed in patients with normal eGFR at baseline. Currently, the KDIGO guidelines[1] recommend protein restriction of 0.8 g/kg/day in patients with eGFR <30 mL/min/ 1.73 m^2 and recommend avoiding excess protein intake of >1.3 g/kg/day in patients with CKD at risk of progressing.

KDIGO and KDOQI[1,16] recommend sodium restriction <2 g/day. Patients with CKD often have impairments in sodium handling. This leads to increased BP, glomerular hyperfiltration, and albuminuria and dampens the response to RAAS blockade. These restrictions may not be applicable to patients with hypotension, salt wasting nephropathies, and prior hemodynamic AKI.

Prevention of AKI

CKD is the most important risk factor for AKI and AKI is now recognized as a risk factor for development of CKD. Patients with CKD are at higher risk of developing AKI, when admitted to the hospital, exposed to iodinated contrast, and when undergoing major surgery. The risk increases with decline in eGFR, increasing albuminuria and with comorbid hypertension or diabetes mellitus. AKI was previously conceptualized as a reversible event. A 2011 meta-analysis of patients with and without AKI found that patients with AKI had higher risks of developing CKD (hazard ratio [HR] 8.8, 95% CI: 3.1–25.5), ESRD (HR 3.1, 95% CI: 1.9–5.0) and mortality (HR 2.0, 95% CI 1.3–3.1) than patients without AKI.[42]

Prevention of hospitalization and infections and avoidance of nephrotoxins (nonsteroidal anti-inflammatory drugs, iodinated contrast) and appropriate dosing of medications based on eGFR is paramount to reduce risk of AKI. Proton pump inhibitors are associated with acute interstitial nephritis and incident and progressive CKD as well as ESRD and should be used judiciously.[43]

Hemodynamic changes also affect kidney function. Attention should be made to prevention of overdiuresis or volume contraction to prevent AKI and chronic prerenal azotemia as an additional factor for progressive CKD. Alternatively, patients with cardiorenal syndrome have a worse prognosis compared to patients with normal renal function and may benefit from more aggressive diuresis. "Sick Day Rules" is a program developed by the UK National Health System that helps guide patients to temporarily stop potentially nephrotoxic drugs (nonsteroidal anti-inflammatory drugs, ACEI/ARB, diuretics, and metformin) when ill to prevent AKI.

Referral to Specialist and RRT Planning/ Multidisciplinary Team Approach

There has been focus on earlier nephrology referrals, since an alarmingly high number of patients are started on RRT within 3 to 6 months of seeing a nephrologist and thus the inability to prevent progression to ESRD and complications of advanced CKD. Earlier referrals improve outcomes of mortality, hospitalization, eGFR decline, initiation of dialysis with an arteriovenous fistula rather than a catheter, increased use of home dialysis therapies, access to pre-emptive kidney transplant, and reduced healthcare costs.

Though most of these studies are retrospective (noninterventional trials), in a 2006 retrospective single-center study from the United Kingdom,[44] they found a significant reduction in eGFR decline from −5.4 mL/min per 1.73 m^2 per year prereferral to −0.35 mL/min per 1.73 m^2 per year, 5-years postreferral to a nephrologist. This emphasizes the importance of preventive medicine, with management of BP, proteinuria, and diabetes before CKD progresses to stage 3 and beyond. Earlier referral also allows for a multidisciplinary approach to CKD with involvement of nurse educators, social workers, dieticians, and referrals to vascular surgeons and transplant centers.

REFERENCES

1. KDIGO CKD Work Group. KDIGO 2012 clinical practice guideline for the evaluation and management of chronic kidney disease. *Kidney Int Suppl.* 2012;3:1–150.
2. Li L, Astor BC, Lewis J, et al. Longitudinal Progression Trajectory of GFR Among Patients With CKD. *Am. J. Kidney Dis.* 2012;59:504–512.
3. Shardlow A, McIntyre NJ, Fluck RJ, McIntyre CW, Taal MW. Chronic kidney disease in primary care: outcomes after five years in a prospective cohort study. *PLoS Med.* 2016;13:e1002128.
4. Tangri N, Stevens LA, Griffith J, et al. A predictive model for progression of chronic kidney disease to kidney failure. *J Am Med Assoc.* 2011;305:1553–1559.
5. Levey AS, Stevens LA, Schmid CH, et al. A New equation to estimate glomerular filtration rate. *Ann Intern Med.* 2009;150:604–612.
6. Ruggenenti P, Perna A, Loriga G, et al. Blood-pressure control for renoprotection in patients with non-diabetic chronic renal disease (REIN-2): multicentre, randomised controlled trial. *Lancet* 2005;365:939–946.
7. Ruggenenti P, Perna A, Gherardi G, Gaspari F, Benini R, Remuzzi G. Renal function and requirement for dialysis in chronic nephropathy patients on long-term ramipril: REIN follow-up trial. *Lancet* 1998;352:1252–1256.
8. Klahr S, Levey AS, Beck GJ, et al. The effects of dietary protein restriction and blood-pressure control on the progression of chronic renal disease. Modification of Diet in Renal Disease Study Group. *N Engl J Med.* 1994;330:877–884.
9. Remuzzi A, Gagliardini E, Sangalli F, et al. ACE inhibition reduces glomerulosclerosis and regenerates glomerular tissue in a model of progressive renal disease. *Kidney Int.* 2006;69: 1124–1130.
10. Ziyadeh FN, Wolf G. Pathogenesis of the podocytopathy and proteinuria in diabetic glomerulopathy. *Curr Diabetes Rev.* 2008;4:39–45.
11. Gröne EF, Gröne HJ. Does hyperlipidemia injure the kidney? *Nat Clin Pract Nephrol.* 2008;4:424–425.
12. Fried LF, Emanuele N, Zhang JH, et al. Combined angiotensin inhibition for the treatment of diabetic nephropathy. *N Engl J Med.* 2013;369(20):1892–1903.
13. Parving HH, Brenner BM, McMurray JJ, et al, Cardiorenal end points in a trial of aliskiren for type 2 diabetes. *N Engl J Med.* 2012;367:2204–2213.
14. Yusuf S, Teo KK, Pogue J, et al. ONTARGET Investigators. Telmisartan, ramipril, or both in patients at high risk for vascular events. *N Engl J Med.* 2008;358(15):1547–1559.
15. Hsu C, McCulloch CE, Darbinian J, Go AS, Iribarren C. Elevated blood pressure and risk of end-stage renal disease in subjects without baseline kidney disease. *Arch Intern Med.* 2005;165:923–928.
16. Taler SJ, Agarwal R, Bakris GL, et al. KDOQI US commentary on the 2012 KDIGO clinical practice guideline for management of blood pressure in CKD. *Am J Kidney Dis.* 2013;62:201–213.
17. James PA, Oparil S, Carter BL, et al. 2014 evidence-based guideline for the management of high blood pressure in adults: report from the panel members appointed to the Eighth Joint National Committee (JNC 8). *J Am Med Assoc.* 2014;311(5):507–520.
18. Wright JT Jr, Williamson JD, Whelton PK; SPRINT Research Group. A randomized trial of intensive versus standard blood-pressure control. *N Engl J Med.* 2015;373(22):2103–2116.
19. Coca SG, Ismail-Beigi F, Haq N, Krumholz HM, Parikh CR. Role of intensive glucose control in development of renal end points in type 2 diabetes mellitus: systematic review and meta-analysis intensive glucose control in type 2 diabetes. *Arch Intern Med.* 2012;172(10):761–769.
20. Action to Control Cardiovascular Risk in Diabetes Study Group, Gerstein HC, Miller ME, et al. Effects of Intensive Glucose Lowering in Type 2 Diabetes. *N Engl J Med.* 2008;358(24): 2545–2559.
21. Patel A, MacMahon S, Chalmers J; ADVANCE Collaborative Group. Intensive blood glucose control and vascular outcomes in patients with type 2 diabetes. *N Engl J Med.* 2008;358:2560–2572.
22. Bomback AS, Kshirsagar AV, Amamoo MA, Klemmer PJ. Change in proteinuria after adding aldosterone blockers to ACE inhibitors or angiotensin receptor blockers in CKD: a systematic review. *Am J Kidney Dis.* 2008;51(2):199–211.

23. Mehdi UF, Adams-Huet B, Raskin P, Vega GL, Toto RD. Addition of angiotensin receptor blockade or mineralocorticoid antagonism to maximal angiotensin-converting enzyme inhibition in diabetic nephropathy. *J Am Soc Nephrol.* 2009;20(12):2641–2650.

24. ClinicalTrials.gov Identifier: NCT02545049.

25. Wanner C, Inzucchi SE, Lachin JM, et al. Empagliflozin and progression of kidney disease in type 2 diabetes. *N Engl J Med.* 2016;375:323–334.

26. Heerspink HJL, Desai M, Jardine M, Balis D, Meininger G, Perkovic V. Canagliflozin Slows Progression of Renal Function Decline Independently of Glycemic Effects. *J Am Soc Nephrol.* 2017;28(1):368–375.

27. Schrier RW, Abebe KZ, Perrone RD, et al.; HALT-PKD Trial Investigators. Blood pressure in early autosomal dominant polycystic kidney disease. *N Engl J Med.* 2014; 371:2255–2266.

28. Torres VE, Abebe KZ, Chapman AB, et al.; HALT-PKD Trial Investigators. Angiotensin blockade in late autosomal dominant polycystic kidney disease. *N Engl J Med.* 2014;371:2267–2276.

29. Torres VE, Chapman AB, Devuyst O, et al. Tolvaptan in patients with autosomal dominant polycystic kidney disease. *N Engl J Med.* 2012;367:2407–2418.

30. Barash I, Ponda MP, Goldfarb DS, Skolnik EY. A pilot clinical study to evaluate changes in urine osmolality and urine camp in response to acute and chronic water loading in autosomal dominant polycystic kidney disease. *Clin J Am Soc Nephrol.* 2010;5:693–697.

31. de Brito-Ashurst I, Varagunam M, Raftery MJ, Yaqoob MM. Bicarbonate supplementation slows progression of CKD and improves nutritional status. *J Am Soc Nephrol.* 2009;20:2075–2084.

32. Dobre M, Yang W, Chen J, et al. Association of serum bicarbonate with risk of renal and cardiovascular outcomes in CKD: a report from the Chronic Renal Insufficiency Cohort (CRIC) study. *Am J Kidney Dis.* 2013;62:670–678.

33. Kanji T, Gandhi M, Clase CM, Yang R. Urate lowering therapy to improve renal outcomes in patients with chronic kidney disease: systematic review and meta-analysis. *BMC Nephrol.* 2015;16:58.

34. Xu X, Qin X, Li Y, et al. Efficacy of folic acid therapy on the progression of chronic kidney disease: the renal substudy of the China Stroke Primary Prevention Trial. *JAMA-Intern Med.* 2016;176(10):1443–1450.

35. Koga S, Ikeda S, Yasunaga T, Nakata T, Maemura K. Effects of nasal continuous positive airway pressure on the glomerular filtration rate in patients with obstructive sleep apnea syndrome.—PubMed—NCBI. *Intern Med.* 2013;52(3):345–349.

36. Elliott S, Tomita D, Endre Z. Erythropoiesis stimulating agents and reno-protection: a meta-analysis. *BMC Nephrol.* 2017;18,14.

37. Nadkarni GN, Uribarri J. Phosphorus and the kidney: what is known and what is needed. *Adv Nutr Int Rev J.* 2014;5:98–103.

38. Chapter 2: Lifestyle and pharmacological treatments for lowering blood pressure in CKD ND patients. *Kidney Int Suppl.* 2012;2(5):347–356.

39. Baigent C, Landray MJ, Reith C, et al.; SHARP Investigators. The effects of lowering LDL cholesterol with simvastatin plus ezetimibe in patients with chronic kidney disease (Study of Heart and Renal Protection): a randomised placebo-controlled trial. *Lancet.* 2011;377(9784):2181–2192.

40. Klahr S, Levey AS, Beck GJ, et al. The effects of dietary protein restriction and blood-pressure control on the progression of chronic renal disease. Modification of diet in renal disease study group. *N Engl J Med.* 1994;330:877–884.

41. Lin J, Fung TT, Hu FB, et al. Association of dietary patterns with albuminuria and kidney function decline in older white women: a subgroup analysis from the Nurses' Health Study. *Am J Kidney Dis.* 2011;57:245–254.

42. Coca SG, Singanamala S, Parikh CR. Chronic kidney disease after acute kidney injury: a systematic review and meta-analysis. *Kidney Int.* 2012;81:442–448.

43. Xie Y, Bowe B, Li T, Xian H, Balasubramanian S, Al-Aly Z. Proton pump inhibitors and risk of incident CKD and progression to ESRD. *J Am Soc Nephrol.* 2016;27(10):3153–3163.

44. Jones C, Roderick P, Harris S, Rogerson, M. Decline in kidney function before and after nephrology referral and the effect on survival in moderate to advanced chronic kidney disease. *Nephrol Dial Transpl.* 2006;21:2133–2143.

13

Renal Artery Stenosis and Revascularization

JOSEPH A. MESSANA AND RAYMOND R. TOWNSEND

INTRODUCTION

Renovascular hypertension refers to an increase in systemic arterial pressure secondary to reduced renal perfusion, usually the result of obstructing renovascular disease. Although renovascular disease is relatively common, a translesional gradient of 10 to 20 mmHg or more is required to stimulate renin secretion, which is a major mediator of the systemic hypertension.[1] Through augmentation of the renin–angiotensin–aldosterone system (RAAS) the kidneys adapt, to a degree, to impaired blood flow by the increase in perfusion pressure. Eventually, stenoses advance to a point where autoregulation fails to compensate reduced renal perfusion, leading to progressive ischemia.[2] The mechanisms of renin-related increases in blood pressure began with the work of Harry Goldblatt[3] who increased blood pressure by placing clips on 1, or both, of the renal arteries of dogs.

Two Kidney 1 Clip

This models human unilateral renal artery stenosis. The clipped kidney secretes renin, which initiates the cascade ending in angiotensin II production and secondary aldosterone stimulation. The contralateral, unclipped kidney experiences elevated pressures due to the effects of RAAS activation generated by the stenotic kidney. The increased perfusion pressure to the unclipped kidney results in a pressure natriuresis with suppression of renin release from the unclipped kidney. This response contracts the blood volume and promotes further renin release from the stenotic kidney in a vicious cycle, and the blood pressure elevation in this instance remains dependent on RAAS activation. In the 2-kidney 1-clip model, renal injury from RAAS system upregulation produces proinflammatory mediators such as vasoconstrictor prostaglandins, nuclear factor kappa B (NF-κB), and profibrotic transforming growth factor beta (TGF-β)[4] and decreases endothelial progenitor cells (EPCs). The 2-kidney 1-clip model responds to RAAS blockade with an angiotensin-converting enzyme inhibitor (ACEI) or an angiotensin receptor blocker (ARB).

One Kidney 1 Clip

This models human bilateral renal artery stenosis or renal artery stenosis in a transplanted kidney. Unlike unilateral disease, when the entire kidney is downstream of a blood flow reducing stenosis, there is impaired natriuresis and an increase in blood volume results with renin activities that return to normal, or low normal, commensurate with the volume increase.

The 1-kidney 1-clip is less responsive to these medications, unless a diuretic is used. When a diuretic is employed, it results in a reduced blood volume, which reinitiates renin secretion from both kidneys. It is at this point of a return to renin secretion that an ACEI or an ARB, coupled with continued diuretic therapy, lowers blood pressure and often results in a reduction in kidney function.

As these vascular lesions progress, the downstream kidney parenchyma responds to ischemia with renal tubular collapse and atrophy.

In both models of renal artery stenosis the ischemic burden propagates oxidative stress, inflammation, and microvessel rarefaction.[5] At the tissue level, this is potentiated by monocyte chemoattractant protein-1 (MCP-1), which promotes further inflammation and fibrosis. When MCP-1 is blocked by the administration of Bindarit, there is significantly less structural remodeling of the poststenotic kidney in animal models.[6]

A central mechanism of kidney function loss in renovascular disease is microvessel rarefaction.

The endothelin-A receptor influences blood vessel density, and antagonism of its receptor in animals with renal artery stenosis promotes microvascular density and renal recovery.[7] Endogenous vascular repair mechanisms become increasingly important after initial or continuous injury, and these are directed by EPCs, which are reduced in patients with atherosclerotic renal artery stenosis (ARAS).[5] Chade and colleagues[8] found that injecting EPCs into the stenotic renal artery of swine-augmented blood vessel proliferation and improved not only endothelial function but also glomerular filtration rate (GFR). EPCs are difficult to collect from peripheral blood, but a better alternative exists with mesenchymal stem cells. Mesenchymal stem cells can be pooled from multiple tissue sources, are easier to culture, and are preferred to EPCs as they more vigorously blunt inflammation and apoptosis by decreasing tumor necrosis factor alpha and MCP-1.[5]

Adaptations to reduced renal blood flow, from atherosclerosis or reductions in perfusion from volume depletion, stimulate adaptive mechanisms involving mitochondrial energy production in this reduced flow situations. These adaptations produce mitochondrial vulnerability when blood flow is rapidly increased, an effect known as reperfusion injury,[9] mediated by the stress induced by free radicals of oxygen. Consequently, preserving mitochondrial function during reperfusion could avoid the damage from reperfusion injury. Experiments in swine demonstrate that Bendavia, a tetrapeptide that prevents oxidation of cardiolipin, can improve GFR at 4 weeks when given at the time of revascularization,[5] presumably through preserving mitochondrial function during the reperfusion period.

Obesity and Renovascular Disease

Obesity exacerbates microvascular rarefaction and potentiates renal cell injury. Obesity leads to release of adipokines, enhanced sodium retention, activation of RAAS, and insulin resistance, all of which can worsen hypertension and renal injury. Obesity is also characterized by increased leptin levels and decreased adiponectin, both of which are correlated to increased sympathetic nervous system activity.[10]

Hyperlipidemia and Renal Parenchyma Injury

Hypercholesterolemia independently incites injury in the renal parenchyma. High-cholesterol diets increase levels of oxidized low-density lipoprotein, which impairs renal vascular dilatation to acetylcholine.[11] Increased levels of oxidized low-density lipoprotein are associated with increased TGF-β, which promotes endothelin production, with vasoconstriction and microvessel rarefaction.[12] In a pig model of renal artery stenosis, statins were found to improve microvascular density and decrease glomerulosclerosis, renal oxidative stress, and fibrosis.[13]

EPIDEMIOLOGY OF RENAL ARTERY STENOSIS

The prevalence of renal artery stenosis varies widely with values around 7% in patients over 65 years old[14] and as high as 20% in referral populations. It is sometimes found incidentally, as in the discovery of fibromuscular dysplasia (FMD) during a transplant donor evaluation or observed during cardiac catheterization or evaluations for aortic aneurysms. Table 13.1 depicts common clinical factors that are important in suspecting the presence of renal artery stenosis. Readers are referred elsewhere for more extensive coverage.[15,16]

Atherosclerotic renal artery stenosis (ARAS) is the most common lesion found in patients with renovascular disease, representing about 90% of cases while FMD is present in the other 10%.[15] The presence of ARAS is associated with reduced survival with mortal events from cardiovascular disease, particularly stroke and congestive heart failure.[17] The presence of atherosclerosis in other vascular beds increases the likelihood of finding it in the kidney arteries.[18] ARAS lesions commonly occur near the ostia of the artery, whereas FMD are more distally located in the kidney arteries.

FMD can affect either the intima, media, or fibrous layers of the artery. The medial variety is the most common and is radiographically associated with a "string of beads." Lesions are commonly in the midportion of the renal artery or near the first arterial bifurcation. Despite being less common, intimal hyperplasia is known to progress to renal ischemia and atrophy. FMD can occur in different arteries particularly the carotid arteries.[19]

FMD case series show renal arteries affected in approximately 70% of cases and cerebral arteries in about 25% of cases. Though multiple vascular beds can be involved at same time, very few studies report this information probably because cerebrovascular FMD is often asymptomatic. We found 1 study indicating that, among 81 patients

TABLE 13.1 COMMON CLINICAL RISK FACTORS FOR RENAL
ARTERY STENOSIS

Factor	Atherosclerotic[a]	Fibromuscular Dysplasia[b]
Age	Older	Younger
Cholesterol	√	–
Cigarette	√	√
Genetic	?	HLA Dw6
Family history of CVD	√	+/–
Hypertension	√	√
Impaired kidney function	√ (Bilateral)	Usually not impaired

[a]Safian RD, Textor SC. Renal-artery stenosis. *N Engl J Med*. 2001;344(6):431–442.
[b]Sang CN, Whelton PK, Hamper UM, et al. Etiologic factors in renovascular fibromuscular dysplasia: a case-control study. *Hypertension*. 1989;14(5):472–479.
CVD = cardiovascular disease.

with renal FMD, 9 (11%) demonstrated concurrent carotid involvement on angiography.[20] FMD affects women more often than men and the right kidney artery more frequently, though kidney function is usually normal. Sometimes it is first detected in pregnancy with new-onset hypertension.

Uncommon Forms of the Renin-Angiotensin System

In addition to FMD and ARAS, renal trauma causing arteriovenous fistulas, renal artery aneurysm, extrinsic compression, systemic vasculitis, arterial occlusion secondary to dissection or thrombosis, or a renal artery embolic event can cause (or emulate) renal artery stenosis.[21]

CLINICAL PRESENTATION OF RENAL ARTERY STENOSIS

Renal artery stenosis can be found incidentally on "drive-by" renal angiography and remain clinically silent, or it can be discovered when searching for an occult cause of end stage renal disease. A dramatic reduction in GFR after introducing antihypertensives, particularly ACEIs or ARBs, is a marker of renal artery stenosis, particularly the bilateral form.[22]

Clinically, renal artery stenosis presents as worsening of pre-existing hypertension with a mild increase in serum creatinine (SCr). Classically, renovascular hypertension (defined as a cure or improvement in diastolic blood pressure a year after corrective surgery assessed off medications[23]) is characterized by short (<1 year) duration of hypertension, abdominal bruits, early

or late age of hypertension onset, fundoscopic findings, azotemia (blood urea nitrogen >20 mg/dL) and hypokalemia (<3.4 mEq/L).[24]

Proteinuria occurs with renal artery stenosis, occasionally secondary to renal artery stenosis alone and improving after revascularization,[25] or it could be a manifestation of concurrent disease, such as focal sclerosing glomerulonephritis or diabetic nephropathy.

"Flash" pulmonary edema is a severe presentation, along with refractory heart failure and acceleration of already treated hypertension with renal decline. Such patients often have either bilateral RAS or a solitary kidney.[26]

Patients with ARAS have a significant cardiovascular disease burden, including coronary artery disease, stroke, and congestive heart failure.[17] The prevalence of target organ damage such as left ventricular hypertrophy and prior heart attack are higher in ARAS than in patients with primary hypertension not due to renovascular disease.[27]

Natural History of Renal Artery Stenosis

Renal artery stenosis progresses at widely variable rates. Some studies suggest there is a 20% to 31% rate of progression over 3 years.[28] In the 1970s, studies showed that atherosclerotic lesion progress to severe levels in 44% to 63% of patients after being followed for 2 to 5 years. Later, this belief was revised by Zierler and colleagues[28] who found a 20% rate of progression over 3 years with only 7% progressing to total occlusion using ultrasound methods to assess renal artery patency. The degree of progression has been mitigated by widespread use of ACEIs, with 1 study suggesting the number of patients with refractory hypertension or progressive renal insufficiency decreased from 21% to 10% with ACEI. Thus, ARAS is not inevitably associated with progressive renal failure.[29]

In FMD, progression rates are less well understood, but progression to occlusion is uncommon.[16]

LABORATORY INVESTIGATION AND DIAGNOSTIC IMAGING

Routine Laboratory Studies

Urinalyses are typically bland. Patients with renal artery stenosis can develop proteinuria as previously discussed. In FMD and unilateral ARAS kidney function is usually normal. In bilateral ARAS creatinine values are often modestly elevated, particularly when treated with a combination of diuretic therapy and RAAS inhibition.

Kidney Function Studies

It was previously thought that performing renin-activity profiling could provide functional information in the context of renal vascular disease. However, evaluating renin activity has been of limited value for multiple reasons. Plasma renin activity changes dramatically with variations in sodium intake, volume status, and in response to many medications. In the past, renal vein renin activity that lateralized (1.5× greater than nonstenotic side) often lead to revascularization; however, randomized trials (as will be noted in the following discussion) have failed to show substantial benefit to revascularization of unilateral stenosis and the use of renin has decreased.

Captopril Renography

Captopril renography uses radioisotopes to estimate blood flow and filtration of each kidney before and after captopril use, along with renal size. Captopril renography has high specificity; thus, it can be applied to populations with low pretest probability. It is less sensitive and specific in the context of renal insufficiency (SCr >2.0 mg/dL). Notably, results are confounded if diuretics and ACEIs are not withdrawn prior to the study. Renography leverages cortical accumulation of the isotope, cortical retention, and excretion to indicate physiologic impairment of kidney blood flow.[30] Some studies found captopril renography

to not be predictive of angiographic findings or revascularization outcomes.[31] Renograms may be asymmetric in the context of ureteral obstruction, previous scarring, and infarction, rendering them less useful predictors of stenosis.

Blood Oxygen Level-Dependent Imaging Magnetic Resonance Imaging

This tool estimates regional renal oxygenation by exploiting the weak magnetic properties of hemoglobin as it shifts between the paramagnetic deoxygenated form and the oxygenated form.[32] Administering furosemide lessens tubular oxygen need and improves the blood oxygen level-dependent oxygenation signal particularly in the medulla. The work of the Mayo group[33,34] using this technology oriented toward identifying stenotic but still salvageable kidney parenchyma through interpreting before and after furosemide administration is ongoing, but limited availability of blood oxygen level-dependent magnetic resonance imaging, and trials showing its utility are limitations.

Kidney Imaging Studies
Doppler Ultrasonography

Ultrasound measures kidney size and assesses blood flow velocity in the aorta and renal arteries. Unilateral renal artery stenosis is supported if kidneys are asymmetric in length with a disparity of 1.5 to 2 cm. Assessment of the prestenotic main renal artery include the peak systolic velocity and the renal-to-aortic ratio. A peak systolic velocity >200 cm/s and a renal-to-aortic ratio >3.5 reflect stenoses of at least 60% with a sensitivity of 71% to 98% and a specificity of 62% to 98%.[1]

Duplex ultrasound parameters also includes the resistance index (RI), reflecting microcirculatory resistance.[35] An RI above 0.8, reflecting lower flows during diastole versus systole, correlated to a lack of response following revascularization in a study of 138 patients with renal artery stenosis.[36] However, at least 1 study noted improvement after revascularization amongst patients even with a RI >0.8.[37] An increased RI also occurs in chronic kidney disease, advanced age, and extremes of heart rate; thus, it is not specific to renal artery stenosis.[35] Though, it is generally accepted that lower resistive indices reflect better-preserved vasculature (Fig. 13.1).

New contrast-enhanced ultrasound utilizing microbubbles shows promise for improved

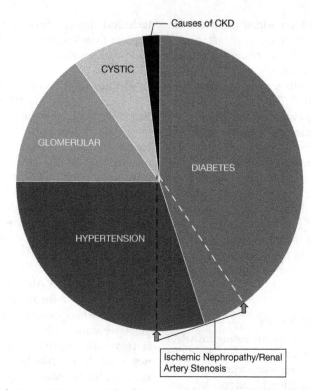

FIGURE 13.1 Pie chart depicting main causes of end-stage renal disease from US Renal Data System 2015 Report. Ischemic nephropathy/renal artery stenosis represents a subset largely of diabetes and hypertension as a cause of end-stage renal disease, with size of pie slice estimated per text in this chapter. CKD = chronic kidney disease.

sensitivity as compared to conventional ultrasound. The microbubbles are a biocompatible membrane shell around a gas and are of 2 varieties: 1 dissipates in 3 minutes, and the other is more persistent and does not undergo glomerular filtration.[35] Ultrasound investigations are attractive given their noninvasive quality and reasonable predictive value. A drawback is false negative studies, which related to operator dependency.

Computed Tomography Angiography

Utilizing helical or multiple detector scanners with intravenous contrast, computed tomography angiography (CTA) can depict vascular lesions reliably with >90% sensitivity and specificity when compared with conventional arteriography, though results are more varied with FMD than ARAS.[38] A shortcoming is the use of a potential nephrotoxin, the iodinated contrast, in an older population with diabetes and chronic kidney disease that is vulnerable to contrast-induced nephropathy. An occasional limitation is reduced visibility of vessel lumens in the setting of advanced vascular calcifications.

Magnetic Resonance Angiography

Magnetic resonance angiography (MRA) is similar to CTA when compared with conventional angiography. MRA studies often use gadolinium to generate images and have sensitivity between 83% and100% and specificity of 92% to 97% for detecting renal artery stenosis.[39] A grave consequence of gadolinium exposure in those with low GFRs is nephrogenic systemic fibrosis, which has limited its use in the United States. Other negatives of this modality include slower image acquisition than CTA, claustrophobia, limitations with implanted ferromagnetic materials, and flow-related artifacts.[35] New advances in MRA without contrast sidestep this issue but tend to be expensive and overestimate the severity of lesions. Most centers rely on MRA or CTA for the bulk of their renovascular disease screening.

Intra-Arterial Angiography

This study remains the gold standard for stenotic lesions and evaluating vascular anatomy. In those detected by "drive-by" angiography, the prevalence of renal artery stenoses of at least 50% in those with hypertension and coronary artery disease is generally 18% to 24%.[40]

There seems to be no added risk from including evaluation of the renal arteries if another vascular bed is being evaluated. Importantly, "visual estimates have poor interobserver variability with a poor correlation to quantitative methods."[35] This is because 2D luminal images do not evaluate renal blood flow, radiolucent atherosclerotic plaque, collateral circulation, and microvascular resistance. This might explain why some patients with >80% stenosis in the CORAL trial had no benefit from stenting. De Bruyne and colleagues[1] utilized a ratio of pressure distal to the stenosis and aortic pressure (P_d/P_a) of 0.90 or less to define which lesions incited increases renin levels and therefore would benefit from revascularization. This ratio correlates to a stenotic gradient of 25 mmHg.

THERAPY

Knowledge of the factors participating in ARAS progression, weight loss and statin use should be integral to a regimen of someone who has ARAS. Moreover, smoking cessation, blood pressure control, exercise, diabetes control, and minimizing alcohol are other lifestyle modifications that can attenuate vascular disease.

An ACEI or ARB are drugs of choice in unilateral stenosis since the pathophysiology is RAAS-mediated and the unaffected kidney can respond to a pressure natriuresis and, in some cases, improve oxidative stress on the parenchyma. A diuretic is usually required for bilateral ARAS or solitary kidney with ARAS to address volume expansion.

A fall in GFR after initiation of RAAS blockade is common, but a large fall such as a doubling in SCr concentration suggests the stenoses are approaching critical levels.

Vascular Intervention

Prior to antihypertensive drug availability, unilateral nephrectomy was utilized when surgeons learned of occlusive vascular disease. This procedure was discredited by Homer Smith in 1956.[41] Emphasis then shifted to surgical repair to restore renal flow. The Cooperative Study of Renovascular Hypertension[42] offered limited support for surgical revascularization but at a cost of high morbidity and mortality. Beginning in the 1980s endovascular procedures like angioplasty, fueled by initial technical success, became exponentially more popular than surgery but lacked control groups and scientific rigor.

Angioplasty in FMD: Blood Pressure Response

Angioplasty remains the intervention of choice for FMD, particularly medial FMD. These lesions are typically distal from the renal artery ostium. Success rates are high (~95%), and repeat angioplasty is often unnecessary, occurring at a rate of approximately 10%. Cure of hypertension, signifying pressures less than 140/90 requiring no antihypertensive medications, have been demonstrated in 35% to 50% of patients.[16]

Angioplasty in ARAS: Blood Pressure Responses

In ARAS, where ostial lesions are frequent, angioplasty alone is often suboptimal, and stenting is frequently added. An expected outcome is not frank clinical cure but rather a less burdensome antihypertensive regimen with decreased pill burden. Some patients have a decrease in both angina and cardiac failure exacerbations. Observational studies have found that after revascularization the typical fall in blood pressure ranges from 25 to 30 mmHg systolic.[43] However, prospective studies do not find the same degree of blood pressure improvement. This disparity in findings has confounded the fervor for opening up arteries and maintaining patency.

Clinical benefit from revascularization appears better if the SCr level is less than 3 mg/dL. Typically, approximately 27% of revascularization generates clinical improvement in renal function, whereas up to 52% of patients have no change in SCr. Unfortunately, 19% to 25% of patients have clinical deterioration following the endovascular procedure.[44] The risk of clinical deterioration occurring in up to one-fourth of patients underscores that the complications from the endovascular procedures can have serious consequences. Although minor issues such as a groin hematoma and pseudoaneurysms occur, the more serious variety of complications include contrast-induced nephropathy, restenosis, atheroembolic disease, retroperitoneal hematomas, renal infarction, thrombosis, and dissection of the aortic, iliac, or renal arteries. Restenosis occurs in up to 30% of patients within the first year.[45]

TABLE 13.2 EFFECTS OF INTERVENTION ON KIDNEY FUNCTION
IN FIBROMUSCULAR DYSPLASIA

Author or STUDY	Year	Intervention[n]	Criteria for Intervention	Duration	Kidney Function Mean+S.D.	
					Start	End
Reiher et al.[a]	2000	Surgery [101]	Renal artery stenosis	Up to 15 years	SCr 1.0+0.4	1.0+0.4
Marekovic et al.[b]	2004	Surgery or PTRA (−)[72]	Hypertension, worsening kidney function	11.2 years	CCr 59+5	78+5
Mousa et al.[c]	2012	PTRA (+/−)[35]	Hypertension, worsening kidney function	Up to 9 years	eGFR 71+6	76+9

[a]Reiher L, Pfeiffer T, Sandmann W. Long-term results after surgical reconstruction for renal artery fibromuscular dysplasia. *Eur J Vasc Endovasc Surg.* 2000;20(6):556–559.

[b]Marekovic Z, Mokos I, Krhen I, Goreta NR, Roncevic T. Long-term outcome after surgical kidney revascularization for fibromuscular dysplasia and atherosclerotic renal artery stenosis. *J Urol.* 2004;171(3):1043–1045.

[c]Mousa AY, Campbell JE, Stone PA, Broce M, Bates MC, Abu Rahma AF. Short- and long-term outcomes of percutaneous transluminal angioplasty/stenting of renal fibromuscular dysplasia over a ten-year period. *J Vasc Surg.* 2012;55(2):421–427.

[d]Levey AS, Greene T, Beck GJ, et al.; Modification of Diet in Renal Disease Study group. Dietary protein restriction and the progression of chronic renal disease: what have all of the results of the MDRD study shown? *J Am Soc Nephrol.* 1999;10(11):2426–2439.

CCr = creatinine clearance. eGFR = estimated glomerular filtration rate.[d] PTRA = percutaneous renal artery angioplasty: (−) no stenting or not stated; (+) stent used in some patients. SCr = serum creatinine (mg/dL)

Intervention in FMD and ARAS for Preserving or Improving Renal Function

Tables 13.2 (FMD) and 13.3 (ARAS) present selected studies that included testing renal function following angioplasty or surgery. We are unaware of any randomized clinical trials comparing angioplasty or surgery to medication in patients with FMD; thus, Table 13.2 presents kidney function data before and after renovascular interventions.

Table 13.3 shows that with current antihypertensive therapy, in conjunction with the availability of other medications (such as statins) and behavioral modifications such as cigarette discontinuation, renal function is not substantially better after intervention for ARAS.

In ASTRAL, 25% of the patients had normal renal function and 40% had close-to-normal renal function, while in CORAL 50% of each cohort had normal kidney function. Both trials were stymied by slow recruitment, which forced CORAL to change its inclusion criteria.[46] A significant concern is that these studies undertook revascularization in patients who were less likely to benefit since they did not meet thresholds for reduced poststenotic blood flow and thus were not capturing the population who could actually

benefit from the procedure. Many patients had already reached blood pressure goals prior to enrollment. In ASTRAL, only 46 of 64 patients randomized to stenting underwent the procedure because their lesions were not hemodynamically significant.

To date, controlled studies of ARAS interventions, with or without stenting, have not shown substantive clinical improvement. Intervening on ARAS remains an individualized decision-making process. Those with advanced degrees of stenosis (>80% luminal narrowing) and those with a rapid rise in creatinine are probably more likely to benefit.

CONCLUSION

ARAS accompanies other vascular diseases,[47] and the difficulty achieving/maintaining blood pressure control and preserving kidney function are considerations determining the value of an intervention. The challenge is to identify those patients with functionally significant stenosis and viable renal parenchyma. Currently imaging and biomarkers only indirectly approximate those who would respond favorably to revascularization. There remains room in the toolbox for new, accurate, prognostic tools in ARAS.

TABLE 13.3 EFFECTS OF ANGIOPLASTY ON KIDNEY FUNCTION IN RANDOMIZED TRIALS OF ATHEROSCLEROTIC RENAL ARTERY STENOSIS INTERVENTION

Author or Study	Year	Intervention[n]:Control[n]	Criteria for stenosis	Duration	Kidney Function (Mean+SD or % Change)			
					INT Start	INT End	CON Start	CON End
Webster et al.[a]	1998	PTRA(−)[25]:Drug Rx[30]	50% with DBP >95 mmHg on 2 meds	3–54 months	Cr[g] 182+108	192+127	148+49	152+49
EMMA[b]	1998	PTRA(+)[23]:Drug Rx[26]	≥75% with DBP >95 on meds; ≥60% if lateralizing findings present	6 months	CCr[k] 1.22+0.42	1.28+0.45	1.22+0.40	1.23+0.33
DRASTIC[c]	2000	PTRA(−)[56]:Drug Rx[50]	>50% stenosis	1 year	CCr 67+23	70+24	60+24	62+27
ASTRAL[d]	2009	PTRA(+)[403]:Drug Rx[403]	RAS and uncertainty how to proceed	5 year	eGFR 40 (5–126)	7.5[i]	40 (7–122)	10.5[i]
STAR[e]	2009	PTRA(+)[62]:Drug Rx[74]	>50% stenosis with CCr <80 mL/min	2 years	CCr 46+16	16%[h]	45+15	22%[h]
CORAL[f,57]	2013	PTRA(+)[459]:Drug Rx[472]	SBP ≥155 mmHg + 80% stenosis; or 60% stenosis with 20 mmHg gradient	43 months	eGFR 58+23	15%[j]	57+22	16%[j]

aWebster J, Marshall F, Abdalla M, et al.; Scottish and Newcastle Renal Artery Stenosis Collaborative Group. Randomised comparison of percutaneous angioplasty vs continued medical therapy for hypertensive patients with atheromatous renal artery stenosis. J Human Hypertens. 1998;12(5):329–335.

bPlouin PF, Chatellier G, Darne B, Raynaud A.; Essai Multicentrique Medicaments vs Angioplastie (EMMA) Study Group. Blood pressure outcome of angioplasty in atherosclerotic renal artery stenosis: a randomized trial. Hypertension. 1998;31(3):823–829.

cvan Jaarsveld BC, Krijnen P, Pieterman H, et al.; Dutch Renal Artery Stenosis Intervention Cooperative Study Group. The effect of balloon angioplasty on hypertension in atherosclerotic renal-artery stenosis. N Engl J Med. 2000;342(14):1007–1014.

dWheatley K, Ives N, Gray R, et al. Revascularization versus medical therapy for renal-artery stenosis. N Engl J Med. 2009;361(20):1953–1962.

eBax L, Woittiez AJ, Kouwenberg HJ, et al. Stent placement in patients with atherosclerotic renal artery stenosis and impaired renal function: a randomized trial. Ann Intern Med. 2009;150(12):840–841.

fCooper CJ, Murphy TP, Cutlip DE, et al.; Coral Investigators. Stenting and medical therapy for atherosclerotic renal-artery stenosis. N Engl J Med. 2014;370(1):13–22.

gSerum creatinine in μmol/L (data shown only for the bilateral intervention [n = 12] and control [n = 16] groups).

hSTAR used a decline of 20% in CCr as the primary outcome.

iResults (in Supplement) reported as increase in serum creatinine (μmol/L) per year.

jCORAL used a decline of 30% in eGFR as a primary renal outcome.

kCCr was reported as mL/sec.

ASTRAL = Angioplasty and Stenting for Renal Artery Lesions. CORAL = Cardiovascular Outcomes in Renal Atherosclerotic Lesions. DRASTIC = Dutch Renal Artery Stenosis Intervention Cooperative Study EMMA = Essai Multicentrique Medicaments vs Angioplastie. STAR = Stent Placement in Patients with Atherosclerotic Renal Artery Stenosis and Impaired Renal Function.PTRA = percutaneous transluminal renal angioplasty: (−) no stenting; (+) stent used in majority of patients. DBP = diastolic blood pressure. RAS = renal artery stenosis. CCr—creatinine clearance (in mL/min). SBP = systolic blood pressure. Cr = creatine. CON = control group. INT—intervention group.

REFERENCES

1. De Bruyne B, Manoharan G, Pijls NH, et al. Assessment of renal artery stenosis severity by pressure gradient measurements. *J Am Coll Cardiol.* 2006;48(9):1851–1855.

2. Textor SC, Lerman L. Renovascular hypertension and ischemic nephropathy. *Am J Hypertens.* 2010;23(11):1159–1169.

3. Goldblatt H. Studies on experimental hypertension. I. The production of persistent elevation of systolic blood pressure by means of renal ischemia. *J Exp Med.* 1934;59(3):347–379.

4. Oliveira-Sales EB, Boim MA. Mesenchymal stem cells and chronic renal artery stenosis. *Am J Physiol Renal Physiol.* 2016;310(1):F6–F9.

5. Lerman LO, Textor SC. Gained in translation: protective paradigms for the poststenotic kidney. *Hypertension.* 2015;65(5):976–982.

6. Zhu XY, Chade AR, Krier JD, et al. The chemokine monocyte chemoattractant protein-1 contributes to renal dysfunction in swine renovascular hypertension. *J Hypertens.* 2009;27(10):2063–2073.

7. Chade AR, Stewart NJ, Peavy PR. Disparate effects of single endothelin-A and -B receptor blocker therapy on the progression of renal injury in advanced renovascular disease. *Kidney Int.* 2014;85(4):833–844.

8. Chade AR, Zhu X, Lavi R, et al. Endothelial progenitor cells restore renal function in chronic experimental renovascular disease. *Circulation.* 2009;119(4):547–557.

9. Nilakantan V, Hilton G, Maenpaa C, et al. Favorable balance of anti-oxidant/pro-oxidant systems and ablated oxidative stress in Brown Norway rats in renal ischemia-reperfusion injury. *Mol Cell Biochem.* 2007;304(1–2):1–11.

10. Zhang X, Lerman LO. Obesity and renovascular disease. *Am J Physiol Renal Physiol.* 2015;309(4):F273–F279.

11. Gradinaru D, Borsa C, Ionescu C, Prada GI. Oxidized LDL and NO synthesis—biomarkers of endothelial dysfunction and ageing. *Mech Ageing Dev.* 2015;151:101–113.

12. Ding G, van Goor H, Ricardo SD, Orlowski JM, Diamond JR. Oxidized LDL stimulates the expression of TGF-beta and fibronectin in human glomerular epithelial cells. *Kidney Int.* 1997;51(1):147–154.

13. Chade AR, Zhu X, Mushin OP, Napoli C, Lerman A, Lerman LO. Simvastatin promotes angiogenesis and prevents microvascular remodeling in chronic renal ischemia. *FASEB J.* 2006;20(10):1706–1708.

14. Hansen KJ, Edwards MS, Craven TE, et al. Prevalence of renovascular disease in the elderly: a population-based study. *J Vasc Surg.* 2002;36(3):443–451.

15. Safian RD, Textor SC. Renal-artery stenosis. *N Engl J Med.* 2001;344(6):431–442.

16. Olin JW, Gornik HL, Bacharach JM, et al. Fibromuscular dysplasia: state of the science and critical unanswered questions: a scientific statement from the American Heart Association. *Circulation.* 2014;129(9):1048–1078.

17. Kalra PA, Guo H, Kausz AT, et al. Atherosclerotic renovascular disease in United States patients aged 67 years or older: risk factors, revascularization, and prognosis. *Kidney Int.* 2005;68(1):293–301.

18. de Mast Q, Beutler JJ. The prevalence of atherosclerotic renal artery stenosis in risk groups: a systematic literature review. *J Hypertens.* 2009;27(7):1333–1340.

19. Chehab BM, Gupta K. Contemporary diagnosis of carotid fibromuscular dysplasia: role of power Doppler and a review of other diagnostic modalities. *Rev Cardiovasc Med.* 2013;14(2-4):e136–e143.

20. Pannier-Moreau I, Grimbert P, Fiquet-Kempf B, et al. Possible familial origin of multifocal renal artery fibromuscular dysplasia. *J Hypertens.* 1997;15(12 Pt 2):1797–1801.

21. Textor SC. Renal arterial disease and hypertension. *Med Clin North Am.* 2017;101(1):65–79.

22. Hricik DE, Browning PJ, Kopelman R, Goorno WE, Madias NE, Dzau VJ. Captopril-induced functional renal insufficiency in patients with bilateral renal-artery stenoses or renal-artery stenosis in a solitary kidney. *N Engl J Med.* 1983;308:373–376.

23. Maxwell MH, Bleifer KH, Franklin SS, Varady PD. Cooperative study of renovascular hypertension: demographic analysis of the study. *J Am Med Assoc.* 1972;220(9):1195–1204.

24. Simon N, Franklin SS, Bleifer KH, Maxwell MH. Clinical characteristics of renovascular hypertension. *J Am Med Assoc.* 1972;220(9):1209–1218.

25. Gu B, Che Q, Li W, et al. Refractory hypertension with massive proteinuria may be reversed in renal artery stenosis patients with low proteinuria selectivity index after stenting. *J Thorac Dis.* 2013;5(4):E158–E161.

26. Pickering TG, Herman L, Devereux RB, et al. Recurrent pulmonary oedema in hypertension due to bilateral renal artery stenosis: treatment by angioplasty or surgical revascularisation. *Lancet.* 1988;2(8610):551–552.

27. Losito A, Fagugli RM, Zampi I, et al. Comparison of target organ damage in renovascular and essential hypertension. *Am J Hypertens.* 1996;9(11):1062–1067.

28. Zierler RE, Bergelin RO, Davidson RC, Cantwell-Gab K, Polissar NL, Strandness DE Jr. A prospective study of disease progression in patients with atherosclerotic renal artery stenosis. *Am J Hypertens.* 1996;9(11):1055–1061.

29. Leertouwer TC, Pattynama PM, van den Berg-Huysmans A. Incidental renal artery stenosis in peripheral vascular disease: a case for treatment? *Kidney Int.* 2001;59(4):1480–1483.

30. Nally JV Jr, Black HR. State-of-the-art review: captopril renography—pathophysiological considerations and clinical observations. *Semin Nucl Med.* 1992;22:85–97.

31. Vasbinder GB, Nelemans PJ, Kessels AG, Kroon AA, De Leeuw PW, van Engelshoven JM. Diagnostic tests for renal artery stenosis in patients suspected of having renovascular hypertension: a meta-analysis. *Ann Intern Med.* 2001;135(6):401–411.

32. Pruijm M, Milani B, Burnier M. Blood oxygenation level-dependent MRI to assess renal oxygenation in renal diseases: progresses and challenges. *Front Physiol.* 2016;7:667.

33. Textor SC, Glockner JF, Lerman LO, et al. The use of magnetic resonance to evaluate tissue oxygenation in renal artery stenosis. *J Am Soc Nephrol.* 2008;19(4):780–788.

34. Gloviczki ML, Glockner JF, Crane JA, et al. Blood oxygen level-dependent magnetic resonance imaging identifies cortical hypoxia in severe renovascular disease. *Hypertension.* 2011;58(6):1066–1072.

35. Odudu A, Vassallo D, Kalra PA. From anatomy to function: diagnosis of atherosclerotic renal artery stenosis. *Expert Rev Cardiovasc Ther.* 2015;13(12):1357–1375.

36. Radermacher J, Chavan A, Bleck J, et al. Use of Doppler ultrasonography to predict the outcome of therapy for renal-artery stenosis. *N Engl J Med.* 2001;344(6):410–417.

37. Zeller T, Muller C, Frank U, et al. Stent angioplasty of severe atherosclerotic ostial renal artery stenosis in patients with diabetes mellitus and nephrosclerosis. *Catheter Cardiovasc Interv.* 2003;58(4):510–515.

38. AbuRahma AF, Yacoub M. Renal imaging: duplex ultrasound, computed tomography angiography, magnetic resonance angiography, and angiography. *Semin Vasc Surg.* 2013;26(4):134–143.

39. Fain SB, King BF, Breen JF, Kruger DG, Riederer SJ. High-spatial-resolution contrast-enhanced MR angiography of the renal arteries: a prospective comparison with digital subtraction angiography. *Radiology.* 2001;218(2):481–490.

40. White CJ. Management of renal artery stenosis: the case for intervention, defending current guidelines, and screening (drive-by) renal angiography at the time of catheterization. *Prog Cardiovasc Dis.* 2009;52(3):229–237.

41. Smith HW. Unilateral nephrectomy in hypertensive disease. *J Urol.* 1956;76(6):685–701.

42. Foster JH, Maxwell MH, Franklin SS, et al. Renovascular occlusive disease: results of operative treatment. *J Am Med Assoc.* 1975;231(10):1043–1048.

43. Burket MW, Cooper CJ, Kennedy DJ, et al. Renal artery angioplasty and stent placement: predictors of a favorable outcome. *Am Heart J.* 2000;139(1 Pt 1):64–71.

44. Textor SC, Wilcox CS. Renal artery stenosis: a common, treatable cause of renal failure? *Annu Rev Med.* 2001;52:421–442.

45. Plouin PF, Chatellier G, Darne B, Raynaud A.; Essai Multicentrique Medicaments vs Angioplastie (EMMA) Study Group. Blood pressure outcome of angioplasty in atherosclerotic renal artery stenosis: a randomized trial. *Hypertension.* 1998;31(3):823–829.

46. Mohan IV, Bourke V. The management of renal artery stenosis: an alternative interpretation of ASTRAL and CORAL. *Eur J Vasc Endovasc Surg.* 2015;49(4):465–473.

47. Textor SC. Current approaches to renovascular hypertension. *Med Clin North Am.* 2009;93(3):717–732.

14

Environmental Toxins and the Kidney

JOSHUA D. KING AND BERNARD G. JAAR

INTRODUCTION

Kidney disease is a global health burden. While the epidemiology of chronic kidney disease (CKD) has been extensively studied, the proportion of kidney disease due to environmental factors is often difficult to determine. In developed countries, diabetes and hypertension are the leading causes of CKD; however, in many developing countries, unknown causes and chronic glomerulonephritis are the main etiologies of CKD.[1] Outside of industrial settings or acute intoxications, the contribution of environmental and occupational nephrotoxins to kidney disease is usually poorly understood or simply unknown.

It is often difficult to define the exact role of individual environmental toxins in contributing to kidney disease. Many toxic agents with in vitro kidney damage have not consistently caused CKD in humans.[2,3] Regardless, exposure to a number of environmental toxic agents have been clearly shown to increase the risk for CKD, even if they cannot be determined to be the principle contributor to kidney disease in many cases.[4,5]

In many developing countries, the exact cause of CKD often remains unclear.[1] Individual toxic causes of CKD and acute kidney injury (AKI), such as nephrotoxic herbal medicines, environmental contaminants such as aristolochic acid, and contamination of foodstuffs with compounds such as melamine are considered to be contributors to the burden of kidney disease in developing countries; however, due to significantly less research in these settings compared to many Western countries, it is not possible to quantify the proportions of AKI or CKD which result from these toxic agents.[1,3,6]

EPIDEMIOLOGY

Determining the exact burden of CKD from environmental causes is probably unfeasible. Toxic agents from the environment are synergistic with traditional risk factors for CKD; patients with hypertension and diabetes with exposure to environmental nephrotoxins generally have higher rates of CKD than patients with only traditional risk factors or environmental exposures alone.[1,7] While occupational exposure to environmental toxicants affect a minority of patients, there is evidence to suggest that low-level exposure to common environmental agents such as lead increase the risk of CKD to varying degrees.[7]

Similarly, the burden of AKI from environmental toxic agents is very difficult to define. Many cases occur in developing countries where the incidence of AKI itself is often poorly characterized, and a definitive diagnosis of AKI related to toxic injury is often not well established. Occupational exposures to nephrotoxicants such as arsine gas, which may cause AKI, are fairly rare. Rates of dietary exposures causing AKI, such as nephrotoxic herbs or mushrooms, are not well characterized. Intentional poisoning (suicidal) exposures due to environmental nephrotoxicants such as agrochemicals are better characterized, but often the nephrotoxicity of these agents is of secondary concern to damage to other vital organ systems.

PATHOGENESIS

While a very large number of environmental and occupational nephrotoxins have been identified, a smaller subset has been clearly implicated in human disease. A list of selected agents may be found in Table 14.1, and the toxicity, common scenarios for exposure, and clinical syndromes for a number of toxic agents are further explored in the following discussion.

Multiple heavy metals have been implicated in kidney disease; Table 14.2 has a partial listing of the most common ones. While the pathogenesis

TABLE 14.1 SELECTED OCCUPATIONAL AND ENVIRONMENTAL TOXIC CAUSES OF CHRONIC KIDNEY DISEASE AND ACUTE KIDNEY INJURY

Glomerulonephritis and vasculitis

Gold salts

Hydrocarbon solvents (toluene, phthalates, others)

Mercury compounds

Silica compounds

Tubulointerstitial nephritis

Aristolochic acid

Arsenic compounds

Cadmium

Hydrocarbons (trichloroethylene, other halogenated > nonhalogenated)

Lead

Uranium

Nephrotoxic acute tubular necrosis

Diethylene glycol

Diquat, paraquat, other herbicides (e.g., glyphosate)

Iron

Orellanine and other mycotoxins

Pennyroyal oil and other herbal derivatives

Acute heme pigment injury (hemolysis)

Arsine

Benzene

Phenol

TABLE 14.2 SELECTED HEAVY METALS IMPLICATED IN KIDNEY DISEASE

Metal	Example Sources	Type(s) of Kidney Disease
Arsenic	Groundwater, folk remedies, manufacturing (plywood, others)	CKD (TIN)
Cadmium	Mining; environmental runoff	CKD (TIN)
Gold	Mining; medications	Glomerular disease
Iron	Acute ingestion	AKI (ATN)
Lead	Paint; moonshine; industrial runoff; battery manufacture	CKD (TIN); proximal tubulopathy
Mercury	Manufacturing (batteries, light bulbs, others); traditional medicines and cosmetics; contaminated fish	AKI (ATN); glomerular disease (membranous nephropathy)
Uranium	Mining; contaminated groundwater; warfare	AKI (ATN); CKD (possible)

CKD = chronic kidney disease. TIN = tubulointerstitial nephritis. AKI = acute kidney injury. ATN = acute tubular necrosis.

of kidney damage from metals is not uniform, tubular damage leading to tubulointerstitial nephritis or acute tubular necrosis is seen with many heavy metals. Glomerular disease may occur with exposure to some metals, such as mercury and gold.

Lead is a well-known nephrotoxicant that primarily targets proximal tubules, causing both tubulointerstitial nephritis and proximal tubular dysfunction such as Fanconi syndrome. Chronic lead poisoning increases the risk for CKD and end stage renal disease (ESRD) and is classically associated with high rates of hypertension and gout.[5] Large-scale studies examining population health and lead exposure, such as the Adult Blood Lead Epidemiology and Surveillance program[5] examining over 50,000 US adult men with blood lead monitoring, found that sustained elevation

in blood lead levels >50 μg/dL increased the risk for ESRD significantly. Lower levels of lead exposure in the general population are also associated with increased risk for CKD and are synergistic with the risks conferred by hypertension and diabetes.[8] With the advent of chelation therapy for acute lead poisoning, acute intoxication is less likely to result in AKI and possibly CKD.[9]

Mercury is found in elemental form (e.g., traditional medications), inorganic form (e.g., mining, industrial exposure), and organic form (e.g., seafood contamination); all types have been associated with CKD.[10,11] Both membranous nephropathy and minimal change disease have been described following mercury exposure.[11] In acute exposure, inorganic forms of mercury have been associated with AKI from acute tubular necrosis.[11]

CKD is clearly associated with long-term exposure to cadmium in industrial and other settings.[12] The most notorious mass cadmium poisoning occurred in Toyama Prefecture, Japan; an epidemic of bone pain and kidney failure was termed "itai-itai" disease, and cadmium pollution from an upstream mining operation was discovered as the cause in the 1950s.[10,12] Cadmium also causes proximal tubular damage and CKD with tubulointerstitial fibrosis on kidney biopsy; these findings are strongly associated with longitudinal cadmium exposure. Nephrolithiasis is also common in patients with chronic cadmium toxicity.[12] Due to cadmium's well-recognized nephrotoxicity, industrial monitoring not only for renal damage (as measured by urine beta-2-microglobulin) but also of blood and urinary cadmium levels are required for workers at risk for cadmium exposure.[10] Patients exposed to both lead and cadmium may be at increased risk from each exposure alone; in the NHANES population (1999–2006), after adjustment for survey year, sociodemographic factors, known CKD risk factors, and blood lead, the odds ratios for albuminuria (≥30 mg/g creatinine), reduced estimated glomerular filtration rate (GFR; <60 mL/minute/1.73 m^2), and both albuminuria and reduced GFR were 1.92 (95% confidence interval [CI]: 1.53–2.43), 1.32 (95% CI: 1.04–1.68), and 2.91 (95% CI: 1.76–4.81), respectively, comparing the highest with the lowest blood cadmium quartiles. The odds ratios comparing participants in the highest with the lowest quartiles of both cadmium and lead were 2.34 (95% CI: 1.72–3.18) for albuminuria, 1.98 (95% CI: 1.27–3.10) for reduced GFR, and 4.10 (95% CI: 1.58–10.65) for both outcomes combined.[7,13]

While uranium has been shown to have proximal tubular toxicity in animal studies, human exposure studies are mixed as to whether chronic uranium exposure is associated with CKD.[3,10] Studies of renal injury markers in populations exposed to uranium through environmental, occupational, and military settings suggest that adverse renal effects may occur. However, studies evaluating GFR in occupational settings did not reveal a significant difference after prolonged exposures.[3]

A number of other heavy metals have been associated with AKI and CKD. The use of gold as a therapeutic agent has been implicated as a cause of glomerular disease in the past.[10] While gold-based medications are rarely used nowadays, gold mining has been associated with risk of exposure to a number of nephrotoxic compounds, most notably silica, mercury, and lead, and therefore may be associated with increased risk for ESRD.[10,14,15]

Exposure to silica compounds has been associated with ESRD. While the mechanism is not entirely clear, chronic inflammation related to fine particles of silica dust has been postulated as the most likely pathophysiologic cause of kidney damage.[14,16] Reviews of workers with industrial exposure to silica have demonstrated an increased risk of kidney disease and hypertension. Animal studies reveal that rodents exposed to silica develop proximal tubular and glomerular damage.[16] Silica exposure is associated with higher rates of systemic autoimmune diseases such as rheumatoid arthritis and scleroderma; similarly, development of antineutrophil cytoplasmic antibody–associated vasculitis with renal involvement has been associated with exposure to silica.[16]

A number of hydrocarbons used in industrial settings have been associated with AKI and, to a lesser extent, CKD. Halogenated hydrocarbons such as trichloroethylene, chloroform, and carbon tetrachloride are converted to nephrotoxic, highly reactive compounds by cytochrome p450 enzymes; these have caused AKI in the setting of industrial exposure and ingestion.[17] Acute exposure to hydrocarbons with a propensity to cause oxidative hemolysis—such as benzene or phenol—can result in AKI from massive heme pigment release with resultant renal tubular injury.[18]

Ingestion of toxic alcohols such as ethylene glycol and diethylene glycol may cause AKI through the generation of nephrotoxic metabolites. In the case of ethylene glycol, metabolism to oxalic acid may result in the formation of calcium oxalate crystals that precipitate within the renal tubules, leading to AKI through obstruction and tubular damage. Other metabolites of ethylene glycol have been demonstrated to be nephrotoxic in animal models, but this has not been definitively proven in humans. Diethylene glycol is metabolized to diglycolic acid, which inhibits the Krebs cycle enzyme succinate dehydrogenase and subsequently causes acute tubular necrosis.[19]

Agrochemicals such as herbicides and pesticides may contribute to CKD in workers with continual exposure, especially in developing countries where regulations limiting more toxic agents or overall exposure limits are lacking. Moreover, pesticides are a common means of suicide by self-poisoning in developing countries;

agents such as paraquat and diquat can cause severe AKI in this setting, the former being more toxic (due primarily to lung injury) and frequently used in suicidal ingestions.[20] Paraquat and diquat both act through generation of reactive oxygen species that cause acute tubular damage with subsequent AKI and may lead to CKD as a result.[20]

Multiple naturally occurring dietary and traditional medicinal compounds have been associated with kidney disease. Herbal medications have been implicated in a large proportion of AKI in sub-Saharan Africa.[1,10] Mushrooms containing orellanine, allenic norleucine, or cyclopeptides are known to cause AKI; allenic norleucine from *Amanita smithiana* species may lead to ESRD.[21]

Aristolochic acid, a compound found in plants of the worldwide *Aristolochia* genus, has been strongly associated with development of CKD from tubulointerstitial nephritis as well as urothelial carcinoma.[4] The so-called Chinese herbal nephropathy, a syndrome of chronic interstitial nephritis linked to ingestion of Chinese herbal medications in diet clinics, has been shown to be principally caused by aristolochic acid. Aristolactam-DNA adducts have been demonstrated in patients with this herbal nephropathy and are likely pathogenetic of both CKD and urothelial carcinoma.[4] The index cases of Balkan endemic nephropathy, a similar syndrome of CKD due to chronic interstitial nephritis with a high rate of development of urothelial carcinoma in northwest Bulgaria, are likely due to contamination of flour with aristolochic acid.[22]

In much of the developing world, food additives are often unregulated or poorly regulated. Epidemics of kidney disease due to food additives are either known or thought to have occurred in countries with less stringent monitoring practices. The same can be said for pharmaceutical additives; substitution of diethylene glycol for glycerol as a "syrup" in liquid medicine formulations has led to notorious epidemics of death, nephrotoxicity, and neurotoxicity in countries including China, Panama, Haiti, and India. In 1937, over 100 deaths occurred in the United States due to the addition of diethylene glycol to sulfanilamide, an antibiotic; one year later, the Food and Drug Administration was empowered to avoid similar future tragedies.[23]

Melamine, a nitrogenous compound synthesized from urea, has caused epidemic of CKD and nephrolithiasis as a result of widespread contamination of milk in 2008, affecting predominantly children 3 years of age or less in China and Hong Kong. Clinical manifestations in affected children included nephrolithiasis, hematuria, proteinuria, and, less commonly, oliguric kidney damage with hypertension and edema.[6]

There is evidence to suggest that some percentage of interstitial nephritis of unknown cause, particularly in developing countries, may be attributed to environmental (dietary and otherwise) or occupational exposure to nephrotoxicants.[1] Countries such as Sudan, Egypt, and others have a relatively large prevalence of CKD due to interstitial nephritis of unknown causes, much more so than most developed countries. It has been postulated that herbal medicines, persistence of heavy metals in the environment (e.g., the widespread groundwater contamination with arsenic in Bangladesh), and agrochemicals may be significant contributors to CKD in developing countries.[1,10]

CKD of uncertain etiology (CKDu) refers to a growing number of seemingly epidemic cases of CKD that cannot be attributed to traditionally common risk factors for CKD such as diabetes mellitus, hypertension, or infectious agents such as hepatitis viruses or human immunodeficiency virus.[24] Most of these cases are clustered in the tropical belt in countries such as Nicaragua, El Salvador, and Sri Lanka, and reports have been increasing in the past decade; CKDu in Central America is largely synonymous with the term "Mesoamerican nephropathy." Renal biopsy findings are generally similar, with glomerulosclerosis, tubular atrophy, and interstitial fibrosis. At present, CKDu appears to be an occupational disease given a much higher prevalence in men engaged in agricultural work. While nontoxicological causes such as heat-related illness have been posited, as have nonenvironmental factors such as nonsteroidal anti-inflammatory drugs and fructose, a number of other potential toxic causes including pesticides have varying degrees of support from epidemiological data.[24]

CLINICAL PRESENTATION

CKD from environmental causes often presents insidiously, with a relatively asymptomatic rise in serum creatinine. Kidney biopsy may reveal tubulointerstitial disease or, less commonly, glomerular disease depending on the particular toxin(s) involved. Relatively few environmental toxic agents have clearly identifiable clinical syndromes, with some exceptions.

Some characteristic examples include chronic lead toxicity, which may (less commonly) be accompanied by a particularly severe tophaceous form of gout termed "saturnine gout;" melamine intoxication leading to kidney stones as well as renal damage; and aristolochic acid toxicity leading to kidney tumors as well as CKD.

Unlike CKD from environmental factors, the cause of AKI can often be attributed to a specific exposure (e.g., herbal medicine, mushrooms, arsine gas exposure), although the individual toxic agent(s) may or may not be known.

Due to the very large number of potential environmental toxins, testing should be directed toward known or strongly suspected exposures based on patient history.

TREATMENT AND MANAGEMENT CONSIDERATIONS

The first principle of treating kidney disease due to environmental or occupational toxins is to remove the patient from exposure to the toxic agent. This may involve removal from the workplace, remediation of the home environment, or, in selected cases of acute ingestion, gastrointestinal decontamination and even hemodialysis. After removal from the source of toxic exposure, antidotal therapy or medication can be considered. While most types of CKD due to environmental exposure have no specific medical therapy other than usual management of CKD and related complications, chelation may be considered for certain heavy metal exposures, preferably with the support of an occupational medicine physician with toxicology expertise or medical toxicologist. AKI due to environmental or occupational toxins may have more specific therapies.

Workers at risk for occupational exposure may benefit from ongoing monitoring. Those working with certain heavy metals, such as lead, mercury, and cadmium, are required to have longitudinal measurements of blood and/or urine metal concentrations as well as appropriate markers of renal damage (e.g., urine beta-2-microglobulin, serum creatinine, etc.).[7,10]

Chelation of metals may have a role in selected cases of heavy metal-associated kidney disease; it should be noted that this treatment option remains controversial and is not universally accepted. While evidence suggests that chelation for lead and mercury-induced kidney disease may be helpful, chelation for cadmium may worsen outcomes.[7,10] Consideration of chelation should be discussed with an occupational

TABLE 14.3 CHELATING AGENTS USED TO TREAT SELECTED HEAVY METALS

Metal	Chelator of Choice	Alternate Agent(s)
Arsenic	Dimercaprol	DMPS (non-US)
Cadmium	None, chelation generally worsens toxicity	None
Gold	Dimercaprol	None
Iron	Deferoxamine	None
Lead	Succimer; dimercaprol + EDTA (severe)	D-penicillamine
Mercury (inorganic)	Dimercaprol	Succimer; DMPS
Uranium	Bicarbonate	None

EDTA = ethylenediamine tetraacetic acid.
DMPS = 2,3-Dimercapto-1-propanesulfonic acid.

medicine physician with toxicology expertise or medical toxicologist experienced in treating heavy metal toxicity. Table 14.3 has a list of chelating agents most often used for treatment of heavy metal toxicity.

CONSIDERATION IN RENAL REPLACEMENT THERAPY

Many environmental toxicants are poorly removed by extracorporeal therapies, with some notable exceptions. In cases of acute ingestion, paraquat is amenable to extracorporeal removal via hemodialysis and/or hemoperfusion; however, this must generally occur within a few hours to influence clinical outcomes.[20] Toxicants causing acute hemolysis, such as arsine or copper, may be removed via exchange transfusion.[18]

It is rare that chronic exposure to environmental agents with nephrotoxic activity would result in concentrations large enough to consider hemodialysis; most of these agents would be poorly amenable to hemodialysis due to low circulating free plasma concentrations. Heavy metals causing kidney disease are not removed by hemodialysis to a clinically important extent.

CONSIDERATIONS IN KIDNEY TRANSPLANTATION

In addition to direct nephrotoxicity from environmental factors, recipients of renal transplant are also at risk for interference with or enhanced toxicity of their immunosuppressive medications. For example, as an inducer of cytochrome P450 enzymes, St. John's wort has caused acute rejection in kidney transplant patients due to increased metabolism of tacrolimus.[25] The exact content of many herbal and traditional medications, particularly those in the developing world, is often unknown; these substances therefore have unknown potential for possibly deleterious interference with drug metabolism and excretion and should be best avoided.

Exposure to certain nephrotoxins, such as aristolochic acid, melamine, or cadmium, increases the risk for kidney or lower urinary tract malignancy. While official cancer screening guidelines for exposure to most environmental nephrotoxins do not exist, patients with significant exposure to aristolochic acid are at relatively high risk for urothelial cancer, and strong consideration should be given to regular cancer screening.[22] This applies to patients with organ transplants as well, who may be at even higher risk due to increased cancer risk from immunosuppressive agents.

CONCLUSION

Environmental and occupational toxins exposure contribute greatly to CKD for a small number of people (e.g., industrial metal workers) and likely contribute in small degrees to a great number of people (e.g., low-level lead exposure). In developing countries, environmental causes of CKD likely play a larger role than is appreciated, and increased public health efforts are likely warranted to limit their impact. As treatment for kidney disease due to environmental and occupational toxins is often significantly limited, close attention to preventative care to those at risk for acute or CKD due to these toxic agents is very important.

REFERENCES

1. Jha V, Garcia-Garcia G, Iseki K, et al. Chronic kidney disease: global dimension and perspectives. *Lancet.* 2013;382(9888):260–272.
2. Shelley R, Kim NS, Parsons P, et al. Associations of multiple metals with kidney outcomes in lead workers. *Occup Environ Med.* 2012;69(10):727–735.
3. Arzuaga X, Rieth SH, Bathija A, Cooper GS. Renal effects of exposure to natural and depleted uranium: a review of the epidemiologic and experimental data. *J Toxicol Environ Health B Crit Rev.* 2010;13(7-8):527–545.
4. Debelle FD, Vanherweghem JL, Nortier JL. Aristolochic acid nephropathy: a worldwide problem. *Kidney Int.* 2008;74:158–169.
5. Chowdhury R, Darrow L, McClellan W, Sarnat S, Steenland K. Incident ESRD among participants in a lead surveillance program. *Am J Kidney Dis.* 2014;64(1):25–31.
6. Hau AK, Kwan TH, Li PK. Melamine toxicity and the kidney. *J Am Soc Nephrol.* 2009;20(2):245–250.
7. Sommar JN, Svensson MK, Björ BM, et al. End-stage renal disease and low level exposure to lead, cadmium and mercury: a population-based, prospective nested case-referent study in Sweden. *Environ Health.* 2013;12:9.
8. Tsaih SW, Korrick S, Schwartz J, et al. Lead, diabetes, hypertension, and renal function: the normative aging study. *Environ Health Perspect.* 2004;112(11):1178–82.
9. Thurtle N, Greig J, Cooney L, et al. Description of 3,180 courses of chelation with dimercaptosuccinic acid in children ≤5 y with severe lead poisoning in Zamfara, northern Nigeria: a retrospective analysis of programme data. *PLoS Med.* 2014;11(10):e1001739.
10. Soderland P, Lovekar S, Weiner DE, Brooks DR, Kaufman JS. Chronic kidney disease associated with environmental toxins and exposures. *Adv Chronic Kidney Dis.* 2010;17(3):254–264.
11. Li SJ, Zhang SH, Chen HP, et al. Mercury-induced membranous nephropathy: clinical and pathological features. *Clin J Am Soc Nephrol.* 2010;5(3):439–444.
12. Piscator M. Long-term observations on tubular and glomerular function in cadmium-exposed persons. *Environ Health Perspect.* 1984; 54:175–179.
13. Navas-Acien A, Tellez-Plaza M, Guallar E, Muntner P, Silbergeld E, Jaar B, Weaver V. Blood cadmium and lead and chronic kidney disease in US adults: a joint analysis. *Am J Epidemiol.* 2009;170(9):1156–1164.
14. Calvert GM, Steenland K, Palu S. End-stage renal disease among silica-exposed gold miners: a new method for assessing incidence among epidemiologic cohorts. *J Am Med Assoc.* 1997;277(15):1219–1223.
15. Yard EE, Horton J, Schier JG, et al. Mercury exposure among artisanal gold miners in Madre de Dios, Peru: a cross-sectional study. *J Med Tox.* 2012;8:441–448.
16. Vupputuri S, Parks CG, Nylander-French LA, et al. Occupational silica exposure and chronic kidney disease. *Ren Fail.* 2012;34(1):40–46.
17. Yaqoob M, Bell GM. Occupational factors and renal disease. *Ren Fail.* 1994;16(4):425–434.

18. Pakulska D, Czerczak S. Hazardous effects of arsine: a short review. *Int J Occup Med Environ Health*. 2006;19(1):36–44.

19. Landry GM, Dunning CL, Conrad T, Hitt MJ, McMartin KE. Diglycolic acid inhibits succinate dehydrogenase activity in human proximal tubule cells leading to mitochondrial dysfunction and cell death. *Toxicol Lett*. 2013;221(3):176–184.

20. Gil HW, Hong JR, Jang SH, Hong SY. Diagnostic and therapeutic approach for acute paraquat intoxication. *J Korean Med Sci*. 2014;29(11):1441–1449.

21. Goldfrank LR. Mushrooms. In: Hoffman RS, Howland MA, Lewin NA, Nelson LS, Goldfrank LR, eds. *Goldfrank's Toxicologic Emergencies*. 10th ed. New York, NY: McGrawHill; 2014.

22. De Broe ME. Chinese herbs nephropathy and Balkan endemic nephropathy: toward a single entity, aristolochic acid nephropathy. *Kidney Int*. 2012;81(6):513–515.

23. Wiener SW. Toxic Alcohols. In: Hoffman RS, Howland MA, Lewin NA, Nelson LS, Goldfrank LR. *Goldfrank's Toxicologic Emergencies*. 10th ed. New York, NY: McGrawHill; 2014.

24. Weaver VM, Fadrowski JJ, Jaar BG. Global dimensions of chronic kidney disease of unknown etiology (CKDu): a modern era environmental and/or occupational nephropathy? *BMC Nephrol*. 2015;16:145.

25. Hebert MF, Park JM, Chen YL, Akhtar S, Larson AM. Effects of St. John's wort (Hypericum perforatum) on tacrolimus pharmacokinetics in healthy volunteers. J *Clin Pharmacol*. 2004;44(1):89–94.

15

Perioperative Renal Protection

SAPNA SHAH AND VIJAY LAPSIA

INTRODUCTION

Acute kidney injury (AKI) is a serious post-operative complication with significant implications on morbidity and mortality. It is estimated to occur in 5% of all hospital admissions, and postoperative AKI is the second most common cause of renal injury among all hospitalized patients.[1] Its occurrence is seen most often following cardiac, vascular, and major abdominal procedures. The most consistent preoperative risk factor contributing to AKI is pre-existing renal impairment. Both general and regional anesthesia can cause reversible decreases in renal blood flow, glomerular filtration rate (GFR), urinary flow, and sodium excretion. These changes are mediated by autonomic and hormonal responses to physiologic stressors like surgery and anesthesia.[2] Postoperative complications including mortality, fluid and electrolyte derangements, infection, sepsis, and gastrointestinal hemorrhage are more commonly seen in patients with chronic kidney disease (CKD) and end-stage renal disease (ESRD).[3] Despite this increased risk, surgical procedures, especially pertaining to vascular access, are common in patients with CKD and ESRD. The mainstay of postoperative AKI prevention is the maintenance of perioperative blood volume with adequate cardiac output. Strategies should consequently be employed to protect perioperative renal function to prevent acute complications and long-term renal injury.

ACUTE KIDNEY INJURY IN THE SURGICAL SETTING

The kidneys are essential for maintaining intravascular volume, controlling the composition of body fluids, eliminating toxins, and modulating hormones. Renal blood flow, normally 20% to 25% of cardiac output, is strictly controlled through autoregulation. This internal adaptive mechanism, largely driven by prostaglandin-mediated myogenic responses of the afferent glomerular arterioles in response to changes in blood pressure, occurs between mean arterial blood pressures of 80 and 180 mmHg. Outside of these autoregulation limits, renal blood flow becomes pressure dependent and glomerular filtration ceases when the mean arterial pressure is less than 40 to 50 mmHg. Both surgery and anesthesia alter renal physiology and normal protective mechanisms and may result in complications such as perioperative fluid overload, hypovolemia, or AKI.[2]

It was previously thought that patients die with, and not of, AKI in critical illness. This belief stemmed from the impression that renal function can be replaced by dialysis; however, despite the use of renal replacement therapy, mortality remains high in patients with hospital-acquired AKI. Renal injury itself, independent of patient's severity of illness, is a prognostic indicator of increased overall mortality.[4] It should therefore not be considered a treatable consequence of serious illness but as a grave complication. All tactics must thus be exercised to protect the kidneys from injury in the perioperative period.

Although data are limited regarding the incidence and consequences of hospital-acquired AKI, it is known that even a small change in serum creatinine is associated with a marked increase in mortality, length of stay, and cost, even after adjustment for severity of illness and CKD. In cardiac surgery, the development of AKI, defined as a 50% increase in serum creatinine, is the strongest risk factor for death. While a small increase in serum creatinine (defined as 0–0.5 mg/dL) is associated with a nearly 3-fold increase in 30-day mortality, larger increases (>0.5 mg/dL) are associated with a greater than 18-fold increase in mortality.[5] Although more pronounced and studied following cardiac surgery, the implications of AKI on increased mortality can also be seen in noncardiac surgeries. Clinicians should be cautious and avoid any precipitating factors for further renal impairment in patients even in whom small alterations in renal function become apparent, previously thought to be fluctuations within the normal range.

The perioperative period results in significant physiologic stresses with multiple potential adverse effects. Fluid shifts, toxin exposures, hormonal alterations, and hemodynamic changes all occur in the perioperative period and can contribute to the development of AKI.[6] The best advice to date for prevention of AKI is unfortunately empirical: avoid hypotension, dehydration, and exposure to nephrotoxins. As a result, anesthesiologists attempt to maintain renal blood flow by a variety of strategies, such as intravenous hydration, tight control of blood pressure, and administration of vasoactive substances. Intraoperative urine output is monitored closely as one measure of success with this goal.[2]

A careful understanding of risk factors may help to reduce the incidence of AKI. Several studies have been performed in both cardiac and general surgery patient populations carefully reviewing risk factors for AKI in the perioperative period. While different in a few aspects, many risk factors are similar between all surgical types: advanced age, diabetes mellitus, active congestive heart failure, hypertension, preexisting CKD, and need for emergent surgery.[7] In cardiac and vascular surgery, additional risk factors include time on cardiopulmonary bypass, need for intra-aortic balloon pump, and aortic cross-clamping.[8] In general surgery, additional risk factors include intraperitoneal surgery, presence of ascites, and preoperative liver dysfunction.[7] The pneumoperitoneum introduced during laparoscopy can result in an abdominal compartment syndrome. The increase in intra-abdominal pressure can produce oliguria in proportion to insufflation pressures secondary to central venous compression, renal parenchymal compression, decreased cardiac output, and increases in plasma levels of renin, aldosterone, and antidiuretic hormone.[2]

Recently risk prediction models for AKI have been proposed for both general and cardiac surgery.[7,8] After cardiac surgery, the risk for AKI is highest among patients with poor cardiac performance defined as those with New York Heart Association class 4 and pulmonary rales, advanced atherosclerotic disease and preexisting CKD.[8] After general surgery, a risk index for AKI has been proposed. This risk model includes age >56 years, male sex, active congestive heart failure, hypertension, emergency surgery, intraperitoneal surgery, CKD (mild defined as preoperative creatinine 1.2–1.9 mg/dL and moderate as >2 mg/dL), and diabetes mellitus. Compared with 0 to 2 risk factors, the presence of 3, 4, 5, and 6 or more risk factors increased the hazard ratio of AKI to 3.1, 8.5, 15.4, and 46.2 respectively.[7] These calculators can be used to provide patients with education and risk estimates and to target high-risk subgroups for postoperative observation and interventions aimed at reducing risk.

Various pharmacological agents have also been used to optimize renal perfusion and tubular function in patients undergoing surgery. These most often include medications such as dopamine and its analogues, calcium channel blockers, diuretics, angiotensin-converting enzyme inhibitors (ACEIs), N-acetyl cysteine, atrial natriuretic peptide, sodium bicarbonate, antioxidants, and erythropoietin. Although initially encouraging, a systematic review of the literature did not find any reliable evidence to suggest these interventions during surgery can protect the kidneys from injury.[9]

Most perioperative AKI is caused by renal hypoperfusion or acute tubular necrosis (ATN). A prolonged prerenal state due to hypotension, hypovolemia, decreased circulating blood volume, and cardiac dysfunction can precipitate ischemic ATN. Other operative factors associated with ischemic ATN include prolonged cardiac bypass time, aortic cross-clamp time, and cold-ischemic time of a donor graft in renal transplantation. ATN may also be due to injury by nephrotoxins such as aminoglycosides, calcineurin inhibitors, iodinated radiocontrast agents, and rhabdomyolysis from trauma, compartment syndromes, or prolonged lithotomy position.[10] Some of these events are predictable preoperatively and may be prevented or ameliorated by optimal hemodynamic support and avoidance of nephrotoxins.

Although their combined weight is less than 1% of total body weight, the kidneys normally receive 20% to 25% of cardiac output per minute, resulting in the highest tissue perfusion in the body. Decreased cardiac output not only directly lowers renal blood flow but also activates renal vasoconstrictors to maintain systemic perfusion.

TABLE 15.1 SUMMARY
OF RECOMMENDATIONS FOR THE
PREVENTION OF ACUTE KIDNEY INJURY
IN THE SURGICAL SETTING

- Renal blood flow is regulated by prostaglandin-mediated myogenic responses of the afferent glomerular arterioles in response to changes in blood pressure.
- Common risk factors for AKI include advanced age, diabetes mellitus, congestive heart failure, hypertension, and pre-existing CKD.
- Avoidance of prolonged hypotension, hypovolemia, decreased circulating blood volume, and decreased cardiac output can decrease renal hypoperfusion and acute tubular necrosis.
- Any intervention, especially volume loading, that restores cardiac output and systemic perfusion improves renal perfusion.
- It remains unresolved whether crystalloids or colloids are the preferred fluid to use for volume resuscitation; however, carbohydrate-based artificial colloids such as hydroxyeythl starch and dextran are associated with AKI and should be avoided.
- Patients with decreased effective circulating volume should not be given medications that inhibit vasodilatory prostaglandins (NSAIDs, ACEIs, or ARBs).
- Currently no pharmacologic agents are proven to be efficacious in reducing perioperative AKI.

AKI = acute kidney injury. CKD = chronic kidney disease. NSAID = nonsteroidal anti-inflammatory drugs. ACEI = angiotensin converting enzyme inhibitors. ARBs = angiotensin II receptor blockers.

Any intervention restoring cardiac output and systemic perfusion therefore improves renal perfusion. Volume loading to prevent hypovolemia is probably the most effective preventive measure against AKI, guided by central venous pressure or pulmonary wedge pressure monitoring. Volume loading will increase renal blood flow, reduce vasoconstrictive stimuli, and potentially limit exposure to nephrotoxic stimuli by improving urine flow. Standard recommendations suggest that fluids and vasoactive drugs should be titrated to mean arterial pressure of 60 mmHg; however, these guidelines underestimate mean renal arterial pressures in patients with baseline hypertension and limit autoregulation mechanisms. It is also important not to administer excessive fluid perioperatively to avoid complications such as pulmonary edema, intra-abdominal hypertension, and poor wound healing because of subcutaneous edema.[11] It remains unresolved whether crystalloids or colloids are the preferred fluids to use. Crystalloids can be given initially to maintain adequate preload. However, in patients with severe hypovolemia and capillary leak due to severe inflammation, colloids may be used. When choosing colloid solutions, it should also be noted that while albumin is renal protective, carbohydrate-based artificial colloids such as hydroxyethyl starch and dextran are frequently associated with AKI and should be avoided.[12] Patients with decreased effective circulating volume should not be given nonsteroidal anti-inflammatory drugs, ACEIs, or angiotensin II receptor blockers, which inhibit vasodilatory prostaglandins. Prostaglandins act as a protective mechanism to maintain glomerular filtration in periods of hypotension or shock.

In summary, identifying patients at risk for perioperative AKI and optimizing renal function prior to surgery is crucial to reduce postoperative AKI. Currently, no pharmacological agents are proven to be efficacious in preventing perioperative acute renal failure, especially in patients with normal preoperative renal function. The most important strategy is to ensure adequate intravascular volume to maintain sufficient renal perfusion. Modification of surgical techniques such as endovascular repair of aortic aneurysm, reducing aortic cross-clamp time, and off-pump coronary artery bypass graft are promising measures in reducing the incidence of perioperative AKI and its associated morbidity and mortality. If AKI significantly increases the risk of death, in certain settings it may be best to defer procedures, such as major surgery or radiocontrast administration, that can cause AKI (Tables 15.1 and 15.2).

CHRONIC KIDNEY DISEASE IN THE SURGICAL SETTING

The world-wide prevalence of CKD is high and is increasing rapidly. In 2010, 26 million American adults had CKD, and millions of others are at increased risk.[13] CKD is also an independent risk factor for cardiovascular disease (CVD). As renal function declines, total mortality, CVD, and hospitalizations all increase. Even moderately decreased estimated GFR and low levels of albuminuria can predict all-cause mortality and CVD in the general population.[14] Despite the increased morbidity and mortality among CKD patients in surgery, their need for surgery continues to

TABLE 15.2 SUMMARY OF RECOMMENDATIONS FOR CHRONIC KIDNEY DISEASE/END-STAGE RENAL DISEASE PATIENTS IN THE SURGICAL SETTING

- The presence of any residual renal function is associated with decreased mortality, reduced intradialytic weight gain, and improved solute clearance in dialysis patients.
- Assessment of cardiac risk and optimization of volume status is imperative prior to surgery, especially in CKD patients as cardiovascular disease is the major cause of death in ESRD patients.
- Chronic beta blocker is associated with reduced myocardial infarction, cardiac revascularization and atrial fibrillation. Given acutely, beta blockers can cause bradycardia, hypotension, stroke, and death.
- Aspirin therapy for primary prevention of CVD should be held for 5 to 7 days prior to surgery due to increased bleeding risk.
- In patients with CKD, statin therapy should be initiated to decrease atherosclerotic events; however the utility of statin therapy is not clear in ESRD patients and is consequently not routinely recommended.
- ACEIs and ARBs should be held on the day of noncardiac surgery to reduce the risk of perioperative death, stroke, or myocardial injury.
- The optimal volume status prior to surgery is dependent on the type of surgery and the estimate of anticipated fluid administration during surgery.
- The serum potassium concentration acceptable prior to surgery depends on the urgency of the surgery.
- In the perioperative period, CKD patients should be optimized by maintaining hematocrit levels >3% through the use of erythropoietin and administration of ddAVP.
- Access planning should be considered and planned preoperatively, potential future fistula sites should be avoided.

CKD = chronic kidney disease. ESRD = end-stage renal disease. CVD = cardiovascular disease. ACEI = angiotensin converting enzyme inhibitors.

rise. With diminished renal reserve, they are more sensitive to complications of surgery and are at increased risk for perioperative electrolyte abnormalities, infection, anemia, and hemodynamic instability. This becomes most evident in patients with ESRD. Given these findings, it is not surprising that the presence of any residual renal function is associated with a lower mortality risk, reduced intradialytic weight gain, and improved solute clearance in dialysis patients.[15]

Cardiovascular diseases and cardiac complications are the major causes of death in patients with ESRD. CKD patients have accelerated atherosclerosis, likely in the setting of impaired endothelial function, low-grade inflammation, altered lipoprotein metabolism, and hypertension, which likely contributes to their high CVD burden. Furthermore, left ventricular hypertrophy is an independent factor associated with poor survival in dialysis patients, and it occurs due to a combination of increased systemic blood pressure and volume overload.[16] Left ventricular hypertrophy is associated with myocardial fibrosis and abnormalities of myocardial relaxation, both of which contribute to diastolic dysfunction and arrhythmias. Assessment of cardiac risk and optimization of volume status is imperative prior to any surgery, especially so in the CKD population. Cardiac revascularization in high-risk patients prior to surgery may decrease intraoperative cardiac risk and enhance survival in patients with CKD.

Preoperative and intraoperative hypertension is common in patients with CKD as a result of anxiety, catecholamine response to stress following surgery, and baseline hypertension. Strategies to reduce perioperative AKI include management of chronic medications that may impact renal hemodynamics in the perioperative period. Chronic beta-blocker use, titrated to an effect 30 days prior to surgery, is superior to acute beta-blocker blockade and associated with reduced myocardial infarction, cardiac revascularization, and atrial fibrillation.[17] If given acutely prior to surgery, beta-blockers are associated with increased incidence of bradycardia, hypotension, stroke, and death. In patients without long-term indications for therapy, preoperative beta-blockers should not be initiated to improve perioperative outcomes.[18]

In regard to antiplatelet therapy, while aspirin may not be useful for primary prevention of atherosclerotic disease in dialysis patients, its use is warranted following myocardial infarction and its prevalence high given the association with CKD patients with CVD. Prior to surgery, the use of low-dose aspirin is associated with increased bleeding with no benefit on outcomes including composite death or myocardial infarction. It should consequently be held 5 to 7 days prior to surgery and not started prior to noncardiac surgery in those not taking aspirin.[19]

Patients with chronic kidney disease should receive statin therapy to decrease major future atherosclerotic events. Perioperative statin therapy is associated with lower all-cause mortality, stroke, composite myocardial infarction, and death but had no difference in all-cause mortality or incidence of kidney injury.[20] The utility of statins in ESRD is not clear, and prior studies have failed to show any benefit in statin therapy in prevention of CVD events in that population.[21,22] Evidence supports avoiding the routine use of statins in this patient population and instead reserving them for patients with elevated cholesterol levels or those with recent CVD events.[23]

Pertaining to ACEIs in CKD, current guidelines suggest that withholding ACEIs and angiotensin II receptor blockers on the day of a noncardiac surgery may reduce the risk of perioperative death, stroke, or myocardial injury in patients who take these medications chronically.[24] In ESRD patients, ACEIs have been shown to dramatically decrease mortality and are continued through the perioperative period.[25]

Patients with CKD are unable to adapt to large variations in salt intake and have impaired ability to concentrate or dilute their urine in response to fluctuations in systemic blood pressure. This impaired ability to excrete sodium, in addition to chronic anemia and often placement of arteriovenous fistula, predisposes patients to volume overload and becomes more relevant as CKD progresses.[3] The optimal volume status prior to surgery is dependent on the type of surgery and the estimate of anticipated fluid administration during surgery. If patients are hypervolemic prior to surgery or receive large volumes of fluid, pulmonary edema can develop immediately postoperatively. If patients are hypovolemic prior to surgery, they have increased rates of hypotension during surgery as a result of anesthesia-induced vasodilation and fluid shifts. Preventative strategies for postoperative complications regarding volume status in CKD patients thus involve achieving euvolemia prior to surgery and a careful discussion between nephrologists, surgeons, and anesthesiologists regarding volume status goals prior to procedures.

Hyperkalemia is one of the most dreaded and dangerous complications of CKD and ESRD in relation to surgery. Plasma potassium usually remains normal until stage 5 CKD due to increase in potassium secretion per functioning nephron and increased output in the stool; however, in the operative period, patients with CKD are at increased risk.[3] Hyperkalemia may be precipitated by blood transfusions, tissue breakdown, acidosis, beta-blockers, ACEIs, heparin, rhabdomyolysis, and the use of Ringer lactate solution. The potassium concentration acceptable prior to surgery depends on the urgency of the surgery. Although no recommendations exist for safe preoperative potassium values, 1 study suggests avoiding general anesthesia in patients with CKD who have a potassium level above 5.5 mEq/L. The type of surgery with respect to blood loss, fluid shifts, and acid-base disturbances all affect the rate of rise of serum potassium concentration.

CKD and ESRD patients are prone to hematologic complications due to 2 opposing mechanisms: bleeding and clotting. Anemia, platelet dysfunction, and hemodialysis itself all contribute to the pathogenesis behind bleeding in renal patients. Impaired adhesiveness and abnormal endothelial interactions both contribute to platelet defects seen in advanced renal failure. Multiple treatment strategies including renal replacement therapy, desmopressin, erythropoietin, estrogen, and cryoprecipitate have been used in the treatment of platelet dysfunction associated with CKD, but studies comparing their effectiveness are limited. Either hemodialysis or peritoneal dialysis can partially correct bleeding time in most uremic patients, although it is unclear whether the procedure actually decreases active bleeding or the risk of major bleeding. Desmopressin (ddAVP), an analog of antidiuretic hormone with little vasopressor activity, acts by stimulating the release of high molecular weight multimers of von Willebrand factor from endothelial cells. Simple and rapidly acting, it is often the first-line therapy used to treat bleeding associated with uremia; however, stores of von Willebrand factor may be depleted after repeated administration causing tachyphylaxis. Erythropoietin improves platelet function by correcting anemia and also directly increasing the number of GPIIb/IIIa receptors on platelets.[26] The improvement in platelet function persists for as long as the hemoglobin remains elevated (bleeding time is reduced because of displacement of platelets such that they are closer to the vascular endothelium). Conjugated estrogen has also been shown to decrease bleeding in both male and female CKD patients. It is thought to improves platelet reactivity by decreasing generation of nitric oxide, is dose dependent, and can be given intravenously, orally, subcutaneously, or transdermal. Finally, plasma extract rich in factor VIII, von Willebrand factor, fibrinogen, and fibronectin can cause rapid resolution of bleeding in uremic patients, but its use is also associated with infectious complications and, consequently, is often only given in life-threatening bleeding. The recommended options to protect CKD and ESRD patients prior to surgery from perioperative bleeding complications is by maintaining hematocrit levels greater than 30% through the use of erythropoietin and administering ddAVP in the perioperative period.[27]

Patients with CKD may also have difficult vascular access; however, safe surgery cannot be performed without reliable intravenous access in both the operative room and during the recovery period. Access should be considered and planned preoperatively as current or potential future fistula sites should be avoided. Use of the internal jugular veins is strongly favored over the subclavian veins because of the catastrophic consequences of catheter-induced subclavian venous stenosis, which may preclude any future vascular access on the ipsilateral side.[28]

Dialysis is usually scheduled 12 to 24 hours prior to surgery. Patients with peritoneal dialysis who are undergoing abdominal surgery should be switched to hemodialysis until wound healing is complete. For those undergoing nonabdominal surgery, peritoneal dialysis should be continued as much as possible.

CONCLUSION

Strategies to maintain renal protection are crucial for caring for patients with CKD in the perioperative setting to prevent complications and avoid progression of CKD. Although evidence is limited, in part due to the variability in defining AKI and the many comorbidities associated with CKD, some recommendations have persisted. First, patients with CKD should be identified through risk assessment and preoperative laboratory testing to clearly understand risk prior to surgery. Second, maintenance of hemodynamic stability and intravascular volume is crucial for patients with CKD to prevent further deterioration. Third, tight glycemic control is associated with less renal impairment and better survival for patients with CKD. To improve renal outcomes, nonemergent procedures should be postponed, renal function and volume status optimized, and nephrotoxic drugs avoided.[29]

REFERENCES

1. Hou SH, Bushinsky DA, Wish JB, Cohen JJ, Harrington JT. Hospital-acquired renal insufficiency: a prospective study. *Am J Med.* 1983;74:243–248.
2. Wasnick J, Butterworth J, Mackey D. Renal Physiology and Anesthesia. In: Butterworth JF, IV, Mackey DC, Wasnick JD, eds. *Morgan & Mikhail's Clinical Anesthesiology.* 5th ed. New York, NY: McGraw-Hill; 2013: Chapter 29.
3. Craig RG, Hunter JM. Recent developments in the perioperative management of adult patients with chronic kidney disease. *Br J Anaesth.* 2008;101:296–310.
4. Menitz PG, Krenn CG, Steltzer H, et al. Effect of acute renal failure requiring renal replacement therapy on outcome in critically ill patients. *Crit Care Med.* 2002;30:2051–2058.
5. Lassnigg A, Schmid ER, Hiesmayr M, et al. Impact of minimal increases in serum creatinine on outcome in patients after cardiothoracic surgery: do we have to revise current definitions of acute renal failure? *Crit Care Med.* 2008;36(4):1129–1137.
6. Brienza N, Giglio MT, Marucci M. Preventing acute kidney injury after noncardiac surgery. *Curr Opin Crit Care.* 2010;16:353–358.
7. Kheterpal S, Tremper KK, Heung M, et al. Development and validation of an acute kidney injury risk index for patients undergoing general surgery: results from a national data set. *Anesthesiology.* 2009;110:505–515.
8. Chertow GM, Lazarus JM, Christiansen CL, et al. Preoperative renal risk stratification. *Circulation.* 1997;95:878–884.
9. Zacharias M, Mugawar M, Herbison GP, Walker RJ, Hovhannisyan K, Sivalingam P, Conlon NP. Interventions for protecting renal function in the perioperative period. *Cochrane Db Syst. Rev.* 2013;(9):CD003590. doi: 10.1002/14651858. CD003590.pub4
10. Tang IY. Prevention of peroperative acute renal failure: what works? *Best Pract Res Clin Anesthesiol.* 2004;18(1):91–111.
11. Holte K, Sharrock NE, Kehlet H. Pathophysiology and clinical implications of perioperative fluid excess. *Br J Anaesth.* 2002;89(4):622–632.
12. Mutter TC, Ruth CA, Dart AB. Hydroxyethyl starch (HES) versus other fluid therapies: effects on kidney function. *Cochrane Db Sys Rev.* 2013;23(7):CD007594.

13. Chronic kidney disease (CKD). National Kidney Foundation. http://www.kidney.org/kidneyDisease/ ckd/index.cfm

14. Athyros VG, Hatzitolios AI, Karagiannis A, et al.; IMPERATIVE Collaborative Group. Improving the implementation of current guidelines for the management of major coronary heart disease risk factors by multifactorial intervention: the IMPERTIVE renal analysis. *Arch Med Sci.* 2011,7:984–992.

15. Shermin D, Bostom AG, Laliberty P, Dworkin LD. Residual renal function and mortality risk in hemodialysis patients. *Am J Kidney Dis.* 2001;38 (1):85–90.

16. Silberberg JS, Barre PE, Prichard SS, Sniderman AD. Impact of left ventricular hypertrophy on survival in end-stage renal disease. *Kidney Int.* 1989;36(2):286–290.

17. Ellenberger C, Tait G, Beattie WS. Chronic β blockade is associated with a better outcome after elective noncardiac surgery than acute β blockade: a single-center propensity-matched cohort study. *Anesthesiology.* 2011;114(4): 817–823.

18. Devereaux PJ, Yang H, Yusuf S, et al.; POISE Study Group. Effects of extended-release metoprolol succinate in patients undergoing non-cardiac surgery (POISE trial): a randomized controlled trial. *Lancet.* 2008;371(9627):1839–1847.

19. Devereaux PJ, Mrkobrada M, Sessler DI, et al.; POISE-2 Investigators. Aspirin in patients undergoing noncardiac surgery. *N Engl J Med.* 2014; 370(16):1494–1503.

20. Antoniou GA, Hajibandeh S, Hajibandeh S, Vallabhaneni SR, Brennan JA, Torella F. Meta-analysis of the effects of statins on perioperative outcomes in vascular and endovascular surgery. *J Vasc Surg.* 2015;61(2):519–532.

21. Wanner C, Krane V, März W, et al.; German Diabetes and Dialysis Study Investigators. Atorvastatin in patients with type 2 diabetes mellitus undergoing hemodialysis. *N Engl J Med.* 2005;353(3):238–248.

22. Fellström BC, Jardine AG, Schmieder RE, et al.; AURORA Study Group. Rosuvastatin and cardiovascular events in patients undergoing hemodialysis. *N Engl J Med.* 2009;360(14):1395–1407.

23. Nemerovski CW1, Lekura J, Cefaretti M, Mehta PT, Moore CL. Safety and efficacy of statins in patients with end-stage renal disease. *Ann Pharmacother.* 2013;47(10):1321–1329.

24. Roshanov PS, Rochwerg B, Patel A, et al. Withholding versus continuing angiotensin-converting enzyme inhibitors or angiotensin II receptor blockers before noncardiac surgery: an analysis of the vascular events in noncardiac surgery patients cohort evaluation prospective cohort. *Anesthesiology.* 2017;126 (1):16–27.

25. Efrati S, Zaidenstein R, Dishy V, et al. ACE inhibitors and survival of hemodialysis patients. *Am J Kidney Dis.* 2002;40(5):1023–1029.

26. Osikov MV. Effect of erythropoietin on free radical oxidation and glycoprotein expression in platelets under conditions of chronic renal failure. *Bull Exp Biol Med.* 2014;157(1):25–27.

27. Kaw D, Malhotra D. Hematology: issues in the dialysis patient. *Sem Dialy.* 2006;19(4):317–322.

28. Friedman, AL. Management of the surgical patient with end-stage renal disease. *Hemodial Int.* 2003;7(3):250–255.

29. Meersh M, Schmidt C, Zarbock A. Patient with chronic renal failure undergoing surgery. *Curr Opinion Anesthesiol.* 2016;29 (3):413–420.

16

Renal Protection in Critically Ill Patients

RYAN W. HAINES AND JOHN R. PROWLE

EPIDEMIOLOGY OF ACUTE KIDNEY INJURY IN THE INTENSIVE CARE UNIT

Since the development and widespread adoption of consensus definitions of acute kidney injury (AKI),[1] over the last years there has been increased recognition of the incidence of even mild AKI. The current KDIGO AKI classification[1] incorporates creatinine changes, urine output data, and need for renal replacement therapy (RRT) to define and stage AKI (Table 16.1). AKI affects more than 50% of patients admitted to the intensive care unit (ICU)[2,3] and is strongly associated with short-term risk of death during critical illness. Our increasing awareness of AKI has been accompanied by recognition of the association of AKI with long-term complications and increased healthcare costs in the community.[2,4,5]

Patients with severe AKI requiring RRT in ICU have been shown to have mortality over 50% during their acute hospitalization and, if they survive, remain at increased risk of mortality and chronic RRT in the longer term[6,7]. However, adverse long-term effects aren't confined to dialysis-requiring AKI; even small rises in creatinine, classified as KDIGO stage 1, have been linked with worse mortality up to 10 years post discharge.[8] In particular, epidemiological research has identified an association with AKI in the ICU and worsening long-term renal function leading to the concept of AKI and CKD as interconnected syndromes and of CKD as a potential mediator of the increased mortality in this population.[9-14]

Importantly, AKI is a clinical syndrome not a unique disease entity. AKI cases in the ICU are of mixed etiology and varying severity. The commonest associations of AKI complicating critical illness are sepsis, major surgery, cardiogenic shock, hypovolemia, and nephrotoxin exposure.[15]

However, these conditions often co-exist and occur on the background of predisposing risk factors, the most significant of which are older age and pre-existing CKD.[10]

PREVENTION VERSUS TREATMENT OF AKI

Despite better definition and early recognition of AKI and proliferation of research, the prevention and treatment of AKI has remained limited to supportive care and prevention of secondary kidney injury with no evidence for any specific interventions to alter the course of AKI. Consequently, AKI-associated mortality in the ICU has remained largely static.[16] Importantly, a large proportion of critical care patients already have established or evolving AKI at ICU admission. Often, even if patients do not have AKI by current definitions, they may already have established subclinical kidney injury. It takes time for creatinine to rise after an abrupt change in glomerular filtration rate (GFR), and the rate of these changes are dependent not only on the severity of renal dysfunction but on acute and chronic determinants of muscle mass and creatinine generation, which will be reduced with older age and chronic illness and may be further decreased in acute illness.[17,18] Therefore, apparently mild AKI may represent significant renal dysfunction particularly in the acutely unwell, highlighting the importance of early recognition of AKI risk factors. This may explain the failure of interventions targeted at altering the course of AKI and emphasizes the importance of treatment of the underlying etiology, such as sepsis, and avoidance of secondary kidney injury.

The delay in creatinine-based diagnosis has led to the search for AKI biomarkers more sensitive to tubular injury early in the time-course of AKI.[19,20] Such biomarkers would enrich a group

TABLE 16.1 KIDNEY DISEASE IMPROVING GLOBAL OUTCOMES (KDIGO) 2012 CRITERIA FOR DIAGNOSIS AND STAGING OF ACUTE KIDNEY INJURY IN ADULTS

Stage	Serum Creatinine	Urine Output
1	increase ≥ 26 µmol/L within 48 hours or increase ≥1.5 to 1.9 X reference SCr	<0.5 mL/kg/hr for >6 consecutive hrs
2	increase ≥ 2 to 2.9 X reference SCr	<0.5 mL/kg/hr for >12 hrs
3	increase ≥3 X reference SCr or increase of ≥ 26 µmol/L to ≥354 µmol/L or commenced on renal replacement therapy regardless of stage	<0.3 mL/kg/hr for >24 hrs or anuria for 12 hrs

SCr = serum creatinine.
Source: Kidney Disease Improving Global Outcomes. KDIGO clinical practice guideline for acute kidney injury: section 2. AKI definition. *Kidney Int Suppl.* 2012;2(1):19–36.

of patients who might benefit from early initiation of reno-protective measures or targeted interventions. Despite many years of research, there is continued uncertainty regarding the clinical application of AKI biomarkers.[19,21] However, recently, urinary biomarkers insulin-like growth factor-binding protein 7 and tissue inhibitor of metalloproteinases-2 have been used to select high-risk cardiac surgery patients to receive a bundle of kidney-directed care (Fig. 16.1)[22] involving hemodynamic optimization and avoidance of nephrotoxins which reduced the short-term incidence of post-operative AKI.[23] While these results require extensive validation, they do suggest a potential role for novel biomarkers in risk stratification for protective intervention,[22] and it is likely that further studies following this template may alter practice and provide an evidence-base for novel AKI diagnostics in the next few years. However, at present, given the difficulty in establishing early diagnosis and near ubiquitous nature of AKI risk factors in critical illness, renal protection in the ICU remains focused on secondary prevention of further kidney injury and supportive management of the wider effects of multiorgan dysfunction.

NONDIALYTIC MANAGEMENT OF AKI IN CRITICAL ILLNESS

As indicated, no specific treatments exist proven to modify the clinical course of the common causes of AKI complicating critical illness. However, while less common, consideration of diagnoses such as urinary outflow obstruction, systemic vasculitis, or thrombotic microangiopathy in patients presenting with AKI and critical illness should not be neglected as disease-specific management strategies would then be indicated. A thorough clinical history and examination, with appreciation of atypical features, such as complete anuria, disproportionate severity of AKI to the clinical context, renal dysfunction that precedes the systemic illness, and major proteinuria and hematuria are the most important steps in recognizing a specific renal diagnosis, directing specialist investigations and appropriate referral.

In the most common situation of critical illness-associated tubular injury, delay in diagnosis and imprecision around severity of AKI contributes to the uncertainty faced by clinicians. Current management strategies (Fig. 16.2) based on low-grade evidence and expert consensus[1] add to this uncertainty. Within this framework, careful titration of hemodynamic interventions with fluid and vasoactive drugs to maintain "adequate" blood pressure and cardiac output, alongside the avoidance of exposure to unnecessary nephrotoxins are the cornerstone of management.

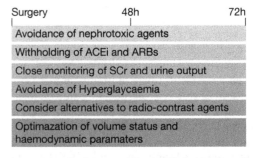

FIGURE 16.1 The "KDIGO care bundle" to reduce the risk of acute kidney injury among high-risk patients who have undergone cardiac surgery. ACEIs = angiotensin converting enzyme inhibitors. ARBs = angiotensin II receptor blockers. SCr = serum creatinine. From Kellum JA. Acute kidney injury: AKI: the myth of inevitability is finally shattered. *Nat Rev Nephrol.* 2017;13(3):140–141.

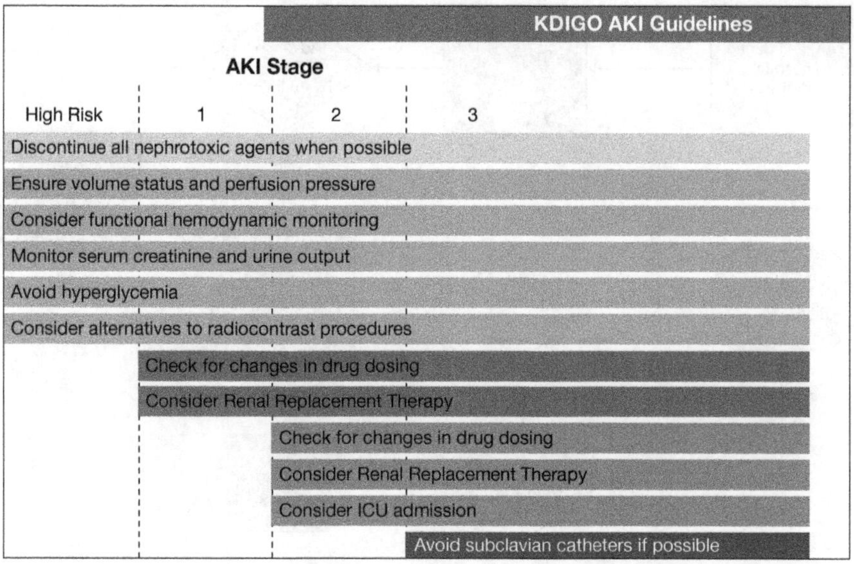

FIGURE 16.2 Summary of Kidney Disease Improving Global Outcomes (KDIGO) 2012 recommendations for the management of patients with or at risk of acute kidney injury (AKI). Recommendations are predominantly based on expert recommendation for close monitoring, supportive hemodynamic management, and avoidance of secondary organ injury. From: Kidney Disease Improving Global Outcomes. KDIGO clinical practice guideline for acute kidney injury: section 2. AKI definition. *Kidney Int Suppl.* 2012;2(1):19–36.

Fluid Therapy

Fluid volume resuscitation to maintain renal blood flow is considered an essential intervention in preventing further renal damage in many clinical scenarios. However, with improved knowledge on the pathophysiology of AKI, other processes such as inflammation have proven to be as important as global renal ischemia limiting the potential treatment effect of fluid therapy.[24] In line with this observation, in 3 large goal-direct therapy trials in sepsis, no proven benefit of protocolled fluid resuscitation and inotrope use was seen in the incidence of AKI or need for RRT.[25] Furthermore, traditional targets for fluid resuscitation such as lactate and central venous pressure have not been shown to consistently improve renal perfusion, especially in sepsis.[26,27] Indeed, ongoing administration of fluid and the development of a positive fluid balance may be associated with renal harm by the development of renal interstitial edema and venous congestion, limiting renal blood flow and oxygen delivery.[28,29] In this context, the CLASSIC trial[30] has recently demonstrated the feasibility and safety of a more restrictive fluid resuscitation regime for critically ill patients with septic shock. Importantly, while not a primary outcome in that study, there was a significantly lower number of patients with worsening AKI with more restrictive fluid resuscitation. This finding suggests that, in contrast to traditional clinical instincts, optimal renal protection may be worsened by overzealous use of intravenous fluids (Fig. 16.3).

The composition of intravenous fluids administered prior to ICU admission and within the ICU is an important consideration in renal protection. Evidence has mounted against the use of hydroxyethyl starch solutions in patients with or at risk of AKI.[31] However, there remains debate regarding the relative merits of colloids versus crystalloids in general. Overall, within the timescale of critical illness, there are few proven benefits of colloids over crystalloid, and both fluids were shown to leave the circulation within hours with little difference in the amount of fluids required when compared in a blinded fashion.[32,33] The use of balanced versus unbuffered crystalloid solutions is another area of debate. Interventional and observational studies have shown decreased incidence of AKI and need for RRT with balanced solutions.[34,35] The physiological basis for the potential harm of unbuffered crystalloids, most commonly 0.9% sodium chloride, is the development of hyperchloremia and associated metabolic acidosis. However, the SPLIT study,[36] a cluster randomized trial of buffered versus

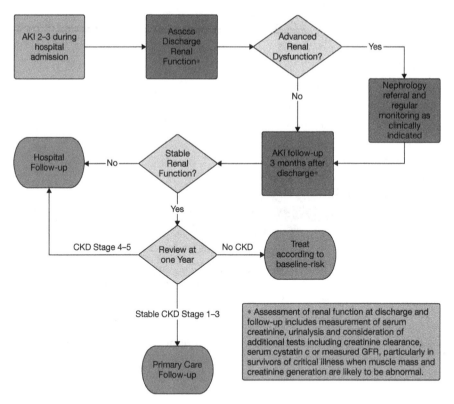

FIGURE 16.3 Potential scheme for follow-up of acute kidney injury (AKI) stages 2 and 3 complicating critical illness. Serial assessments at 3 months and 1 year after AKI are required to establish the presence and severity of chronic kidney disease (CKD) and establish prognosis. In most cases, long-term follow-up and treatment can be achieved outside of specialist nephrology services following CKD management guidelines. GFR = glomerular filtration rate. From Forni LG, Darmon M, Ostermann M, et al. Renal recovery after acute kidney injury. *Intensive Care Med.* 2017;43(6):855–866.

unbuffered crystalloids use in the ICU, did not show any increase in the need for RRT with use of 0.9% saline. A limitation of the SPLIT study is the relatively small volumes of fluid administered to most patients, and further trials are ongoing in this area.[37]

Vasopressor Therapy in AKI

The administration of vasopressors such as norepinephrine is a routine response to hypotension in the ICU. Historical concerns about the damage such drugs could inflict on renal tissue by reducing renal perfusion do not appear sustained when targeting mean arterial pressures (MAPs) up to 75 mmHg.[38] In patients with existing hypertension, targeting a higher MAP of 80 to 85 mmHg during vasodilatory shock has been shown to improve renal outcomes but not overall survival.[39] Thus, when setting blood pressure targets for vasopressors, tailored therapy

accounting for the patients pre-existing medical conditions and the clinical context may be beneficial. However, in younger patients and those without pre-existing hypertension, there is little evidence to support pursuing a MAP >65. Further studies are planned and ongoing to examine the benefits of a higher MAP in patients with chronic hypertension and to better define ideal blood pressure targets for the general critical care population.[40] Finally, while higher blood pressure targets are conceivably of benefit in lowing risk of severe AKI, no MAP targets have been identified that render survival benefits to patients requiring RRT, particularly if higher doses of vasopressors are required.

Specific Pharmacological Interventions for AKI

Despite demonstration of no renal protective benefit from for low "renal-dose" dopamine in critically ill patients in 2000,[41] many other pharmacological interventions targeting the renal circulation or inflammatory mechanisms have been developed and tested, with no clear evidence of clinical effectiveness even when used in the optimal contexts.[42-44] More recently, the early use of vasopressin over norepinephrine septic shock with vasodilatory hypotension has been examined in a multicenter randomized controlled trial (RCT). While there was no difference in the primary renal outcome, there was significantly less use of RRT in the vasopressin group than in the norepinephrine group.[45] A benefit of the ionodilatory calcium sensitizer, levosimendan, in reducing the incidence of AKI was suggested in a meta-analysis of studies in cardiac surgery.[46] However, in a large multicenter RCT of levosimendan in sepsis, there was no difference in renal outcomes.[47] Thus, currently there is no clear evidence to suggest benefit of any specific vasopressors or inotropes to achieve hemodynamic targets in patients with or at risk of AKI in the ICU.

Management of Potential Nephrotoxins

Consensus guidelines recommend avoidance of nephrotoxins in patients with or at risk of AKI, while some agents such as nonsteroidal anti-inflammatories or antihypertensive targeting the renin–angiotensin–aldosterone system can simply be omitted, other agents such as nephrotoxic antimicrobial and radiological contrast may be required for treatment of the primary condition. A risk–benefit analysis will need to consider necessary nephrotoxic treatment and its alternatives in the context of the illness. For antibiotics such as aminoglycoside and glycopeptides, appropriate therapeutic drug monitoring is essential to ensure adequate therapy and minimize toxicity. A particular problem during critical illness is difficulty in determining the current level of renal function for initial dosing as formula-based approaches to estimation of GFR or creatinine clearance are invalid in critical illness both due to lack of steady state and reduction in creatinine production. Use of filtration markers such as Cystatin C, which is less confounded by metabolic changes associated with critical illness, has been shown to improve achievement of target vancomycin concentrations in the ICU, potentially improving both therapeutic efficacy while minimizing nephrotoxicity.[48] In the case of intravenous contrast, the evidence for effective interventions in the critically ill population is very limited. In general, it is suggested that nonurgent contrast-enhanced investigations or interventions not be delayed for potential preventative measures of uncertain benefit.[49] Indeed, given the multiple AKI risk factors present in most ICU patients, the significance of contrast-associated nephropathy may be overstated in the critically ill[50] and more general patient population.[51] Correcting hypovolemia or dehydration using isotonic crystalloids is the only recommended renal protective measure for patients receiving intravascular contrast media during critical illness.[49] Importantly this does not mean that all patients should be given fluids, unlike the outpatient populations where this evidence base was established, most critically ill patients and those with AKI in particular, are overhydrated and intravenous fluids prophylaxis should not be at the expense of significant worsening of fluid overload.

RENAL PROTECTION IN SPECIFIC CAUSES OF AKI IN THE ICU

Rhabdomyolysis

There are multiple causes of rhabdomyolysis in critically ill patients involving damage to muscle tissue from both traumatic and nontraumatic insults.[52] AKI occurs in 13% to 50% of patients with rhabdomyolysis[52,53]; however, multiple mechanisms may underlie the development of AKI, including myoglobin related intrarenal vasoconstriction, direct tubular toxicity, and tubular obstruction as well as other AKI etiologies including hypovolemia and systemic inflammation. A creatine kinase level of greater than 5,000 U/L is widely agreed as an indicator for significant muscle injury.[54] However, such findings are relatively common in the critically ill, with only a minority suffering overt clinical rhabdomyolysis.

Once rhabdomyolysis is suspected, a careful search should be undertaken to remove the underlying cause and limit further muscle injury. This might involve surgical decompression of a compartment syndrome or withdrawal of a precipitating drug. Protocolled fluid replacement is the mainstay of nonspecific renal protective treatment, albeit without strong prospective evidence, aiming to replace fluid sequestered into damaged muscle and to dilute the nephrotoxic effects of myoglobin.[55,56] Typical goals of fluid administration are to maintain a high urine output (greater than 2mL/kg/h ideal body weight) and to achieve an alkaline urine (pH greater than 6) to limit the toxicity of myoglobin.[56,57] Importantly, while fluid treatment is considered beneficial, given the established adverse effects of fluid overload if oliguria is refractory to medical therapy, intravenous fluid should be ceased and RRT used to control fluid balance if clinically indicated. Finally, there is limited evidence for the use of RRT beyond treating the traditional complications of AKI.[58] The efficient removal of myoglobin (17.8 kDa protein) by using highly permeable membranes or absorptive techniques is an area of ongoing research but is not an established therapy.[59]

Liver Disease and Hepatorenal Syndrome

Hepatorenal syndrome (HRS) is a unique form of AKI that has specific clinical challenges and treatment options. The underlying pathophysiology of HRS is complex with vasomotor and non-vasomotor components.[60] Clinically divided into type 1 (acute onset) and type 2 HRS (progressive course), the diagnosis traditionally hinges on the presence of cirrhosis and strict exclusion of other causes of AKI such as shock. More recently, however, there has been a move toward a broader consideration of AKI in advanced liver disease accepting the multiple and overlapping etiologies of AKI.[61,62] Consequently management of AKI in liver disease involves many of the broad strategies for AKI in the critically ill alongside consideration of specific interventions. One area is the specific focus on renal perfusion where—for example, in type 1 HRS—there is evidence for the use of terlipressin[63,64] (available in Europe, but not currently in the United States) or other vasopressors[65] in combination with intravascular volume expansion with 20% albumin to reduce pathological splanchnic vasodilatation, improve renal function, and possibly reduce mortality. As terlipressin has potentially significant side effects, notably organ ischemia, therapy should be monitored closely and discontinued if there is no response. Finally, in patients with tense ascites, the role of elevated intra-abdominal pressure (IAP) should be considered, as outlined more generally in the following discussion, with therapeutic paracentesis alongside appropriate volume expansion with albumin being a potential therapeutic option.[66]

Increased Intra-Abdominal Pressure

Intra-abdominal hypertension is defined as a sustained IAP of greater than 12 mmHg. Its presence has been shown to reduce microcirculatory flow through venous congestion and negatively impact the function of abdominal organs including the kidney.[67] Studies have shown an independent association between raised IAP and AKI.[68] Clinicians need to be alert to those patients most at risk of raised IAP including abdominal surgery, trauma, ileus, pancreatitis abdominal wall burns, and gross fluid overload in general. Measurement of IAP via the bladder remains the recommended approach to confirm a diagnosis in high-risk patients, but it requires careful positioning and sedation to achieve accurate readings.[69] Treatment may be medical, with vasopressors to maintain abdominal perfusion pressure and diuretics or ultrafiltration to treat fluid overload and reduce venous congestion, or surgical, with abdominal decompression. In abdominal compartment syndrome, defined by the presence of an IAP greater than 20 mmHg and new organ failure, surgical intervention should be strongly considered.[69]

RENAL REPLACEMENT THERAPY

RRT is required in 8% to 12% of critically ill patients, with both intermittent hemodialysis (IHD) and continuous RRT (CRRT) in use across the world.[3] CRRT is the recommended modality of choice for hemodynamically unstable patients in ICU in the latest consensus guidelines.[1,70] Despite lack of evidence for benefit of CRRT over IHD in terms of survival or renal outcomes in small randomized trials, in practice, it is very difficult to effectively treat the sickest critically ill patients with an intermittent therapy. Furthermore, there is now extensive epidemiological evidence from multicenter prospective observational studies[71,72] and meta-analysis of observational data[73] that first use of IHD to treat AKI in the ICU is associated with an increased risk of nonrecovery of renal function and progression to end-stage renal disease in survivors. It is hypothesized intermittent episodes of relative hypovolemia during IHD cause recurrent injury to the injured and recovering kidney, compromising long-term recovery. However, in the absence of multicenter prospective randomized studies, the exact benefits of CRRT over IHD, if any, remain controversial, and some centers do report good results from IHD in selected patients.[74] As well as modality, there is still a wide variation in its timing and delivery of RRT in the ICU. Balancing the need for RRT to treat AKI and its complications, such as fluid overload, with the risks associated with an invasive intervention remains a topic of debate. The only large multicenter RCT[75] examining RRT timing based on AKI diagnostic criteria did not demonstrate benefit from earlier RRT; however, such benefit has been suggested in a single center study[76] with other trials ongoing. Other aspects of RRT and their effect on renal outcome are summarized in Table 16.2. Overall, a number of aspects of RRT provided in the ICU have been hypothesized to

TABLE 16.2 RENAL REPLACEMENT THERAPY CHARACTERISTICS THAT MIGHT AFFECT RECOVERY FROM ACUTE KIDNEY INJURY AS ADJUDGED BY THE ACUTE DISEASE QUALITY INITIATIVE EXPERT CONSENSUS WORKGROUP

RRT Characteristic	Effect on Renal Recovery	Effect on Patient Recovery
Modality (intermittent, prolonged intermittent, continuous, peritoneal)[a]	Intermittent RRT might delay recovery	No effect
Fluid purity and quality standards	Dialysate purity might affect recovery	No effect
Membrane type[b]	Bioincompatible membranes might delay recovery	Bioincompatible membranes might affect recovery
Anticoagulation	No reported effect on recovery	Uncertain effect
Haemodynamic stability[c]	Hypotension might delay recovery	Uncertain effect
Mode of solute clearance (diffusion or convection)[d]	No evidence of effect	No evidence of effect
Ultrafiltration rate	Rapid fluid removal might delay recovery by causing hypotension	No data
Fluid Balance[e]	A positive fluid balance during RRT might delay recovery	A positive fluid balance during RRT might delay recovery
Dialysate temperature	A cooler dialysate sodium concentrations might minimize hypotension and thereby promote recovery	No data
Dialysate composition	Higher dialysate temperature might minimize hypotension and thereby promote recovery	No data
Effect of RRT on other care parameters	RRT might affect drug dosing, nutritional support, and nephrotoxin accumulation, which might affect recovery	RRT might affect drug dosing, nutritional support, and nephrotoxin accumulation, which might affect recovery
RRT components (e.g., access, circuit, fluid composition)	Possible adverse effect	Unknown
Dose/intensity (i.e., small solute, clearance)[f]	Level 1 evidence that intensity of solute control does not affect recovery	Level 1 evidence that intensity of solute control does not affect recovery

[a]Only association studies; one RCT.
[b]Bioincompatible membranes are no longer in use.
[c]Based on association.
[d]Small underpowered RCTs.
[e]independent association.
[f]No effect of small solute control in two large RCTs.
RRT = renal replacement therapy. RCT = randomized controlled trial.
Source: Chawla LS, Bellomo R, Bihorac A, et al. Acute kidney disease and renal recovery: consensus report of the Acute Disease Quality Initiative (ADQI) 16 Workgroup. *Nat Rev Nephrol*. 2017;13(4):241–257.

be associated with improved renal outcomes via improved hemodynamic stability during therapy and avoidance of secondary renal injury in recovery (Table 16.2). However, it is unlikely that high-quality mortality data from randomized trials will come available to guide many important aspects of RRT, such as choice of modality, as the size of properly powered studies would be unfeasible.[73] Thus, many treatment recommendations are likely to remain based on physiological arguments and epidemiological evidence. In these arguments, the deleterious effects of fluid accumulation and fluid overload on both renal outcomes and mortality are of key importance.[77] The role of CRRT in more precisely controlling fluid balance in ICU patients is an emerging area. Evidence in pediatric population suggests a harmful effect of allowing 10% to 20% fluid accumulation from admission to ICU with the suggestion that in this context the degree of fluid overload is a valid trigger for RRT initiation.[78]

DIAGNOSIS OF LONG-TERM RENAL DYSFUNCTION

Attention to renal protection for the critically ill patient with AKI should not cease at ICU discharge. Despite growing evidence on the link between AKI and CKD, long-term follow-up of patients after AKI in critical care is limited.[79] The role of outpatient follow-up should extend beyond renal function measurements and include modification of cardiovascular risk factors and assessment of quality of life indicators—both of which have been shown to be affected in survivors of an AKI episode.[4] However, there is still uncertainty on how to best implement a follow-up strategy.[80] Diagnosing long-term renal dysfunction can be difficult after critical illness as loss of muscle mass and creatinine generation falsely elevates estimated GFR at ICU and hospital discharge.[81-83] Given these concerns, measuring creatinine at least 3 months after hospital discharge should be a minimum in patients with significant AKI in the ICU, irrespective of apparent recovery. Whether this follow-up is performed by primary care physician, intensivist, or nephrologist will depend on resources and the care environment. A proposed pathway to invite all patients with an episode of AKI back to a follow-up clinic 3 to 6 months after hospital discharge, measuring estimated GFR and proteinuria and then discharging or referring patients further depending on their CKD category.[84] However, even this approach may still miss

the longer term increased risk of CKD, and all survivors of AKI stages 2 and 3 should consider ongoing yearly assessment of renal function in primary care. Other renal filtration markers that are less dependent on muscle mass may have a role in this group of patients. Cystatin C, a renal filtration marker less dependent on muscle mass, may improve the diagnosis of CKD[85] particularly after critical illness.[83]

REFERENCES

1. Kidney Disease Improving Global Outcomes. KDIGO clinical practice guideline for acute kidney injury: section 2. AKI definition. *Kidney Int Suppl*. 2012;2(1):19–36.
2. Ostermann M, Chang RW. Acute kidney injury in the intensive care unit according to RIFLE. *Crit Care Med*. 2007;35(8):1837–1843; quiz 1852.
3. Hoste EA, Bagshaw SM, Bellomo R, et al. Epidemiology of acute kidney injury in critically ill patients: the multinational AKI-EPI study. *Intensive Care Med*. 2015;41(8):1411–1423.
4. Chawla LS, Amdur RL, Shaw AD, Faselis C, Palant CE, Kimmel PL. Association between AKI and long-term renal and cardiovascular outcomes in United States veterans. *Clin J Am Soc Nephrol*. 2014;9(3):448–456.
5. Kerr M, Bedford M, Matthews B, O'Donoghue D. The economic impact of acute kidney injury in England. *Nephrol Dial Transplant*. 2014;29(7):1362–1368.
6. De Corte W, Dhondt A, Vanholder R, et al. Long-term outcome in ICU patients with acute kidney injury treated with renal replacement therapy: a prospective cohort study. *Crit Care*. 2016;20(1):256.
7. Wald R, Quinn RR, Luo J, et al. Chronic dialysis and death among survivors of acute kidney injury requiring dialysis. *J Am Med Assoc*. 2009;302(11):1179–1185.
8. Linder A, Fjell C, Levin A, Walley KR, Russell JA, Boyd JH. Small acute increases in serum creatinine are associated with decreased long-term survival in the critically ill. *Am J Respir Crit Care Med*. 2014;189(9):1075–1081.
9. Jones J, Holmen J, De Graauw J, Jovanovich A, Thornton S, Chonchol M. Association of complete recovery from acute kidney injury with incident CKD stage 3 and all-cause mortality. *Am J Kidney Dis*. 2012;60(3):402–408.
10. Chawla LS, Eggers PW, Star RA, Kimmel PL. Acute kidney injury and chronic kidney disease as interconnected syndromes. *N Engl J Med*. 2014;371(1):58–66.
11. Horne KL, Packington R, Monaghan J, Reilly T, Selby NM. Three-year outcomes after acute kidney

injury: results of a prospective parallel group co-hort study. *BMJ Open.* 2017;7(3):e015316.

12. Walcher A, Faubel S, Keniston A, Dennen P. In critically ill patients requiring CRRT, AKI is asso-ciated with increased respiratory failure and death versus ESRD. *Ren Fail.* 2011;33(10):935–942.

13. Chertow GM, Burdick E, Honour M, Bonventre JV, Bates DW. Acute kidney injury, mortality, length of stay, and costs in hospitalized patients. *J Am Soc Nephrol.* 2005;16(11):3365–3370.

14. Hoste EAJ, Clermont G, Kersten A, et al. RIFLE criteria for acute kidney injury are associated with hospital mortality in critically ill patients: a cohort analysis. *Crit Care.* 2006;10(3):R73.

15. Uchino S, Kellum JA, Bellomo R, et al. Acute renal failure in critically ill patients: a multi-national, multicenter study. *J Am Med Assoc.* 2005;294(7):813–818.

16. Hoste EA, Clermont G, Kersten A, et al. RIFLE criteria for acute kidney injury are associated with hospital mortality in critically ill patients: a cohort analysis. *Crit Care.* 2006;10(3):R73.

17. Schetz M, Gunst J, Van den Berghe G. The impact of using estimated GFR versus creatinine clear-ance on the evaluation of recovery from acute kidney injury in the ICU. *Intensive Care Med.* 2014;40(11):1709–1717.

18. Pickering JW, Ralib AM, Endre ZH. Combining creatinine and volume kinetics identifies missed cases of acute kidney injury following cardiac ar-rest. *Crit Care.* 2013;17(1):R7.

19. Ostermann M, Joannidis M. Biomarkers for AKI improve clinical practice: no. *Intensive Care Med.* 2015;41(4):618–622.

20. Pickkers P, Ostermann M, Joannidis M, et al. The intensive care medicine agenda on acute kidney injury. *Intensive Care Med.* 2017;43(9):1198–1209.

21. Endre ZH, Walker RJ, Pickering JW, et al. Early in-tervention with erythropoietin does not affect the outcome of acute kidney injury (the EARLYARF trial). *Kidney Int.* 2010;77(11):1020–1030.

22. Kellum JA. Acute kidney injury: AKI: the myth of inevitability is finally shattered. *Nat Rev Nephrol.* 2017;13(3):140–141.

23. Meersch M, Schmidt C, Hoffmeier A, et al. Prevention of cardiac surgery-associated AKI by implementing the KDIGO guidelines in high risk patients identified by biomarkers: the PrevAKI randomized controlled trial. *Intensive Care Med.* 2017;43(11):1551–1561.

24. Lipcsey M, Bellomo R. Septic acute kidney in-jury: hemodynamic syndrome, inflammatory dis-order, or both? *Crit Care.* 2011;15(6):1008.

25. Kellum JA, Chawla LS, Keener C, et al. The Effects of Alternative Resuscitation Strategies on Acute Kidney Injury in Patients with Septic Shock. *Am J Respir Crit Care Med.* 2016;193(3):281–287.

26. Di Giantomasso D, May CN, Bellomo R. Vital organ blood flow during hyperdynamic sepsis. *Chest.* 2003;124:1053–1059.

27. Ruokonen E. Regional blood flow and ox-ygen transport in septic shock. *Crit Care Med.* 1993;21:1296–1303.

28. Firth JD, Raine AE, Ledingham JG. Raised venous pressure: a direct cause of renal sodium retention in oedema? *Lancet.* 1988;1(8593):1033–1035.

29. Legrand M, Dupuis C, Simon C, et al. Association between systemic hemodynamics and septic acute kidney injury in critically ill patients: a retrospective observational study. *Crit Care.* 2013;17(6):R278.

30. Hjortrup PB, Haase N, Bundgaard H, et al. Restricting volumes of resuscitation fluid in adults with septic shock after initial manage-ment: the CLASSIC randomised, parallel-group, multicentre feasibility trial. *Intensive Care Med.* 2016;42(11):1695–1705.

31. Haase N, Perner A, Hennings LI, et al. Hydroxyethyl starch 130/0.38-0.45 versus crys-talloid or albumin in patients with sepsis: system-atic review with meta-analysis and trial sequential analysis. *Brit Med J.* 2013;346:f839.

32. Jungheinrich C, Neff TA. Pharmacokinetics of hydroxyethyl starch. *Clin Pharm.* 2005;44(7):681–699.

33. Finfer S, Bellomo R, Boyce N, et al. A compar-ison of albumin and saline for fluid resuscita-tion in the intensive care unit. *N Engl J Med.* 2004;350(22):2247–2256.

34. Shaw AD, Bagshaw SM, Goldstein SL, et al. Major complications, mortality, and resource utilization after open abdominal surgery: 0.9% saline compared to Plasma-Lyte. *Ann Surg.* 2012;255(5):821–829.

35. Yunos NM, Bellomo R, Hegarty C, Story D, Ho L, Bailey M. Association between a chloride-liberal vs chloride-restrictive intravenous fluid adminis-tration strategy and kidney injury in critically ill adults. *J Am Med Assoc.* 2012;308(15):1566–1572.

36. Young P, Bailey M, Beasley R, et al. Effect of a Buffered Crystalloid Solution vs Saline on Acute Kidney Injury Among Patients in the Intensive Care Unit: The SPLIT Randomized Clinical Trial. *J Am Med Assoc.* 2015;314(16):1701–1710.

37. Semler MW, Self WH, Wang L, et al. Balanced crystalloids versus saline in the intensive care unit: study protocol for a cluster-randomized, multiple-crossover trial. *Trials.* 2017;18(1):129.

38. Redfors B, Bragadottir G, Sellgren J, Sward K, Ricksten SE. Effects of norepinephrine on renal perfusion, filtration and oxygenation in

vasodilatory shock and acute kidney injury. *Intensive Care Med.* 2011;37(1):60–67.

39. Asfar P, Meziani F, Hamel JF, et al. High versus low blood-pressure target in patients with septic shock. *N Engl J Med.* 2014;370(17):1583–1593.

40. Lamontagne F, Meade MO, Hébert PC, et al. Higher versus lower blood pressure targets for vasopressor therapy in shock: a multicentre pilot randomized controlled trial. *Intensive Care Med.* 2016;42(4):542–550.

41. Bellomo R, Chapman M, Finfer S, Hickling K, Myburgh J. Low-dose dopamine in patients with early renal dysfunction: a placebo-controlled randomised trial. Australian and New Zealand Intensive Care Society (ANZICS) Clinical Trials Group. *Lancet.* 2000;356(9248):2139–2143.

42. Park JH, Shim JK, Song JW, Soh S, Kwak YL. Effect of atorvastatin on the incidence of acute kidney injury following valvular heart surgery: a randomized, placebo-controlled trial. *Intensive Care Med.* 2016;42(9):1398–1407.

43. Bove T, Zangrillo A, Guarracino F, et al. Effect of fenoldopam on use of renal replacement therapy among patients with acute kidney injury after cardiac surgery: a randomized clinical trial. *J Am Med Assoc.* 2014;312(21):2244–2253.

44. Garg AX, Kurz A, Sessler DI, et al. Perioperative aspirin and clonidine and risk of acute kidney injury: a randomized clinical trial. *J Am Med Assoc.* 2014;312(21):2254–2264.

45. Gordon AC, Mason AJ, Thirunavukkarasu N, et al. Effect of early vasopressin vs norepinephrine on kidney failure in patients with septic shock: the VANISH randomized clinical trial. *J Am Med Assoc.* 2016;316(5):509–518.

46. Zhou C, Gong J, Chen D, Wang W, Liu M, Liu B. levosimendan for prevention of acute kidney injury after cardiac surgery: a meta-analysis of randomized controlled trials. *Am J Kidney Dis.* 2016;67(3):408–416.

47. Gordon AC, Perkins GD, Singer M, et al. Levosimendan for the prevention of acute organ dysfunction in sepsis. *N Engl J Med.* 2016;375(17):1638–1648.

48. Frazee E, Rule AD, Lieske JC, et al. Cystatin c-guided vancomycin dosing in critically ill patients: a quality improvement project. *Am J Kidney Dis.* 2017;69(5):658–666.

49. Joannidis M, Druml W, Forni LG, et al. Prevention of acute kidney injury and protection of renal function in the intensive care unit: update 2017: expert opinion of the Working Group on Prevention, AKI section, European Society of Intensive Care Medicine. *Intensive Care Med.* 2017;43(6):730–749.

50. Cely CM, Schein RM, Quartin AA. Risk of contrast induced nephropathy in the critically ill: a prospective, case matched study. *Crit Care.* 2012;16(2):R67.

51. Wilhelm-Leen E, Montez-Rath ME, Chertow G. Estimating the risk of radiocontrast-associated nephropathy. *J Am Soc Nephrol.* 2017;28(2):653–659.

52. Bosch X, Poch E, Grau JM. Rhabdomyolysis and acute kidney injury. *N Engl J Med.* 2009;361(1):62–72.

53. Delaney KA, Givens ML, Vohra RB. Use of RIFLE criteria to predict the severity and prognosis of acute kidney injury in emergency department patients with rhabdomyolysis. *J Emerg Med.* 2012;42(5):521–528.

54. Brancaccio P, Lippi G, Maffulli N. Biochemical markers of muscular damage. *Clin Chem Lab Med.* 2010;48(6):757–767.

55. Better OS. The crush syndrome revisited (1940–1990). *Nephron.* 1990;55(2):97–103.

56. Beilstein CM, Prowle JR, Kirwan CJ. Automated fluid management for treatment of rhabdomyolysis. *Int J Nephrol.* 2016;2016:2932593.

57. Brochard L, Abroug F, Brenner M, et al. An official ATS/ERS/ESICM/SCCM/SRLF statement: prevention and management of acute renal failure in the ICU patient: an international consensus conference in intensive care medicine. *Am J Respir Crit Care Med.* 2010;181(10):1128–1155.

58. Zeng X, Zhang L, Wu T, Fu P. Continuous renal replacement therapy (CRRT) for rhabdomyolysis. *Cochrane Db Sys Rev.* 2014(6):CD008566.

59. Ronco C. Extracorporeal therapies in acute rhabdomyolysis and myoglobin clearance. *Crit Care.* 2005;9(2):141–142.

60. Adebayo D, Morabito V, Davenport A, Jalan R. Renal dysfunction in cirrhosis is not just a vasomotor nephropathy. *Kidney Int.* 2015;87(3):509–515.

61. Salerno F, Gerbes A, Ginès P, Wong F, Arroyo V. Diagnosis, prevention and treatment of hepatorenal syndrome in cirrhosis. *Gut.* 2007;56(9):1310–1318.

62. Nadim MK, Kellum JA, Davenport A, et al. Hepatorenal syndrome: the 8th International Consensus Conference of the Acute Dialysis Quality Initiative (ADQI) Group. *Crit Care.* 2012;16(1):R23.

63. Gluud LL, Christensen K, Christensen E, Krag A. Terlipressin for hepatorenal syndrome. *Cochrane Db Sys Rev.* 2012(9):CD005162.

64. European Association for the Study of the L. EASL clinical practice guidelines on the management of ascites, spontaneous bacterial peritonitis,

and hepatorenal syndrome in cirrhosis. *J Hepatol.* 2010;53(3):397–417.

65. Sharma P, Kumar A, Shrama BC, Sarin SK. An open label, pilot, randomized controlled trial of nora-drenaline versus terlipressin in the treatment of type 1 hepatorenal syndrome and predictors of response. *Am J Gastroenterol.* 2008;103(7):1689–1697.

66. Umgelter A, Reindl W, Wagner KS, et al. Effects of plasma expansion with albumin and paracen-tesis on haemodynamics and kidney function in critically ill cirrhotic patients with tense ascites and hepatorenal syndrome: a prospective uncon-trolled trial. *Crit Care.* 2008;12(1):R4.

67. Malbrain ML, Cheatham ML, Kirkpatrick A, et al. Results from the International Conference of Experts on Intra-Abdominal Hypertension and Abdominal Compartment Syndrome: I. Definitions. *Intensive Care Med.* 2006;32(11):1722–1732.

68. Sugrue M, Jones F, Deane SA, Bishop G, Bauman A, Hillman K. Intra-abdominal hypertension is an independent cause of postoperative renal im-pairment. *Arch Surg.* 1999;134(10):1082–1085.

69. Kirkpatrick AW, Roberts DJ, De Waele J, et al. Intra-abdominal hypertension and the abdom-inal compartment syndrome: updated con-sensus definitions and clinical practice guidelines from the World Society of the Abdominal Compartment Syndrome. *Intensive Care Med.* 2013;39(7):1190–1206.

70. Truche AS, Darmon M, Bailly S, et al. Continuous renal replacement therapy versus intermittent he-modialysis in intensive care patients: impact on mortality and renal recovery. *Intensive Care Med.* 2016;42(9):1408–1417.

71. Bonnassieux M, Duclos A, Schneider AG, et al. Influence of initial renal replacement therpay mo-dality on renal recovery at hospital discharge. *Crit Care Med.* 2018;46(2):e102–e110.

72. Wald R, Shariff SZ, Adhikari NK, et al. The as-sociation between renal replacement therapy modality and long-term outcomes among crit-ically ill adults with acute kidney injury: a retrospective cohort study. *Crit Care Med.* 2014;42(4):868–877.

73. Schneider AG, Bellomo R, Bagshaw SM, et al. Choice of renal replacement therapy modality and dialysis dependence after acute kidney in-jury: a systematic review and meta-analysis. *Intensive Care Med.* 2013;39(6):987–997.

74. Liang KV, Sileanu FE, Clermont G, et al. Modality of RRT and recovery of kidney function after AKI in patients surviving to hospital discharge. *Clin J Am Soc Nephrol.* 2016;11(1):30–38.

75. Gaudry S, Hajage D, Schortgen F, et al. Comparison of two strategies for initiating renal replacement therapy in the intensive care unit: study protocol for a randomized controlled trial (AKIKI). *Trials.* 2015;16:170.

76. Zarbock A, Kellum JA, Schmidt C, et al. Effect of early vs delayed initiation of renal replace-ment therapy on mortality in critically ill patients with acute kidney injury. *J Am Med Assoc.* 2016;315(20):2190.

77. Prowle JR, Echeverri JE, Ligabo EV, Ronco C, Bellomo R. Fluid balance and acute kidney injury. *Nat Rev Nephrol.* 2010;6(2):107–115.

78. Sutherland SM, Zappitelli M, Alexander SR, et al. Fluid overload and mortality in chil-dren receiving continuous renal replacement therapy: the prospective pediatric continuous renal replacement therapy registry. *Am J Kidney Dis.* 2010;55(2):316–325.

79. Siew ED, Peterson JF, Eden SK, et al. Outpatient nephrology referral rates after acute kidney in-jury. *J Am Soc Nephrol.* 2012;23(2):305–312.

80. Commissioning for Quality and Innovation (CQUIN) Guidance 2015/16. NHS England; 2016. https://www.england.nhs.uk/wp-content/uploads/2015/03/9-cquin-guid-2015-16.pdf

81. Puthucheary ZA, Rawal J, McPhail M, et al. Acute skeletal muscle wasting in critical illness. *J Am Med Assoc.* 2013;310(15):1591–1600.

82. Prowle JR, Kolic I, Purdell-Lewis J, Taylor R, Pearse RM, Kirwan CJ. Serum creatinine changes associated with critical illness and detection of persistent renal dysfunction after AKI. *Clin J Am Soc Nephrol.* 2014;9(6):1015–1023.

83. Ravn B, Prowle JR, Martensson J, Martling CR, Bell M. Superiority of serum cystatin c over creatinine in prediction of long-term prog-nosis at discharge from ICU. *Crit Care Med.* 2017;45(9):e932–e940.

84. Forni LG, Darmon M, Ostermann M, et al. Renal recovery after acute kidney injury. *Intensive Care Med.* 2017;43(6):855–866.

85. Shlipak MG, Coresh J, Gansevoort RT. Cystatin C versus creatinine for kidney function-based risk. *N Engl J Med.* 2013;369(25):2459.

17

Obstructive Uropathies

PRIYA DESHPANDE AND SHUCHITA SHARMA

INTRODUCTION

Obstructive uropathy is the term used for the structural or functional changes in the urinary tract that affect the urinary outflow. This impaired flow of urine may or may not result in renal disease. In case of unilateral obstruction in a patient with 2 normal kidneys, there may be little or no significant change in kidney function. However, bilateral obstruction or unilateral obstruction in a solitary functioning kidney can result in significant renal failure. Obstructive uropathy and hydronephrosis are not synonymous as the latter term refers only to the dilatation of the urinary tract, and one can be present in the absence of the other.

EPIDEMIOLOGY

Obstructive uropathy is a common problem and can occur at any age. It can commonly be seen in patients of all ages and gender with cancer. In children, it is more commonly seen in boys, and usually results from congenital urinary tract abnormalities. In patients in their second or third decade of life, obstructive uropathy can result from ureteral obstruction due to nephrolithiasis, more commonly seen in men, or due to pregnancy and other gynecological causes in women. The prevalence again increases in men over the age of 60 due to prostatic enlargement.

ETIOLOGY AND PATHOGENESIS

The causes of obstructive uropathy can be very varied and classified in different ways, such as acute or chronic, complete or partial, and upper or lower urinary tract obstruction. Here, we classify the etiology of obstructive uropathy based on causes that are either intrinsic or extrinsic to the urinary tract (Table 17.1).

Intrinsic Causes of Urinary Obstruction

Intrinsic causes can be further divided into intraluminal and extraluminal/intramural obstruction.

Urinary flow can be obstructed intraluminally due to renal tubular obstruction from precipitation of crystals or proteins such as Bence Jones proteins in myeloma or uric acid crystals in tumor lysis syndrome. Similarly, papillary necrosis and sloughing of papillary tissue can result in intraluminal obstruction. Macroscopic hematuria from renal cysts, tumors, or arteriovenous malformations resulting in blood clots can also result in a similar picture.

One of the most common reasons to develop obstruction is nephrolithiasis, which usually results in acute unilateral urinary tract obstruction. Commonly seen renal stones are calcium oxalate and calcium phosphate. Others less commonly seen are uric acid stones, struvite stones, and cysteine stones.

Extraluminal causes include structural obstruction from intramural tumors, infections, ureteral strictures secondary to radiotherapy, prior surgeries or infections and scarring, or as a result of iatrogenic ureteral disruption or ligation. It can also occur as a result of structural obstruction of the lower urinary tract from urethral strictures, benign or malignant tumors of the bladder, bladder calculi, or bladder and/or urethral trauma.

Functional disorders of the upper or lower urinary tract such as vesicoureteral junction dysfunction and neurogenic bladder (secondary to neurologic disorders like multiple sclerosis, Parkinson's disease, and spinal injuries or from medications like anticholinergics and levodopa) can also result in significant urinary obstruction.

TABLE 17.1 ETIOLOGY OF OBSTRUCTIVE UROPATHY

Intrinsic Causes

Intraluminal
- Stones (calcium oxalate, calcium phosphate, uric acid, cysteine, struvite)
- Crystals (uric acid)
- Proteins (Bence Jones)
- Blood clots secondary to gross hematuria

Extraluminal
- Intramural tumors
- Intramural infections
- Iatrogenic ureteral disruption or ligation
- Urethral strictures
- Bladder tumors
- Bladder calculi
- Urethral or bladder trauma
- Vesicoureteral junction dysfunction
- Neurogenic bladder (Neurologic disorders or medications)

Extrinsic Causes
- Benign prostatic hyperplasia
- Cancer of the surrounding structures (Prostate cancer, cervical cancer, ovarian tumors, lymphatic tumors
- Pregnancy
- Inflammation of the surrounding structures (Crohn's disease, pancreatitis, appendicitis, diverticulitis
- Large aneurysm of aorta or iliac vessels
- Retroperitoneal fibrosis
- Retroperitoneal tumors

Extrinsic Causes of Urinary Obstruction

The most common reason for extrinsic compression of the urinary tract in men is prostatic enlargement from benign prostate hypertrophy or prostate cancer resulting in partial or complete urethral obstruction. In women of childbearing age, the gravid uterus compressing the ureters can cause mild unilateral or bilateral obstruction. In most cases, this is asymptomatic and self-limited and resolves after delivery.

Tumors or cysts from the surrounding structures such as cervical cancer, prostatic cancer, ovarian tumors, and lymphatic tumors can cause obstruction of urinary flow at the level of ureters or urethra. Similarly, inflammation in the surrounding organs, such as Crohn's disease, pancreatitis, appendicitis, and diverticulitis, can also result in compression of the urinary tract.

Large aneurysms of the nearby vessels such as aorta or iliac vessels can be another big culprit.

Retroperitoneal disease in the form of retroperitoneal fibrosis, tumors such as lymphomas and sarcomas, and enlarged lymph nodes can all result in obstruction of the urinary tract.

PATHOPHYSIOLOGY

Urinary tract obstruction results in morphological and histopathologic changes in the kidneys. Initial changes are characterized by enlargement and edema of the kidney along with dilatation of the calyces, pelvis, and tubules. These changes are reversible initially, but if left untreated or inadequately treated, they will eventually cause irreversible damage to the kidneys and urinary tract. Untreated obstruction results in permanent dilatation of the renal pelvis and thinning of the renal cortex and medulla. Microscopic examination of the kidney tissue can show tubulointerstitial fibrosis and obliteration of the glomeruli.

Obstruction of the urinary tract can cause changes in both the glomerular filtration rate (GFR) and tubular function. GFR has been shown to decline progressively with complete ureteral obstruction. These changes have been best studied in animal models. In a rat model with temporary, complete unilateral obstruction, the decrease in fraction of total GFR was much faster than the decrease in total renal blood flow to the affected kidney.[1] Removal of obstruction in the same model resulted in improvement in GFR; however, the degree of improvement was based on the duration of obstruction.[1]

The fall in the GFR is thought to be due to both the decrease in single-nephron GFR as well as decrease in the number of functioning nephrons. Angiotensin II and thromboxane A2 have been shown to play an important role in the marked decrease of the plasma flow to nephron during obstruction.[2] In a rat model, when the animals were pretreated with angiotensin-converting enzyme inhibitors and thromboxane synthase inhibitors 48 hours prior to and during obstruction, the relief of short-term obstruction resulted in normalization of kidney function.[2] Furthermore, recent studies have shown that complete unilateral ureteral obstruction results in morphological changes in renal vasculature, most likely due to vascular remodeling.[3] The molecular mechanisms of these alterations are not entirely clear.

An interstitial infiltrate, predominantly of macrophages, has been shown to play a key role in acute functional changes and the late morphological changes that occur as a result of ureteral obstruction.[4] Also, studies have shown that ureteral obstruction even for relatively short periods of time can result in permanent loss of nephrons, and the return of GFR to normal is mostly due to hyperfiltration in the remaining nephrons.[5]

The changes in tubular function manifest as changes in water excretion and ability to maintain electrolyte balance. There is marked inability to concentrate urine post-obstruction, and this abnormality may persist for a few months even after release of obstruction.[6] Some of the factors that have been thought to cause this abnormality are unresponsiveness of the collecting duct to vasopressin, a reduction in number of sodium transporters, and a loss of tonicity in the medulla.[6]

Urinary tract obstruction also results in defects of urinary acidification and changes in handling of potassium.[6] These defects are most likely due to reduced activity of the NA-K-ATPase pump due to tubular injury and hyporeninemic hypoaldosteronism (type IV RTA) with marked increase in bicarbonate excretion from abnormalities of the H+- ATPase activity in the intercalated cells. The relief of complete obstruction results in marked increase in potassium excretion mostly from increased delivery of sodium to the distal tubule and increased sodium–potassium exchange. The recovery of tubular function, however, is usually much slower than improvement in GFR.

CLINICAL MANIFESTATIONS

Patients presenting with obstructive uropathy manifest symptoms based on the area of obstruction. Those with upper urinary tract obstruction (especially secondary to a ureteral stone) may develop flank or lower back pain, which is thought to result from stretching of the renal capsule or the collecting system. Pain associated with nephrolithiasis in the lower part of the urinary tract may radiate to the groin. Renal calculi can cause hematuria from mechanical trauma to the epithelium. Hematuria can also be associated with neoplasms of the urinary tract and can be micro- or macroscopic.

In case of bilateral obstruction or unilateral, the patients can be oliguric or anuric and further develop constitutional symptoms such as nausea and vomiting. There can be associated fever if the obstruction is associated with infection, such as pyelonephritis or an infected calculus. This is usually an emergency, and rapid diagnosis and treatment with minimally invasive elimination of infectious foci leads to improved outcomes in patients.

Patients with lower urinary tract obstruction may not report any change in their voiding but only have suprapubic pain or fullness.

On clinical exam, patients with upper urinary tract obstruction may have costovertebral angle tenderness. Patients with lower urinary tract obstruction may have a palpable bladder. Obstructive uropathy is associated with hypertension because of increased blood volume and activation of the renin–angiotensin–aldosterone system.[7]

Abnormal laboratory data may include elevated serum blood urea nitrogen and creatinine levels particularly if there is bilateral obstruction. Hyperkalemia can result from defects in urinary acidification and potassium handling. Urinalysis may reveal hematuria, pyuria, mild proteinuria, and /or infection. Urinary electrolytes, especially after prolonged obstruction, reflect the inability of the tubules to absorb sodium and concentrate urine.

DIAGNOSIS

The diagnosis of obstructive uropathy requires a high index of suspicion and, depending on its nature, can be confirmed clinically and/ or with an imaging modality.

The first question that needs to be asked is, Is the patient in acute kidney injury as a result of the obstruction? A thorough review of the clinical history (especially regarding onset and patient's ability to urinate), clinical exam (e.g., palpable bladder, costovertebral angle tenderness), and relevant lab results (i.e., serum creatinine level and electrolytes) can help answer this question. Some patients with urinary obstruction develop significant acute kidney injury with electrolyte derangements (severe hyperkalemia, severe acidosis) necessitating urgent treatment or even the initiation of renal replacement therapy.

After the patient's renal function is assessed, we have to ask, Why is this patient obstructed and at what level? This question can be answered using clinical and imaging tools. For upper urinary tract lesions, the following imaging modalities can be used: intravenous pyelogram (IVP), renal and bladder sonogram, computed tomography (CT), magnetic resonance imaging (MRI), and nuclear scintigraphy.

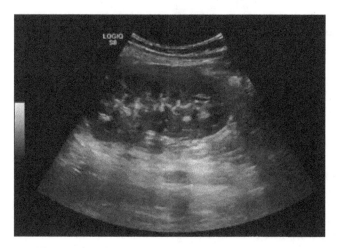

FIGURE 17.1 A normal left kidney as seen by ultrasound.

IVP was heralded as the "gold standard" for the diagnosis of unilateral renal obstruction secondary to nephrolithiasis. However, given the risks of exposure to contrast (especially in the setting of allergy or renal impairment) and urinary tract infections, the use of IVP has been largely replaced by ultrasound and CT.

Sonography is one of the safest and least expensive studies to provide imaging of the upper and lower urinary tract. It has a sensitivity of 98% and specificity of 75% for detecting urinary obstruction.[8]

For lower urinary tract imaging, a bladder ultrasound can be used to rule out urinary retention secondary to bladder outflow obstruction. This can help avoid unnecessary bladder catheterizations.

Sonographic imaging of the upper urinary tract is essentially used to rule out hydronephrosis (Figs. 17.1 and 17.2). Hydronephrosis is graded from I to IV:

Grade I: slight dilation of the renal pelvis without extension into the calyces

Grade II: dilation of both the renal pelvis and the calyces without any cortical thinning

Grade III: the same characteristics as Grade II along with cortical thinning

Grade IV: massive dilation of renal pelvis and calyces and severe cortical thinning.

The degree of cortical thinning may correlate with chronicity of the urinary obstruction.[9]

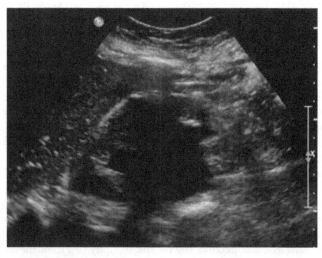

FIGURE 17.2 Severe hydronephrosis of the right kidney.

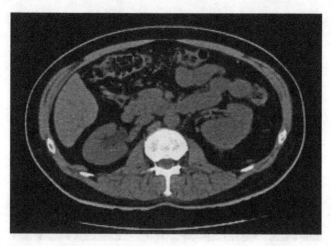

FIGURE 17.3 Patient with right-sided hydronephrosis.

However, there are limitations to using renal ultrasound as the imaging modality. First, ultrasound may not demonstrate early stages of obstruction. Sufficient time needs to elapse for the obstruction to cause dilatation of the upper urinary tract and collection of urine in the kidney, demonstrating hydronephrosis. Second, caution must be exercised when using ultrasound for the detection of hydronephrosis as there is a risk of false positives. Parapelvic renal cysts are frequently mistaken for hydronephrosis. A study conducted by Ellenbogen et al.[10] comparing ultrasonography to excretory urography showed that ultrasound correctly identified hydronephrosis in nearly 100% of cases, but there was a false positive rate of 25%. False positives can also occur due to blood vessels in the renal sinuses, but these can be differentiated from hydronephrosis using renal Doppler.[8]

CT detects urinary tract dilation and obstruction earlier than ultrasonography (Figs. 17.3 and 17.4). An unenhanced CT is useful in visualizing calculi, which appear radio-dense (Fig. 17.5). This study should be reserved for patients who are clinically suspected of having an obstructive stone. Ureteral stones result in findings such as ureterectasis, dilation of the pelvocalyceal system, and sometimes renal enlargement. Perinephric fat stranding can be seen as well and directly correlates with the severity of the obstruction.[11] The composition of the stones can be determined using a dual energy CT scan.[12]

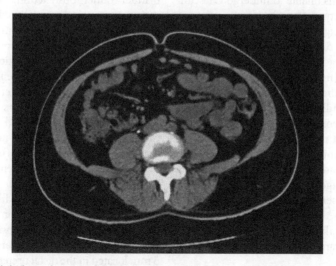

FIGURE 17.4 Nephrolith (hyperdense) in the right ureter.

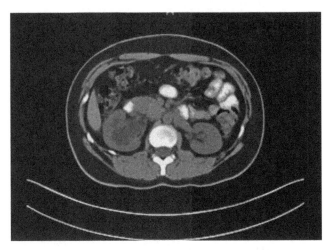

FIGURE 17.5 Patient with severe right-sided hydronephrosis secondary to congenital uretero-pelvic junction obstruction.

CT urogram has become another preferred modality for imaging the urinary tract and has replaced IVP. The CT urogram is a physiologic study that consists of 3 phases: unenhanced (to help locate calculi), enhanced (to detect renal masses), and delayed (excretory phase to visualize urothelium) imaging. However, this study must be used with caution in patients with renal impairment or with allergy to contrast.

In patients who cannot receive iodinated contrast, MRI either with or without gadolinium may be another option to visualize the upper and lower urinary tracts. However, MRI is a poor study for identifying calculi, and gadolinium should be used cautiously in patients with renal impairment. MRI, although expensive, can be used in populations unable to undergo CT scanning, such as pregnant women.

Nuclear scintigraphy is another tool that can be used to diagnose obstruction. The 2 most common radiotracers that are used are Tc99m-MAG3 (mercaptoacetyltriglycine) or Tc99m-DTPA (dietylenetriaminepentacetate), and they are rapidly taken up and excreted by the urinary system. After the intravenous administration of a radiotracer, a series of renal images are obtained as the gamma camera detects emitted radiation. This is followed by a second set of images obtained after the administration of furosemide. These images capture the movement of the radiotracer through each kidney (i.e., uptake and excretion), and this generates renogram curves to determine renal function.[13]

Urodynamic studies can serve to diagnose obstruction of the lower urinary tract, mainly bladder outlet obstruction. An elevated postvoid residual on bladder ultrasound may indicate problems with bladder wall contraction or obstruction of the bladder outlet. Urodynamic studies further evaluate bladder compliance, urinary flow rate, and detrusor muscle pressure upon voiding.[8]

TREATMENT

Prompt diagnosis and treatment of obstructive uropathy results in alleviation of symptoms and may help with preserving renal function.

For patients presenting with acute lower urinary tract obstruction symptoms secondary to bladder outlet obstruction, bladder catheterization serves to decompress the bladder. Once symptoms are alleviated, patients may benefit from medical management for the cause of obstruction. For instance, patients with benign prostatic hyperplasia may benefit from 5-alpha reductase inhibitors (finasteride) and alpha-1A-adrenoreceptor inhibitors (tamsulosin) to help reduce prostate size and relax the smooth muscle around the bladder neck and prostate, thereby allowing for better urine flow. Similarly, in a patient with neurogenic bladder, self-catheterization multiple times a day may be required to decompress the bladder.[8,14,15]

Identification of the lesion is paramount in treating upper urinary tract obstruction. If the obstruction is secondary to ureteral calculi less than 5 mm located in the distal ureter, then intravenous and oral hydration along with pain control may help with spontaneous passage of the stone. Alpha-1A-adrenoreceptor inhibitor (tamsulosin) is often used for medical management and passage of small stones. Larger stones, especially those in the proximal ureter, are more difficult to pass and may require interventions such as shock wave lithotripsy, percutaneous nephrolithotomy, or even laparoscopic stone removal. Tamsulosin has also been shown to be a safe and effective therapy for passage of renal and ureteral stones after shock wave lithotripsy.[16] Sometimes ureteral stents are placed to maintain patency of the ureter.[8,14]

Percutaneous nephrostomy is considered when there is an upper urinary tract obstruction. This procedure is used particularly in the setting of acute kidney injury or if there is an infection above the level of ureteral obstruction (pyonephrosis).[14] After the placement of a percutaneous nephrostomy and decompression of the kidney, further studies can be performed to locate the exact area of the obstruction and further management.[14]

After relief of a chronic obstruction, patients may experience postobstructive diuresis. Urine production more than 200 mL per hour for 2 hours or more than 3 L in 24 hours following bladder decompression is considered postobstructive diuresis.[17] The polyuria can be accompanied by electrolyte derangements (i.e., hypokalemia, hypomagnesemia) and hypovolemia. Patients with postobstructive diuresis need volume replacement (either oral or intravenous depending on severity). For intravenous replacement, typically half normal saline is used, and half of the daily urine volume is replaced. However, excessive volume replacement may exacerbate the diuresis. Typically postobstructive diuresis is self-limiting and lasts 24 hours.[17,18]

CONCLUSION

Obstructive uropathy remains a considerable cause for acute kidney injury. Thus, prompt diagnosis and treatment with effective relief of obstruction is important in preventing long-term and permanent damage to the kidneys.

REFERENCES

1. Provoost AP, Molenaar JC. Renal function during and after a temporary complete unilateral ureteral obstruction in rats. *Invest Urol.* 1981; 18(4):242–246

2. Purkerson ML, Klahr S. Prior inhibition of vasoconstrictors normalizes GFR in postobstructed kidneys. *Kidney Int.* 1989; 25(6):1305–1314

3. Li WQ, Dong ZQ, Zhou XB et al. Renovascular morphological changes in a rabbit model of hydronephrosis. *J Huazhong Univ Sci Tevhnolog Med Sci.* 2014; 34(4):575–581

4. Harris KP, Schreiner GF, Klahr S. Effect of leukocyte depletion on the function of the postobstructed kidney in the rat. *Kidney Int.* 1989; 36(2):210–245.

5. Bander SJ, Buerkert JE, Martin D, Klahr S. Long-term effects of 24-hr unilateral ureteral obstruction on renal function in the rat. *Kidney Int.* 1985; 28(4): 614–620.

6. Klahr S, Harris K, Purkerson ML. Effects of obstruction on renal functions. *Pediatr Nephrol.* 1988; 2(1):34–42.

7. Michael B. Obstructive uropathy. In: Edgar V. Lerma, Mitchell H. Rosner, Mark A. Perazella, eds. *Current Diagnosis and Treatment: Nephrology and Hypertension.* New York, NY: McGraw-Hill; 2009.

8. Greenberg A, ed. *Primer on Kidney Diseases.* Philadelphia, PA: Saunders/Elsevier; 2009.

9. O'Neill, W Charles. *Atlas of renal ultrasonography.* Phildelphia: Saunders, 2001.

10. Ellenbogen, PH, W Scheible, LB Talner and GR Leopold. Sensitivity of gray scale ultrasound in detecting urinary tract obstruction. *Am J Roentgenol.* 1978;130:731–733.

11. Han NY, Sung DK, Kim MK, Park BJ, Sim KC, Cho SB. Perirenal fat stranding on CT: is there an association with bladder outlet obstruction? *Brit J Radiol.* 2016;1063:20160195.

12. Haley WE, Ibrahim el-SH, Qu M, et al. The clinical impact of accurate cystine calculi characterization using dual-energy computed tomography. *Case Rep Radiol.* 2015 (2015):801021.

13. Taylor A, Schuster DM, Alazraki NP. *A Clinician's Guide to Nuclear Medicine.* Reston, VA: Society of Nuclear Medicine; 2006.

14. Feehally J, Floege J, Johnson RJ. *Comprehensive Clinical Nephrology.* Philadelphia, PA: Mosby Elsevier; 2007.

15. Beckman TJ, Mynderse LA. Evaluation and medical management of benign prostatic hyperplasia. *Mayo Clin Proc.* 2005;80:1356–1362.

16. Zheng S, Liu LR, Yuan HC, Wei Q. Tamsulosin as adjunctive treatment after shockwave lithotripsy in patients with upper urinary tract stones: a systematic review and meta-analysis. *Scand J Urol Nephrol.* 2010;44(6):425–432.

17. Halbgewachs C, Domes T. Postobstructive diuresis: pay close attention to urinary retention. *Can Fam Physician.* 2015;61.2:137–142.

18. Gonzalez CM. Pathophysiology, diagnosis, and treatment of the postobstructive diuresis. In: McVary KT, ed. *Management of Benign Prostatic Hypertrophy.* New York, NY: Humana Press; 2004: 35–45.

18

Nephron-Sparing Surgery

STEFANO PULIATTI, NANCY FERRARI, BERNARDO ROCCO,
GIAMPAOLO BIANCHI, AND SALVATORE MICALI

INTRODUCTION

Renal carcinoma has an enormous epidemiological importance. Due to the exceptional advancement of diagnostic techniques, it is possible to obtain advanced diagnosis, precise descriptions of the dimensions of the site, the morphological characteristics of these neoformations, and the component of healthy renal parenchyma not involved by the tumor. Thus, the removal of a whole kidney to eliminate, in most of the cases, a new tumor formation of a few centimeters, known in its characteristics prior to the presurgery staging, is now considered to be more and more an archaic treatment.

Urological surgery has moved toward nephron-sparing surgery (NSS) removal with oncological safety and good results, for functional masses up to 7 cm of diameter (T1). Recent advances in surgical technology allows these procedures to be performed via laparoscopic or robot-assisted techniques.

EPIDEMIOLOGY

Renal cell carcinoma (RCC) accounts for 2% to 3% of all cancers, with a higher incidence rate in Western countries. Since the 1990s, there has been a continuing increase in the incidence of RCC in Europe, except in Denmark and Sweden. In previous decades, an annual increase of this pathology by 2% was recorded worldwide, with an increase in the mortality rate in Europe until the 1990s. In 2012, 84,400 new cases of RCC and 34,700 deaths related to kidney cancer were registered.[1-3] In North America, in 2012, the International Agency for Research on Cancer[4] reports an incidence of 63,822 kidney cancer cases.

ETIOPATHOGENESIS

RCC is the most common solid lesion of the kidney and accounts for 90% of these forms of malignant kidney tumor. It is a predominant pathology in men (1.5:1), with a peak incidence between 60 to 70 years of age. Among the various risk factors for the occurrence of this tumor, the most important ones are poor lifestyle, smoking, hypertension, and obesity. Many other risk factors have been described, such as eating habits or occupational exposure to specific carcinogens, but they are not supported by sufficient scientific evidence. Moderate alcohol consumption has been described in the literature as a protective factor, although it still has not been well clarified as to which mechanism is responsible for the action.[5]

CLINICAL PRESENTATION, DIAGNOSIS, AND STAGING

In most cases, patients with kidney tumors are asymptomatic, and the finding of the pathology is incidental. The classic symptom triad that was once characteristic of kidney cancer—that is, flank pain, hematuria, and palpable abdominal mass—now is found in only about 6% of cases. Accordingly, the physical examination has a marginal role in the diagnosis of RCC.[5]

The large-scale use of radiological techniques, such as sonography and computed tomography (CT), has resulted in the increase of the number of incidental diagnoses of RCC, allowing the detection of smaller and smaller masses and at earlier stages.

RCC presents as a solid mass on sonography, hyperechoic, sometimes cystic with septations. This framework needs a second-level diagnosis confirmation, such as CT of the abdomen with contrast or magnetic resonance imaging. These

TABLE 18.1 BOSNIAK CLASSIFICATION SYSTEM

Bosniak Category	Features	Workup
I	A simple benign cyst with a hairline-thin wall that does not contain septa, calcification, or solid components. It has the same density as water and does not enhance with contrast medium.	Benign
II	A benign cyst that may contain a few hairline-thin septa. Fine calcification may be present in the wall or septa. Uniformly high-attenuation lesions <3 cm in size, with sharp margins but without enhancement.	Benign
IIF	These cysts may contain more hairline-thin septa. Minimal enhancement of a hairline-thin septum or wall can be seen. There may be minimal thickening of the septa or wall. The cyst may contain calcification, which may be nodular and thick, but there is no contrast enhancement. There are no enhancing soft tissue elements. This category also includes totally intrarenal, nonenhancing, high attenuation renal lesions >3 cm in size. These lesions are generally well-marginated.	Follow-up. A small proportion are malignant (about 5%).
III	These lesions are indeterminate cystic masses that have thickened irregular walls or septa in which enhancement can be seen.	Surgery or follow-up. Over 50% of the lesions are malignant.
IV	These lesions are clearly malignant cystic lesions that contain enhancing soft-tissue components.	Surgical therapy recommended. Mostly malignant tumor.

Source: Ljungberg B, Cowan NC, Hanbury DC et al. EAU guidelines on renal cell carcinoma: the 2010 update. *Eur Urol*. 2010;58:398–406.

tests, besides giving additional information on the nature of the mass in the kidney, allow us to draw specific evidence about its extent on the site, the possible extrarenal spread and possible lymph node metastases or distant ones.

CT has a sensitivity of 90% for tumors of diameter less than 3 cm and over 97% for larger tumors.

The renal masses are divided into solid masses and cystic masses. The Bosniak classification system is widely used to classify cystic renal masses; it divides them into 5 categories on the basis of CT images, which allow us to predict the risk of malignancy of the mass itself (Table 18.1).

Select masses not well characterized radiologically, such as small masses (which could benefit from active surveillance), with metastases (to choose the best therapeutic approach), the masses to be subjected to ablative therapies, one might need to perform a percutaneous kidney biopsy. The biopsy is not absolutely necessary prior to a surgical procedure in patients with favorable diagnosis.

Histological Diagnosis

The renal masses can be distinguished from a pathology standpoint as benign or malignant renal tumors.

Among the most frequent benign tumors, the following subtypes are included: papillary adenoma, fibroma or hamartoma, angiomyolipoma, and oncocytoma.

Among the malignant renal tumors, RCC represents more than 90% of these tumors and is classified as nonpapillary or clear cell, papillary, and chromophobe.

There are other less frequent malignant renal tumors, including variants of sarcomatoid RCC, cancer of the collecting ducts of Bellini, multilocular clear cell RCC, and others.

TNM Staging

TNM system is universally used for renal carcinoma anatomic staging.

Since 1987, TNM system has undergone constant changes, up to the latest version of 2010 (Tables 18.2 and 18.3).[6,7]

TABLE 18.2 TNM CLASSIFICATION

Stage	Classification
	Primary tumors (T)
Tx	Primary tumor cannot be assessed
T0	No evidence of primary tumor
T1	Tumor ≤7cm in greatest dimension, limited to the kidney
T1a	Tumor ≤4cm in greatest dimension, limited to the kidney
T1b	Tumor >4 cm but ≤7 cm in greatest dimension, limited to the kidney
T2	Tumor >7 cm in greatest dimension, limited to the kidney
T2a	Tumor >7 cm but ≤10 cm in greatest dimension, limited to the kidney
T2b	Tumor >10 cm, limited to the kidney
T3	Tumor extends into major veins or perinephric tissues but not into the ipsilateral adrenal gland and not beyond the Gerota's fascia
T3a	Tumor grossly extends into the renal vein or its segmental (muscle-containing) branches, or tumor invades perirenal and/or renal sinus fat but not beyond the Gerota's fascia
T3b	Tumor grossly extends into the vena cava below the diaphragm
T3c	Tumor grossly extends into the vena cava above the diaphragm or invades the wall of the vena cava
T4	Tumor invades beyond the Gerota's fascia (including contiguous extension into the ipsilateral adrenal gland)
	Regional lymph node (N)
Nx	Regional lymph nodes cannot be assessed
N0	No regional lymph node metastasis
N1	Metastasis in regional lymph node(s)
	Distant metastasis (M)
M0	No distant metastasis
M1	Distant metastasis

Prognostic Factors

The factors that affect the prognosis of kidney cancer can be divided into anatomical, histological, clinical, and molecular. The anatomical factors such as tumor size, angioinvasion, renal capsule and adrenal invasion, great vessels involvement, lymph node involvement, and distant metastases are generally gathered in the TNM classification system.

The Fuhrman nuclear grade is the histological classification system of kidney cancer that is more widely accepted, along with the differentiation of subtypes of RCC. In this classification, there are 4 nuclear grades defined in order of increasing nuclear size, irregularity, and nucleolar prominence. This classification has proven to be an important predictor of distant metastasis after nephrectomy.[8]

Clinical factors basically represent the general condition of the patient, the pain, and the presence of cachexia or blood dyscrasias.

TABLE 18.3 TNM STAGE GROUPING

TNM Stage Grouping	Tumor (T)	Lymph Nodes (N)	Metastasis (M)
Stage I	T1	N0	M0
Stage II	T2	N0	M0
Stage III	T3	N0	M0
	T1, T2, T3	N1	M0
Stage IV	T4	Any N	M0
	Any T	Any N	M1

Numerous molecular biomarkers have been extensively studied, such as vascular endothelial growth factor, the hypoxia inducible factor, p53, and cadherins. To date, studies have not shown any improvement in predictions, and their use is not recommended for routine clinical practice.

TREATMENT AND MANAGEMENT CONSIDERATION OF NEPHRON-SPARING SURGERY

Evolution of the RCC Treatment

In 1969, Robson et al.[9] presented radical nephrectomy (RN) as a treatment of choice for localized RCC.

The spread and qualitative improvement of radiological diagnostic tests, such as sonography and CT, have gradually allowed to discover renal masses of ever smaller dimensions and increasingly at early stages. This has resulted in a significant increase in the incidence of tumors of the kidney, with a significant reduction in the size of the detected masses. Early diagnosis and the detection of small masses has allowed us to seek less invasive treatments of RN, which enable preservation of the renal parenchyma not affected by the tumor.

Since 1980, partial nephrectomy (PN) became a more accepted alternative to RN.[10] In the following years, NSS has shown, thanks to long-term analysis, the same oncological outcomes compared to the RN. In addition, its preservation capacity for healthy renal parenchyma, has resulting in increased overall survival and reduction of the development of major comorbidities.[11]

Alongside the preservation of the renal parenchyma, kidney surgery minimally invasive techniques were developed, and in 1990 the first laparoscopic nephrectomy was successfully performed by Clayman et al.[12] Based on these experiences, in 1993, the first cases of laparoscopic PN were performed by McDougall et al.[13] and Winfield et al.[14] Finally, in 2006 Gettman et al.[15] described the first experience of robotic-assisted PN.

The pace in development of NSS and keyhole surgery has led to several benefits for the patient in terms of preservation of renal function, minimizing complications associated with reduction of kidney function, decreasing hospital length of stay, and postoperative pain. The direct consequence of these surgical advances has been a significant societal cost saving.

In accordance with the guidelines of the European Association of Urology and the American Society of Urology, PN is the gold standard for renal cancer in clinical stage T1, particularly the degree of recommendation is a level A in the T1a and level B in the T1b. Data have shown that, since 2007, 13% of new masses for diagnoses measure less than 2 cm, 37% less than 3 cm, and 60% less than 4 cm.[5,16] The vast majority of renal masses are then diagnosed in stage T1 and may use a NSS approach.

Renal cysts classified as Bosniak ≥type III must be treated as RCC. Therefore, if their size is in stage T1, they can also consider the use of NSS treatment. Additionally, NSS may be beneficial in the following cases in which performing a RN would mean leaving the patient anephric with end-stage renal disease and force the patient to dialysis:

- solitary kidney patients for unilateral renal agenesis
- solitary kidney patients from prior nephrectomy
- patients with bilateral RCC that would otherwise require bilateral nephrectomy
- patients with unilateral RCC, but the other kidney is at great risk of reduced kidney function due to nephrolithiasis, chronic pyelonephritis, and diseases such as chronic ureteral reflux and diabetes, among others.[17]

Features of the NSS

As described in the previous paragraph, the strong indication for NSS exists for lesions in stage T1. In these cases, NSS has been shown to have a cancer-specific survival and disease-free survival comparable to the RN.[18,19]

NSS is not significantly different from RN in regards to hospitalization, rate of transfusion, blood loss, and rate of perioperative complications. The significant advantages of the NSS compared to RN are

- smaller reduction in kidney function.
- greater patient satisfaction, recorded through quality-of-life questionnaires.
- reduced risk of chronic cardiovascular diseases.[18,20–22]

There are, however, cases in which NSS is best avoided. RN is the curative treatment of choice in the presence of advanced local growth cancers, if the partial resection is not possible due to the unfavorable location of the tumor and when there is a significant deterioration of the patient's health.

There are nephrometric systems developed with the aim of standardizing the choice of an approach rather than another alternative for elective NSS. The 3 most commonly used systems are the R.E.N.A.L. (radius, exophytic/endophytic properties, nearness of tumor to collecting system or sinus, anterior/posterior, and hilar tumor touching the main renal artery or vein and location relative to polar lines), PADUA (preoperative aspects and dimensions used for an anatomical classification), and C-index (concordance index).[23] They provide guidance on the basis of information obtained from second-level radiological surveys and scores in relation to location, size, and morphology of the neoformation. They are predictive of perioperative complications of PN that can be standardized and can, therefore, affect the decision to perform an RN or a NSS technique.[5] The development of more sophisticated imaging devices and future editing and reconstructive software might represent more consistent tools to provide a better nephrometric prediction.

Indication for the Associated Procedures

Ipsilateral adrenalectomy is recommended only if there is clinical evidence of preoperative involvement of the adrenal gland. If the renal mass was approachable via NSS, but there was involvement of the ipsilateral adrenal gland, it is mandatory to perform a RN. In exceptional cases, the execution of a frozen section of the adrenal gland may be performed to assess the possible malignancy of the mass.[24]

Lymph node dissection is not recommended in cases of localized tumor without evidence of lymph node invasion.[5]

Classification of NSS Interventions

Several types of interventions are included within the general concept of NSS, each with unique characteristics and with specific indications:

- **Enucleation**: removal of single tumor mass, separated from the remaining parenchyma due to its pseudocapsule. In this case, there is a complete sparing of the surrounding renal parenchyma.
- **Enucleoresection**: removal of the lesion along with a few millimeters of thickness of the surrounding healthy parenchyma (Fig. 18.1, open enucleo-resection).
- **PN**: removal of at least 1 cm in peritumoral parenchyma.
- **Polar resection**: complete removal of the renal pole (upper or lower) in which the tumor is contained.
- **Heminephrectomy**: removal of half renal parenchyma, containing the tumor.
- **Subtotal nephrectomy**: removal of more than half of the renal parenchyma in which the tumor is contained.

Depending on the general clinical characteristics of the patient and the neoformation to be treated, one can decide which intervention strategy is the best.

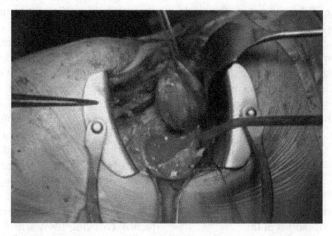

FIGURE 18.1 Open enucleoresection.

NSS Techniques: Open, Laparoscopic, and Robotic

For many years, open surgery was the best approach for NSS and will most likely remain for many surgeons the approach they have more confidence with to treat complex masses. Open surgery can cause disfigurements, possible abdominal pain, and herniations in the lumbar and abdominal area, which can adversely affect the patient's quality of life. Another limit of open surgery is the long hospitalization and slow recovery after surgery.[24]

In an effort to overcome these limitations, minimally invasive techniques such as laparoscopy and robotic surgery were developed.

Several studies show that the laparoscopic PN has oncological results equivalent to the open technique.

The considerable advantages of the laparoscopic approach are

- Reduction of bleeding during surgery
- Reduction of hospitalization time after surgery
- Faster convalescence
- Reduction of postoperative pain[24]

The limitations are:

- Long learning curve of laparoscopic PN for the surgeon
- Technical difficulties related to a 2D view
- Nonintuitive instrument control
- Increase in surgical time
- Increase of warm ischemia time, because of the longer time it takes to remove the mass and do the suture of the parenchyma

These considerations have limited the widespread use of this NSS technique to only a few specialized centers.[24,25]

The robotic-approach PN proved from the start to be a promising method, able to overcome the technical difficulties of laparoscopic PN. Many studies show that the robotic-approach PN has extended the indication to a NSS of complex renal masses, more extensive, endophytic and hilar.

The advantages of robotics are:

- 3D viewing,
- Intuitive instrument control,
- Avoiding the vibrations of the surgeons' hand

- Triangulation of the same with greater scope for action
- Fast learning curve.

Gill et al.[28] reported that to achieve adequate learning in laparoscopy that would allow an ischemia time of less than 30 minutes, at least 565 procedures were needed, while with the robot-assisted technique, the same result was achieved after 30 procedures. In all these methods, and of great importance, is the possibility of using intraoperative ultrasound probes, which allow an adequate and precise localization of the tumor, optimizing resection and reducing the risk of positive surgical margins.

Techniques of Preservation of Renal Function in NSS

After establishing that the NSS oncological results are similar to those of the RN, the surgeon has as secondary objective, the maintenance of renal function, while attempting to minimize the loss of nephronic mass.

It is well known that the loss of renal function after NSS is a multifactorial process linked to nonmodifiable causes (age, comorbidities, presurgery renal function, and contralateral kidney function) and modifiable factors, such as the ischemia time and the nephronic mass that one can save, always keeping in mind that the primary objective is the complete eradication of the tumor.[27]

The factors on which the surgeon can act are mainly

- Amount of renal tissue to be removed
- Ischemia time
- Remaining renal parenchyma hemostasis modalities following tumor resection

The amount of renal tissue removed to obtain the complete excision of the tumor will be the predictive indicator of the extent of preserved renal function. The ischemia time is another crucial factor. The greater the extension of the mass, greater is its vascularization, and, therefore, it may be necessary for renal artery clamping during the excision phase of the mass and in the reconstructive phase of the parenchyma.[26]

The reduction of intraoperative bleeding allows to maintain an optimal operating field, thus facilitating the intervention and consequently reducing the warm ischemia time. The latter is responsible for nephron loss. Studies

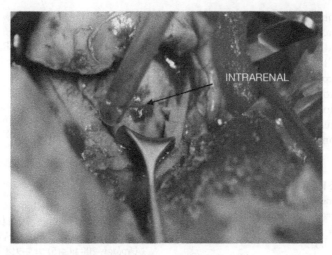

INTRARENAL

FIGURE 18.2 "Cold ischemia" nephron-sparing surgery.

have shown that by reducing ischemic time one obtains better results in preserving renal function. It is well known that in patients with normal renal function, a warm ischemia time up to 25 to 30 minutes is well tolerated with no significant damage on postoperative renal function. If in the past it was not uncommon to exceed the warm ischemia time, in recent years, time is thoroughly maintained in range.[26]

In the case of very complex masses it may be indicated to perform an intervention of NSS with "cold ischemia" (Fig. 18.2), by the apposition of ice within the surgical field, with the aim of minimizing nephron damage even in case of ischemic times >30 minutes. Because each minute of ischemia can be crucial in determining the extent of renal damage, new techniques have been introduced gradually with the aim to reduce the ischemic time.

Another option is to proceed with a laparoscopic PN without clamping the renal artery. This technique is called "zero ischemia" PN (without ischemia); however, it has been shown that there was no statistically significant improvements in postoperative renal function but a higher burden of intraoperative bleeding. Patients who may benefit from this technique are those with an already impaired renal function preoperatively.[26] Gill et al.[28] and Nguyen[29] have reduced ischemia time during laparoscopic PN from 31 minutes to 20 minutes, using the technique of fast unclamping.

Other studies have been conducted on the use of pharmacological intraoperative hypotension and a selective clamping of the arteries (selective clamping). Gill et al.[28] have developed a microvascular superselective dissection technique, with selective devascularization of the tumor. No adequate results on the benefits of this technique in terms of preservation of renal function have, however, been reported.

The markers generally used in urological studies for the determination of renal damage are represented by the measurement of the renal function and the glomerular filtration rate. These markers can be affected by biases related to the contralateral kidney function. More reliable results but more difficult to realize would be provided from obtaining a renal scintigraphy before and after the PN.[27]

After removal of the renal mass, the remaining parenchyma may suffer from decreased renal function, from induced ischemia through too deep sutures or through incorrect orientation. Several techniques are being investigated and proposed selective sutures or hemostasis, using absorbable clips, on the perforating vessels from the healthy parenchyma that supply blood to the tumor. Some more aggressive investigators have reported series in which a suture has not been used but only bipolar coagulation and hemostatic materials.[30]

CONCLUSION

For tumors in stage T1, it is indicated and highly recommended that they be removed by NSS. NSS preserves functional renal tissue, lowers complications compared to RN, and reduces the risks to which a patient with solitary kidney is subjected to. More and more centers are equipped with the latest technology, including the Da Vinci robot, which allows the execution of minimally invasive surgery, reducing pain, comorbidities, and hospital length of stay following surgery. All these improvements in care lead to reduced expenses and hence a reduction in societal costs following surgery. Techniques of NSS continue to be improved in an effort to reduce renal ischemia and minimize the loss of kidney function as a result of the surgical procedure.

REFERENCES

1. European Network of Cancer Registries. *EUROCIM Version 4.0: European Incidence Database V2.3, 730 Entity Dictionary.* Lyon, France: ENCR; 2001.
2. Levi F, Ferlay J, Galeone C, et al. The changing pattern of kidney cancer incidence and mortality in Europe. *BJU Int.* 2008;101: 949–958.
3. Ferlay J., Steliarova-Foucher E, Lortet-Tieulent J, et al. Cancer incidence and mortality patterns in Europe: estimates for 40 countries in 2012. *Eur J Cancer*, 2013;49:1374–1403.
4. Ferlay J, Soerjomataram I, Ervik M, et al. GLOBOCAN 2012 v1.0, Cancer incidence and mortality worldwide: IARC CancerBase No. 11; 2012. http://gco.iarc.fr/today/online-analysis-multi-barsmode=population&mode_population=continents&population=900&sex=0&cancer=21&type=0&statistic=0&prevalence=0&color_palette=default
5. Ljungberg B, Cowan NC, Hanbury DC et al. EAU guidelines on renal cell carcinoma: the 2010 update. *Eur Urol.* 2010;58:398–406.
6. Edge SB, Byrd DR, Compton CC, et al. *AJCC Cancer Staging Manual.* 7th ed. New York, NY: Springer-Verlag; 2010.
7. NCCN Clinical Practice Guidelines in Oncology: Kidney Cancer. V 2.2014. National Comprehensive Cancer Network; 2014. http://www.nccn.org/professionals/physician_gls/pdf/kidney.pdf
8. Fuhrman SA, Lasky LC, Limas C. Prognostic significance of morphologic parameters in renal cell carcinoma. *Am J Surg Pathol.* 1982;6(7):655–663.
9. Robson CJ, Churchill BM, Anderson W. The results of radical nephrectomy for renal cell carcinoma. *J Urol.* 1969;101(3):297–301.
10. Benway BM, Bhayani SB. Surgical outcomes of robot-assisted partial nephrectomy. *BJU Int.* 2011;108(6 Pt 2):955–961.
11. Pettus JA, Jang TL, Thompson RH, Yossepowitch O, Kagiwada M, Russo P. Effect of baseline glomerular filtration rate on survival in patients undergoing partial or radical nephrectomy

for renal cortical tumors. *Mayo Clin Proc.* 2008;83(10):1101–1106.
12. Clayman RV, Kavoussi LR, Soper NJ, et al. Laparoscopic nephrectomy: initial case report. *J Urol.* 1991;146(2):278–282.
13. McDougall EM, Clayman RV, Chandhoke PS, et al. Laparoscopic partial nephrectomy in the pig model. *J Urol.* 1993;149(6):1633–1636.
14. Winfield HN1, Donovan JF, Godet AS, Clayman RV. Laparoscopic partial nephrectomy: initial case report for benign disease. *J Endourol.* 1993;7(6):521–526.
15. Gettman MT, Blute ML, Chow GK, Neururer R, Bartsch G, Peschel R. Robotic-assisted laparoscopic partial nephrectomy: technique and initial clinical experience with DaVinci robotic system. *Urology.* 2004;64(5):914–918.
16. Benway BM1, Bhayani SB, Rogers CG, et al. Robot assisted partial nephrectomy versus laparoscopic partial nephrectomy for renal tumors: a multi-institutional analysis of perioperative outcomes. *J Urol.* 2009;182(3):866–872.
17. Tsui KH, van Ophoven A, Shvarts O, Belldegrun A. Nephron-sparing surgery for renal cell carcinoma. *Rev Urol.* 1999; 1(4):216–225.
18. Dash A1, Vickers AJ, Schachter LR, Bach AM, Snyder ME, Russo P. Comparison of outcomes in elective partial vs radical nephrectomy for clear cell renal cell carcinoma of 4-7 cm. *BJU Int.* 2006;97(5):939–945.
19. Crépel M, Jeldres C, Perrotte P, et al. Nephron-sparing surgery is equally effective to radical nephrectomy for T1BN0M0 renal cell carcinoma: a population-based assessment. *Urology.* 2010;75(2):271–275.
20. Zhao PT, Richstone L, Kavoussi LR. Laparoscopic partial nephrectomy. *Int J Surg.* 2016;36(Pt C):548–553.
21. Kates M, Badalato GM, Pitman M, McKiernan JM. Increased risk of overall and cardiovascular mortality after radical nephrectomy for renal cell carcinoma 2 cm or less. *J Urol.* 2011;186(4):1247–1253.
22. Weight CJ, Larson BT, Fergany AF, et al. Nephrectomy induced chronic renal insufficiency is associated with increased risk of cardiovascular death and death from any cause in patients with localized cT1b renal masses. *J Urol.* 2010;183(4):1317–1323.
23. Klatte T, Ficarra V, Gratzke C, et al. A literature review of renal surgical anatomy and surgical strategies for partial nephrectomy. *Eur Urol.* 2015;68:980–982.
24. Ramani AP, Abreu SC, Desai MM, et al. Laparoscopic upper pole partial nephrectomy with concomitant en bloc adrenalectomy. *Urology.* 2003;62(2):223–226.

25. Ficarra V, Novara G, Volpe A, Mottrie A. Robot-assisted vs traditional laparoscopic partial nephrectomy: the time for meta-analysis has not yet arrived. *BJU Int.* 2013;112(4):E334–E336.

26. Cha EK, Lee DJ, Del Pizzo JJ. Current status of robotic partial nephrectomy (RPN). *BJU Int.* 2011;108(6 Pt 2):935–941.

27. Porpiglia F, Bertolo R, Amparore D, et al. Evaluation of functional outcomes after laparoscopic partial nephrectomy using renal scintigraphy: clamped vs clampless technique. *BJU Int.* 2015;115(4):606–612.

28. Gill IS, Patil MB, Abreu AL, et al. Zero ischemia anatomical partial nephrectomy: a novel approach. *J Urol.* 2012;187(3):807–814.

29. Nguyen MM, Gill IS. Halving ischemia time during laparoscopic partial nephrectomy. *J Urol.* 2008;179(2):627–632.

30. Antonelli A, Minervini A, Mari A, et al.; RECORD Project-LUNA Foundation. TriMatch comparison of the efficacy of FloSeal versus TachoSil versus no hemostatic agents for partial nephrectomy: results from a large multicenter dataset. *Int J Urol.* 2015;22(1):47–52.

19

Choice of Renal Replacement Therapy

SARA SAMONI AND CLAUDIO RONCO

INTRODUCTION

Acute kidney injury (AKI) is a clinical syndrome characterized by a sudden decrease in kidney function resulting in retention of creatinine, urea, and other waste products and dysregulation of fluids and electrolytes.

The incidence of AKI widely ranges depending on the definition used and the studied population. However, about 5% to 7% of hospitalized patients develop AKI during hospital stay; this incidence is further increased to 25% in critically ill patients admitted to the intensive care unit (ICU). The development of AKI is associated with a high mortality rate, especially when multiorgan failure coexists.[1] In the absence of any effective pharmacologic therapies, severe AKI is usually managed through renal replacement therapy (RRT).[2] Once the initiation of RRT has been decided, physicians must address the vascular access placement and prescribe the modality, the dose, and the anticoagulation of the treatment. As RRT should be tailored to the patient, the initial prescription should be tailored to the patient's current need. Fig. 19.1 shows a suggested algorithm for the management of AKI requiring RRT.

Currently, it is generally accepted that chronic kidney disease (CKD) is the major risk factor for AKI occurrence, and, vice versa, AKI episodes are risk factors for development of CKD. The optimum RRT required to reduce both nonrenal and renal unfavorable outcomes are still a matter of debate. In this chapter, we will discuss the relationship between AKI and CKD, the indications and timing for RRT initiation, and the choice of RRT modality according to the clinical conditions.

THE INTRICATE LINK BETWEEN AKI AND CKD

Prevalence of CKD has progressively risen during the last decades, due to patients' demographic characteristics and availability of medical care.[3] Several studies have demonstrated that CKD is the major risk factor for development of AKI, especially among patients admitted to the ICU.[4] In fact, CKD patients frequently develop an acute worsening of renal function (acute-on-chronic [AoC] kidney disease) during acute illness.[4] The AoC kidney disease might be due to several mechanisms, including failure of autoregulation, abnormal vasodilation, and adverse effects related to diuretics, antihypertensive agents, and/or nephrotoxins.[5] The decrease of renal functional reserve (RFR), which progressively occurs in worsening stages of CKD, may increase the susceptibility to develop AKI.[6] RFR is the capability of kidneys to improve their function in response to various stimuli, and it is generally measured as the degree of rise in glomerular filtration rate (GFR) during a protein loading test. Although the exact mechanism by which GFR increases is not completely understood, some authors hypothesized the existence of a population of "dormant cortical nephrons" not involved in filtration during resting conditions but potentially recruitable in response to a kidney stress. The entity of RFR progressively decreases in the elderly and in worsening stages of CKD. Moreover, RFR may be reduced after an AKI episode, even in cases of complete recovery of renal function.[6] Additionally, organ cross-talk feedbacks due to or associated with CKD lead to nonrenal organ dysfunctions that may contribute to the development of AKI.

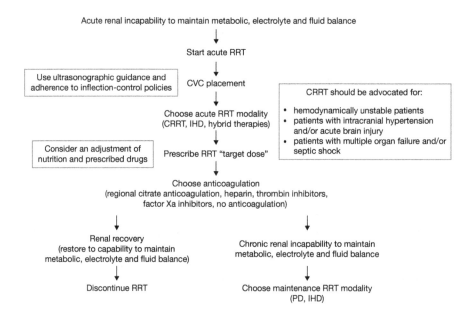

FIGURE 19.1 Algorithm for the management of acute kidney injury requiring renal replacement therapy.

RRT = renal replacement therapy. CVC = central venous catheter. CRRT = continuous renal replacement therapy. IHD = intermittent hemodialysis. PD = peritoneal dialysis.

On the other hand, patients who survive critical illnesses after an AoC kidney disease episode have a high risk for CKD progression.[4] Several studies have demonstrated that, even when renal function is fully recovered after the acute insult, most of patients with AKI have a progression to advanced stages of CKD.[5] Moreover, CKD progression after AKI occurs even in the absence of common risk factors (such as arterial hypertension, diabetes, or cardiovascular disease), with less severity of AKI independent of the cause of AKI.[5] Several pathophysiological mechanisms for the progression of renal damage are under investigation,[5] but the final common pathways appears likely to be maladaptive repair and disordered regeneration.[7]

It is generally accepted that AKI and CKD are closely linked in a highly complex relationship.[5] The development of AKI and the worsening of CKD may recycle several times in the patient life until the onset of end-stage renal disease (ESRD). Schematically, renal function may be considered as the sum of the function of all single nephrons. In this context, the occurrence of AKI episodes reduces the number of functioning nephrons, thus predisposing to CKD. Similarly, CKD patients (with less functioning renal mass) are prone to develop AoC kidney diseases. AoC kidney diseases, and vice versa, by means of a

further reduction in functioning nephrons, contribute to CKD progression to ESRD. Considering renal function as defined above, Fig. 19.2 schematically represents the functioning nephrons loss in AKI and CKD and the link between them.

TIMING OF RRT INITIATION

In the absence of effective pharmacologic therapies, severe AKI is usually managed through RRT.[2] In fact, despite the controversy regarding "optimization" of RRT based on timing, modality, and dose of treatment, avoidance of renal support in an oligoanuric critically ill patient is not an acceptable option.

Over the years, several studies have tried to identify the adequate timing for RRT initiation in patients with AKI. Initial data from retrospective, observational, and small prospective studies performed in the 1960s and 1970s suggested that early initiation of RRT was associated with improved outcome in patients with AKI. In those studies, the level of blood urea or blood urea nitrogen was used to define early or late initiation of RRT. Similar favorable results with early RRT, using the same blood urea nitrogen criteria, were demonstrated in more recent observational studies.[8] Consistent with this hypothesis, when timing of RRT was investigated in relation to ICU admission, a late RRT was associated with

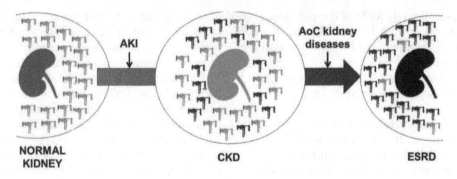

FIGURE 19.2 Link between acute kidney injury and chronic kidney disease. Schematically, renal function may be considered as the sum of the function of all single nephrons. In this context, the occurrence of AKI episodes reduces the number of functioning nephrons, thus predisposing to CKD progression. Similarly, CKD, in which functioning nephrons are less, predisposes to AoC kidney diseases. AoC kidney diseases, vice versa, by means of a further reduction of functioning nephrons, contribute to CKD progression until ESRD. AKI = acute kidney injury. CKD = chronic kidney disease. AoC kidney disease = acute-on-chronic kidney disease. ESRD = end-stage renal disease.

higher mortality, long-term RRT requirement, and hospital length of stay.[9] Additionally, a correlation between late RRT and worst outcomes have also been found when the staging of AKI at RRT initiation was used to classify early versus late treatments.[10] Although results from these studies suggest that early RRT in AKI patients may improve renal and nonrenal outcomes, recent reports offer contrasting results. In fact, in a randomized clinical trial (RCT) of 100 patients with AKI stage 2 (KDIGO criteria and utilizing the novel biomarker neutrophil gelatinase associated lipocalin ≥400 ng/mL), Wald et al. failed to demonstrate significant differences in mortality between the group starting RRT within 12 hours of meeting the inclusion criteria and the group starting RRT according to "classic indications" (e.g., hyperkalemia, acidosis, and severe respiratory failure)[11]. Similar results were achieved by another RCT of 620 critically ill patients in which the prevalent RRT modality was intermittent hemodialysis (IHD). Patients randomized to the "early" arm received RRT within 6 hours of reaching AKI stage 3 while in the "late" arm RRT was only started if clinical indications occurred. In both groups, mortality was around 50% with no significant difference. Importantly, 60% of patients in the "late" arm did not require RRT; in this group, patients who initiated late RRT had the highest mortality.[12]

Although the recommendations are not graded, KDIGO guidelines[2] suggest starting RRT when life-threatening changes in fluid, electrolyte, and acid-base balance occur. In clinical practice, this recommendation is usually observed. In fact, the decision to initiate RRT is commonly based on clinical or biochemical issues such as fluid overload and/or solutes imbalances (azotemia, hyperkalemia, severe acidosis). More precisely, the Acute Dialysis Quality Initiative[13] states that, based on the existing evidence, RRT should be considered when renal capacity cannot guarantee a sufficient metabolic, electrolyte, and fluid balance. Nonetheless, indications and timing of RRT remain controversial and remain among the top priorities in research in this field.[13]

VASCULAR ACCESS

A nontunneled, noncuffed, large-bore, double-lumen dialysis catheter is commonly used for acute RRT in critically ill patients with AKI. The catheter should be placed using ultrasonographic guidance and with adherence to infection-control policies. The central vein should be chosen depending on patient's clinical and instrumental features. KDIGO guidelines, according to the incidence of catheter-related complications for each site, suggest the following order for catheter insertion: (i) right internal jugular vein; (ii) femoral vein; (iii) left internal jugular vein; and (iv) subclavian vein.[2]

CHOICE OF RRT MODALITY

Once RRT initiation has been decided, the most appropriate RRT modality should be selected. The choice of RRT prescription depends not only on patient's need but also organizational characteristics such as availability of technological and human resources and staff experience. Currently, continuous RRT (CRRT) is the prevalent acute RRT modality used in Australia and in most European countries, and its use is increasing in the United States.[14]

There are at least 3 clinical settings in which CRRT should be advocated:

1. **Hemodynamically unstable patients**: The choice of acute RRT modality should primarily take into account patient's hemodynamic status. In fact, it is well known that CRRT guarantees a better dialysis tolerance by means of slower fluid subtraction and absence of fluid shifts due to the rapid solute removal.[2] In hemodynamically stable ICU patients, a Cochrane meta-analysis[15] did not demonstrate a significant difference between CRRT and IHD in terms of mortality. Nonetheless, patients treated with CRRT achieved better hemodynamic parameters.

2. **Patients with intracerebral hemorrhage and/or acute brain injury.** IHD has been associated to further increases in intracerebral pressure; in addition, CRRT has been demonstrated to avoid hyponatremia and thermal losses better than other RRT modalities.[16]

3. **Patients with multiple organ failure and/or septic shock.** When blood purification requirement is accompanied by multiple organ failure or septic shock, CRRT is recommended.[13]

On the contrary, IHD provides adequate metabolic control[15] in hemodynamically stable patients and may be preferred to allow patients mobilization, rehabilitation, and early ICU discharge.[13]

In recent years, the so-called hybrid therapies, such as sustained low efficiency dialysis, extended daily dialysis, and prolonged intermittent RRT have been developed. They may combine advantages from CRRT and IHD and may be viable alternatives for critically ill patients with AKI. The precise role of hybrid techniques warrants further investigation with RCTs.[17]

DOSE OF RRT

What constitutes the most adequate RRT dose for any specific patient is not known. However, a significant correlation exists between RRT dose and survival in both intermittent and CRRT in the general population.[18] Dose identifies the volume of blood cleared of waste products and toxins by the extracorporeal circuit per unit of time.[18] Over the years, several different definitions and formulas to calculate RRT dose have been used, leading to problems in both clinical practice and research activities. Recent consensus[18] recommends that once the initiation of RRT has been decided, the "target dose" should be prescribed by physicians on the basis of specific clinical conditions. During the treatment, considering the flow rates in the extracorporeal circuit, a "current dose" may be estimated. During downtime, when the machine treatment is stopped (e.g., because of machine alarms, circuit clotting, radiological exams, etc.), the current dose is zero. The total amount of downtime during the treatment influences the "average effective delivered dose," which is the measured clearance delivered to the patient. To reduce the discrepancies between the target dose and the average effective delivered dose the "target machine dose" can be modified during the treatment.[18]

Several studies have tried to define the most optimal dose, which is the lowest dose associated with the best patient outcome. Previous studies reported that a dose of 35 mL/k/h correlate with a lower mortality rate.[19] However, 2 large RCTs recently failed to confirm these findings.[20,21] Based on this evidence, the current KDIGO guidelines recommend achieving an effluent volume corresponding to a target dose of 20 to 25 mL/kg/h for CRRT in patients with AKI.[2] One must be cognizant that the target dose is dynamic and can be modified according to patient needs. The next steps in the decision tree following the choice of RRT modality and prescription are nutritional and drug dosage adjustments.[2] Although there are no available recommendations, an in-depth knowledge of dialysis techniques and pharmacokinetics may help physicians prescribe drugs at adequate dose and intervals. Additionally, monitoring the plasma level of drugs, when available, may contribute to further personalization of therapy and prevention of under or overdosing.

ANTICOAGULATION

A correlation between membrane dysfunction and solute clearance during RRT has been clearly demonstrated. In particular, by the time that membrane fouling (accumulation of undesirable foreign matter causing clogging of pores or coating of surfaces and inhibiting or limiting the function) occurs and clearance of urea falls by 20%, the clearance of larger solutes may have already been impaired.[22] In this context, considering middle molecular weight molecules as the solute target to be removed, an adequate sieving coefficient for these molecules should be maintained over a long period of time. Unfortunately, membrane fouling is not easily measurable in clinical practice. However, systemic and regional anticoagulation, as well as heparin-grafted membranes, can reduce filter clotting and membrane fouling and improve dialysis delivery.

Anticoagulation (and filter patency) should ensure optimal dialysis delivery without compromising patient safety. The current KDIGO guidelines[2] suggest using regional citrate anticoagulation in all patients without contraindications and with either high or low risk of bleeding. Major contraindications for the use of citrate include severe liver dysfunction and the shock with muscle hypoperfusion due to the risk for citrate accumulation.[2] The administration of unfractioned heparin into the RRT circuit remains the most used anticoagulation. In patients with heparin-induced thrombocytopenia, heparin must be discontinued, and direct thrombin inhibitors (i.e., argatroban) or factor Xa inhibitors (i.e., danaparoid or fondaparinux) or no anticoagulation should be considered during RRT.[2]

RECOVERY FROM AKI AND RISK TO DEVELOP CKD

Recovery from AKI may be full, partial, or none. Varying severity of CKD including ESRD requiring maintenance RRT may persist. The exact rate as well as the pathophysiological mechanisms leading to progression of renal damage are still under investigation. It is generally agreed that the final common pathways are likely maladaptive repair and disordered regeneration.[7]

Although some studies found a lower proportion of ESRD requiring maintenance RRT in patients initially treated with CRRT,[23] a recent large single-center retrospective study[24] showed no difference in renal recovery rate between CRRT and IHD used as initial RRT modality. Discontinuation of RRT should be considered when renal recovery is able to guarantee a sufficient metabolic, electrolyte, and fluid balance.[13] Some markers have been proposed to individualize the right timing for RRT weaning. Among these, the most used in clinical practice are serum creatinine levels with a constant dialysis dose and urine output. Recently, daily urine urea excretion (24-hour urine urea) and daily urine creatinine excretion (24-hour urine creatinine) have been demonstrated to have good reliability in predicting successful RRT weaning.[25] The right timing for RRT discontinuation, as well as the decision to start RRT should be individualized based on the demand capacity of a specific patient.[13]

TRANSITION BETWEEN DIFFERENT RRT MODALITIES

There is a progressive increase in the number of ESRD patients admitted to the ICU with acute critical illnesses, driven in part by changing patient demographics and the increasing availability of maintenance RRT such as IHD and peritoneal dialysis (PD).[1] In fact, IHD and PD patients are more prone to repeated hospital and ICU admissions.[1] When an IHD or PD patient is admitted to the ICU, a transition from maintenance to the most appropriate RRT modality, based on patient's current clinical conditions, may be required.[26] Considerations about indications for CRRT in ESRD patients do not differ from those prevailing among the general population. The use of PD in unstable patients, despite being theoretically appropriate, has some limitations (e.g., risk of infection, potential interference with mechanical ventilation, lower efficiency, unpredictability of fluid removal). Patients who recover from critical illnesses, can progressively restart their previous maintenance RRT regimen. An exception is represented by cases in which the acute event (i.e., abdominal injury) caused an extensive loss of peritoneal surface prevents the PD performance.

Conversely, patients who do not recover renal function after an AoC kidney disease episode and require maintenance RRT, PD, or IHD should be addressed, according to patients' clinical and individual needs.[26]

CONCLUSION
- AKI is a clinical syndrome characterized by a sudden decrease in kidney function that frequently occurs in ICU patients, dramatically increasing mortality rates.
- CKD is the major risk factor for AKI occurrence, and, vice versa, AKI episodes are risk factors for CKD development.
- Severe AKI is usually managed through RRT. Acute RRT should be considered

when renal capacity cannot guarantee a sufficient metabolic, electrolyte, and fluid balance.

- Once the initiation of RRT has been decided, physicians must address the vascular access placement and prescribe the modality, the dose, and the anticoagulation of the treatment.
- A nontunneled, double-lumen dialysis catheter, placed in a central vein using ultrasonographic guidance and with adherence to infection-control policies, is commonly used for acute RRT.
- Acute RRT prescriptions depend on both patient's need and organizational characteristics. In hemodynamically unstable patients, acute brain injury and/or impaired intracranial compliance (determines the ability of the intracranial compartment to accommodate an increase in volume without a large increase in intracranial pressure), and multiple organ failure or septic shock, CRRT should be advocated.
- In all other cases, IHD provides an adequate metabolic control and may be preferred to allow patients mobilization, rehabilitation, and ICU discharge.
- The precise role of the so-called hybrid therapies should be further investigated with RCT.
- Dose identifies the volume of blood cleared of waste products and toxins by the extracorporeal circuit per unit of time. A consensus on terminology has recently been achieved.
- Based on evidence, an effluent volume corresponding to a target dose of 20 to 25 mL/kg/h is recommended for CRRT in patients with AKI.
- Despite the recommendation for regional citrate anticoagulation in all patients without contraindications, the administration of unfractioned heparin into the RRT circuit remains the most used anticoagulation.
- RRT should be tailored to the patient's needs.
- Once AKI has resolved, a full, partial, or no renal recovery may occur. Hence, different degrees of CKD may persist.

REFERENCES

1. Uchino S, Kellum J a., Bellomo R, et al. Acute renal failure in critically ill patients. A multinational, multicenter study. *J Am Med Assoc.* 2005;294(7):813–818.
2. Kellum J, Lameire N, Aspelin P, et al. KDIGO clinical practice guideline for acute kidney injury. *Kidney Int Suppl.* 2012;2(1):1–138.
3. Hill N, Fatoba S, Oke J, et al. Global prevalence of chronic kidney disease: a systematic review and meta-analysis. *PLoS One.* 2016;11(7):1–18.
4. Rimes-Stigare C, Frumento P, Bottai M, Mårtensson J, Martling C-R, Bell M. Long-term mortality and risk factors for development of end-stage renal disease in critically ill patients with and without chronic kidney disease. *Crit Care.* 2015;19(1):383.
5. Lakhmir S. Chawla, Paul W. Eggers, Robert A. Star PLK. Acute kidney injury and chronic kidney disease as interconnected syndromes. *N Eng J Med.* 2014;371(1):58–66.
6. Sharma A, Mucino MJ, Ronco C. Renal functional reserve and renal recovery after acute kidney injury. *Nephron-Clin Pract.* 2014;127(1–4):94–100.
7. Chawla LS, Kimmel PL. Acute kidney injury and chronic kidney disease: an integrated clinical syndrome. *Kidney Int.* 2012;82(5):516–524.
8. Liu KD, Himmelfarb J, Paganini E, et al. Timing of initiation of dialysis in critically ill patients with acute kidney injury. *Clin J Am Soc Nephrol.* 2006;1(5):915–919.
9. Sm B, Uchino S, Bellomo R, et al. Timing of renal replacement therapy and clinical outcomes in critically ill patients with severe acute kidney injury. *J Crit Care.* 2009;24(1):129–140.
10. Shiao CC, Wu VC, Li WY, et al. Late initiation of renal replacement therapy is associated with worse outcomes in acute kidney injury after major abdominal surgery. *Crit Care.* 2009;13(5):R171.
11. Smith OM, Wald R, Adhikari NK, Pope K, Weir MA, Bagshaw SM; Canadian Critical Care Trials Group. Standard versus accelerated initiation of renal replacement therapy in acute kidney injury (STARRT-AKI): study protocol for a randomized controlled trial. Trials 2013;14:320. doi: 10.1186/1745-6215-14-320
12. Gaudry S, Hajage D, Dreyfuss D. Initiation of renal-replacement therapy in the intensive care unit. *N Engl J Med.* 2016;375(19):1899–1902.
13. Ostermann M, Joannidis M, Pani A, et al. Patient selection and timing of continuous renal replacement therapy. *Blood Purif.* 2016;42(3):224–237.
14. Legrand M, Darmon M, Joannidis M. Management of renal replacement therapy in ICU

patients: an international survey. *Intensive Care Med.* 2013;39(1):101–108.

15. Ks R, Adams J, Am M, Muirhead N, Rabindranath K, Macleod AM. Intermittent versus continuous renal replacement therapy for acute renal failure in adults. *Cochrane Db Sys Rev.* 2007;(3):CD003773.

16. Davenport A. Management of acute kidney injury in liver disease. *Contrib Nephrol.* 2010;165:197–205.

17. Neves JB, Rodrigues FB, Castel??o M, Costa J, Lopes JA. Extended daily dialysis versus intermittent hemodialysis for acute kidney injury: a systematic review. *J Crit Care.* 2016;33:271–273.

18. Neri M, Villa G, Garzotto F, et al. Nomenclature for renal replacement therapy in acute kidney injury: basic principles. *Crit Care.* 2016;20(1):318.

19. Ronco C, Bellomo R, Homel P, et al. Effects of different doses in continuous veno-venous haemofiltration on outcomes of acute renal failure: a prospective randomised trial. *Lancet.* 2000;356(9223):26–30.

20. Uchino S, Bellomo R, Morimatsu H, et al.; Beginning and Ending Supportive Therapy for the Kidney (B.E.S.T. Kidney) Investigators. Continuous renal replacement therapy: a worldwide practice survey. *Intensive Care Med.* 2007;33(9):1563–1570.

21. The VA/NIH Acute Renal Failure Trial Network. Intensity of renal support in critically ill patients with acute kidney injury. *Lancet.* 2008;359(1):7–20.

22. Pasko DA, Churchwell MD, Salama NN, Mueller BA. Longitudinal hemodiafilter performance in modeled continuous renal replacement therapy. *Blood Purif.* 2011;32(2):82–88.

23. Schneider AG, Bellomo R, Bagshaw SM, et al. Choice of renal replacement therapy modality and dialysis dependence after acute kidney injury: a systematic review and meta-analysis. *Intensive Care Med.* 2013;39(6):987–997.

24. Liang K V., Sileanu FE, Clermont G, et al. Modality of RRT and recovery of kidney function after AKI in patients surviving to hospital discharge. *Clin J Am Soc Nephrol.* 2016;11(1):30–38.

25. Viallet N, Brunot V, Kuster N, et al. Daily urinary creatinine predicts the weaning of renal replacement therapy in ICU acute kidney injury patients. *Ann Intensive Care.* 2016;6(1):71.

26. De Rosa S, Samoni S, Villa G, Ronco C. Management of chronic kidney disease patients in the intensive care unit: mixing acute and chronic illness. *Blood Purif.* 2017:151–162.

20

Preserving Residual Kidney Function

MITEN J. DHRUVE AND JOANNE M. BARGMAN

INTRODUCTION

As patients with chronic kidney disease (CKD) progress to end-stage kidney disease and dialysis, it is humbling to note the high rates of morbidity and mortality that they encounter. In an effort to provide optimal care for these patients, it is crucial to appreciate the many benefits of residual kidney function (RKF) in these patients. This chapter focuses on these benefits and outlines several strategies to help preserve this function.

Maiorca et al.[1] was one of the first groups to document survival benefit of RKF in dialysis patients. In 1995, they studied 102 dialysis patients (68 on peritoneal dialysis [PD] and 34 on hemodialysis [HD]) and noted that for every 1mL/min increase in glomerular filtration rate (GFR), there was a 40% reduction in risk of death.[1] A larger study by Diaz-Buxo et al.[2] looking at 1,603 PD patients also observed similar findings, with RKF strongly associated with survival among PD patients. Interestingly, peritoneal clearance was not associated with survival. These findings were strengthened by the reanalysis of the CANUSA study,[3] where we observed a 36% decrease in the relative risk of death for every 250 mL increase in 24-hour urine volume. Once again, the addition of peritoneal solute clearance or ultrafiltration did not affect the risk of death. The Netherlands Cooperative Study on the Adequacy of Dialysis[4] group also demonstrated a 12% reduction in mortality for every 1mL/min increase in residual GFR. With these different studies all showing similar findings, it is convincing that RKF is strongly associated with survival in patients on PD. It is worthy to note that this association also appears to extend to those on HD. Shemin and colleagues[5] were one of the first investigators to document a protective benefit of RKF on mortality in HD patients with an odds ratio for death of 0.44. Similarly, in the study by Termorshuizen et al.[6] every 1 unit increase in renal Kt/V_{urea} resulted in an astounding 66% decrease in relative risk of death.

The mechanism of the reduction in mortality, however, remains elusive. One explanation proposed is that preserved residual urine output leads to better volume control and, thus, reduction of hypertension, sympathetic overdrive, and left ventricular hypertrophy. This correlation has been borne out in the study by Wang et al.[7] who showed that in 158 PD patients, loss of RKF was strongly associated with increase in left ventricular hypertrophy. Moreover, patients with left ventricular mass index in the upper 50th percentile had higher rates of death and cardiovascular mortality. Another equally intriguing explanation of reduction of mortality is the reduction in inflammation and oxidative stress. Several studies looking at the value of C-reactive protein as an indicator of inflammation have found it to be a strong predictor of cardiovascular mortality in dialysis patients. In the hemodialysis population specifically, patients with RKF had lower C-reactive protein levels in addition to reduced mortality.[8] Furthermore, it has been suggested that more RKF may be correlated to more middle and large molecular weight solute clearance, better erythropoietin production, and vitamin D production.[5] Although several limitations exist with the previous studies, RKF and outcome remain an intriguing correlation. Conversely, a counterargument by Misra et al.[9] proposes that results may be confounded by informative censoring, which occurs when the reason for patient dropout is related to underlying GFR. This study performed a reanalysis of CANUSA and described a significantly lower GFR in patients who either died or were transferred to HD compared to those who completed the study. They argue that exclusion of these patients selects an intrinsically healthier patient cohort leading to skewed data set.[9] Nonetheless, the mortality benefits described by the previously mentioned studies is noteworthy.

In addition to the survival benefit, reduction of left ventricular hypertrophy, decreased inflammation, and better middle and large molecule clearance, RKF is associated with improved quality of life (QOL) and reduced dietary restriction. The NECOSAD group[4] and the CHOICE study group[8] both demonstrated improved QOL, especially in domains of physical functioning, vitality, kidney disease-specific symptoms, and effect of kidney disease on daily life and sleep disorders. Some of this improvement in QOL was felt to be due to a more relaxed diet and achievement of better phosphate control in patients with RKF.

Finally, with peritonitis being associated with increased morbidity and mortality and the leading cause of technique failure, it is notable that RKF is associated with lower risk of peritonitis and increased length of time to first peritonitis.[10]

After appreciating the importance of RKF in dialysis patients, it is imperative that we do everything we can to preserve it. The following discussion addresses different ways to preserve RKF in this population.

HOW TO PRESERVE RKF

Avoid Hemodialysis

There is a growing body of evidence that now highlights the rapidity of decline in RKF in HD compared to PD. One of the earliest studies was a retrospective analysis of 57 HD and 58 continuous ambulatory peritoneal dialysis (CAPD) patients. It was observed that the rate of decline of RKF was twice as fast in HD compared to PD patients.[11] This finding was confirmed by Moist et al.[12] who studied 811 incident HD patients and 1,032 incident PD patients. After adjustment for baseline GFR and other confounders, PD was associated with a 64% lower risk of anuria at 1-year follow-up. Some of proposed mechanisms include hemodynamic instability in HD patients, bio-incompatible dialysis membranes, and inflammation and oxidative stress due to exposure to the extracorporeal HD circuit.

We have recently reported a retrospective analysis of 77 incident PD patients and found that the rate of decline in RKF in the first year of PD was lower than in the year preceding start of dialysis.[13] This recapitulated a study from a decade earlier in a smaller number of patients.[14] Possible explanations for this phenomenon include the importance of removal of uremic toxins that could otherwise propagate further kidney injury, gentle offloading of hyperfiltration in the remnant kidneys, and avoidance of large hemodynamic fluctuations compared to conventional HD.[13] With all these benefits of PD on RKF, it is easy to understand why a "PD first" approach is widely advocated.

Incremental Dialysis

Even though PD fares better at preventing loss of RKF, there is still a slow progression to anuria in these patients. Some of this decline has been postulated to be due to glucose degradation end-products absorbed from conventional PD solutions, systemic inflammation, and increased ultrafiltration causing hypotension. There are now studies looking at the benefits of incremental PD. In this form of dialysis, incident patients with RKF are initiated on 3 dialysis exchanges or fewer per day. As RKF decreases over time, the PD prescription is increased to achieve adequate clearance. In a recent study by Sandrini et al.[15], 29 patients were started on incremental PD, defined as 1 or 2 dwells per day on CAPD while 76 were on standard "full" PD—3 to 5 dwells per day. RKF in the incremental PD group remained stable while it decreased in the standard group. Similarly, a recent randomized controlled trial studied 139 patients randomized to either 3 or 4 exchanges a day. They noted that after 24 months there was no difference in urine volume, survival, or peritonitis.[16] Due to the potential benefits of incremental dialysis, a growing number of institutions, including ours, now follow a similar approach while closely monitoring patients for clinical signs and symptoms of inadequate clearance.

A similar strategy is also being employed in the HD population. With this approach, patients with RKF are started on twice weekly treatments. This, however, remains controversial with some observational data showing improved survival when compared to conventional 3× per week HD while other studies have shown similar or even reduced survival.[17,18]

CAPD or Automated PD

Much debate exists regarding the effects of CAPD versus automated PD (aPD) on RKF. Observational studies have demonstrated a faster decline in RKF in patients on aPD as compared to CAPD. This is postulated to be due to increased overnight ultrafiltration by aPD contemporaneous with the nocturnal dip in blood pressure. These 2 events would then propagate hypoperfusion injury on already-damaged kidneys, leading to loss of RKF. Unfortunately, reports on this question are small and observational in nature, making it difficult to draw any solid conclusions.[19]

Avoid Peritonitis

Peritonitis is the leading cause of technique failure and also contributes significantly to morbidity and mortality. It is also an important cause of RKF loss, and patients who have peritonitis demonstrate a greater slope of RKF decline. Shin et al.[20] showed that the higher peritonitis group (>0.86 episode/patient/year) had an RKF slope of −0.12 mL/min/month while the lower peritonitis group (<0.86 episode/patient/year) had an RKF slope of −0.07 mL/min/month, $p < 0.0001$. One proposed mechanism is the increase in systemic inflammatory cytokines during peritonitis. These are subsequently filtered by the kidneys, leading to more renal injury. Intensive patient training, aseptic technique, application of antibacterial ointment to PD exit site, and use of antibiotic prophylaxis during procedures such as colonoscopy, endoscopy, dental procedures, and gynecological procedures are some steps that can be taken to prevent peritonitis.

Avoid Nephrotoxic Agents

Dialysis patients with RKF should receive similar advice provided to CKD patients with progressive renal failure. Specifically, they should be advised to avoid radiocontrast agents, nonsteroidal antiinflammatory medications, aminoglycosides, and other nephrotoxic agents. Most programs recognize the importance of avoiding nephrotoxins, but prophylaxis prior to use of radiocontrast dyes remains controversial. Most studies have failed to demonstrate a significant benefit with the use of N-acetylcysteine in dialysis patients.[21] Despite this, we would recommend avoidance of radiocontrast dye if at all possible, adequate preprocedure hydration, reduced volume of dye, and use of N-acetylcysteine due to a conceivable benefit and minimal side effect profile.

The effect of aminoglycosides on RKF are also debatable. Nephrotoxicity is hypothesized to be secondary to tubular accumulation. This, however, is not correlated in a large observational trial by Badve et al.[22] In this paper, 1,075 patients who received aminoglycosides as initial empiric antibiotic for peritonitis had a rate of decline in RKF similar to the control group. Furthermore, the rate of RKF loss was also similar for patients who were exposed to multiple courses of aminoglycosides. The major limitation with this study has to do with its observational design. Apart from a high dropout rate, there is also lack of information on compliance and aminoglycoside levels. Due to the uncertainty, we avoid aminoglycoside antibiotics in patients with RKF or administer a short duration of therapy with modification to a less nephrotoxic antibiotic based on sensitivity profiles if at all possible.

Use of Biocompatible Solutions

As mentioned previously, it has been suggested that exposure to different components in conventional PD solutions could lead to a more rapid decline in RKF. The high glucose and low pH PD solutions are metabolized into reactive carbonyl compounds and advanced glycation end products that influence glomerular structure and function, leading to glomerulosclerosis. To combat this, there are now several neutral pH, low-glucose degradation product (GDP) solutions that have been developed and studied. Icodextrin PD solution is composed of a large group of polydispersed polymers, which are poorly absorbed through the capillaries and thus retained in the peritoneal space for longer periods of time than dextrose. A double-blind randomized study compared it to glucose-based solutions and found higher ultrafiltration rates. Loss of RKF was also significantly less in the icodextrin group as compared to the dextrose group.[23] One proposed explanation is that icodextrin was selectively initiated in hypervolemic patients rather than euvolemic patients. This resulted in ultrafiltration to normovolemia rather than to volume depletion. We use icodextrin in patients who are extracellular fluid volume expanded, and closely follow with frequent volume assessments.

Other neutral pH, low-glucose degradation product solutions have been studied. Gambrosol Trio, a low glucose degradation product solution, was noted to be associated with a decreased decline in RKF when compared to standard dextrose solutions.[24] Unfortunately, this study had small numbers, high dropout rates, and increased angiotensin converting enzyme inhibitor (ACEI) use in the intervention group. Balance, another biocompatible solution also has a neutral pH, is lactate buffered and has low concentrations of glucose degradation products. In a multicenter open randomized crossover study, 86 patients were randomized to use of Balance solution or standard dextrose solution. The Balance arm had higher urine volume but a decrease in peritoneal ultrafiltration compared to the standard group. This finding, however, did not meet statistical significance.[25] Furthermore, the reduced ultrafiltration with Balance may have been wholly or partly responsible for the increased urinary output. Two recent large multicenter randomized controlled trials studies, the Trio trial[26] and balANZ trial[27] showed opposite results. The Trio trial noted that patients on the biocompatible solution had a slower decline in RKF. There was, however, a high dropout rate, and, interestingly, the treatment group had significantly higher rates of peritonitis. The balANZ trial did not detect any statistically significant difference in rate of RKF decline but did find a longer time to first peritonitis event. Once again, this study suffered a high dropout rate with enrollment of only 55% of the intended patient population.[28]

With these data, it is difficult to make a strong case for the use of biocompatible solutions, which also come bearing a substantially increased cost in many centers and may be associated with a reduction in ultrafiltration.

Renal Angiotensin System Blockade

The renin–angiotensin–aldosterone system (RAAS) is known to play several crucial roles, including blood pressure control. It is also known to increase inflammation and fibrosis through upregulation of key transcription factors such as NF-kB. RAAS inhibition has been a mainstay of therapy in a variety of renal diseases and function by decreasing angiotensin II and consequently aldosterone. This leads to a decrease in GFR due to the decrease in efferent arteriolar constriction and a reduction in intraglomerular pressure. It is expected that the GFR may decrease by up to 30% at initiation of RAAS inhibition. Despite this decrease in GFR, there are several important benefits of this therapy both in the CKD and the dialysis population.

Suzuki et al.[29] performed a prospective randomized open label study with 34 patients. The treatment group received valsartan therapy while the control group received other antihypertensive therapy. Patients in valsartan arm had a significantly slower decline in RKF up to 2 years from study initiation. Li et al.[30] also conducted a randomized study with 60 PD patients to assess effects of ramipril. The treatment group, however, had more diabetic patients and a lower baseline GFR than the control group. Over 12 months, residual GFR had declined by 2.07 mL/min in treatment group as compared to 3.00 mL/min in control group ($p = 0.03$). There was also a decreased rate of progression to anuria in treatment group compared to control.[30] Unfortunately, both these studies, although randomized, were limited by small numbers.

In the HD literature, there have been conflicting results regarding effect of ACEI/angiotensin receptor blockade (ARB) on RKF. However, a recent randomized trial by Kjaergaard et al.[31] showed that patients on ARB had an increased urine volume after 12 months of treatment. This finding however was not statistically significant. The major issue with this study was that of the 41 patients that were randomized, 11 patients dropped out in each arm of the study, leaving a small cohort of patients at the end of study.

Despite the shortcomings of the aforementioned studies, RAAS blockade by either ARB or ACEI is strongly suggested in dialysis patients with RKF. Apart from the beneficial effects on RKF and decrease in inflammation and fibrosis, ARB/ACEI are known to have both cardioprotective and peritoneal membrane preservation qualities. Furthermore, we have also previously shown that use of ACE/ARB in PD population was correlated with a 62% reduced risk of death.[32]

Use of Diuretics

One of primary concerns in dialysis patients remains extracellular fluid expansion. This usually leads to prescription of higher glucose concentration peritoneal dialysate or increased ultrafiltration on hemodialysis. Both of these therapies come at a significant cost, including increased glucose load to patients as well as increased possibility of hypotension from acute volume shift. Diuretics can help mitigate these risks by increasing urine volume and, therefore, allowing the patient increased fluid and salt intake. Medcalf et al.[33] in 2001 published a randomized open label study in which 61 patients were randomized to either furosemide 250 mg daily or no diuretic. After 1 year, urine volume in control group had decreased by approximately 300 mL/24 hours while it remained stable in diuretic group. Decline in urinary urea and creatinine clearance was similar in both groups. Despite this benefit, diuretics remain underutilized in most centers.

Comparatively in the HD literature, there exists very little high-quality evidence to support diuretic use. One observational study looked at 16,420 HD patients in Dialysis Outcomes and Practice Patterns[34] study and noted that patients on diuretics had lower interdialytic weight gain, twice the probability of retaining RKF, and decreased episodes of hyperkalemia.

With the previously stated benefits, we would recommend that patients with RKF be maintained on diuretics and they be titrated as required to help attain adequate volume control.

Preservation of Transplant Renal Function

Patients with a kidney transplant are subjected to several immunosuppressive medications that carry significant side effects. These medications are known to increase the risk of infections and malignancy. Many physicians, therefore, will decrease or stop immunosuppressive medications as soon as patients with a transplanted kidney progress to dialysis. Jassal et al.,[35] however, argue that continuation of immunosuppressive medications will slow the rate of loss of transplant RKF. This paper used a decision analysis with 2 treatment options: remain on predialysis immunosuppressive medications or gradual taper of steroids with a discontinuation of all immunosuppressive agents. This study reported that the life expectancy for patients not on immunosuppressive therapy was 5.3 years compared to 5.8 years in treatment group mainly due to preservation of RKF of transplanted kidney. This benefit outweighed the risks associated with the medications including malignancy and infection. Interestingly, this analysis was performed with cyclosporine as the immunosuppressive medication, which leads to possibility that there might be greater benefit if nonnephrotoxic immunosuppressive agents such as mycophenolate mofetil were used. It still is important that the patient be informed of the adverse effects and close monitoring for malignancy be performed when continuing the patient on these medications.

Low Protein Diet

In the CKD population, it is usually recommended to decrease dietary protein intake. This is felt to decrease the nitrogen load on the kidneys and reduce hyperfiltration. Protein restriction, however, has not been well studied in the dialysis population. One of the major studies performed was a randomized controlled trial by Jiang et al.[36] Sixty patients were randomized to either a low (0.6 g–0.8 g/kg), keto acid supplemented low (0.6–0.8 g/kg), or high (1.0–1.2 g/kg) protein diet. The keto acid supplemented group maintained a stable eGFR and urine output while both indices declined in the other groups. Unfortunately, the low protein group was unable to lower their dietary protein to desired levels. Due to the inability to achieve target dietary protein intake and small numbers, it is hard to draw any strong conclusions. Furthermore, malnutrition is an issue in dialysis patients due to uremia, systemic inflammation, polypharmacy, and frequent nausea, and this makes it difficult and impractical to implement a low protein diet in these patients.

CONCLUSION

RKF is strongly associated with benefits in survival, morbidity and QOL in dialysis patients. Practices such as incremental dialysis, avoidance of interim hemodialysis in those choosing PD, avoidance of peritonitis and nephrotoxic medications, use of RAAS blockade, and maintenance of transplant kidney function are all methods that can be implemented to help protect this vital function.

REFERENCES

1. Maiorca R, Brunori G, Zubani R, et al. Predictive value of dialysis adequacy and nutritional indices for mortality and morbidity in CAPD and HD patients: a longitudinal study. *Nephrol Dial Transplant*. 1995;10(12):2295–2305.
2. Diaz-Buxo JA, Lowrie EG, Lew NL, Zhang SM, Zhu X, Lazarus JM. Associates of mortality among peritoneal dialysis patients with special reference to peritoneal transport rates and solute clearance. *Am J Kidney Dis*. 1999;33(3):523–534.
3. Bargman JM, Thorpe KE, Churchill DN; Group CPDS. Relative contribution of residual renal function and peritoneal clearance to adequacy of dialysis: a reanalysis of the CANUSA study. *J Am Soc Nephrol*. 2001;12(10):2158–2162.
4. Termorshuizen F, Korevaar JC, Dekker FW, et al. The relative importance of residual renal function compared with peritoneal clearance for patient survival and quality of life: an analysis of the Netherlands Cooperative Study on the Adequacy of Dialysis (NECOSAD)-2. *Am J Kidney Dis*. 2003;41(6):1293–1302.
5. Shemin D, Bostom AG, Laliberty P, Dworkin LD. Residual renal function and mortality risk

in hemodialysis patients. *Am J Kidney Dis.* 2001;38(1):85–90.

6. Termorshuizen F, Dekker FW, van Manen JG, et al. Relative contribution of residual renal function and different measures of adequacy to survival in hemodialysis patients: an analysis of the Netherlands Cooperative Study on the Adequacy of Dialysis (NECOSAD)-2. *J Am Soc Nephrol.* 2004;15(4):1061–1070.

7. Wang AY, Wang M, Woo J, et al. Inflammation, residual kidney function, and cardiac hypertrophy are interrelated and combine adversely to enhance mortality and cardiovascular death risk of peritoneal dialysis patients. *J Am Soc Nephrol.* 2004;15(8):2186–2194.

8. Shafi T, Jaar BG, Plantinga LC, et al. Association of residual urine output with mortality, quality of life, and inflammation in incident hemodialysis patients: the Choices for Healthy Outcomes in Caring for End-Stage Renal Disease (CHOICE) study. *Am J Kidney Dis.* 2010;56(2):348–358.

9. Misra M, Vonesh E, Churchill DN, Moore HL, Van Stone JC, Nolph KD. Preservation of glomerular filtration rate on dialysis when adjusted for patient dropout. *Kidney Int.* 2000;57(2):691–696.

10. Han SH, Lee SC, Ahn SV, Lee JE, Kim DK, Lee TH, et al. Reduced residual renal function is a risk of peritonitis in continuous ambulatory peritoneal dialysis patients. *Nephrol Dial Transplant.* 2007;22(9):2653–2658.

11. Lysaght MJ, Vonesh EF, Gotch F, et al. The influence of dialysis treatment modality on the decline of remaining renal function. *ASAIO Trans.* 1991;37(4):598–604.

12. Moist LM, Port FK, Orzol SM, et al. Predictors of loss of residual renal function among new dialysis patients. *J Am Soc Nephrol.* 2000;11(3):556–564.

13. He L, Liu X, Li Z, et al. Rate of decline of residual kidney function before and after the start of peritoneal dialysis. *Perit Dial Int.* 2016;36(3):334–339.

14. Berlanga JR, Marron B, Reyero A, Caramelo C, Ortiz A. Peritoneal dialysis retardation of progression of advanced renal failure. *Perit Dial Int.* 2002;22(2):239–242.

15. Sandrini M, Vizzardi V, Valerio F, et al. Incremental peritoneal dialysis: a 10 year single-centre experience. *J Nephrol.* 2016;29(6):871–879.

16. Yan H, Fang W, Lin A, Cao L, Ni Z, Qian J. Three versus 4 daily exchanges and residual kidney function decline in incident CAPD patients: a randomized controlled trial. *Am J Kidney Dis.* 2017;69(4):506–513.

17. Mathew A, Obi Y, Rhee CM, et al. Treatment frequency and mortality among incident hemodialysis patients in the United States comparing incremental with standard and more frequent dialysis. *Kidney Int.* 2016;90(5):1071–1079.

18. Hanson JA, Hulbert-Shearon TE, Ojo AO, et al. Prescription of twice-weekly hemodialysis in the USA. *Am J Nephrol.* 1999;19(6):625–633.

19. Bieber SD, Burkart J, Golper TA, Teitelbaum I, Mehrotra R. Comparative outcomes between continuous ambulatory and automated peritoneal dialysis: a narrative review. *Am J Kidney Dis.* 2014;63(6):1027–1037.

20. Shin SK, Noh H, Kang SW, et al. Risk factors influencing the decline of residual renal function in continuous ambulatory peritoneal dialysis patients. *Perit Dial Int.* 1999;19(2):138–142.

21. Kshirsagar AV, Poole C, Mottl A, et al. N-acetylcysteine for the prevention of radiocontrast induced nephropathy: a meta-analysis of prospective controlled trials. *J Am Soc Nephrol.* 2004;15(3):761–769.

22. Badve SV, Hawley CM, McDonald SP, et al. Use of aminoglycosides for peritoneal dialysis-associated peritonitis does not affect residual renal function. *Nephrol Dial Transplant.* 2012;27(1):381–387.

23. Davies SJ, Woodrow G, Donovan K, et al. Icodextrin improves the fluid status of peritoneal dialysis patients: results of a double-blind randomized controlled trial. *J Am Soc Nephrol.* 2003;14(9):2338–2344.

24. Haag-Weber M, Kramer R, Haake R, et al. Low-GDP fluid (Gambrosol trio) attenuates decline of residual renal function in PD patients: a prospective randomized study. *Nephrol Dial Transplant.* 2010; 25(7): 2288–2296.

25. Williams JD, Topley N, Craig KJ, et al. The Euro-Balance Trial: the effect of a new biocompatible peritoneal dialysis fluid (balance) on the peritoneal membrane. *Kidney Int.* 2004;66(1):408–418.

26. Sikaneta T, Wu G, Abdolell M, et al. The Trio Trial—a randomized controlled clinical trial evaluating the effect of a biocompatible peritoneal dialysis solution on residual renal function. *Perit Dial Int.* 2016;36(5):526–532.

27. Martin Wilkie. The balANZ study—strengthening the evidence for neutral-pH solutions low in glucose degradation products. *Perit Dial Int.* 2012;32(5):489–492.

28. Johnson DW, Brown FG, Clarke M, et al. Effects of biocompatible versus standard fluid on peritoneal dialysis outcomes. *J Am Soc Nephrol.* 2012;23(6):1097–1107.

29. Suzuki H, Kanno Y, Sugahara S, Okada H, Nakamoto H. Effects of an angiotensin II receptor blocker, valsartan, on residual renal function in patients on CAPD. *Am J Kidney Dis.* 2004;43(6):1056–1064.

30. Li PK, Chow KM, Wong TY, Leung CB, Szeto CC. Effects of an angiotensin-converting enzyme inhibitor on residual renal function in patients receiving peritoneal dialysis: a

randomized, controlled study. *Ann Intern Med.* 2003;139(2):105–112.

31. Kjaergaard KD, Peters CD, Jespersen B, et al. Angiotensin blockade and progressive loss of kidney function in hemodialysis patients: a randomized controlled trial. *Am J Kidney Dis.* 2014;64(6):892–901.

32. Fang W, Oreopoulos DG, Bargman JM. Use of ACE inhibitors or angiotensin receptor blockers and survival in patients on peritoneal dialysis. *Nephrol Dial Transplant.* 2008;23(11): 3704–3710.

33. Medcalf JF, Harris KP, Walls J. Role of diuretics in the preservation of residual renal function in patients on continuous ambulatory peritoneal dialysis. *Kidney Int.* 2001;59(3):1128–1133.

34. Bragg-Gresham JL, Fissell RB, Mason NA, et al. Diuretic use, residual renal function, and mortality among hemodialysis patients in the Dialysis Outcomes and Practice Pattern Study (DOPPS). *Am J Kidney Dis.* 2007;49(3):426–431.

35. Jassal SV, Lok CE, Walele A, Bargman JM. Continued transplant immunosuppression may prolong survival after return to peritoneal dialysis: results of a decision analysis. *Am J Kidney Dis.* 2002;40(1):178–183.

36. Jiang N, Qian J, Sun W, et al. Better preservation of residual renal function in peritoneal dialysis patients treated with a low-protein diet supplemented with keto acids: a prospective, randomized trial. *Nephrol Dial Transplant.* 2009;24(8):2551–2558.

An Appreciation of Dimitrios G. Oreopoulos, MD, an Early Advocate for "*Nephroprevention*"

Joanne M. Bargman

The nephrology community is well-acquainted with the works of Dimitrios Oreopoulos, particularly his seminal contributions to, and championing of, peritoneal dialysis. What perhaps is less appreciated is that he was very involved in many other aspects of medicine.

He received a PhD in calcium and stone metabolism and continued to publish incisive papers in this area in high-ranking journals. He also founded the journal *Humane Medicine* to publish papers on the social-, ethical-, and humanities-driven aspects of patient care. His interest in the patient experience served as a prescient forerunner to the current focus on patient-centered outcomes.

Two decades ago, he became increasingly convinced that the focus in nephrology was weighted almost exclusively on the therapeutics side, and there was a dearth of research and commentary about preventing renal disease. Dr. Oreopoulos decided to put together an international conference with "nephroprevention" as the theme.

He proceeded, essentially single-handedly, to find sponsors, invite the speakers, book the hotels, and bring this unique conference to fruition. The first "Prevention in Renal Disease" meeting took place in Toronto in 2002. The meeting was a success, and the reputation built over time. The conference continued annually for a decade and hosted both speakers and attendees from around the world. He would sit at the side of the room all day, clearly enjoying the experience. I would trudge home exhausted at the end of the day, but Dimitrios, energized, would take fellows and speakers out for Greek food and socializing.

Dimitrios Oreopoulos was ahead of his time in so many aspects of medicine, and with publication of this book about prevention in renal medicine, it is a fitting opportunity to remember and salute his contribution.

SECTION IV

Drugs and Kidney Function

21

Principles of Drug Therapy in Reduced Kidney Function

TIMOTHY NGUYEN, TRAN TRAN, AND THOMAS DOWLING

INTRODUCTION

It is estimated that the overall prevalence of chronic kidney disease (CKD) in the general population, where estimated glomerular filtration rate (eGFR) is less than 60 mL/min/1.73 m^2, is approximately 14%.[1-3] This high rate of kidney disease is particularly alarming in adults 65 years and older, who often receive multiple medications. Here, the potential for inappropriately high doses of medications can lead to a higher risk of adverse effects.[2] Most drugs are excreted by the kidney and drug dosage adjustments are likely required in renal impairment to avoid accumulation and exposure-related toxicity, particularly if the drug is associated with nephrotoxicity.

Kidney disease affects physiological changes and alterations in the pharmacokinetics (PK) and the pharmacodynamics (PD) of many drugs.[4] Glomerular filtration rate (GFR) is considered the best overall index of kidney function. The rate of decline in GFR with normal aging is believed to occur at approximately 1 mL/min/year after the age of 40.[1,2,5,6] Kidney function can be assessed by using endogenous and exogenous markers such as serum creatinine (SCr), inulin, and cystatin C; radionuclide-labeled estimated equations for creatinine clearance (Clcr) such as Cockcroft-Gault (C-G); and estimated equations for GFR such as the Modification of Diet in Renal Disease (MDRD) study equation, and the Chronic Kidney Disease Epidemiology Collaboration Epidemiology (CKD-EPI) study equation. Table 21.1 gives example of common methods of kidney function assessment and their clinical applications.[4,7-14] The most accurate measures include urine collection methods (such as a 24-hour urine creatinine collection) and qualitative confirmatory diagnostic approaches such as kidney biopsy.[1,2,7-10]

Appropriate dose adjustment of drugs that rely on the kidney for elimination is a critical step in preventing drug adverse events. Many medications are cleared by the kidneys and require special dosing considerations in CKD.[12,15-17] The C-G formula has been the most commonly employed guide for drug dosing, since it has been used during drug development and is often included in the Food and Drug Administration (FDA) approved drug label.[11] However, newer equations that were designed to estimate GFR, such as the MDRD and CKD-EPI study equations, appear to offer improved accuracy at estimating GFR when compared to C-GClcr equation.[8-10,18] Improper use and dosing of medications can, therefore, be prevented when a systematic approach is used prior to initiating drug therapy or adjusting drug doses when kidney function is altered.[12,15-17]

EPIDEMIOLOGY AND MECHANISM

Many factors can contribute to the development or worsening of CKD progression, including drugs and co-existing chronic diseases. Age-related decline in kidney function and drug–drug interactions are also considerations that may alter the renal elimination of drugs. As the kidney function declines, so does the clearance of renally cleared drugs or drug metabolites. PK drug characteristics changes, and commonly electrolyte disturbances may change sensitivity to pharmacological and toxic effects. The kidney's endocrine and metabolic functions are compromised in CKD, necessitating therapy, and multiple drugs can lead to drug interactions. Approximately 50% of all drugs or their metabolites are excreted by the kidneys.[12,15-16] Medication dosage reduction is needed in CKD if >30% of a drug or active metabolite appears unchanged in the urine,

TABLE 21.1 EXAMPLE OF COMMON METHODS OF KIDNEY FUNCTION ASSESSMENT AND THEIR CLINICAL APPLICATIONS

Tools	Clinical Utility	Comments
Cockroft-Gault (CG) (CG) Clcr = (140—age) (IBW, kg)/(72 × Scr) Female × 0.85	Estimates Clcr Often use for drug dosing	Takes into account age, body mass, and gender Underestimates GFR in geriatric patients Since it relies on patient's body weight, an overestimation of Clcr is expected if total body weight substantially exceeds lean body mass, as in obese and edematous patients, where GFR prediction inaccuracy is more often encountered.
MDRD Four-variables MDRD study equations (abbreviated): GFR (mL/min/1.73 m^2) = $186 \times [P_{cr}]^{-1.154} \times [Age]^{-0.203} \times [0.742$ if female$] \times [1.210$ if AA$]$	Estimates GFR Used to classify stages of CKD Commonly used in older people with eGFR <60 mL/min/1.73 m^2 Takes into account age, gender and race	May erroneously categorize some healthy persons as having CKD Have been shown to give a more accurate assessment of GFR than does measured Clcr or calculated Clcr from CG equation Has not been validated in subjects older than 70 years of age May overestimate the prevalence of CKD in elderly patients MDRD equation was developed from a population of patients with CKD, but underestimates GFR in healthy populations

CKD-EPI Collaboration
GFR = $a \times (SCr/b)^c \times (0.993)^{age}$
	Estimates GFR
	The variable a takes on the following values on the basis of race and sex:
	• Black
	 • Women = 166
	 • Men = 163
	• White/other
	 • Women = 144
	 • Men = 141
	• The variable b takes on the following values on the basis of sex:
	 • Women = 0.7
	 • Men = 0.9
	• The variable c takes on the following values on the basis of sex and creatinine measurement:
	 • Women
	  • SCr ≤0.7 mg/dL = −0.329
	  • SCr >0.7 mg/dL = −1.209
	 • Men
	  • SCr ≤0.9 mg/dL = −0.411
	  • SCr >0.9 mg/dL = −1.209
		May overestimate the prevalence of CKD in elderly patients

AA = African American. CG = Cockroft-Gault. CKD = chronic kidney disease. CKD-EPI = chronic kidney disease epidemiology. Clcr = creatinine clearance. CysC = cystatin C. GFR = glomerular filtration rate. IBW = ideal body weight. MDRD = modification of diet in renal disease. Pcr = plasma creatinine. SCr = serum creatinine.

Source: Matzke GR, Comstock T. Influence of renal disease and dialysis on pharmacokinetics. In: Evans W, Schentag J, Burton M, eds. *Applied Pharmacokinetics: Principles of Therapeutic Drug Monitoring*. Baltimore, MD: Lippincott, Williams & Wilkens; 2005: 187–212; Cockroft DW, Gault MH. Prediction of creatinine clearance from serum creatinine. *Nephron*. 1976;16:31–41; Levey AS, Bosch JP, Lewis JB, et al.; Modification of Diet in Renal Disease Study Group. A more accurate method to estimate glomerular filtration rate from serum creatinine: a new prediction equation. *Ann Intern Med*. 1999;130:461–470; Levey AS, Stevens LA, Schmid CH, et al.; Chronic Kidney Disease Epidemiology Collaboration (CKD-EPI). A new equation to estimate glomerular filtration rate. *Ann Intern Med*. 2009;150:604–612; Levey AS, Coresh J, Greene T, et al. Using standardized serum creatinine values in the modification of diet in renal disease study equation for estimating glomerular filtration rate. *Ann Intern Med*. 2006;145:247–254; Dowling TC, Matzke GR, Murphy JE, Burkart GJ. Evaluation of renal drug dosing: prescribing information and clinical pharmacist approaches. *Pharmacotherapy*. 2010;30(8):776–786; Olyaei AJ, Steffl JL. A quantitative approach to drug dosing in chronic kidney disease. *Blood Purif*. 2011;31:138–145. Matzke GR, Frye RF. Drug therapy individualization for patients with renal insufficiency. In: DiPiro JT, Talbert RL, Yee GC, et al. *Pharmacotherapy: A Pathophysiologic Approach*. McGraw Hill.

medications have a narrow therapeutic index, or drugs have decreased renal clearance.[12,16,17] Elimination of drugs is most obviously affected by CKD but PK parameters (e.g., absorption, distribution, and metabolism) of drugs may also be altered even if they are not primarily excreted by the kidney.

Kidney disease and complications of kidney disease such as cardiovascular disease may contribute to alteration in drug absorption (Table 21.2). Examples of factors that can impact PK properties are absorption, distribution, metabolism, and excretion in kidney disease.[4,16,17] Alterations in drug absorption (change in gastric pH due to antacid drugs), gastrointestinal motility (hypermotility/hypomotility), vomiting and diarrhea secondary to CKD treatment, and alterations in volume of distribution (Vd; protein/tissue binding, altered body composition). Vd of many drugs is increased due to fluid overload, decreased protein binding, or altered tissue binding. Metabolism via hepatic route is also affected by CKD (e.g., cytochrome P450, P-glycoprotein). Variation in fluid condition is common in kidney disease; for example, critically ill patients often require large volume of intravenous fluids for various illnesses (e.g., shock) and may lead to edema. This increased in Vd may lead to a reduction in serum drug concentrations. The increase in the apparent Vd is associated with decrease in protein binding affinity and may affect the unbound fraction of many acidic drugs. For example, phenytoin

drug concentration is significantly higher in severe kidney disease patient compares to patients without kidney disease.[4,16,17]

Kidney disease also affects the metabolism of some drugs, and accumulation of both metabolite and the parent compound may occur. Adequate studies in this field are lacking, and due to the nature of kidney disease and the exposure to these mechanisms, serum drug concentration of both parent compound and metabolite may be distinctly different. The clinical response may be different as well. This makes it difficult to predict drug responses in a given clinical setting. It is often difficult to predict drug clearance due to many factors, including patients' state of kidney function: acute kidney injury (AKI) versus CKD. Furthermore, drugs and medications are eliminated to various degrees by the different forms of dialysis; e.g., hemodialysis [HD], peritoneal dialysis [PD], continuous renal replacement therapy [CRRT]).

In HD, drug clearance is influenced by various factors including molecular weight of the drug, protein binding, Vd, solubility, pore size, dialysis membrane (high-flux/low-flux), filter surface area, and flow rates. HD drug clearance is reduced by low-flux membranes and drugs with large Vd and extensive protein binding.[13] PD usually has low-efficiency drug clearance; small Vd and low protein binding are cleared well.[13] The clearance is usually less efficient compared to HD. Other options also should be considered such as CRRT and kidney transplantation. In CRRT, the rate of drug removal is dependent on the sieving coefficient and ultrafiltrate volume should be taken into consideration.

ESTIMATION OF KIDNEY FUNCTION

The GFR is the single best test to assess overall renal function. It cannot be measured directly, and several factors can cause interpatient variability including body size/body surface area (BSA; approximately 8% higher in males), annual age-related decline (approximately 0.75–7 mL/min/1.73 m²), pregnancy, protein intake, and drugs, among other factors. SCr has limitations including variability among individuals and assay methodology.[1,11,13,19] Most of the equations in use are dependent on SCr, which, by default, assumes creatinine production and excretion are at steady state. Renal function may not accurately be reflected by performing these calculations in populations with rapidly changing renal function

---

TABLE 21.2 EXAMPLES OF FACTORS THAT CAN IMPACT PHARMACOKINETIC PROPERTIES (ABSORPTION, DISTRIBUTION, METABOLISM AND EXCRETION) IN KIDNEY DISEASE

Gastric pH

Protein binding

Volume of distribution

Hepatic metabolism (e.g., cytochrome P450)

Glycoprotein (P-glycoprotein)

Source: Matzke GR, Comstock T. Influence of renal function and dialysis on drug disposition. In: Michael E Burton, Leslie M Shaw, Jerome J Schentag and William E Evans. *Applied Pharmacokinetics & Pharmacodynamics Principles of Therapeutic Drug Monitoring*. 2006. Lippincott, Williams & Wilkens. 187–212; Aymanns C, Keller F, Maus S, et al. Review on pharmacokinetics and pharmacodynamics and the aging kidney. *Clin J Am Soc Nephrol*. 2010;5:314–327; Verbeeck RK, Musuamba FT. Pharmacokinetics and dosage adjustment in patients with renal dysfunction. *Eur J Clin Pharmacol*. 2009;65:757–773.

such as the acutely ill and is an inherent weakness of this strategy. However, assessing renal clearance via estimation of Clcr or eGFR is the current standard to guide drug dosing and predict drug concentration.[1,11,13,19]

The estimated Clcr (eClcr) and eGFR are commonly derived using these equations: C-G Clcr,[7] MDRD eGFR,[8] and CKD-EPI eGFR[9] (see Table 21.1). The C-G Clcr was developed in 1976, and it is an estimate of the Clcr, which approximates the GFR. However, creatinine undergoes both glomerular filter and tubular secretion; therefore, Clcr will tend to overestimate GFR. The C-G Clcr equation utilizes a patient's age in years, sex, SCr in mg/dL, and weight in kilogram. The study included 249 people with approximately 96% being male[7]; therefore, there are limitations associated with this formula. Older adults usually have lower muscle mass and decreased protein intake in their diet, possibly resulting in falsely decreased SCr levels.[1-2] This, in turn, may lead to an inaccurate estimation of the Clcr or GFR. Additionally, the original study in 1976 used actual body weight to calculate Clcr. Since then, additional modifications to the formula have been made to suggest that using ideal body weight or adjusted body weight in individuals with greater than 30% of their ideal body weight may yield more accurate estimates of renal function.[11,14] Furthermore, manufacturer labeling for certain drugs such as dabigatran, dofetilide, eptifibatide, premetrexed, phentermine, topiramate, rivaroxaban, and zoledronic acid specifically recommend using actual body weight when calculating Clcr,[19-24] although this is rare.

In 1998, the FDA included the C-G Clcr as an example of estimating Clcr in its publication, "Guidance for Industry: Pharmacokinetics in Patients with Impaired Renal Function—Study Design, Data Analysis, and Impact on Dosing and Labeling."[25] As a result, dosing recommendations in FDA-approved product labeling are commonly based on PK studies using the C-G Clcr formula. An updated draft guidance to the aforementioned document was released in 2010, which now includes examples of both the C-G Clcr and the MDRD eGFR; however, the use of the MDRD equation in renal impairment PK studies is not easily ascertainable without reviewing individual studies for each specific drug.[26] Due to the inaccuracies of the MDRD equation at GFR levels above 60 mL/min/1.73 m[2], the National Institute of Diabetes and Digestive and Kidney Disease[27] recommended the CKD-EPI equation

instead. Standardization in this area will be beneficial in informing future studies and clinical practice.

It is important to note that the MDRD and CKD-EPI equations provided estimates of measured GFR using a BSA-standardized unit of mL/min/1.73 m[2], in contrast to the C-G Clcr, which estimates Clcr in mL/min. This is based on the original intention of the MDRD and CKD-EPI studies, which was to develop equations based on patients who received a measured iothalamate GFR reported in mL/min/1.73 m[2]. The MDRD was developed in 1999 from 628 patients with CKD.[8] Originally, the formula utilized 6 variables: SCr, age, ethnicity, gender, blood urea nitrogen, and albumin levels. Currently, the 4-variable formula is most commonly used, which includes the SCr, age, ethnicity, and gender.[10] Due to the influence of body mass, the estimated GFR or Clcr may lead to inaccuracy of the GFR in overweight and underweight individuals and especially in older adults with lower body mass. Recent studies have shown that the MDRD equation significantly underestimates kidney function in individuals with GFR >60 mL/min/1.73 m[2], which limits its widespread application.[8] For this reason, the reporting of eGFR in clinical labs is limited to GFR values <60 mL/min/1.73 m[2].

The CKD-EPI formula[9] was derived in 2009 using 12,150 patients from diverse populations to create a more accurate formula than the MDRD when utilizing it in patients with GFR >60 mL/min/1.73 m[2]. A subpopulation of 8,254 participants was used for development of the formula, and 3,896 participants were used for the purpose of external validation. The CKD-EPI equation involves a multipart calculation, based on different subpopulations, including race and sex. The formula also uses the variables of SCr and age to determine GFR. Although this formula has been shown to be superior to the MDRD formula, it did not perform well in older adults.[18] Some data showed that the CKD-EPI creatinine equation was more accurate in individuals with eGFR >60 mL/min/1.73 m[2], while other showed that the MDRD equation was more accurate in those with GFRs <60 mL/min/1.73 m[2].[28]

The National Kidney Education Disease Program (NKEDP) reported a large simulation study comparing eClcr and eGFR calculated from standardized creatinine levels to each other and to the gold standard measurement of GFR. The NKEDP reported few differences in drug dosing for most drugs tested in majority of patients and suggested, based on the simulation study, either equation can be used to estimate kidney function.[29,30] The NKEDP suggested other considerations such as using a single kidney estimate to guide detection, evaluation, management of CKD, and drug dosing for consistent high-quality healthcare and utilizing either eGFR or eClcr for drug dosing with consideration for very large or small patients (in such cases, the eGFR can be reported in terms of mL/min using adjusted for BSA). Both the MDRD and CKD-EPI equations estimated GFR adjusted for BSA.[30]

Despite the extensive research performed in this area, assessments of renal function and dose adjustment recommendations should not be used alone for the purpose of therapeutic drug monitoring but should also be accompanied by clinical judgment. Imprecision associated with the limitations of these equations places a higher potential for toxicity and treatment failure, particularly for vulnerable populations such as those in critical care, at outlier extremes in weight or size, with multiple comorbid conditions affecting drug PK properties (absorption, distribution, metabolism, excretion), and meeting exclusion criteria for available drug PK studies.

Renal dose adjustment cutoffs for drugs do not always correspond to GFR ranges for Kidney Disease Outcome Quality Initiatives (KDOQI) stages (Table 21.3). End-stage kidney disease

TABLE 21.3 NATIONAL KIDNEY FOUNDATION KDOQI GUIDELINES: STAGES OF CHRONIC KIDNEY DISEASE: GUIDANCE FROM KDOQI TO CLASSIFY KIDNEY FUNCTION ACCORDING TO FIVE STAGES OF CKD AND DEFINED IN PART BY EGFR

CKD Stages	Estimated GFR (mL/min/1.73 m²)
1	≥90
2	60 to 89
3	Stage 3a: 45 to 59
	Stage 3b: 30 to 44
4	15 to 29
5	Less than 15

CKD = chronic kidney disease. GFR = glomerular filtration rate. KDOQI = Kidney Disease Outcomes Quality Initiative. NKF = National Kidney Foundation.
Source: National Kidney Foundation. K/DOQI clinical practice guidelines for chronic kidney disease: evaluation, classification, and stratification. *Am J Kidney Dis*. 2002;39(2 Suppl 1):S1–266.

patients on dialysis represents an additional complexity to drug dosing as the extent to which various dialysis modalities remove drugs must also be considered. Some drugs may require supplemental doses or a paradoxical dose increase relative to those with normal renal function to compensate for the extent of drug removed via dialysis.

GENERAL DRUG DOSING CONSIDERATION

Recommended adjustments in renal impairment typically take the form of reducing the dose (e.g., decrease dose by 50%) while keeping the same dosing interval, maintaining the same dose while extending the dosing interval (e.g., dosing every 24 hours instead of every 12 hours), or changing both the dose and interval.[11,12,14] With the exception of drugs that require therapeutic drug monitoring such as vancomycin or aminoglycosides for which trough and/or peak concentration levels help guide a modified dosing strategy, most dose adjustments for renal impairment are based on Clcr, which can be found in tertiary drug references and manufacturer package inserts and are informed by data from PK studies.[19-24,31-34] Infrequently, use in renal impairment may not be established based on the lack of PK studies, and, therefore, the use of the drug in this population is typically not recommended. There are very few exceptions where PK studies are not necessary in renal impairment because drug dose adjustments are unlikely; these include drugs administered as a single dose, drugs primarily eliminated by the lungs, and monocolonal antibodies. Otherwise, for most acute and chronic drugs excreted predominantly by the kidney (i.e., >30% drug unchanged), dose adjustments are usually appropriate if the drugs could reasonably be used to treat patients who have concomitant CKD or renal impairment.[12,16,17] This rule, however, is not all-inclusive as many drugs primarily metabolized and removed through hepatic pathways may also require dose adjustment despite bypassing the kidney. This is because renal dysfunction can also alter hepatic and gut metabolism independently of drug elimination, which can have implications on drug efficacy and toxicity. Worth noting is endoxaban, a new oral anticoagulant approved in 2015 for atrial fibrillation and venous thromboembolism that is contraindicated in patients with a Clcr greater than 95 mL/min.[35] This represents a historically uncommon scenario for which drug appropriateness for indications other than CKD may now need to be more routinely evaluated for patients without renal impairment.

SUCCINCT DRUG DOSING CONSIDERATION

Loading Dose

The Vd is altered in kidney disease and an initiating loading dose is recommended for many drugs, particularly those that have hydrophilic properties.

Maintenance Dose

Patient factors, fluid volume status, kidney function status (e.g., AKI, CKD), are essential in determining appropriate maintenance drug dose.

Therapeutic Drug Monitoring

Drugs that have narrow therapeutic concentrations and potential for causing toxicity should be closely monitored.

SUCCINCT PRESCRIBING PRINCIPLES IN CKD SHOULD BE CONSIDERED

- Evaluate for decreased renal clearance.
- Obtain history, eClcr/eGFR.
- Consider kidney function: AKI versus CKD.
- Altered PK drug characteristics.
- Consider stable serum drug concentrations, adverse effects, and patient convenience.
- Monitor drug response, clinically evidence of drug toxicity, and efficacy.
- Adjust regimen based on efficacy/toxicity and change in renal function as appropriate.
- Dose adjustments can be made by reducing the dose, increasing the dosing interval, or a combination of the two.
- In patients with drug toxicities from accumulation, consider extracorporeal removal of drugs: HD versus PD versus CRRT.
- Use Key Clinical Practice Guidelines: National Kidney Foundation,[30] KDOQI,[36] European Renal Best Practice,[37] Kidney Disease Improving Global Outcomes,[38] and Canadian Society of Nephrology.[39]
- Examples of commonly used tertiary drug dosing references include Micromedex

(DrugDex, Greenwood Village, CO),[31] Lexi-Comp (Lexi-Drugs Online, Hudson, OH),[32] Epocrates Rx (San Mateo, CA),[33] and Dialysis of Drugs.[34]

CONCLUSION

The increasing prevalence of kidney disease requires an increased awareness of the need for drug dose adjustments in this special population. Estimating kidney function by various assessment methods is important and applying good prescribing practice is important for limiting drug toxicities and improving the care of the patients we serve.

REFERENCES

1. Levey AS, Coresh J, Balk E, et al. National Kidney Foundation practice guidelines for chronic kidney disease: evaluation, classification, and stratification. *Ann Intern Med.* 2003;139:137–147.
2. Nguyen T, Goldfarb D. The older adult patients and kidney function. *Consult Pharm.* 2012;27:431–444.
3. Kidney Disease Statistics for the United States. National Institute of Diabetes and Digestive and Kidney Disease. https://www.niddk.nhi.gov/health-information/health-statistics/Pages/Kidney-disease-statistics-united-states.aspx.
4. Matzke GR, Comstock T. Influence of renal disease and dialysis on pharmacokinetics. In: Evans W, Schentag J, Burton M, eds. *Applied Pharmacokinetics: Principles of Therapeutic Drug Monitoring.* Baltimore, MD: Lippincott, Williams & Wilkens; 2005: 187–212.
5. Weinstein J, Anderson S. The aging kidney: physiological changes. *Adv Chronic Kidney Dis.* 2010;17:302–307.
6. Kaplan C, Pasternack B, Shah H, et al. Age-related incidence of sclerotic glomeruli in human kidneys. *Am J Pathol.* 1974;80:227–234.
7. Cockcroft DW, Gault MH. Prediction of creatinine clearance from serum creatinine. *Nephron.* 1976;16:31–41.
8. Levey AS, Bosch JP, Lewis JB, et al.; Modification of Diet in Renal Disease Study Group. A more accurate method to estimate glomerular filtration rate from serum creatinine: a new prediction equation. *Ann Intern Med.* 1999;130:461–470.
9. Levey AS, Stevens LA, Schmid CH, et al.; Chronic Kidney Disease Epidemiology Collaboration (CKD-EPI). A new equation to estimate glomerular filtration rate. *Ann Intern Med.* 2009;150:604–612.
10. Levey AS, Coresh J, Greene T, et al. Using standardized serum creatinine values in the

modification of diet in renal disease study equation for estimating glomerular filtration rate. *Ann Intern Med.* 2006;145:247–254.

11. Dowling TC, Matzke GR, Murphy JE, Burkart GJ. Evaluation of renal drug dosing: prescribing information and clinical pharmacist approaches. *Pharmacotherapy.* 2010;30(8):776–786.

12. Olyaei AJ, Steffl JL. A quantitative approach to drug dosing in chronic kidney disease. *Blood Purif.* 2011;31:138–145.

13. American Kidney Foundation. KDOQI clinical practice guidelines for chronic kidney disease: evaluation, classification, and stratification. *Am J Kidney Dis.* 2002;39(2 Suppl 1):S1–26.

14. Matzke GR, Frye RF. Drug therapy individualization for patients with renal insufficiency. In: DiPiro JT, Talbert RL, Yee GC, et al. *Pharmacotherapy: A Pathophysiologic Approach.* New York, US: McGraw Hill; 2016.

15. Corsonello A, Pedone C, Corica F, et al. Concealed renal insufficiency and adverse drug reactions in elderly hospitalized patients. *Arch Intern Med.* 2005;165:790–795.

16. Aymanns C, Keller F, Maus S, et al. Review on pharmacokinetics and pharmacodynamics and the aging kidney. *Clin J Am Soc Nephrol.* 2010;5:314–327.

17. Verbeeck RK, Musuamba FT. Pharmacokinetics and dosage adjustment in patients with renal dysfunction. *Eur J Clin Pharmacol.* 2009;65:757–773.

18. Willems JM, Vlasveld T, den Elzen WP, et al. Performance of Cockcroft-Gault, modification of diet in renal disease, and chronic kidney disease epidemiology collaboration in estimating prevalence of renal function and predicting survival in the oldest old. *BMC Geriatrics.* 2013;13:113.

19. Tikosyn (dofetilide) Pfizer; March 2016. https://www.pfizer.com/products/product-detail/tikosyn

20. Integrilin (eptifibatide). Whitehouse Station, NJ: Merck; April 2014. http://www.merck.com/product/usa/pi_circulars/i/integrilin/integrilin_pi.pdf

21. Alimta (pemetrexed). Eli Lilly; June 2018. http://pi.lilly.com/us/alimta-pi.pdf

22. Qsymia. VIVUS; March 2018. https://qsymia.com/hcp/include/media/pdf/prescribing-information.pdf

23. Xarelto (rivaroxaban). Janssen Pharmaceuticals; October 2017. http://www.janssenlabels.com/package-insert/product-monograph/prescribing-information/XARELTO-pi.pdf

24. Reclast (zoledronic acid). Novartis Pharmaceuticals; July 2017. https://www.pharma.us.novartis.com/sites/www.pharma.us.novartis.com/files/reclast.pdf?

25. Pharmacokinetics in patients with impaired renal function—study design, data analysis, and impact on dosing and labeling. Center for Drug Evaluation and Research, US Food and Drug Administration. Guidance for Industry; May 1998. http://www.fda.gov/downloads/Drugs/GuidanceComplianceRegulatoryInformation/Guidances/UCM072127.pdf

26. Pharmacokinetics in patients with impaired renal function—study design, data analysis, and impact on dosing and labeling. Center for Drug Evaluation and Research, US Food and Drug Administration. Guidance for Industry; March 2010. https://www.fda.gov/downloads/Drugs/GuidanceComplianceRegulatoryInformation/Guidances/UCM204959.pdf

27. MDRD for adults (conventional units). National Institute of Diabetes and Digestive and Kidney Diseases Health Information Center. https://www.niddk.nih.gov/health-information/health-communication-programs/nkdep/lab-evaluation/gfr-calculators/adults-conventional-unit/Pages/adults-conventional-unit.aspx

28. Earley A, Miskulin D, Lamb EJ, et al. Estimating equations for glomerular filtration rate in the era of creatinine standardization. *Ann Intern Med.* 2012;56:785–795.

29. CKD & drug dosing: information for providers. National Institute of Diabetes and Digestive and Kidney Diseases Health Information Center; April 2015. https://www.niddk.nih.gov/health-information/health-communication-programs/nkdep/a-z/ckd-drug-dosing/Pages/CKD-drug-dosing.aspx

30. www.kidney.org

31. Micromedex (DrugDex, Greenwood Village, CO)

32. Lexi-Comp (Lexi-Drugs Online, Hudson, OH). https://online.lexi.com/lco/action/home

33. Epocrates Rx (San Mateo, CA). https://online.epocrates.com/

34. Mason NA, Bailie GR. *Dialysis of Drugs.* Renal Pharmacy Consultants, LLC; 2018. www.renalpharmacyconsultants.com

35. Savaysa (edoxaban). Daiichi Sankyo; January 2015. https://www.accessdata.fda.gov/drugsatfda_docs/label/2015/206316lbl.pdf

36. Professional guidelines. National Kidney Foundation; 2017. https://www.kidney.org/professionals/guidelines

37. European Renal Best Practices; 2018. http://www.european-renal-best-practice.org

38. KDIGO guidelines. KIDGO; 2018. https://kdigo.org/guidelines

39. https://www.csnscn.ca/committees/clinical-practice-guidelines

22

Acute Kidney Injury from Therapeutic Agents

DAPHNE KNICELY, MICHAEL J. CHOI, AND SUMESKA THAVARAJAH

INTRODUCTION

Many agents used for therapeutic and diagnostic purposes can be nephrotoxic. Drug-induced nephrotoxicity accounts for up to 20% of hospital-acquired acute kidney injury (AKI).[1] The adverse renal effects are often related to the agent's mechanism of action. Inherent properties that predispose the kidney to injury include the large proportion of cardiac output perfusing the kidney and the high concentrations of medications and relative hypoxia in some portions of the kidney.[1-4] Genetic polymorphisms, age, gender, pre-existing chronic kidney disease (CKD), and AKI itself are factors that impact patient susceptibility. We examine a few common agents that are associated with nephrotoxicity in the inpatient setting with a focus on risk factors for injury and potential preventative strategies as there may be no alternative medications.

CONTRAST-INDUCED NEPHROPATHY

Contrast-induced nephropathy (CIN) is an AKI following administration of iodinated radiocontrast agents and is the third most frequent cause of in hospital AKIs.[5-7] The incidence of CIN varies depending on the population, being 0.6% to 11% in the general population and as high as 50% in those with CKD, diabetes mellitus, heart failure, advanced age, or use of other nephrotoxic medications.[6-8] For the minority of patients who require renal replacement therapy, there is an associated increased cost of hospitalization and increased mortality.[5] Patients with CIN who do not require renal replacement therapy are also at a greater risk for death, prolonged hospitalization, and early and late cardiovascular events.[7,9]

CIN is defined as AKI developing within 24 to 72 hours after intravascular (arterial or venous) contrast is administered. AKI typically peaks on day 3 to 5 and then returns to baseline renal function within 2 weeks.[7,10] CIN is usually nonoliguric and typically does not require dialysis. Unlike most other intrinsic causes of AKI, the fractional excretion of sodium may be <1%.

The mechanisms of injury for CIN include direct tubular cellular toxicity and decreased renal perfusion due to contrast-induced vasoconstriction caused by activation of adenosine and endothelin.[10,11] CIN represents a form of acute tubular necrosis (ATN), which is often nonoliguric. Non iso-osmolar contrast agents have higher osmolality than plasma, and this osmotic effect within the tubular lumen causes increased salt and water delivery to the loop of Henle, which activates tubuloglomerular feedback. This decreases glomerular filtration rate (GFR) to prevent excess renal sodium loss. Increased water reabsorption increases interstitial pressure which compresses the vasa recta leading to medullary hypoxemia. Non iso-osmolar radiocontrast agents can also increase viscosity and derange red blood cell deformability leading to increased resistance to flow. Local tissue ischemia triggers activation of reactive oxygen species, which further contributes to renal tubule damage.[12] Direct toxic effects in renal tubular epithelial and mesangial cells result in cell death through increased cellular DNA fragmentation and down regulation of signaling molecules involved in cell survival.[10,13]

Risk factors for CIN include pre-existing CKD stage 3 or greater, age >70 years old, diabetes mellitus (type 1 or 2) with renal dysfunction, nephrotoxic drug use (nonsteroidal anti-inflammatory drugs [NSAIDs], cyclosporine, aminoglycosides, etc.), pre-procedure hemodynamic instability, volume depletion, and other comorbidities that might affect renal perfusion (such as hypertension and congestive heart

≥ Stage 3 chronic kidney disease

Age >70 years

Diabetes

Nephrotoxic drug use

Pre-procedure hemodynamic stability

Volume depletion

Co-morbid conditions that decrease renal perfusion

failure; Table 22.1).[5,7,8] There is a correlation between baseline renal dysfunction (with diabetes) and risk of CIN.[5] Diabetes mellitus without renal impairment is presently felt unlikely an independent CIN risk factor[7,8] In hemodynamically unstable patients, it is recommended, if possible, to delay radiocontrast administration until the patient is stable.[8] Nephrotoxic medications should be discontinued prior to any radiocontrast study. Similarly, it is recommended that diuretic therapy be discontinued prior to radiocontrast studies, if possible,[7] as forced euvolemic diuresis protocols are associated with a significantly increased risk of CIN. There is controversy as to whether intravenous contrast has the same nephrotoxicity as intra-arterial contrast.[10]

There is conflicting data on CIN risk associated with use of angiotensin converting enzyme inhibitors and angiotensin receptor blockers, renal transplantation, multiple myeloma, and cirrhosis. Theoretically, removing renin–angiotensin–aldosterone system (RAAS) blockade would help maintain glomerular filtration with contrast-induced preglomerular vasoconstriction.[9] While there is insufficient evidence to recommend discontinuation of angiotensin converting enzyme inhibitors and angiotensin receptor blockers in all patients prior to radiocontrast administration, it might be reasonable to hold RAAS blockade prior to contrast administration and resume them post procedure.[7,9]

Radiocontrast agents are classified as high-osmolar (>500 mOsm/kg), low-osmolar (320–500 mOsm/kg), and iso-osmolar (280–290 mOsm/kg). High-osmolar agents are considered a risk factor for CIN but are no longer widely used. No conclusions regarding a significant clinical difference in CIN risk have been determined for low versus iso-osmolar agents.[13] Differing

guidelines suggest that volume of radiocontrast affects CIN risk, but this has been brought into question. One study demonstrated that >100 mL of iodinated radiocontrast was associated with an increased risk of CIN; however, another study demonstrated that <250 mL of radiocontrast agent was associated with a relatively low risk. In general, it is recommended to use as little radiocontrast volume as possible for acceptable imaging quality. Low-osmolar radiocontrast agents are reasonable for moderate risk patients, and iso-osmolar radiocontrast agents are often used in the highest risk patients.[9] Repeated exposures should be delayed for 48 hours and 72 hours for those with higher CIN risk if possible.[8]

CIN prevention involves screening for pre-existing renal impairment.[7] When a serum creatinine result is not available, it is recommended to perform a simple questionnaire or dipstick testing for urine protein to identify renal impairment.[7] There are risk assessment models available, which can be used for counseling about the risks of the procedure and selecting prophylactic interventions.[7,14,15]

Extracellular volume expansion with intravenous isotonic sodium chloride or sodium bicarbonate may counteract intrarenal hemodynamic alterations and direct toxic effects in those who are at risk of CIN.[7,8] Sodium bicarbonate might decrease the generation of free radicals in addition to volume expansion to prevent CIN. Study results conflict on sodium bicarbonate benefit with possible errors in preparation of sodium bicarbonate. Guidelines recommend either solution for volume expansion and prevention of CIN.[7,8,10] There is no agreed upon standard for the optimal rate or duration of infusion for CIN prevention (e.g., 1–1.5 mL/kg/hour for at least 6 hours pre- and postprocedure or fluids 1 hour preprocedure to 3–6 hours postprocedure).[7,8] The amount of fluid administered should be determined after careful evaluation of the patient's volume status. There might be some benefit of oral volume expansion, but there is not enough evidence to support its use over intravenous volume expansion.[7–9]

N-acetylcysteine (NAC) is low cost and relatively safe and may provide benefit through antioxidant effects by scavenging of free radicals and through nitric oxide-dependent vasodilation and improved medullary oxygenation.[8] Studies suggest there might be a protective effect of NAC with intravenous isotonic crystalloids prior to renal injury, but results are inconsistent.[16] Oral

NAC has shown significant benefit for CIN in some studies compared to control, but intravenous NAC has not shown a significant improvement.[16] It is recommended by nephrology clinical practice guidelines for CIN prevention[10]; however, due to conflicting studies, NAC is not routinely administered for CIN prevention.

Statins (3-hydroxy-3-methylglutaryl-coenzyme A reductase inhibitors) appear to protect against the development of CIN. Statins inhibit the uptake of radiocontrast by renal tubular cells, reduce endothelial dysfunction and oxidative stress, decrease inflammation, decrease mesangial cell proliferation, and protect podocytes.[9] A meta-analysis[17] suggested that short-term use can prevent CIN even in high-risk patients. It is unclear if high- versus low-dose statins have a better effect on preventing CIN.

INTRAVENOUS IMMUNOGLOBULIN-INDUCED OSMOTIC NEPHROSIS

Intravenous immunoglobulin (IVIG) contains sterile highly purified human immunoglobulins, mainly IgG, and a stabilizing substance (glucose, maltose, sucrose, sorbitol, glycine, or albumin).[18] IVIG products contain a "black box" warning about the risk of AKI.[19]

Sucrose-containing immunoglobulin preparations were present in 74% to 90% of the reported AKI cases.[18] Sucrase is not present to metabolize sucrose on the brush border of proximal tubules.[19] Sucrose on entering the tubular epithelial cells via pinocytosis is incorporated into lysosomes leading to an osmotic gradient with epithelial cell swelling and cytoplasmic vacuolization of mainly proximal tubules.[18–21] This narrows the tubular lumen, which causes injury and degeneration of the proximal tubular epithelium.[18,19]

In general, reports of AKI with sucrose-free IVIG are relatively rare.[21] Maltose-based IVIG has been found to cause osmotic nephrosis but is typically less severe than sucrose-based IVIG perhaps because maltase is present along proximal tubule brush borders to degrade maltose.[21] Maltose-induced AKI might occur through inhibition of maltase or with a high tubular load of maltose, which overwhelms the metabolic capacity of the epithelial brush border. Mannitol-based IVIG-induced AKI has been reported and is postulated to occur through renal vasoconstriction caused by high levels of mannitol or concomitant administration of other nephrotoxic agents.

AKI due to IVIG causes osmotic nephrosis, characterized by vacuolization of mainly proximal tubules. Oliguric AKI usually develops about 3 to 5 days after initiation of IVIG. On average, there is renal function recovery within 7 to 15 days after IVIG cessation. Renal replacement therapy may be required in 32% to 40% of cases.[19,20] Management of IVIG-induced osmotic nephrosis is essentially supportive.[18]

The risk factors for IVIG-induced AKI include pre-existing AKI or CKD, kidney transplant, age >65 years old, diabetes mellitus, volume depletion, sepsis, paraproteinemia, and simultaneous use of other nephrotoxic medications. Patients with renal impairment and/or kidney transplant have the greatest risk.[18–21] Patients with risk factors for osmotic nephrosis should not be given sucrose-based IVIG. If no other option is available, then it is recommended to decrease the dose, concentration, and/or rate of administration of the IVIG to reduce the risk of AKI.[18–20] For those patients with risk factors, hydration is recommended, but there are specific guidelines regarding fluid type and duration are not currently available. Renal function is checked prior to initial infusion and then again in 5 days with careful monitoring of urine output throughout the infusion period. If AKI develops, IVIG should be discontinued.[19]

AMINOGLYCOSIDE NEPHROTOXICITY

Aminoglycosides are highly potent and bactericidal antibiotics. Examples include gentamicin, tobramycin, and amikacin. AKI continues to be the major dose-limiting toxicity of aminoglycosides. The risk of AKI with aminoglycosides has led some clinicians to limit aminoglycosides as a therapeutic option with the risk of AKI being as high as 25% in some case series.[7,20]

Aminoglycosides should be used for as short a period of time as possible. Repeated administration of aminoglycosides over days or weeks can result in the accumulation of aminoglycosides within the renal interstitium and proximal tubular epithelial cells, leading to a higher incidence of AKI.[7] Aminoglycosides are taken up through megalin receptors in proximal tubule epithelial cells, become concentrated in the proximal tubule, and then bind to acidic phospholipids within the lipid bilayer causing aggregation and inhibition of phospholipase activity.[22] This leads to myeloid body formation, impaired protein synthesis, degradation of mitochondrial function, and culminates in apoptosis and necrosis of tubular epithelial cells.[22,23] Early signs of AKI include increased urinary excretion of calcium, magnesium, proteins, and other organic anions, potentially leading to hypocalcemia, hypomagnesemia, and tubular proteinuria. As the damage continues, increased urine excretion of potassium and sodium can be seen along with increases in serum creatinine. Aminoglycosides cause an increase in intracellular calcium levels, leading to mesangial contraction and decreased GFR. There is a reduction in renal blood flow secondary to increases in renal vascular resistance with increased endothelin-1 and thromboxane A2.[22]

Aminoglycoside-associated nephrotoxicity is characterized as nonoliguric AKI. There is a slow rise in serum creatinine and a hypo-osmolar urine about 5 days after treatment starts. AKI from aminoglycosides is usually not the sole reason for AKI. Recovery of AKI usually occurs after drug discontinuation.[22]

Risk factors for aminoglycoside-associated nephrotoxicity are age >65 years old, pre-existing AKI or CKD, diabetes mellitus, concomitant use of other nephrotoxic medications, prolonged aminoglycoside use, elevated aminoglycoside levels, repeated exposures to separate courses of aminoglycosides over a short interval, and sepsis with intravascular volume depletion and rapid alterations in fluid dynamics.[7,22,23]

It is recommended that aminoglycosides be administered as a single daily dose rather than multiple daily doses to limit aminoglycoside uptake in renal tubular cells while preserving the therapeutic value of these agents. Drug level monitoring is recommended when multiple daily dosing is used for more than 24 hours. Aminoglycoside levels are variable, and subtle changes in the volume of distribution, renal blood flow, and GFR can affect renal handling of aminoglycosides and alter the risk of nephrotoxicity. The therapeutic drug concentration maximum should be at least 10-fold greater than the minimum inhibitory concentration of the infectious disease. The trough level should be undetectable by 18 to 24 hours to limit accumulation of aminoglycosides in renal tubular cells.[7] Drug-level monitoring is recommended with single daily dosing for more than 48 hours as well with at least a single peak measurement with a therapeutic goal of 10-fold greater than the minimum inhibitory concentration of the infectious disease. Some clinicians recommend at least 1 or a weekly trough level obtained at either 12, 18, or 24 hours after the aminoglycoside dose, which should be below the limits of detection of the assay at these time intervals.[7] Aminoglycosides should be administered in patients who are volume replete.

VANCOMYCIN NEPHROTOXICITY

The nephrotoxicity from vancomycin has evolved over the last 6 decades. Early preparations of the medication contained impurities leading to a brown appearance, resulting in the nickname "Mississippi mud."[24] The impurities were thought to cause the nephrotoxicity associated with the medications.[25] As the quality of vancomycin formulations improved, the incidence of nephrotoxicity decreased from 25% to 30% to 5% to 7%.[26] Animal studies suggest a combination of vancomycin-induced oxidative stress in proximal renal tubular cells, mitochondrial dysfunction, and apoptosis contribute to AKI.[27] Oxidative phosphorylation induces free oxygen radicals and decreases the activity of antioxidative enzymes.[28,29] Superoxide production by vancomycin depolarizes the mitochondrial membrane. Release of cytochrome C and activation of caspases 9 and 3 contribute to apoptosis.[29,30] The accumulation of the drug in the proximal tubule cells may lead to renal tubular ischemia and acute tubulointerstitial damage.[24] The predominant injury based on recent biopsy findings seems to be acute interstitial nephritis (AIN) with some cases of nephrotoxic ATN. However, recently Loque et al.[31] described obstructive tubular casts composed of vancomycin aggregates and uromodulin in biopsy samples of AKI after intravenous administration of vancomycin. Risk factors for nephrotoxicity include elevated vancomycin trough levels of >20 mg/dL, duration of therapy >7 days, doses of >4 g/day, and use of concomitant nephrotoxic agents.[31-35] The presence of AKI, underlying CKD, obesity altering the volume of distribution, older age, and comorbidities contribute to the risk of vancomycin nephrotoxicity. Targeting trough levels of 15 to 20 mg/dL is important for minimizing toxicity. Frequent monitoring of drug levels especially in the setting of AKI is essential. In light of the previously described tubular obstruction findings, adequate volume repletion should be part of prevention strategies. Animal studies have studied cilastatin to minimize toxicity by reducing cellular uptake of vancomycin and interfering with apoptosis.[30,36]

AMPHOTERICIN

Amphotericin B is an antifungal agent used for severe systemic mycoses infection. It is a polyene antifungal agent that is insoluble in water. It is solubilized with deoxycholate and administered in electrolyte-free solutions. This agent kills fungi by binding cholesterol in the cellular membrane thus increasing membrane permeability. This causes back diffusion of hydrogen ions and sodium entry through membrane pores resulting in activation of mitogen-activated kinases and increased intracellular calcium concentration, which may cause tubular injury.[37] In addition to the toxic injury, there is an ischemic injury from the renal vasoconstriction and reduction in blood flow.[38] Tubular epithelial cells, especially in the medulla, are susceptible to this injury resulting in ATN and tubular dysfunction. Up to 80% of individuals receiving the medication will have renal injury, which limits treatment.[39,40] Amphotericin can also cause hypomagnesemia, hypokalemia, nephrogenic diabetes insipidus, and renal tubular acidosis.[37] Discontinuation of amphotericin in most cases will lead to recovery of GFR, but decreased concentrating ability, magnesium wasting, and potassium wasting are often persistent despite medication discontinuation. Predisposing factors for amphotericin B nephrotoxicity include volume depletion, use of other agents that may cause ATN, underlying CKD, and cumulative dose above 5 g.[10] Preventative measures incorporate aggressive fluid resuscitation to counteract the renal vasoconstriction.[38] Alternative dosing regimens have been attempted to minimize toxicity, including continuous infusions, alternate day dosing, or 2 to 4 hour infusions.[41,42] Continuous infusion dosing may result in lower systemic doses potentially reducing efficacy. Alternative formulations such as amphotericin B colloidal, amphotericin B lipid complex, and liposomal amphotericin B have been developed to minimize side effects. The alternative preparations have lower rates of nephrotoxicity.[10] A double-blind randomized study involving 18 centers demonstrated lower rates of nephrotoxicity when comparing alternative formulations to standard amphotericin B (42.3% with amphotericin B, 14.1% with liposomal amphotericin B, and 14.8% with amphotericin B lipid complex).[30,43] Use of daily oral NAC 600 mg twice a day for the prevention of ATN injury from amphotericin has shown some benefit.[44] In a randomized trial comparing placebo and NAC co-administered with amphotericin B, the NAC group demonstrated fewer episodes of AKI (34.78%) versus placebo (65.22%), which was statistically significant but with significantly increased adverse events such as nausea and vomiting.[44]

NONSTEROIDAL ANTI-INFLAMMATORY DRUGS

NSAIDs are commonly implicated in drug-induced renal injury with an estimated 2.5 million cases per year.[44] The frequency of complications is partially due to the ability to take the medications without a prescription, leading to complications from medication interactions or use in the setting of comorbidities. In the United States, it is estimated that 30 billion over-the-counter doses of NSAIDs are taken every year.[45] NSAIDs use has been associated with hemodynamic effects leading to prerenal injury, hypertension, ischemic ATN, and papillary necrosis. NSAIDs can cause acute or chronic interstitial nephritis, electrolyte abnormalities such as hyperkalemia or hyponatremia, and secondary glomerular diseases such as minimal change disease and membranous nephropathy.[46,47] The beneficial effects of NSAIDs through reduction of inflammation by inhibition of prostaglandins are the primary mechanism for the hemodynamic renal complications. Prostaglandins E2 and I2 increase afferent glomerular vasodilation to maintain renal perfusion. Inhibition of prostaglandins impair vasodilation especially in the setting of volume depletion or decreased cardiac output or with RAAS blockade. NSAID-induced hemodynamic changes promote prerenal and ischemic ATN episodes. Prostaglandins also stimulate renin- and angiotensin-mediated aldosterone release.[48] With NSAIDs use, the inhibition of prostaglandin leads to hyporeninemic hypoaldosteronism manifested by a tendency to hyperkalemia and metabolic acidosis. NSAIDs use can result in sodium retention causing hypertension and edema. NSAIDs block the effect of prostaglandins, which normally inhibit loop of Henle and cortical-collecting tubule sodium reabsorption and also block prostaglandins ability to inhibit ADH mediated water reabsorption in the collecting tubules[49] NSAIDs have been associated with acute, subacute, and chronic papillary necrosis. The papillary and medullary regions have increased dependence on prostaglandin-induced vasodilation for adequate blood flow and, therefore, are more susceptible to ischemia with NSAIDs use.[50] AIN is an inflammatory reaction to NSAIDs in the renal interstitium, leading to edema and tubulitis from lymphocytic and eosinophilic infiltration. The presence of rash, peripheral eosinophilia, and eosinophiluria are usual features of an allergic AIN but are commonly absent from NSAID-induced AIN. The usual AKI time course is within weeks or months of exposure. Chronic interstitial nephritis may occur with long-time exposure to NSAIDs and manifested as a slowly worsening of renal function. This class of medications is also associated with minimal change disease, often with AIN. The proposed mechanism involves cyclooxygenase inhibition, leading to conversion of arachidonic acid to leukotriene and activation of T helper cells, which infiltrate glomeruli and cause podocyte injury.[51,52]

Older age, pre-existing renal disease, volume depleted states, diuretic use, RAAS blockade, higher NSAIDs doses, chronic use, and heart failure are identified as risk factors for renal injury.[53,54] The incidence of renal injury is not affected by which NSAID is used.[53] Preventative measures include avoidance of the agents when the estimated GFR is <30 mL/min/1.73m^2, in volume depleted states, and in the setting of heart failure. Long-term chronic use is not recommended in those with hypertension or CKD.[55] Management of NSAID-induced renal injury involves stopping the medications and ensuring adequate volume status. In the setting of interstitial nephritis and glomerular injury, immunosuppressive agents may be considered in addition to cessation of agents.

CONCLUSION

There are many therapeutic agents that cause renal toxicity that often become the limiting factor in the agent's use. Often, there are no alternative agents available, so recognition of the risk factors for nephrotoxicity and incorporation of preventative measures are critical. Many of the adverse effects are due to the drug's inherent mechanism of action. Close monitoring of renal function is required to determine proper dosing and identifying early AKI.

REFERENCES

1. Mehta RL, Pascual MT, Soroko S, et al.; Program to Improve Care in Acute Renal Disease. Spectrum of acute renal failure in the intensive care unit: the PICARD experience. *Kidney Int.* 2004;66(4):1613–1621.

2. Perazella MA. Renal vulnerability to drug toxicity. *Clin J Am Soc Nephrol.* 2008;3(3):844–861.

3. Lee W, Kim RB. Transporters and renal drug elimination. *Annu Rev Pharmacol Toxicol.* 2004;44:137–166.

4. Khrunin AV, Moisseev A, Gorbunova V, Limborska S. Genetic polymorphisms and the efficacy and toxicity of cisplatin based chemotherapy in ovarian cancer patients. *Pharmacogenomic J.* 2010;10(1):54–61.

5. Andreucci M, Faga T, Riccio E, et al. The potential use of biomarkers in predicting contrast-induced acute kidney injury. *Int J Nephrol Renovasc Dis.* 2016;9:205–221.

6. Au TH, Bruckner A, Mohuiddin SM, Hilleman DE. The prevention of contrast-induced nephropathy. *Ann Pharmacother.* 2014;48(10):1332–1342.

7. Sharfuddin, Asif A, Weisbord SD, Palevsky PM, Molitoris BA. Acute kidney injury. In: Skorecki K, Chertow GM, Marsden PA, Taal MW, Yu ASL, eds. *Brenner and Rector's The Kidney.* 10th ed. Philadelphia, PA: Elsevier; 2016: 30, 1044–1099

8. Tao SM, Wichmann JL, Schoepf UJ, et al. Contrast-induced nephropathy in CT: incidence, risk factors and strategies for prevention. *Eur Radiol.* 2016;26(9):3310–3318.

9. Aubry P, Brillet G, Catella L, et al. Outcomes, risk factors, and health burden of contrast-induced acute kidney injury: an observational study of one million hospitalizations with image-guided cardiovascular procedures. *BMC Nephrol.* 2016;17(1):167.

10. Kidney Disease: Improving Global Outcomes (KDIGO) Acute Kidney Injury Work Group. KDIGO clinical practice guideline for acute kidney injury. *Kidney Int Supp.* 2012;2:1–138.

11. Abbas FM, Julie BM, Sharma A, Halawa A. "Contrast nephropathy" in renal transplantation: is it real? *World J Transplant.* 2016;6(4):682–688.

12. Persson PB, Hansell P, Liss P. Pathophysiology of contrast medium-induced nephropathy. *Kidney Int.* 2005;68(1):14–22.

13. Eng J, Wilson RF, Subramaniam RM, Zhang A, et al. Comparative effect of contrast media type on the incidence of contrast-induced nephropathy: a systematic review and meta-analysis of observational studies. *Eur J Int Med.* 2015;285–291.

14. Mehran R, Aymong ED, Nikolesky E, et al. A simple risk score for prediction of contrast induced nephropathy after percutaneous coronary intervention: development and initial validation. *J Am Coll Cardiol.* 2004;44:1393–1399.

15. McCullough PA, Choi JP, Feghali GA, et al. Contrast-induced acute kidney injury. *J Am Coll Cardiol.* 2016;68(13):1465–1473.

16. Wang N, Qian P, Kumar S, et al. The effect of N-acytylcysteine on the incidence of

contrast-induced kidney injury: a systemic review and trial sequential analysis. *Int J Cardiol.* 2016;209:319–327.

17. Li H, Wang C, Liu C, et al. Efficacy of short-term statin treatment for the prevention of contrast-induced acute kidney injury in patients undergoing coronary angiography/percutaneous coronary intervention: a meta-analysis of 21 randomized controlled trials. *Am J Cardiovasc Drugs.* 2016;16(3):201–219.

18. Lakshmanadoss U, Balakrishnan E, DiSalle, MR. Sucrose nephropathy following IV immunoglobulin. *J Basic Clin Pharm.* 2010; 1(2):125–127.

19. Berger M. Adverse effects of IgG therapy. *J Allergy Clin Immunol Pract.* 2013; 1(6):558–566.

20. Cheng MJ, Christmas C. Special considerations with the use of intravenous immunoglobulin in older persons. *Drugs Aging.* 2011;28(9):729–736.

21. Dickenmann M, Oettl T, Mihatsch MJ. Osmotic nephrosis: acute kidney injury with accumulation of proximal tubular lysosomes due to administration of exogenous solutes. *Am J Kidney Dis.* 2008;51(3):491–503.

22. Vicente-Vicente L, Casanova AG, Hernández-Sánchez MT, et al. A systematic meta-analysis on the efficacy of pre-clinically tested nephroprotectants at preventing aminoglycoside nephrotoxicity. *Toxicology.* 2017;377:14–24.

23. Wargo KA, Edwards J D. Aminoglycoside-induced nephrotoxicity. *J Pharm Pract.* 2014;27(6):573–577.

24. Mergenhagen KA, Borton AR. Vancomycin nephrotoxicity: a review. *J Pharm Pract.* 2014;27(6):545–553.

25. Bamgbola O. Review of vancomycin induced renal toxicity: an update. *Ther Adv Endocrinol Metab.* 2016;7(30):136–147.

26. Farber BF, Moellering RC Jr. Retrospective study of the toxicity of preparations of vancomycin from 1974 to 1981. *Antimicrob Agents Chemother.* 1983;23:138–141.

27. Oktem F, Arslan M, Ozguner F, et al. In vivo evidence suggesting the role of oxidative stress in pathogenesis of vancomycin-induced nephrotoxicity: protection by erdostein. *Toxicology.* 2005;215:227–233.

28. Nishino Y, Takemura S, Miniamiyama Y, et al. Targeting superoxide dismutase to renal proximal tubule cells attenuates vancomycin-induced nephrotoxicity in rats. *Free Radic Res.* 2003;37:373–379.

29. Arimura Y, Yano T, Hirano M, et al. Mitochondrial superoxide production contributes to vancomycin-induced renal tubular cell apoptosis. *Free Radic Biol Med.* 2012;52:1865–1873.

30. Humanes B, Jado J, Comano S, et al. Protective effects of cilastatin against vancomycin-induced

nephrotoxicity. *Biomed Res Int.* 2015. Article ID 704382

31. Luque Y, Louis K, Jouanneau C, et al. Vancomycin-Associated Cast Nephropathy. *J Am Soc Nephrol.* 2017; 28(6):1723–1728.

32. Hanrahan TP, Kotapati C, Roberts MJ, et al. Factors associated with vancomycin nephrotoxicity in the critically ill. *Anaesth Intensive Care.* 2015; 43(5): 594–599.

33. Bosso JA, Nappi J, Rudisill C, et al. Relationship between vancomycin trough concentrations and nephrotoxicity: a prospective multicenter trial. *Antimicrob Agents Chemother.* 2011;55 (12): 5475–5479.

34. Lodise TP, Lomasetro B, Graves J, et al. Larger vancomycin doses (at least 4 grams per day) are associated with an increased incidence of nephrotoxicity. *Antimicrob Agents Chemother.* 2008;52(4):1330–1336.

35. Jeffers MN, Isakow W, Doherty JA, et al. A retrospective analysis of possible renal toxicity associated with vancomycin in patients with health care- associated methicillin-resistant Staphylococcus aureus pneumonia. *Clin Ther.* 2007;29(6):1107–1115.

36. Toyoguchi T, Takashis S, Hosoya J, et al. Nephrotoxicity of vancomycin and drug interaction study with cilastatin in rabbits. *Antimicrobial Agents Chemother.* 1997;41(9):1985–1990.

37. Rocha PN, Kobayashi D, Almeida LC, et al. Incidence, predictors, and impact on hospital mortality of amphotericin B nephrotoxicity defined using newer acute kidney injury diagnostic criteria. *Antimicrobial Agents and Chemother.* 2015;59(8):4759–4769.

38. Heidemann HT, Gerkens JF, Jackson EK, Branch RA. Effect of aminophylline on renal vasoconstriction produced by amphotericin B in the rat. *Arch Pharmacol.* 1983;324:148–152.

39. Pathak A, Pien FD, Carvalho L. Amphotericin B use in a community hospital, with special emphasis on side effects. *Clini Infect Dis.* 1998;26:334–338.

40. Safdar A, Ma J, Saliba F, et al. Drug induced nephrotoxicity caused by amphotericin B lipid complex and liposomal amphotericin B. *Medicine.* 2010;89(4):236–244.

41. Ullmann AJ. Nephrotoxicity in the setting of invasive fungal diseases. *Mycoses.* 2008;35(Suppl 1):25–30.

42. de Rosa FG, Bargiacchi O, Audagnotto S, et al. Continous infusion of amphotericin B deoxycholate: does decreased nephrotoxicity couple with time-dependent pharmacodynamics? *Leuk Lymphoma.* 2006;47:1964–1966.

43. Techapornroong M, Suankratay C. Alternate day versus once- daily administration of amphotericin

B in the treatment of cryptococcal meningitis: randomized controlled trial. *Scand J Infect Dis.* 2007;39:896–901.

44. Karimzadeh I, Khalili H, Sagheb MM, Farsaei S. A double blinded placebo-controlled, multicenter clinical trial of N-acetylcysteine for preventing amphotericin B induced nephrotoxicity. *Expert Opin Drug Metab Toxicol.* 2015;11(9):1345–1355.

45. Singh G, Triadafilopoulos G. Epidemiology of NSAID induced gastrointestinal complications. *J Rheumatol.* 1999;26 (Suppl 56):18–24.

46. Rahman S, Malcoun A. Nonsteroidal antiinflammatory drugs, cyclooxygenase-2, and the kidneys. *Prim Care Clin Office Pract.* 2014;41:803–821.

47. Pazhayattil GS, Shirali AC. Drug-induced impairment of renal function. *Int J Nephrol Renovasc Dis.* 2014;7:457–468.

48. Schneider V, Levesque LE, Zhang B, et al. Association of selective and conventional nonsteroidal anti-inflammatory drugs with acute renal failure: a population-based, nested case control analysis. *Am J Epidemiol.* 2006;164(9):881–889.

49. Kramer HJ, Glanzer K, Dusing R. Role of prostaglandins in the regulation of renal water excretion. *Kidney Int.* 1981;19(6):851–859.

50. Atta MG, Whelton A. Acute papillary necrosis induced by ibuprofen. *Am J Ther.* 1997;4:55–60.

51. Perazella MA, Markowitz GS. Drug-induced acute interstitial nephritis. *Nat Rev Nephrol.* 2010;6:461–470.

52. Clive DM, Stoff JS. Renal syndromes associated with nonsteroidal anti-inflammatory drugs. *N Engl J Med.* 1984;310(9):563–572.

53. Levin ML. Patterns of tubulointerstitial damage associated with nonsteroidal anti-inflammatory drugs. *Semin Nephrol.* 1988;8:55–61.

54. Huerta C, Castellsague J, Varas-Lorenzo C, and Garcia Rodriguez LA. Nonsteroidal anti-inflammatory drugs and risk of ARF in the general population. *Am J Kid Dis.* 2005;45(3):531–539.

55. Ungprasert P, Cheungpasitporn W, Crowson CS, Matteson EL. Individual non-steroidal anti-inflammatory drugs and risk of acute kidney injury: a systematic review and meta-analysis of observational studies. *Eur J Int Med.* 2015;26:285–291.

23

Immunological Agents in the Treatment of Glomerulonephritis

SAMIRA FAROUK AND JONATHAN WINSTON

INTRODUCTION

Glomerulonephritis (GN) is the second most common cause of end-stage renal disease worldwide and, in the United States, the third leading cause behind diabetes and hypertension. GN can be defined as a range of disorders, often immune-mediated, which cause inflammation within the glomerulus and other parts of the kidney.[1] A primary role of the immune system in the pathogenesis of most cases of GN is well described. We now understand that mechanisms of immune-mediated glomerular injury include glomerular antibody deposition leading to an immune response, complement cascade activation, and T and B cell activation.[1,2] Immunological or immunosuppressive therapies to decrease the activity of the immune system for treatment of glomerular disease have evolved significantly over time and continue to change today in response to robust clinical trials and better understanding of disease mechanisms.

As early as 1950, physicians hypothesized that postinfectious GN may result from glomerular deposition of an antigen-antibody complex. Remission was induced by administration of a potent immunosuppressive agent, nitrogen mustard.[3] By 1957, the histologic lesion of "idiopathic nephrotic syndrome" was first described.[4] Knowing that glucocorticoids decrease inflammation by binding to steroid receptors and inhibit the gene expression of inflammatory markers,[5] a small prospective study of 20 patients was performed. The majority of patients with idiopathic nephrotic syndrome responded to corticosteroid or corticotropin therapy,[6] thus heralding the modern age of immunosuppressant therapy for GN. A larger prospective multicenter study in 1981 supported the findings, showing that 8

weeks of corticosteroid therapy led to a dramatic reduction in proteinuria in 93.1% of children with minimal change nephrotic syndrome.[7]

Beginning in the 1970s, several studies at the National Institutes of Health suggested that the steroid-sparing agents such as the DNA-alkylating agent cyclophosphamide (CYC) and purine analog azathioprine (AZA) could benefit patients with systemic lupus erythematosus. A small, randomized control trial at the National Institutes of Health in lupus nephritis patients compared treatment regimens with various combinations of CYC, AZA, and glucocorticoids. In this study, patients treated with CYC alone had a median survival of 15 years and minimal progression to end-stage renal disease, while those treated with glucocorticoids and AZA had a median survival of only 10 years.[8] A similarly designed study utilizing longer duration of therapy published in 1996 showed highest rates of renal remission in lupus nephritis patients after treatment with dual therapy with glucocorticoids and CYC, when compared to monotherapy.[9] Treatment of renal vasculitis disorders like polyarteritis nodosa and granulomatosis with polyangiitis soon followed.[10,11] The 3 major class of drugs for immune-mediated GN—steroids, AZA, and CYC—became the choice of therapy for these disorders. These drugs became the foundation for treatment of other, less specific forms of GN in which treatment, albeit empiric, was considered necessary.

IMMUNOSUPPRESSIVE AGENTS AND USE IN GLOMERULAR DISEASE

Each immunosuppressive agent has a unique mechanism of action by which it decreases the activity, proliferation, or life span of immune cells—ultimately decreasing inflammation. The selection of immunosuppressive agent is a complex process dictated by disease and patient characteristics, disease severity, adverse effects of the agent, and clinical trial data. In the following discussion, we briefly review the use of commonly used immunosuppressive agents in the modern era in selected glomerular diseases and their notable adverse effects (Table 23.1). We will not discuss the indications for treatment or escalation of therapy here.

Lupus Nephritis

As previously described, the treatment of lupus nephritis evolved over the course of 30 years from steroids alone, to the addition of CYC to the steroid regimen. Over the last 20 years, clinical trials have studied the efficacy of numerous other immunosuppressive agents including mycophenolate mofetil (MMF; inhibitor of de novo purine synthesis), rituximab (monoclonal antibody against B-cell surface protein CD20), tacrolimus (a calcineurin inhibitor [CNI]), and abatacept (CTLAIg-4 fusion protein). In 2010,

TABLE 23.1 MECHANISM OF ACTION AND NOTABLE ADVERSE EFFECTS OF IMMUNOLOGICAL AGENTS COMMONLY CURRENTLY USED FOR GLOMERULONEPHRITIS

Agent (Discovery of IS Activity)	Mechanism of IS Action	Notable Adverse Effects
Nitrogen Mustard (1949)	Inhibit gene expression of inflammation-associated molecules (i.e., cytokines, chemokines)[a]	Diabetes mellitus, CNS effects, Cushing's syndrome, skin changes, hypertension, peptic ulcern[b]
Cyclophosphamide (1959)	DNA alkylating agent	Bone marrow suppression, infertility, hemorrhagic cystitis[c]
Azathioprine (1959)	Inhibits intracellular purine synthesis	Bone marrow suppression, leukopenia, pancreatitis, hypersensitivity reaction[d]
Cyclosporine (1976)	Calcineurin inhibitor	Diabetes mellitus, gingival hypertrophy, hirsutism, GI effects, nephrotoxicity, neurotoxicity, hypertension, malignancy[e]
Tacrolimus (1987)	Calcineurin inhibitor	Diabetes mellitus, alopecia, nephrotoxicity, neurotoxicity, hypertension, GI effects, malignancy[e]
Mycophenolate mofetil (1991)	Inhibits IMPDH and de novo purine synthesis[f]	Leukopenia, GI effects[g]
Rituximab (1997)	Monoclonal antibody against B-cell surface protein CD20[18h]	Infusion reaction, cytokine release syndrome, HBV reactivation[i]
Sirolimus (1999)	Inhibitor of mTOR	Myelosuppression, pneumonitis, GI effects, proteinuria

[a]Baldwin DS. Effect of nitrogen mustard on clinical course of glomerulonephritis. *Arch. Intern. Med.* 1953;92:162.
[b]Schäcke H, Döcke WD, Asadullah K. Mechanisms involved in the side effects of glucocorticoids. *Pharmacol Ther.* 2002;96:23–43.
[c]Gershwin ME. Cyclophosphamide: use in practice. *Ann Intern Med.* 1974;80:531–540.
[d]Pearson DC, May GR, Fick G, Sutherland LR. Azathioprine for maintaining remission of Crohn's disease. *Cochrane Database Syst Rev.* 2000;(2):CD000067.
[e]Jose M. The CARI guidelines. Calcineurin inhibitors in renal transplantation: adverse effects. *Nephrology (Carlton)* 2007;12 Suppl 1:S66–S74.
[f]Allison AC, Eugui ES. Mycophenolate mofetil and its mechanisms of action. *Immunopharmacology.* 2000;47(2–3):85–118.
[g]Silverman Kitchin JE, Pomeranz MK, Pak G, Washenik K, Shupack JL. Rediscovering mycophenolic acid: a review of its mechanism, side effects, and potential uses. *J Am Acad Dermatol* 1997;37:445–449.
[h]Maloney DG, Grillo-López AJ, White CA, et al. IDEC-C2B8 (Rituximab) anti-CD20 monoclonal antibody therapy in patients with relapsed low-grade non-Hodgkin's lymphoma. *Blood* 1997;90:2188–2195.
[i]Tsutsumi Y, Kanamori H, Mori A, et al. Reactivation of hepatitis B virus with rituximab. *Expert Opin Drug Saf.* 2005;4(3):599–608.
IS = immunosuppression. CNS = central nervous system. GI = gastrointestinal. IMPDH = inosine 5'-monophosphate dehydrogenase. HBV = hepatitis B virus. mTOR = mechanistic target of rapamycin.

the Aspreva Lupus Management[12] study, an international randomized control trial of 370 patients, found that MMF and intravenous CYC had similar overall efficacy for short-term induction therapy for lupus nephritis. However, Hispanics and black patients had a lower response to intravenous CYC—though this finding was statistically significant only for Hispanic patients. In 2010, a meta-analysis of randomized controlled trials confirmed the finding of similar efficacy of MMF compared to CYC and also found that MMF was more effective than AZA.[13] While a small study of Chinese patients has shown similar efficacy between a tacrolimus regimen compared to CYC[22] studies of rituximab and abatacept have not shown a benefit compared to placebo thus far.[14,15]

Today, the combination of and either MMF or CYC and glucocorticoids remains the primary therapeutic strategy for lupus nephritis. The decision to use MMF or CYC, typically intravenous to minimize toxicity, is based on a discussion between the nephrologist and the patient given the significantly different adverse effect profiles. Prophylaxis for *Pneumocystis* pneumonia should be considered for patients receiving prolonged therapy with high doses of glucocorticoids, as the risk of pneumonia increases significantly after 8 weeks of therapy with an equivalent dose of 20 mg prednisone or higher.[16]

Primary/Idiopathic Membranous Nephropathy

The combination of glucocorticoids and CYC or CNI have also been shown to be effective in inducing remission of idiopathic MN.[17,18] While chlorambucil-based regimens have been found to be equally effective, CYC regimens are preferred in clinical practice because of lower toxicity of CYC. CNI in combination with glucocorticoids have also been shown to be effective in inducing remission, though higher relapse rates occurred in the CNI group of an RCT comparing cyclosporine and prednisone to prednisone plus placebo.[18] The first randomized trial of rituximab in 75 patients for primary membranous nephropathy showed an increase in serum albumin at 6 months and an increased rate of proteinuria remission, which was seen at a median time of 7 months.[19] These results have not yet been replicated.

Primary/Idiopathic Focal Segmental Glomerulosclerosis

While there are no randomized control trials for the initial treatment of primary focal segmental glomerulosclerosis (FSGS), glucocorticoids are the mainstay of treatment despite the fact that only a small percentage of patients will achieve complete and stable remission with steroids alone.[20] Given the high side effect profile of glucocorticoids, limited studies have also looked at CNIs (cyclosporin A and tacrolimus) as an alternative primary therapy. When used as an initial therapy, tacrolimus has been shown to be effective in inducing partial remission.[21]

Cyclosporine has been studied extensively in steroid-resistant FSGS and has also been shown to induce significantly higher partial and complete remission when compared to placebo and chlorambucil.[22,23] Though no randomized studies have been done, cases and observational studies have showed some efficacy of other immunological agents including MMF, CYC, rituximab, adrenocorticotropic hormone gel, and abatacept.[24]

Antineutrophilic Cytoplasmic Antibody-Associated Vasculitis

Long-term mortality for antineutrophil cytoplasmic antibodies (ANCA) associated vasculitis remains high despite current therapeutic options.[25] Randomized trials over the last decade have compared the efficacy of induction therapy with intravenous versus oral CYC (CYCLOPS trial[26]) and CYC versus rituximab (RAVE[27] and RITUXIVAS[28] trials). The results of these trials revealed that intravenous CYC is noninferior to oral CYC, and induction with rituximab is noninferior to CYC—though the relapse rates are higher. Glucocorticoids should be initiated as part of induction therapy and tapered by 4 to 6 months. Though one small non-blinded clinical trial showed possible efficacy for MMF as induction therapy, this strategy has not yet been tested in large, randomized clinical trials. Options for maintenance therapy include MMF, AZA, rituximab, or methotrexate.

Plasmapheresis, or plasma exchange, is an important adjunctive therapy for ANCA-associated vasculitis. The MEPEX trial published in 2007 demonstrated that plasma exchange could be beneficial for renal recovery for those patients with severe renal dysfunction (creatinine greater than 5.8 mg/dL), though there was no improvement in long term mortality when compared to high-dose methylprednisolone.[29] The role for plasma exchange will become clearer after the completion of the PEXIVAS trial (Clinicaltrials. gov identifier: NCT00987389), a randomized trial in which patients will receive plasma exchange and standard or low-dose glucocorticoids or no plasma exchange and standard or low-dose glucocorticoids. Plasma exchange should also be utilized in the presence of pulmonary hemorrhage and antiglomerular basement membrane antibodies.

An exciting, more targeted therapy for ANCA-associated vasculitis is the C5a receptor inhibitor, avacopan (CCX168). In a phase 2 randomized, clinical trial, avacopan allowed for decreased dosing of glucocorticoids with similar outcomes, including remission rates and vasculitis activity scores. Those patients treated with avacopan and decreased glucocorticoids also reported higher quality of life.

Complement and Glomerular Disease

Though complement activation in glomerular disease has traditionally been associated with auto-antibody associated diseases processes, the complement system has now been implicated in other glomerular diseases such as FSGS and thrombotic microangiopathies.[30] In addition to the C5a receptor antagonist avacopan previously described, other complement system inhibitors have emerged.

Eculiziumab is an anti-C5 monoclonal antibody that inhibits the terminal complement effector pathway, thus inhibiting all complement pathways. It has been now approved for use in the treatment of atypical hemolytic uremic syndrome. A longer acting anti-C5 monoclonal antibody (ALXN1210) is now being tested in a clinical trial (Clinicaltrials. gov identifier: NCT02949128). OMS721, a novel inhibitor of mannan-binding lectin-associated serine protease-2 is also being tested in a phase 1 clinical trial (Clinicaltrials. gov identifier: NCT02682407). AMY-101 is a C3 inhibitor also being evaluated for use in glomerular diseases (Clinicaltrials.gov identifier: NCT03316521).

It is likely that novel complement inhibitors will continue to be developed and tested in the future, further expanding the arsenal of more targeted glomerular disease therapies.

Rituximab in Refractory Glomerular Diseases

Refractory diseases can be challenging for the nephrologist. Both CYC and rituximab have shown to be efficacious in the treatment of various refractory glomerular diseases. Rituximab induces apoptosis of both mature and immature B cells

(importantly, not antibody-secreting plasma cells) and thus has been a therapy of interest in glomerular disease.[31] It has been used in both steroid-resistant and steroid-dependent minimal change disease and FSGS, including recurrent of FSGS in the transplanted kidney. Though a randomized trial has not yet been done, rituximab has been effective in the treatment of idiopathic or primary membranous nephropathy, with reductions in phospholipase A2 receptor titers as well as sustained remission.[31] Randomized trials have also shown that there may be a role for rituximab in the treatment of refractory lupus nephritis.

THE FUTURE

As our understanding of the mechanisms of glomerular diseases improves, new therapeutic targets are discovered, and disease-specific immunological agents emerge both in nephrology and other disciplines, novel targeted therapies are certain to evolve. The goal has always been increased efficacy with more tolerable side effect profiles.

Signaling of tyrosine kinase pathways may represent a new, targeted therapy for immune-mediated GN. Tyrosine kinase pathways have been implicated in ANCA vasculitis, lupus nephritis, and antiglomerular basement membrane disease. Targeting these pathways may allow for safer and more effective of selected glomerular diseases.[32]

Numerous clinical trials are ongoing to study various immunological agents in the treatment of different glomerular diseases. While some test the agents that have been successful in other diseases in a different disease, other trials are evaluating novel agents such as monoclonal antibodies. For example, a study of belimumab, the monoclonal antibody that inhibits the B-cell activating factor, in idiopathic membranous nephropathy patients has recently completed, and results are pending (Clinicaltrials.gov identifier: NCT01610492). The results of trials such as this, will allow for the advancement of glomerular disease treatments, and ideally develops therapies that are more efficacious with fewer toxicities.

Selected upcoming trials include (by Clinicaltrials.gov identifier and name):

NCT02216747: Low Dose Steroids in the Treatment of Nephrotic Syndrome Relapse

NCT03157037: An Open-Label Phase II Study to Evaluate the Efficacy and Safety of IdeS in Anti-GBM Disease

NCT00977977: Rituximab Plus Cyclosporine in Idiopathic Membranous Nephropathy

NCT03095118: Daratumumab in the Treatment of PGNMID and C3GN

NCT00354198: Efficacy of Pentoxifylline on Rapidly Progressive Glomerulonephritis

NCT00843856: Mycophenolate Mofetil and Tacrolimus Versus Tacrolimus for the Treatment of Idiopathic Membranous Glomerulonephritis (IMG) (MTAC)

NCT00001789: BG9588 (Anti-CD40L Antibody) to Treat Lupus Nephritis

NCT02093533: Eculizumab in Primary MPGN (EAGLE)

NCT00275613: Pilot Study of Rituximab for Membranoproliferative Glomerulonephritis

NCT00050713: Sirolimus Therapy for Idiopathic and Lupus Membranous Nephropathy

REFERENCES

1. Chadban SJ, Atkins RC. Glomerulonephritis. *Lancet.* 2005;365:1797–1806.

2. Tipping PG, Kitching AR. Glomerulonephritis, Th1 and Th2: what's new? *Clin. Exp. Immunol.* 2005;142:207–215.

3. Baldwin DS. Effect of nitrogen mustard on clinical course of glomerulonephritis. *Arch. Intern. Med.* 1953;92:162.

4. Jennette JC, D'Agati VD, Olson JL, Silva FG. *Heptinstall's Pathology of the Kidney.* Philadelphia, PA: Lippincott Williams & Wilkins; 2014.

5. van der Velden VH. Glucocorticoids: mechanisms of action and anti-inflammatory potential in asthma. *Mediators Inflamm.* 1998;7(4):229–237.

6. Goodman HC, Baxter JH. The nephrotic syndrome; clinical observations on therapy with prednisone and other steroids. *J Am Med Assoc.* 1957;165:1798–1808.

7. The primary nephrotic syndrome in children: identification of patients with minimal change nephrotic syndrome from initial response to prednisone: a report of the International Study of Kidney Disease in Children. *J Pediatr.* 1981;98(4):561–564.

8. Steinberg AD. The treatment of lupus nephritis. *Kidney Int.* 1986;30:769–787.

9. Gourley MF, Austin HA 3rd, Scott D, et al. Methylprednisolone and cyclophosphamide, alone or in combination, in patients with lupus nephritis: a randomized, controlled trial. *Ann Intern Med.* 1996;125:549–557.

10. Hoffman GS, Kerr GS, Leavitt RY, et al. Wegener granulomatosis: an analysis of 158 patients. *Ann Intern Med.* 1992;116:488–498.

11. Leib ES, Restivo C, Paulus HE. Immunosuppressive and corticosteroid therapy of polyarteritis nodosa. *Am J. Med.* 67, 941–947 (1979).

12. Appel GB, Contreras G, Dooley MA, et al. Mycophenolate mofetil versus cyclophosphamide for induction treatment of lupus nephritis. *J Am Soc Nephrol.* 2009;20:1103–1112.

13. Henderson LK, Masson P, Craig JC, et al. Induction and maintenance treatment of proliferative lupus nephritis: a meta-analysis of randomized controlled trials. *Am J Kidney Dis.* 2013;61:74–87.

14. Chen W, Tang X, Liu Q, et al. Short-term outcomes of induction therapy with tacrolimus versus cyclophosphamide for active lupus nephritis: A multicenter randomized clinical trial. *Am. J. Kidney Dis.* 2011;57:235–244.

15. Rovin BH, Furie R, Latinis K, et al. Efficacy and safety of rituximab in patients with active proliferative lupus nephritis: the Lupus Nephritis Assessment with Rituximab study. *Arthritis Rheum.* 2012;64:1215–1226.

16. Limper AH, Knox KS, Sarosi GA, et al. An official American Thoracic Society statement: treatment of fungal infections in adult pulmonary and critical care patients. *Am J Respir Crit Care Med.* 2011;183:96–128.

17. Ponticelli C, Zucchelli P, Passerini P, et al. A 10-year follow-up of a randomized study with methylprednisolone and chlorambucil in membranous nephropathy. *Kidney Int.* 1995;48:1600–1604.

18. Cattran DC, Appel GB, Hebert LA, et al. Cyclosporine in patients with steroid-resistant membranous nephropathy: a randomized trial. *Kidney Int.* 2001;59:1484–1490.

19. Dahan K, Debiec H, Plaisier E, et al. Rituximab for severe membranous nephropathy: a 6-month trial with extended follow-up. *J Am Soc Nephrol.* 2017;28:348–358.

20. Meyrier A. Nephrotic focal segmental glomerulosclerosis in 2004: an update. *Nephrol Dial Transplant.* 2004;19:2437–2444.

21. Duncan N, Dhaygude A, Owen J, et al. Treatment of focal and segmental glomerulosclerosis in adults with tacrolimus monotherapy. *Nephrol Dial Transplant.* 2004;19:3062–3067.

22. Heering P, Braun N, Müllejans R, et al. Cyclosporine A and chlorambucil in the treatment of idiopathic focal segmental glomerulosclerosis. *Am J Kidney Dis.* 2004;43:10–18.

23. Cattran DC, Appel GB, Hebert LA, et al. North America Nephrotic Syndrome Study

Group. A randomized trial of cyclosporine in patients with steroid-resistant focal segmental glomerulosclerosis. *Kidney Int.* 1999;56:2220–2226.

24. Beer A, Mayer G, Kronbichler A. Treatment strategies of adult primary focal segmental glomerulosclerosis: a systematic review focusing on the last two decades. *BioMed Res. Int.* 2016;419:2578.

25. Luqmani R, Suppiah R, Edwards CJ, et al. Mortality in Wegener's granulomatosis: a bimodal pattern. *Rheumatol.* 2011;50:697–702.

26. de Groot K, Harper L, Jayne DR, et al. Pulse versus daily oral cyclophosphamide for induction of remission in antineutrophil cytoplasmic antibody-associated vasculitis: a randomized trial. *Ann Intern Med.* 2009;150:670–680.

27. Stone JH, Merkel PA, Spiera R, et al. Rituximab versus cyclophosphamide for ANCA-associated vasculitis. *N Engl J Med.* 2010;363:221–232.

28. Jones RB, Tervaert JW, Hauser T, et al. Rituximab versus Cyclophosphamide in ANCA-Associated Renal Vasculitis. *N Engl J Med.* 2010;363:211–220.

29. Jayne DRW, Gaskin G, Rasmussen N, et al. Randomized trial of plasma exchange or high-dosage methylprednisolone as adjunctive therapy for severe renal vasculitis. *J Am Soc Nephrol.* 2007;18:2180–2188.

30. Angeletti A, Reyes-Bahamonde J, Cravedi P, Campbell KN. Complement in non-antibody-mediated kidney diseases. *Front. Med.* 2017;4:99.

31. Ejaz AA, Asmar A, Alsabbagh MM, Ahsan N. Rituximab in immunologic glomerular diseases. *mAbs* 2012;4:198–207.

32. Ma TKW, McAdoo SP, Tam FWK. Targeting the tyrosine kinase signalling pathways for treatment of immune-mediated glomerulonephritis: from bench to bedside and beyond. *Nephrol Dial Transplant.* 2017;32:i129–i138.

24

NSAIDs and the Kidney

LILI CHAN AND TONIA KIM

INTRODUCTION

The incidence of acute kidney injury (AKI) is rising, and it is well-established that AKI and chronic kidney disease (CKD) are interconnected processes. Nonsteroidal anti-inflammatory drugs (NSAIDs) are commonly used analgesic medications, accounting for approximately 98 million prescriptions in 2012. More than 29 million adults report that they are regular users, with higher use seen with increasing age.[1] Multiple adverse drug reactions have been identified including cardiovascular, gastrointestinal, and genitourinary systems. While NSAIDs pose a small threat to patients with normal renal function, in the susceptible patient they can affect the kidney in multiple ways including AKI, minimal change disease, membranous nephropathy, and interstitial nephritis. NSAIDs also affects sodium excretion, fluid balance, and blood pressure. In this chapter, we will review the different renal pathologies associated with NSAIDs, mechanisms of NSAID-induced kidney injury and prevention strategies.

EPIDEMIOLOGY

While the incidence of NSAID-induced renal toxicity requiring physician intervention is relatively low (between 1%–5%), given the prominent use of NSAIDs, this represents a large number of individuals at risk.[2] Those with existing renal insufficiency, the elderly, and those predisposed to dehydration (individuals on diuretics, alcohol abusers) are more likely to have NSAID induced renal toxicity. In a group of elderly patients exposed to NSAIDS, the incidence of renal toxicity was as high as 12%.[3] There are several different types of renal toxicities associated with NSAID use, the most common of which is ischemic AKI. We will discuss each type in this chapter.

CLINICAL SYNDROMES

Ischemic Acute Kidney Injury

The mechanism of action of NSAIDs is due the inhibition of prostaglandin synthesis via COX inhibition in several potential ways: (i) rapid reversible competitive inhibition, (ii) rapid reversible noncompetitive inhibitions, and (iii) irreversible time-dependent inactivation (Fig. 24.1).[4] There are 2 forms of cyclooxygenase (COX): COX-1, which is constitutively expressed, and COX-2, which is induced by cytokines and other inflammatory mediators. There are currently 2 classes of NSAIDs available in the market: those that are nonselective and inhibit both COX-1 and COX-2, and selective inhibitors, which are COX-2 selective.

A brief discussion of glomerular filtration rate (GFR) is essential to understanding the effects of NSAIDs. GFR is dependent on several factors. As blood flows through the afferent arteriole, glomerular hydrostatic pressure exerts an outward force, which favors filtration while glomerular oncotic pressure opposes filtration. Bowman's space hydrostatic pressure also opposes filtration (Fig. 24.2). A normal glomerulus is depicted in Fig. 24.3A. When there is a reduction in absolute or effective circulation, there is an increase in catecholamines and activation of the renin–angiotensin–aldosterone system (RAAS), which leads to vasoconstriction within the renal vasculature (efferent arteriole vasoconstriction > afferent arteriole vasoconstriction). This vasoconstriction is countered by a compensatory release of prostaglandins, which enables adequate renal perfusion, by causing afferent arteriole vasodilation (Fig. 24.3B). Therefore, the use of NSAIDS that block prostaglandins will lead to a decrease in renal blood flow and GFR (Fig. 24.3C). Particularly important is the

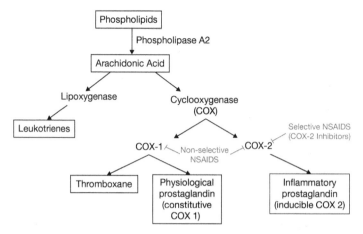

FIGURE 24.1 Mechanism of action of nonsteroidal anti-inflammatory drugs (NSAIDs).

inhibition of prostaglandin-mediated dilation of the afferent renal arteriole.[5] RAAS inhibitors lead to a decreased angiotensin II effect, which blocks the vasoconstriction of the efferent arteriole and afferent arteriole and causes vasodilation of the efferent arteriole more than vasodilation of afferent arteriole, resulting in a reduced filtration pressure. (Fig. 24.3D) Therefore, NSAID use with medications such as diuretics and/or RAAS inhibitors (Fig. 24.3E), which decrease renal perfusion, will increase the risk for AKI. One study found an adjusted rate ratio of 1.64 with triple therapy including NSAIDs, diuretics, and RAAS inhibitors.[5] While this change is fully reversible

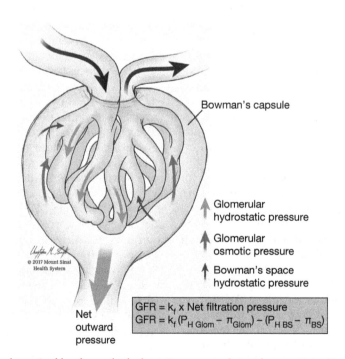

FIGURE 24.2 GFR is determined by glomerular hydrostatic pressure, glomerular osmotic pressure, Bowman's space hydrostatic pressure, and Bowman's space oncotic pressure, which is negligible. GFR = glomerular filtration rate. kf = filtration coefficient. PH glom = glomerular hydrostatic pressure. πglom = glomerular osmotic pressure; PH BS = Bowman's space hydrostatic pressure, πBS = Bowman's space oncotic pressure.

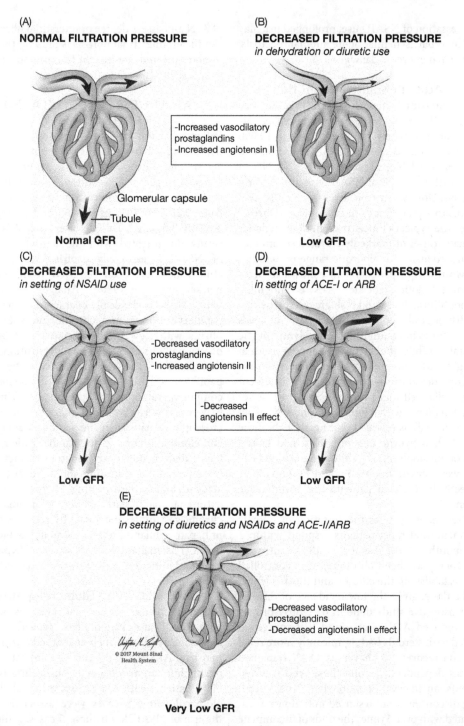

FIGURE 24.3 (A) Filtration pressure under normal circumstances. (B) Decreased filtration pressure during dehydration or diuretic use which is associated with increased angiotensin II, which causes vasoconstriction of efferent arterioles > afferent arterioles and a release of vasodilatory prostaglandins (acting on afferent arterioles), which mitigates the extent of afferent vasoconstriction. (C) Decreased filtration pressure during NSAID use, which inhibits vasodilatory prostaglandins and increases angiotensin II. (D) Decreased filtration pressure during ACEI or ARB use, which leads to decreased angiotensin II effect, leading to vasodilation of efferent arterioles > afferent arterioles. (E) Decreased filtration pressure during dehydration/diuretics and NSAIDs and ACEI/ARB, use which causes both a decreased release of vasodilatory prostaglandins and angiotensin II effect. ACEI = angiotensin converting enzyme inhibitor. ARB = angiotensin receptor blocker. GFR = glomerular filtration rate. NSAID = nonsteroidal anti-inflammatory drug.

after cessation of NSAID use, prolonged use may lead to renal ischemia, acute tubular necrosis, and permanent renal damage.[6]

Acute Interstitial Nephritis

Acute interstitial nephritis (AIN) is an uncommon form of NSAID nephrotoxicity, affecting approximately 1 of every 5,000 to 10,000 patients. In one case series, NSAIDs accounted for 11% of all biopsy-proven AIN.[6,7] AIN can occur within 1 week of NSAID use and as early as 2 days. However, it typically arises after several months to 1 year after initiation of NSAID treatment. The typical clinical presentation includes the acute onset of markedly elevated serum creatinine, edema, and nephrotic range proteinuria (in two-thirds of patients).[6] In contrast to beta-lactam antibiotic associated AIN, eosinophilia, eosinophiluria, fever, and rash are often absent.

Histological exam of renal biopsies demonstrates interstitial edema and lymphocytic infiltrate. While the glomeruli appear normal on light and immunofluorescence, electron microscopy demonstrates blunting and effacement of epithelial cell foot processes. In a case series of 133 patients with biopsy-proven AIN of all causes, urinalysis revealed that nearly half of the patients had pyuria, and one-third had hematuria or eosinophiluria.[7] White and red blood cell casts were present in only 3% and 1% of patients respectively; 0.2% of patients had bland urine sediment.

Treatment includes the cessation of NSAID treatment, and most patients respond within 1 to 3 months. [6,8] The use of steroids is controversial. There have been no randomized controlled trials establishing the efficacy and this likely will not be done, given the low incidence of disease. A retrospective study done in 61 biopsy-proven drug-induced AIN cases found that the group treated with steroids had significantly more renal function recovery: 3.8% versus 44.4% remained dialysis dependent. Among those who received steroids, an interval of more than 7 days from drug discontinuation to steroid initiation was associated with over 6 times the odds of incomplete renal recovery, adjusted odds ratio of 6.6 (confidence interval 95%: 1.3–33.6).[9] Many clinicians will consider the use of steroids if there is no improvement in renal function after removal of the offending agent or if there is severe interstitial nephritis present. When considering steroid treatment, experts suggest performing a renal biopsy prior to initiation of therapy to confirm diagnosis of AIN and assess degree of interstitial fibrosis. If significant interstitial fibrosis is present, the likelihood of significant benefit to immunosuppression is reduced.[10]

ANALGESIC-ASSOCIATED NEPHROPATHY

Patients who develop analgesic-associated nephropathy have a history of continuous analgesic abuse over many years; a minimum of 5 years is generally required.[11] There is high variability in prevalence of this disease, ranging from 0.23% to 10% in the US and as high as 36% in Belgium.[6] This disease process is classically documented with the use of mixtures of NSAIDS, especially aspirin and phenacetin, which has been removed from the US market since the 1980s.[11] Analgesic-associated nephropathy is classically characterized by renal papillary necrosis and chronic interstitial nephritis with slow progression to renal failure, occasionally in association with transitional cell carcinoma of the uroepithelium.[11] The renal papillary necrosis is best seen on noncontrast computed tomography scanning.[12] Urinalysis may reveal sterile pyuria or macroscopic or microscopic hematuria in the setting of sloughing and elimination of necrotic papilla. Patients also have tubulomedullary dysfunction characterized by impaired concentrating ability, renal tubular acidosis, and sodium wasting. There may also be extrarenal manifestations such as anemia from chronic gastrointestinal losses from gastric ulcers or hepatocellular injury.[13] Treatment is avoidance of NSAIDs, management of associated hypertension, and initiation of dialysis when needed.

Minimal Change Glomerulopathy

Minimal change disease has been associated with NSAID use. Patients have typical signs of nephrotic syndrome such as marked edema and may have AKI. It often occurs with interstitial nephritis but can also occur by itself. In a review of 55 patients with acute onset minimal change glomerulopathy, 5 cases were associated with the use of NSAIDS. Of these 5 cases, 2 did not have evidence of interstitial nephritis.[14] In another series of 24 patients with NSAID-induced nephrotic syndrome, 2 patients had minimal change disease without interstitial nephritis on biopsy.[15] Evaluation of urine sediment may reveal granular casts, pyuria, hematuria, and renal tubular cells. In the same series, proteinuria ranged from 2.6 to 26.2 g, and peak creatinine ranged from 0.8 to 14.8 mg/dL. Five of the 24 patients required temporary dialysis. Histologically, the lesion is identical to that of idiopathic minimal change, with normal light microscopy findings and diffuse effacement of foot processes on electron microscopy.[16]

The exact mechanism is currently unclear, but given that it recurs after re-exposure, there is likely some cell-meditated hypersensitivity reaction. The release of permselectivity promoting factors from inflammatory cells may be causal. Additionally, some compounds have direct toxicity to the glomerular epithelial cells.[16] Treatment includes cessation of NSAID use. One series documented 100% recovery, with 80% of patients obtaining remission within 15 days.[14,15] The benefits of steroids in this situation is not clearly defined.[16]

Membranous Nephropathy

While nephrotic syndrome associated with NSAID use is typically due to minimal change disease, a small subset also have membranous nephropathy. In a series from the Mayo Clinic,[17] 13 out of 125 patients with early stage membranous nephropathy were identified as NSAID-associated membranous nephropathy based on clinical criteria. Onset of symptoms is rapid and can present anywhere from 4 weeks to 3 years of therapy. In the same series, 92% of patients had nephrotic syndrome, with mean proteinuria of 10.2 g/day.

While phospholipase A2 receptor staining is generally positive only in idiopathic membranous, 3 out of 4 cases of NSAID associated membranous nephropathy were positive.[18] It is currently unclear if this could represent the concurrence of 2 diseases or if the altered inflammatory response and formation of auto-antibodies plays a role. There was rapid improvement in proteinuria after cessation of NSAIDs and a decrease to less than 1 g/day, on average, by 25 weeks.[17]

Blood Pressure Effects

NSAIDs lead to elevated blood pressure in both normotensive and hypertensive individuals, with the most marked effects seen in patients with controlled hypertension. The pathophysiology is thought to be related to decreased sodium excretion, increased fluid retention, and increased total peripheral vasoconstriction.[19] However, there is marked variability on the blood pressure effects of different NSAIDS; one meta-analysis documented changes in mean arterial pressure

from 0.49 mmHg for piroxicam compared to 3.74 mmHg for naproxen.[20,21] NSAID use in combination with antihypertensive treatment must be done with caution, because, depending on the antihypertensive treatment, there will be different effects on blood pressure induced by NSAID use. The smallest increase in systolic blood pressure is seen in patients who are on calcium channel blockers, as compared to beta-blockers, diuretics, and angiotensin converting enzyme inhibitors.[22]

CONSIDERATIONS IN KIDNEY TRANSPLANTATION

Kidney transplant patients are generally maintained on immunosuppression with calcineurin inhibitors such as cyclosporine or tacrolimus. In rats, it has been demonstrated that cyclorsporine and tacrolimus lower renal COX-2 expression, even in the face of lower salt intake or combination of low salt and RAAS blockade.[23] Therefore, the addition of NSAIDs will result in further vasoconstriction and lead to a decline in renal blood flow and glomerular filtration rate. It is recommended that patients with renal transplants on calcineurin inhibitors should avoid the use of NSAIDS.

PREVENTION STRATEGIES

While NSAID use in healthy persons is associated with low risk of renal toxicity, the risk is increased in patients with CKD or those on RAAS blocking agents and diuretics. There are currently no effective treatments, other than avoidance, for prevention of NSAID-associated renal disease. As many susceptible persons may not be aware of their risk, it is imperative that careful review of medications, including over-the-counter medications, be performed.

Jang et al.[24] evaluated the effect of a pharmacy-based community education intervention program in adults at high risk for NSAID induced AKI and found that 48% of participants reported taking NSAIDS, while only 14% of patients had kidney function determined prior to initiation of therapy. Sixty-seven percent of participants reported that the intervention encouraged them to limit their use of NSAIDS. There are several approaches to counseling patients regarding the risks of AKI, ranging from educational pamphlets to flagging prescription bags of high-risk patients, which indicates the need for direct counseling.[25] Therefore, we urge that, regardless of method, all patients, especially those with risk factors for developing kidney complications, should be counseled on the importance of limiting NSAID use as this has been demonstrated to be an easy and effective prevention strategy.

As one of the mechanisms for NSAID-induced renal injury is through the inhibition of prostaglandins, several studies have evaluated the role of misoprostol, an oral prostaglandin E analogue. One study done in 12 female volunteers, 6 who were normotensive and 6 who were hypertensive on thiazide diuretics, found that treatment with misoprostol blunted the decrease in GFR caused by indomethacin.[26] In another study, 25 patients with CKD secondary to type II diabetes were treated with indomethacin and either misoprostol or placebo. Those in the misoprostol group had significantly higher inulin clearance than those who were given placebo at 1.5 and 2 hours after indomethacin dose. Similar results are found in the elderly and in patients with cirrhosis.[27,28] The most common side effect of misoprostol is minor gastrointestinal symptoms, none of which required cessation of the drug.[26,27] However, given the short half-life of misoprostol, the small sample size of current studies, and the lack of long-term follow-up, misoprostol is currently not routinely used for prevention of NSAID-induced kidney injury.

While there are currently no accepted medications for prevention of NSAID-induced kidney injury, one potential target is inhibition of glycogen synthase kinase 3 beta (GSK3β). GSK3β inhibition is thought to ameliorate NSAID-induced AKI by inducing COX 2 expression. Bao et al.[29] treated mice with either vehicle or 4-benzyl-2-methyl-1,2,4-thiadiazolidine-3,5-dione (TDZD-8), a GSK3β inhibitor, and then treated them with diclofenac. While the mice treated with the vehicle developed elevation in serum creatinine, treatment with the GSK3β inhibitor preserved renal function. However, studies so far are limited to animal studies only, and there are no current drugs on the market that effect this pathway.

CONCLUSION

NSAIDS are commonly used and widely available analgesic medications used around the world. The use of NSAIDs can lead to several renal disorders, the most common of which is acute ischemic renal injury. Without effective medications for prevention or treatment, focus should be on increasing awareness of NSAID-associated AKI especially in high-risk groups such as patients who are elderly, hypertensive, and those on diuretics.

REFERENCES

1. Wehling M. Non-steroidal anti-inflammatory drug use in chronic pain conditions with special emphasis on the elderly and patients with relevant comorbidities: Management and mitigation of risks and adverse effects. *Eur J Clin Pharmacol.* 2014;70(10):1159–1172.
2. Whelton A. Drugs : Physiologic Foundations and Clinical Implications. 1999;106(5):13S–24S.
3. Gurwitz JH, Avorn J, Ross-Degnan D, et al. Nonsteroidal anti-inflammatory drug—associated azotemia in the very old. *J Am Med Assoc.* 1990;264(4):471–475.
4. Conaghan PG. A turbulent decade for NSAIDs: Update on current concepts of classification, epidemiology, comparative efficacy, and toxicity. *Rheumatol Int.* 2012;32(6):1491–1502.
5. Dreischulte T, Morales DR, Bell S, Guthrie B. Combined use of nonsteroidal anti-inflammatory drugs with diuretics and/or renin–angiotensin system inhibitors in the community increases the risk of acute kidney injury. *Kidney Int.* 2015;88101(10):396–403.
6. Murray MD, Brater DC. Renal Toxicity of the Nonsteroidal Anti-Inflammatory Drugs. *Annu Rev Pharmacol Toxieol.* 1993;32:435–465.
7. Muriithi AK, Leung N, Valeri AM, et al. Biopsy-proven acute interstitial nephritis, 1993–2011: a case series. *Am J Kidney Dis.* 2014;64(4):558–566.
8. Porile JL, Bakris GL, Garella S. Acute interstitial nephritis with glomerulopathy due to nonsteroidal anti-inflammatory agents: a review of its clinical spectrum and effects of steroid therapy. *J Clin Pharmacol.* 1990;30(5):468–475.
9. González E, Gutiérrez E, Galeano C, et al. Early steroid treatment improves the recovery of renal function in patients with drug-induced acute interstitial nephritis. *Kidney Int.* 2008;73(8):940–946.
10. Michel DM, Kelly CJ. Acute interstitial nephritis. *J Am Soc Nephrol.* 1998;9(3):506–515.
11. De Broe ME, Elseviers MM. Analgesic nephropathy. *N Engl J Med.* 1998;338(7):446–452.
12. Elseviers MM, De Schepper A, Corthouts R, et al. High diagnostic performance of CT scan for analgesic nephropathy in patients with incipient to severe renal failure. *Kidney Int.* 1995;48(4):1316–1323.
13. Nanra RS, Stuart-Taylor J, De Leon AH, White KH. Analgesic nephropathy: Etiology, clinical syndrome, and clinicopathologic correlations in Australia. *Kidney Int.* 1978;13:79–92.
14. Warren G V, Korbet SM, Schwartz MM, Lewis EJ. Minimal change glomerulopathy associated with nonsteroidal antiinflammatory drugs. *Am J Kidney Dis.* 1989;13(2):127–130.

15. Feinfeld DA, Olesnicky L, Pirani CL, Appel GB. Nephrotic syndrome associated with use of the nonsteroidal anti-inflammatory drugs. Case report and review of the literature. *Nephron.* 1984;37(3):174–179.

16. Glassock RJ. Secondary minimal change disease. *Nephrol Dial Transpl.* 2003;18(6):52–58.

17. Radford MG, Holley KE, Grande JP, et al. Reversible membranous nephropathy associated with the use of nonsteroidal anti-inflammatory drugs. *J Am Med Assoc.* 1996;276(6):466–469.

18. Nawaz FA, Larsen CP, Troxell ML. Membranous nephropathy and nonsteroidal anti-inflammatory agents. *Am J Kidney Dis.* 2013;62(5):1012–1017.

19. Johnson AG. NSAIDs and increased blood pressure: what is the clinical significance? *Drug Saf.* 1997;17(5):277–289.

20. Mulkerrin EC, Clark BA, Epstein FH. Increased salt retention and hypertension from non-steroidal agents in the elderly. *QJM.* 1997;90(6):411–415.

21. Pope JE, Anderson JJ, Felson DT. A meta-analysis of the effects of nonsteroidal anti-inflammatory drugs on blood pressure. *Arch Intern Med.* 1993;153(4):477–484.

22. White WB. Cardiovascular effects of the cyclooxygenase inhibitors. *Hypertension.* 2007;49(3):408–418.

23. Hörl WH. Nonsteroidal anti-inflammatory drugs and the kidney. *Pharmaceuticals.* 2010;3(7):2291–2321.

24. Min Jang S, Cerulli J, Grabe DW, et al. NSAID-avoidance education in community pharmacies for patients at high risk for acute kidney injury, Upstate New York, 2011. *Acute Kidney Inj Prev Chronic Dis.* 2011;11:E220.

25. Pai AB. Keeping kidneys safe: the pharmacist's role in NSAID avoidance in high-risk patients. *J Am Pharm Assoc.* 55(1):e15–e23.

26. Weir MR, Klassen DK, Hall PS, et al. Minimization of Indomethacin-Induced Reduction in Renal Function by Misoprostol. *J Clin Pharmacol.* 1991;31(8):729–735.

27. Nesher G, Sonnenblick M, Dwolatzky T. Protective effect of misoprostol on indomethacin induced renal dysfunction in elderly patients. *J Rheumatol.* 1995;22(4):713–716.

28. Ackerman Z, Cominelli F, Reynolds TB. Effect of misoprostol on ibuprofen-induced renal dysfunction in patients with decompensated cirrhosis: results of a double-blind placebo-controlled parallel group study. *Am J Gastroenterol.* 2002;97(8):2033–2039.

29. Bao H, Ge Y, Zhuang S, Dworkin LD, Liu Z, Gong R. Inhibition of glycogen synthase kinase-3β prevents NSAID-induced acute kidney injury. *Kidney Int.* 2012;81(7):662–673.

25

Contrast and the Kidney

AYUB AKBARI AND SWAPNIL HIREMATH

INTRODUCTION

Contrast media, which usually contain barium, iodine, or gadolinium, are extremely useful for delineating internal tissues in medical imaging for ease for diagnosis and interventions. Indeed, iodinated contrast media are one of the most widely used pharmaceutical agents worldwide (estimated a decade ago at more than 80 million doses worldwide).[1] At the same time, they are widely quoted to be the most common cause of iatrogenic acute kidney injury (AKI) and the third most common cause of AKI in the hospital.[2]

In most cases of contrast-induced AKI (CI-AKI), kidney dysfunction is mild and transient and detected by small changes in serum creatinine. Clinically significant important kidney injury is much less common, especially among individuals with normal kidney function. Given its association with longer hospital stay and long-term morbidity and mortality, preventing CI-AKI—which is, after all, an iatrogenic condition—remains an important goal. In this chapter we will discuss the diagnosis, epidemiology, pathophysiology, and management with a focus on prevention of CI-AKI.

EPIDEMIOLOGY

Overall Incidence

The actual incidence of AKI after a contrast-enhanced imaging test varies in the literature from as low as 1% to as high as 30% and depends on the nature and dose of the contrast administered and the underlying risk in the population studied.[3–8] In addition, these estimates may be confounded by the fact that many of these AKI episodes may be contrast-associated rather than contrast-induced (Fig. 25.1).[9]

Computed Tomography Scans versus Angiography

The risk of CI-AKI varies with the route of administration of the contrast agent, with the risk being lower with intravenous versus intraarterial administration of contrast. With elective angiography, typically about 10% to 15% patients develop AKI (as defined by a rise in creatinine within 48 hours of exposure); however, the incidence of severe AKI requiring dialysis is much lower at less than 1%. The incidence of AKI after intravenous administration of contrast (i.e., contrast-enhanced computed tomography [CT] scans) is believed to be much lower. A prospective study reported it to be 2.5% overall with the risk sequentially increasing as the underlying baseline kidney function decreased.[10] However, other studies have questioned whether the true incidence of contrast nephropathy after intravenous contrast is this high, given that there is underlying fluctuation in serum creatinine levels.[11] Recent studies, which incorporate propensity-matched controls who did not receive contrast, make a reasonable case that there is little additional increase in AKI after intravenous contrast administration when adjusted for the underlying baseline risk of AKI.[12,13] Given that there is possible selection bias in such observational studies (i.e., patients at high risk of AKI may not receive contrast and may be overrepresented in controls), the debate whether intravenous contrast causes CI-AKI at all still continues. Since this question cannot be answered by a randomized trial and observational studies will always have limitations, it is reasonable to continue with prophylactic measures when using intravenous contrast in patients with advanced chronic kidney disease (CKD).

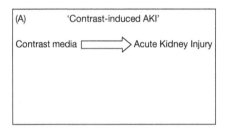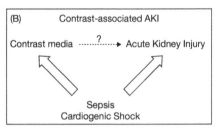

FIGURE 25.1 (A) The occurrence of acute kidney injury after a contrast-enhanced imaging leads to a diagnosis of contrast-induced acute kidney injury. (B) Assessment of confounding (e.g., presence of sepsis or cardiogenic shock), which lead to contrast imaging, suggests this may often be contrast-associated acute kidney injury, with the causative role of contrast being unclear.

Risk Factors

The most important underlying risk factor for development of CI-AKI is CKD. The incidence is <1% in unselected general population but is reported to be as high as 20% to 30% with decreased kidney function and other cumulative risk factors.[14] Among patients undergoing percutaneous coronary intervention, the risk of AKI has been reported[14] to be just under 20% when the baseline kidney function was glomerular filtration rate (GFR) <60 mL/min/1.73m², compared to less than 1% in unselected populations.[15] For outpatient CT scans with iodinated contrast, the risk has been reported to increase from 2.4% (with GFR 45–59 mL/min/1.73m²) to 11.1% (for GFR 30–44 mL/min/1.73m²) in one study[16] and at 0% (GFR 45–59 mL/min/1.73m²), 2.9% (GFR 30–44 mL/min/1.73m²), and 12.1% (GFR <30 mL/min/1.73m²) in another study.[10] Protocol-driven prophylactic measures and other factors may have played a role in achieving the lower risk (i.e., 2.9% vs. 11.1% in the GFR 30–44 mL/min/1.73m² subgroup) in the latter case. To reiterate, these risk estimates do not imply causation and refer to the biochemical definition of CI-AKI, the need for renal replacement therapy (RRT) being much lower at all levels of kidney function.

Other risk factors described in the literature include diabetes, older age, cirrhosis, proteinuria, and other comorbid conditions including congestive heart failure, hypotension, volume depletion, and concomitant administration of other nephrotoxic agents (e.g., nonsteroidal anti-inflammatory drugs). Several risk scores have been published, some of which include procedural variables such as dose of contrast and are hence less useful for planning prophylaxis.[17–19] A validated risk score, which uses preprocedural variables and predicts risk of AKI

as well as AKI requiring dialysis, is shown in Table 25.1.[18]

Metformin, a commonly used medication to control blood sugar in patients with diabetes, is often considered to be a risk factor for CI-AKI (since the package insert advises withholding it at least 48 hours before a contrast imaging test), but this is misleading. In patients who develop AKI, there is a higher incidence of metformin-associated lactic acidosis, which is associated with high fatality rate. But it only occurs in a fraction of those patients who are not only taking metformin but also either have unstable kidney function at baseline or do develop severe CI-AKI and in whom the recognition of kidney failure does not result in discontinuation of metformin.[20,21]

For dialysis-dependent patients, either on peritoneal dialysis (where they often do have significant residual kidney function) or on hemodialysis, contrast imaging does not seem to cause a decline in the residual kidney function.[22,23] There is no role for early or intensive dialysis to remove contrast material in these patients.

MECHANISM OF KIDNEY INJURY

Decreased renal blood flow, tubular cell damage, and tubular obstruction are the most commonly described pathways to AKI occurring after contrast administration.[24] Coronary angiography and left ventriculography has been shown to cause a decrease in renal blood flow measured directly using renal artery catheterization.[25] In addition, animal data suggest differential vasoconstriction of afferent more than efferent arteriole leading to decreased GFR.[26] The vasoconstriction also occurs in the renal medulla, via decreased blood flow in the vasa recta.[27] Tissue hypoxia can then result in free radical release, leading to oxidant

TABLE 25.1 A VALIDATED RISK SCORE TO ASSESS RISK OF ACUTE KIDNEY INJURY AFTER A PERCUTANEOUS CORONARY INTERVENTION

	Points		Converting Points to Risk			
	AKI	AKI-D	AKI	Risk (%)	AKI-D	Risk (%)
Age, y						
<50	0		0	1.9	0	0.03
50 to 59	2		5	2.6	1	0.05
60 to 69	4		10	3.6	2	0.09
70 to 79	6		15	4.9	3	0.15
80 to 89	8		20	6.7	4	0.27
>90	10		25	9.2	5	0.48
			30	12.4	6	0.84
Prior 2 weeks HF	11	2	35	16.5	7	1.5
GFR < 30	18	5	40	21.7	8	2.6
GFR 30–45	8	3	45	27.9	9	4.4
GFR 45–60	3	1	50	35.1	10	7.6
Diabetes	7	1	55	43.0	11	12.6
Prior heart failure	4		>60	51.4	12	20.3
Prior CVD	4				13	31.0
NSTEMI/unstable angina	6	1				
STEMI	15	2				
Prior cardiogenic shock	16					
Prior cardiac arrest	8	3				
Anemia	10					
IABP	11					

AKI = acute kidney injury. AKI-D = AKI requiring dialysis. HF = heart failure. NSTEMI = non-ST elevation myocardial infarction. IABP = intra-aortic balloon pump.
Source: Tsai TT, Patel UD, Chang TI, et al. Validated contemporary risk model of acute kidney injury in patients undergoing percutaneous coronary interventions: insights from the National Cardiovascular Data Registry Cath-PCI Registry. *J Am Heart Assoc.* 2014;3(6):e001380; used under the Creative Commons Attribution Non-Commercial License.

damage to the tubular cells from reactive oxygen species.[27] Tubular filtration of relatively higher osmolar contrast media also results in osmotic diuresis, increasing medullary oxygen consumption and exacerbating the medullary hypoxia. Lastly, reabsorption of water leaves a high concentration of viscous contrast material in the tubules, which can result in intratubular physical obstruction.[24]

CLINICAL PRESENTATION

Diagnosis

Classical CI-AKI definitions, as an absolute increase of 0.5 mg/dL (44 μmol/L) or a relative increase of 25% in serum creatinine within 72 hours in the absence of another cause,[28] are being replaced with the Acute Kidney Injury Network and Kidney Disease: Improving Global Outcomes classifications, as an absolute increase of 0.3 mg/dL (26.4μmol/L) or relative increase of 50% within 48 hours.[28,29] These milder forms of AKI, as previously defined, are important to identify and prevent, since they not only result in longer hospital stay but also because they are associated with increased long-term morbidity and mortality.[30,31] These definitions, however, are mainly used for research purposes and are likely to evolve further, with the advent of biomarkers such as neutrophil gelatinase-associated lipocalin or Nephrocheck° (a combination of tissue inhibitor of metalloproteinases-2 and insulin-like growth factor binding protein 7).[32]

Patients with CI-AKI are generally asymptomatic but have an acute rise in serum creatinine concentration within 24 to 72 hours after administration of the contrast agent.[33] The kidney failure is usually nonoliguric in milder cases, but oliguria is a hallmark when a patient is developing severe AKI needing RRT.[34] Further clinically significant deterioration is unlikely if the serum creatinine concentration does not increase by more than 0.5 mg/dL (44 μmol/L) within 24 hours.[33] To make an unequivocal diagnosis of CI-AKI, other potential causes of AKI must be ruled out, which is not always possible since they often coexist. Patients receiving contrast-enhanced tests often have sepsis, are on nephrotoxic agents, or may be volume contracted.[35,36] Embolic renal disease from cholesterol emboli is rarely diagnosed and often masquerades as CI-AKI. The relatively rapid onset (rise of creatinine within 24 hours) and typical course may help differentiate CI-AKI from other causes of AKI. Urinalysis may be unremarkable or may show granular casts, tubular cells, or small amounts of proteinuria. Fractional excretion of sodium is low and is unhelpful in differentiating CI-AKI from a prerenal, volume responsive cause of AKI.[34]

Prognosis

The natural course of CI-AKI is serum creatinine peaking (i.e., nadir of kidney function) between 24 to 72 hours, followed by rapid resolution over the next 5 days. Sometimes resolution may take up to 2 weeks.[33] Overall, very few patients, perhaps less than 1% of patients with CI-AKI, will develop kidney failure that requires dialysis and even smaller proportion (10%–50% of those who need dialysis) will remain dialysis dependent. The minority that remain dialysis dependent consist of a mixture of cases of true CI-AKI along with atheroembolic disease and other causes of AKI, such as ischemic acute tubular necrosis, that often occur in these patients.[35,36]

A large body of literature has emerged showing that an episode of AKI associates with poor long-term outcomes, with faster decline in kidney function, higher rates of subsequent RRT requirement, and higher rates of hospitalization for heart failure and all-cause mortality.[30,37] It is possible that this association may be a marker of patients at high risk for these events and may not be on the causal pathway.[38] If the latter is true, CI-AKI by itself may indeed be a less important

health issue. Future trials showing a parallel decrease in CI-AKI as well as hard clinical outcomes are required to establish more robust evidence for causality.

Prevention

Certainly, the most effective method of preventing CI-AKI is to not give iodinated contrast unless absolutely essential, especially to patients at high risk such as those with advanced kidney disease. However, this approach is not feasible in many instances and may result in therapeutic nihilism (or "renalism") toward CKD patients.[39] For diagnostic purposes, contrast-enhanced magnetic resonance imaging is an option, but unfortunately the risk of nephrogenic systemic fibrosis from gadolinium[40] limits this imaging options with GFR <30 mL/min, though these risks are much lower with the currently used macrocyclic gadolinium compounds.[41] Unfortunately, for cardiac diagnostic or therapeutic intervention, no other option is available but to give iodinated contrast. Given the elective nature of the nephrotoxic insult, which allows for attempting prophylaxis, many different interventions have been tested for CI-AKI prevention, which we address in the following discussion.

Fluid Administration

Peri-procedural volume administration has been the mainstay of preventive treatment for CI-AKI and presumably works by reducing the concentration of the contrast medium in the tubules, improving medullary blood flow (via suppression of vasopressin) and increasing urinary flow itself.[24] Isotonic saline has been shown to be superior to half-normal (0.45%) saline.[15] There has been significant research in the possible superiority of a bicarbonate-based strategy compared to normal saline, under the hypothesis that the resultant alkaline urine in the tubules will decrease free radical formation and subsequent oxidant tubular damage. However, the initial promise from the first trial has been belied by subsequent larger trials and meta-analyses.[42–45] The largest trial on this issue, PRESERVE (Prevention of Serious Adverse Events following Angiography),[46–47] enrolled 5,177 high-risk patients undergoing angiography and reported no benefit with a bicarbonate-based strategy (odds ratio 0.93; 95% confidence interval [CI] 0.72–1.22). Another approach with very promising results relied on using left ventricular end-diastolic pressure (LVEDP) to guide fluid administration in patients undergoing cardiac catheterization, with a relative risk of 0.41 (95% CI 0.22–0.79, $p = 0.005$) for CI-AKI, compared to the standard saline protocol.[48] This trial also showed reduction in clinically meaningful outcomes (i.e., reduction in persistent renal impairment and all-cause mortality at 6 months), though the number of events were small. Another point to be noted is that the intervention group received significantly larger amounts of fluid (mean 1727 mL compared to 812 mL in the control group), questioning the role of LVEDP-guided therapy vis-à-vis more fluid alone. Also, LVEDP measurement is not practical in other settings, such as intravenous contrast administration with CT scans, especially in the outpatient settings. Small trials have tested oral hydration strategies compared to intravenous, and though they may be as effective, the small numbers of events in these trials preclude any definitive recommendations at this stage.[49] Another randomized trial compared intravenous hydration to no hydration and reported no difference in CI-AKI incidence (2.6% vs 2.7%).[50] The population was intermediate risk, including patients with either GFR 30–45 mL/min/1.73m^2 or GFR 45–59 mL/min/1.73m^2 with diabetes or 2 or more additional risk factors, thus excluding patients with the highest risk (GFR <30 mL/min/1.73m^2). Approximately half the patients received contrast by arterial route, and the amount of contrast used was modest (average dose ~ 90 mL).

Despite these limitations, this trial suggests that prophylactic measures may only be needed in very high-risk patients (e.g., GFR <30 mL/min/1.73m^2 or GFR 30–45 mL/min/1.73m^2 with additional risk factors).

Choice and Volume of Contrast Agent

Since the direct kidney damage occurs due to the contrast agent, significant research has been done with respect to the physicochemical properties, specifically ionicity, osmolality, and viscosity of the contrast agent and modifications to decrease CI-AKI (see Table 25.2 for classification of the different types). High-osmolality contrast agents, such as diatrizoate, have been categorically shown to be worse compared to low-osmolality agents and are no longer used in routine clinical practice.[51] In the comparison of low-osmolality contrast agents (iohexol) versus iso-osmolar contrast agents (iodixanol), the first trial showed a significantly lower risk of CI-AKI with iso-osmolar contrast agents,[52] but subsequent larger trials have had different results.[8,53] The results of the systematic reviews and meta-analyses suggest the possibility of a small, nonsignificant benefit with iodixanol but with significant heterogeneity. This heterogeneity has been resolved either by grouping trials based on route of contrast (i.e., lower risk of CI-AKI in intra-arterial contrast imaging with iodixanol use[54]) or by specific contrast agents (i.e., iodixanol resulting

TABLE 25.2 CLASSIFICATION OF IODINATED CONTRAST MEDIA

Ionicity	Relative Osmolarity	Osmolality (mOsm/kg H$_2$O)	Examples
Ionic monomers	High osmolarity	1200–1900	Diatrizoate Iothalamate Metrizoate Iodamide Ioxithalamate
Ionic dimers	Low osmolarity	600	Ioxaglate
Nonionic monomers	Low osmolarity	500–700	Iopamidol Iohexol Iomeprol Iopentol Iopromide Ioversol Ioxitol Metrizamide
Nonionic dimers	Iso-osmolar	290–320	Iodixanol Iotrolan

in less CI-AKI compared to iohexol but not to other low-osmolar agents[55]). The volume of contrast administration also does matter, suggesting lower risk of CI-AKI with lower doses of contrast used. A ratio of the volume (of contrast dose in mL) to creatinine clearance (variously as >2.6 to > 4) has also been reported to be associated with higher risk of CI-AKI, suggesting that the lower the creatinine clearance, the lower should be the volume of contrast used.[56,57]

Prophylactic RRT

Hemodialysis and hemofiltration, done soon after the contrast administration, have been studied for CI-AKI prevention with mixed results.[58] The rationale for doing this is to help remove the offending iodinated contrast material, especially in patients with reduced kidney function who may not be able to clear it quickly. Biologically, however, the iodinated contrast material injected into, say, the coronary circulation or the left ventricle for ventriculography would reach and cause damage to the nephrons within a few cardiac cycles. Therefore, the efficacy of removing contrast after the lapse of the time it takes to set up dialysis is not very plausible. Indeed, the largest trial studying this was emphatically negative.[59,60] Other trials have reported a decrease in the proportion of patients having a decrease in creatinine clearance on the fourth day post contrast[61] or even in in-hospital mortality.[62] These trials are very challenging to interpret given that the hemofiltration or hemodialysis itself would change creatinine clearance directly, and to tease the effect of this from the effect due to CI-AKI attenuation is not possible. In addition, these procedures are accompanied with inherent risks, such as those associated with central line placement and hemodynamic issues with the RRT procedure itself.[58] Current recommendations state that prophylactic RRT should not be used for prophylaxis of CI-AKI.[5,7]

Medications
N-Acetylcysteine

N-acetylcysteine (NAC) can replenish endogenous glutathione, a biological antioxidant and was reported to reduce the risk of CI-AKI in a small trial.[63] However, subsequent trials have provided conflicting results. Heterogeneity with respect to the dose and route of administration and its possible effect on creatinine rather than kidney function made it hard to determine the true efficacy of NAC.[64,65] The Acetylcysteine for

Contrast-Induced Nephropathy Trial,[66] done with 2,308 patients and with measurement not just of CI-AKI on basis of change in creatinine but also with clinical events such as need for RRT and mortality, did not show any benefit of NAC. These patients, however, were at low risk compared to the aforementioned PRESERVE trial.[46] In the latter, again, there was no benefit with NAC (OR 1.02; 95% CI: 0.78–1.33). Oral NAC in doses used for CI-AKI prevention does not have any adverse effects; however, intravenous route may rarely cause anaphylactoid reactions.[67] In addition, though it is not expensive, often times it has been used in place of—rather than in addition to—truly effective prophylactic strategies such as volume expansion.[68]

Diuretics

Diuretics increase urine flow, theoretically reduce medullary oxygen requirement, and may have a diluting effect on the iodinated contrast being filtered into the tubules. Diuretics have been investigated in prevention of CI-AKI. Unfortunately, by themselves, use of furosemide and mannitol has been shown to actually be detrimental[69] and increase the incidence of CI-AKI, which is not entirely unsurprising given the protective effect of volume expansion. More recently, however, the use of furosemide in addition to intravenous fluids (in the RenalGuard® system), dosed to achieve a urine output >300 mL/hour, at which point contrast administration is permitted, and subsequent titration of intravenous fluids (and furosemide as required) to match urine output has been shown to be more effective than hydration alone.[70,71] To note, both the RenalGuard® system, and the LVEDP-guided hydration strategies previously mentioned result in a higher amount of volume administered to the intervention group compared to the controls and allow this to be done in a safe manner without causing volume overload.

Statins

Statins have been found to be protective as compared to placebo, as well as when high-dose (e.g., atorvastatin 80 mg) are compared to low-dose statins in prevention of CI-AKI.[72] However, these trials have been conducted in patients undergoing coronary angiography and/ or interventions and not patients receiving intravenous contrast and typically enrolled limited number of patients with CKD. Therefore, these results cannot be easily translated into patients at high risk of CI-AKI. Lastly, under most current guidelines, the typical patient profile undergoing coronary angiography should be on a statin in the long term and not just for CI-AKI prevention.[73]

Others

Small trials with ascorbic acid, calcium channel blockers, dopamine, fenoldopam, atrial natriuretic peptides, prostaglandin E1, and nonselective endothelin antagonists have all either failed to show any benefit in CI-AKI prevention or have shown benefit in small trials that need replication.[74-78]

MANAGEMENT CONSIDERATIONS

CI-AKI usually is a biochemical diagnosis. In most patients, kidney function returns to baseline within 2 weeks. In severe cases, management is similar to that for AKI from any other cause. Careful control of fluid and electrolyte balance, avoidance of further nephrotoxic insults, attention to nutrition, and surveillance for complications are generally all that is required, although dialysis may be necessary in the occasional patient. Indications for dialysis are no different than in other patients with AKI, taking into account clinical and biochemical factors such as hyperkalemia and volume overload. Prophylactic hemodialysis soon after administration of a contrast agent in patients with high serum creatinine concentrations has had inconsistent effects as previously noted. Dialysis also should not be done for routine removal of contrast medium after imaging in previously dialysis-dependent patients.

CONCLUSION

CI-AKI remains a concern, especially with interventions involving intra-arterial contrast. CI-AKI is not common in the absence of risk factors, and these are generally detectable with a history and physical examination and a determination of a serum creatinine concentration. Since CI-AKI can be associated with other adverse clinical outcomes, preventive measures are advisable, especially with advanced pre-existing kidney disease when there is a risk the patient may require dialysis. Although CI-AKI is associated with later adverse events, causality has not been proven, and the efficacy of preventive measures directed at CI-AKI in preventing these associated events has not been established. At this time, the optimal approach to prevent CI-AKI, summarized in Box 25.1, includes

---

BOX 25.1

ASSESSMENT OF CI-AKI RISK AND USE OF PROPHYLACTIC MEASURES

1. Assess the risk of CI-AKI in a patient requiring a contrast imaging test
   a. Use the NCDR risk score[18] (from Table 25.1) if patient is undergoing a percutaneous coronary intervention
   b. For patients undergoing intravenous contrast administration, consider estimated glomerular filtration rate < 30 mL/min/1.73 m^2 as principal risk factor.
   c. Additional risk factors include:
      i. Older age
      ii. Diabetes mellitus
      iii. Unstable kidney function
2. Assess risk/benefit of the proposed contrast imaging and consider alternative imaging in high risk patients
3. Modify correctable risk factors and hold medications that may act as nephrotoxins
4. Use lowest possible dose of contrast media; consider using iodixanol or a low-osmolar contrast agent (other than iohexol)
5. In high risk patients, correct dehydration, hold diuretics and consider intravenous fluids if no contraindication. Either normal (0.9%) saline or isotonic sodium bicarbonate, started at initial rate of 3 mL/kg/hour at least one hour before and continued at 1 mL/kg/hour for 6 hours later are commonly recommended.
6. In high risk patients, monitor creatinine within 24 to 72 hours postcontrast.

minimizing contrast dose, using either iodixanol or a low-osmolar contrast agent other than iohexol, and using isotonic sodium bicarbonate or saline in very high-risk patients. The AMACING (Prophylactic Hydration to Protect Renal Function from Intravascular Iodinated Contrast Material in Patients at High Risk of Contrast-Induced Nephropathy) trial[50] suggests that in intermediate-risk patients receiving a judiciously modest contrast dose, prophylaxis is unnecessary. Finally, supportive care is indicated if severe CI-AKI does occur.

REFERENCES

1. Katzberg RW, Haller C. Contrast-induced nephrotoxicity: clinical landscape. *Kidney Int Suppl.* 2006;100:S3–S7.
2. Hou SH, Bushinsky DA, Wish JB. Hospital-acquired renal insufficiency: A prospective study. *Am J Med.* 1983;2:243–248.
3. Barrett BJ. Contrast nephrotoxicity. *J Am Soc Nephrol.* 1994;5(2):125–137.
4. Katzberg RW, Barrett BJ. Risk of iodinated contrast material-induced nephropathy with intravenous administration. *Radiology.* 2007;243(3):622–628.
5. Section 4: contrast-induced AKI. *Kidney International Supplements.* 2012;2(1):69–88.
6. McCullough PA, Stacul F, Becker CR, et al. Contrast-Induced Nephropathy (CIN) Consensus Working Panel: executive summary. *Rev Cardiovasc Med.* 2006;7(4):177–197.
7. Owen R, Hiremath, S. Myers A, Fraser-Hill M, Benko A, Barrett B. Canadian Association of Radiologists: consensus guidelines for the prevention of contrast induced nephropathy: update 2011. *Can Assoc Radiol J.* 2014;65(2):96–105.
8. Solomon R, Deray G. How to prevent contrast-induced nephropathy and manage risk patients: practical recommendations. *Kidney Int Suppl.* 2006;100:S51–S53.
9. Vandenberghe W, De Corte W, Hoste EA. Contrast-associated AKI in the critically ill: relevant or irrelevant? *Curr Opin Crit Care.* 2014;20(6):596–605.
10. Kim SM, Cha R, Lee JP, et al. Incidence and outcomes of contrast-induced nephropathy after computed tomography in patients with CKD: a quality improvement report. *Am J Kidney Dis.* 2010;55(6):1018–1025.
11. Bruce RJ, Djamali A, Shinki K, Michel SJ, Fine JP, Pozniak MA. Background fluctuation of kidney function versus contrast-induced nephrotoxicity. *Am J Roentgenol.* 2009(3):711–718.
12. McDonald RJ, McDonald JS, Carter RE, et al. Intravenous contrast material exposure is not an independent risk factor for dialysis or mortality. *Radiology.* Dec 2014;273(3):714–725.
13. McDonald JS, McDonald RJ, Carter RE, Katzberg RW, Kallmes DF, Williamson EE. Risk of intravenous contrast material-mediated acute kidney injury: a propensity score-matched study stratified by baseline-estimated glomerular filtration rate. *Radiology.* 2014;271(1):65–73.
14. Dangas G, Iakovou I, Nikolsky E, et al. Contrast-induced nephropathy after percutaneous coronary interventions in relation to chronic kidney disease and hemodynamic variables. *Am J Cardiol.* 2005;95(1):13–19.
15. Mueller C, Buerkle G, Buettner HJ, et al. Prevention of contrast media-associated nephropathy: randomized comparison of 2 hydration regimens in 1620 patients undergoing coronary angioplasty. *Arch Intern Med.* 2002;162(3):329–336.
16. Weisbord SD, Mor MK, Resnick AL, Hartwig KC, Palevsky PM, Fine MJ. Incidence and outcomes of contrast-induced AKI following computed tomography. *Clin J Am Soc Nephrol.* 2008;3(5):1274–1281.
17. Mehran R, Aymong ED, Nikolsky E, et al. A simple risk score for prediction of contrast-induced nephropathy after percutaneous coronary intervention: development and initial validation. *J Am Coll Cardiol.* Oct 6 2004;44(7):1393–1399.
18. Tsai TT, Patel UD, Chang TI, et al. Validated contemporary risk model of acute kidney injury in patients undergoing percutaneous coronary interventions: insights from the National Cardiovascular Data Registry Cath-PCI Registry. *J Am Heart Assoc.* 2014;3(6):e001380.
19. Brown JR, DeVries JT, Piper WD, et al. Serious renal dysfunction after percutaneous coronary interventions can be predicted. *Am Heart J.* 2008;155(2):260–266.
20. Goergen SK, Rumbold G, Compton G, Harris C. Systematic review of current guidelines, and their evidence base, on risk of lactic acidosis after administration of contrast medium for patients receiving metformin. *Radiology.* 2010;254(1):261–269.
21. Pond GD, Smyth SH, Roach DJ, Hunter G. Metformin and contrast media: genuine risk or witch hunt? *Radiology.* Dec 1996;201(3):879–880.
22. Janousek R, Krajina A, Peregrin JH, et al. Effect of intravascular iodinated contrast media on natural course of end-stage renal disease progression in hemodialysis patients: a prospective study. *Cardiovasc Intervent Radiol.* 2010;33(1):61–66.
23. Weisbord SD, Bernardini J, Mor MK, et al. The effect of coronary angiography on residual renal function in patients on peritoneal dialysis. *Clin Cardiol.* 2006;29(11):494–497.

24. Persson PB, Hansell P, Liss P. Pathophysiology of contrast medium-induced nephropathy. *Kidney Int*. 2005;68(1):14–22.

25. Mockel M, Radovic M, Kuhnle Y, et al. Acute renal haemodynamic effects of radiocontrast media in patients undergoing left ventricular and coronary angiography. *Nephrol Dial Transplant*. 2008;23(5):1588–1594.

26. Liu ZZ, Viegas VU, Perlewitz A, et al. Iodinated contrast media differentially affect afferent and efferent arteriolar tone and reactivity in mice: a possible explanation for reduced glomerular filtration rate. *Radiology*. 2012;265(3):762–771.

27. Heyman SN, Brezis M, Epstein FH, Spokes K, Silva P, Rosen S. Early renal medullary hypoxic injury from radiocontrast and indomethacin. *Kidney Int*. 1991;40(4):632–642.

28. Endre ZH, Pickering JW. Outcome definitions in non-dialysis intervention and prevention trials in acute kidney injury (AKI). *Nephrol Dial Transplant*. 2010;25(1):107–118.

29. Mehta RL, Kellum JA, Shah SV, et al.; Acite Kidney Injury Network. Acute Kidney Injury Network: report of an initiative to improve outcomes in acute kidney injury. *Crit Care*. 2007;11(2):R31.

30. James MT, Ghali WA, Knudtson ML, et al. Associations between acute kidney injury and cardiovascular and renal outcomes after coronary angiography. *Circulation*. 2011;123(4):409–416.

31. Hoste EA, Doom S, De Waele J, et al. Epidemiology of contrast-associated acute kidney injury in ICU patients: a retrospective cohort analysis. *Intensive Care Med*. 2011;37(12):1921–1931.

32. Bihorac A, Chawla LS, Shaw AD, et al. Validation of cell-cycle arrest biomarkers for acute kidney injury using clinical adjudication. *Am J Respir Crit Care Med*. 2014;189(8):932–939.

33. Guitterez NV, Diaz A, Timmis GC, et al. Determinants of serum creatinine trajectory in acute contrast nephropathy. *J Interv Cardiol*. Oct 2002;15(5):349–354.

34. Fang LS, Sirota RA, Ebert TH, Lichtenstein NS. Low fractional excretion of sodium with contrast media-induced acute renal failure. *Arch Intern Med*. 1980;140(4):531–533.

35. Modi KS, Rao VK. Atheroembolic renal disease. *J Am Soc Nephrol*. 2001;12(8):1781–1787.

36. Stratta P, Bozzola C, Quaglia M. Pitfall in nephrology: contrast nephropathy has to be differentiated from renal damage due to atheroembolic disease. *J Nephrol*. 2012;25(3):282–289.

37. James MT, Ghali WA, Tonelli M, et al. Acute kidney injury following coronary angiography is associated with a long-term decline in kidney function. *Kidney Int*. 2010;78(8):803–809.

38. Coca SG, Zabetian A, Ferket BS, et al. Evaluation of Short-Term Changes in Serum Creatinine Level as a Meaningful End Point in Randomized Clinical Trials. *J Am Soc Nephrol*. 2016;27(8):2529–2542.

39. Chertow GM, Normand SL, McNeil BJ. "Renalism": inappropriately low rates of coronary angiography in elderly individuals with renal insufficiency. *J Am Soc Nephrol*. 2004;15(9):2462–2468.

40. Grobner T. Gadolinium--a specific trigger for the development of nephrogenic fibrosing dermopathy and nephrogenic systemic fibrosis? *Nephrol Dial Transplant*. 2006;21(4):1104–1108.

41. Edwards BJ, Laumann AE, Nardone B, et al. Advancing pharmacovigilance through academic-legal collaboration: the case of gadolinium-based contrast agents and nephrogenic systemic fibrosis-a Research on Adverse Drug Events and Reports (RADAR) report. *Br J Radiol*. 2014;87(1042):20140307.

42. Brar SS, Hiremath S, Dangas G, Mehran R, Brar SK, Leon MB. Sodium bicarbonate for the prevention of contrast induced-acute kidney injury: a systematic review and meta-analysis. *Clin J Am Soc Nephrol*. 2009;4(10):1584–1592.

43. Brar SS, Shen AY, Jorgensen MB, et al. Sodium bicarbonate vs sodium chloride for the prevention of contrast medium-induced nephropathy in patients undergoing coronary angiography: a randomized trial. *J Am Med Assoc*. 2008;300(9):1038–1046.

44. Hiremath S, Brar SS. The evidence for sodium bicarbonate therapy for contrast-associated acute kidney injury: far from settled science. *Nephrol Dial Transplant*. 2010;25(8):2802–2804.

45. Merten GJ, Burgess WP, Gray LV, et al. Prevention of contrast-induced nephropathy with sodium bicarbonate: a randomized controlled trial. *J Am Med Assoc*. 2004;291(19):2328–2334.

46. Weisbord SD, Gallagher M, Kaufman J, et al. Prevention of contrast-induced AKI: a review of published trials and the design of the prevention of serious adverse events following angiography (PRESERVE) trial. *Clin J Am Soc Nephrol*. 2013;8(9):1618–1631.

47. Weisbord SD, Gallagher M, Jneid H, et al. Outcomes after angiography with Sodium Bicarbonate and Acetylcysteine. *N Engl J Med*. 2018;378(7):603–614.

48. Brar SS, Aharonian V, Mansukhani P, et al. Haemodynamic-guided fluid administration for the prevention of contrast-induced acute kidney injury: the POSEIDON randomised controlled trial. *Lancet*. 2014;383(9931):1814–1823.

49. Hiremath S, Akbari A, Shabana W, Fergusson DA, Knoll GA. Prevention of contrast-induced acute

kidney injury: is simple oral hydration similar to intravenous? A systematic review of the evidence. *PLoS One.* 2013;8(3):e60009.

50. Nijssen EC, Rennenberg RJ, Nelemans PJ, et al. Prophylactic hydration to protect renal function from intravascular iodinated contrast material in patients at high risk of contrast-induced nephropathy (AMACING): a prospective, randomised, phase 3, controlled, open-label, non-inferiority trial. *Lancet.* 2017;389(10076):1312–1322.

51. Barrett BJ, Carlisle EJ. Metaanalysis of the relative nephrotoxicity of high- and low-osmolality iodinated contrast media. *Radiology.* 1993;188(1):171–178.

52. Aspelin P, Aubry P, Fransson SG, Strasser R, Willenbrock R, Berg KJ. Nephrotoxic effects in high-risk patients undergoing angiography. *N Engl J Med.* 2003;348(6):491–499.

53. Laskey W, Aspelin P, Davidson C, et al. Nephrotoxicity of iodixanol versus iopamidol in patients with chronic kidney disease and diabetes mellitus undergoing coronary angiographic procedures. *Am Heart J.* 2009;158(5):822–828.

54. McCullough PA, Brown JR. Effects of intra-arterial and intravenous iso-osmolar contrast medium (iodixanol) on the risk of contrast-induced acute kidney injury: a meta-analysis. *Cardiorenal Med.* 2011;1(4):220–234.

55. Heinrich MC, Haberle L, Muller V, Bautz W, Uder M. Nephrotoxicity of iso-osmolar iodixanol compared with nonionic low-osmolar contrast media: meta-analysis of randomized controlled trials. *Radiology.* 2009;250(1):68–86.

56. Capodanno D, Ministeri M, Cumbo S, Dalessandro V, Tamburino C. Volume-to-creatinine clearance ratio in patients undergoing coronary angiography with or without percutaneous coronary intervention: implications of varying definitions of contrast-induced nephropathy. *Catheter Cardiovasc Interv.* 2014;83(6):907–912.

57. Tan N, Liu Y, Zhou YL, et al. Contrast medium volume to creatinine clearance ratio: a predictor of contrast-induced nephropathy in the first 72 hours following percutaneous coronary intervention. *Catheter Cardiovasc Interv.* 2012;79(1):70–75.

58. Cruz DN, Goh CY, Marenzi G, Corradi V, Ronco C, Perazella MA. Renal replacement therapies for prevention of radiocontrast-induced nephropathy: a systematic review. *Am J Med.* Jan 2012;125(1):66–78 e63.

59. Cruz DN, Perazella MA, Bellomo R, et al. Extracorporeal blood purification therapies for prevention of radiocontrast-induced nephropathy: a systematic review. *Am J Kidney Dis.* 2006;48(3):361–371.

60. Reinecke H, Fobker M, Wellmann J, et al. A randomized controlled trial comparing hydration therapy to additional hemodialysis or N-acetylcysteine for the prevention of contrast medium-induced nephropathy: the Dialysis-versus-Diuresis (DVD) Trial. *Clin Res Cardiol.* 2007;96(3):130–139.

61. Lee PT, Chou KJ, Liu CP, et al. Renal protection for coronary angiography in advanced renal failure patients by prophylactic hemodialysis. A randomized controlled trial. *J Am Coll Cardiol.* 2007;50(11):1015–1020.

62. Marenzi G, Marana I, Lauri G, et al. The prevention of radiocontrast-agent-induced nephropathy by hemofiltration. *N Engl J Med.* 2003;349(14):1333–1340.

63. Tepel M, van der Giet M, Schwarzfeld C, Laufer U, Liermann D, Zidek W. Prevention of radiographic-contrast-agent-induced reductions in renal function by acetylcysteine. *N Engl J Med.* 2000;343(3):180–184.

64. Gonzales DA, Norsworthy KJ, Kern SJ, et al. A meta-analysis of N-acetylcysteine in contrast-induced nephrotoxicity: unsupervised clustering to resolve heterogeneity. *BMC Med.* 2007;5:32.

65. Hoffmann U, Fischereder M, Kruger B, Drobnik W, Kramer BK. The value of N-acetylcysteine in the prevention of radiocontrast agent-induced nephropathy seems questionable. *J Am Soc Nephrol.* 2004;15(2):407–410.

66. Acetylcysteine for prevention of renal outcomes in patients undergoing coronary and peripheral vascular angiography: main results from the randomized Acetylcysteine for Contrast-Induced Nephropathy Trial (ACT). *Circulation.* 2011;124(11):1250–1259.

67. Yamamoto T, Spencer T, Dargan PI, Wood DM. Incidence and management of N-acetylcysteine-related anaphylactoid reactions during the management of acute paracetamol overdose. *Eur J Emerg Med.* 2014;21(1):57–60.

68. Weisbord SD, Mor MK, Kim S, et al. Factors associated with the use of preventive care for contrast-induced acute kidney injury. *J Gen Intern Med.* 2009;24(3):289–298.

69. Majumdar SR, Kjellstrand CM, Tymchak WJ, Hervas-Malo M, Taylor DA, Teo KK. Forced euvolemic diuresis with mannitol and furosemide for prevention of contrast-induced nephropathy in patients with CKD undergoing coronary angiography: a randomized controlled trial. *Am J Kidney Dis.* 2009;54(4):602–609.

70. Solomon R. Forced diuresis with the RenalGuard system: impact on contrast induced acute kidney injury. *J Cardiol.* 2014;63(1):9–13.

71. Evaluation of RenalGuard® System to reduce the incidence of contrast induced nephropathy in at-risk patients (CIN-RG). 2015; https://clinicaltrials.gov/ct2/show/NCT01456013

72. Thompson K, Razi R, Lee MS, et al. Statin use prior to angiography for the prevention of contrast-induced acute kidney injury: a meta-analysis of 19 randomised trials. *Eurointervention.* 2016;12(3):366–374.

73. Stone NJ, Robinson JG, Lichtenstein AH, et al. 2013 ACC/AHA guideline on the treatment of blood cholesterol to reduce atherosclerotic cardiovascular risk in adults: a report of the American College of Cardiology/American Heart Association Task Force on Practice Guidelines. *J Am Coll Cardiol.* 2014;63(25 Pt B):2889–2934.

74. Bagshaw SM, Ghali WA. Theophylline for prevention of contrast-induced nephropathy: a systematic review and meta-analysis. *Arch Intern Med.* 2005;165(10):1087–1093.

75. Sadat U, Usman A, Gillard JH, Boyle JR. Does ascorbic acid protect against contrast-induced acute kidney injury in patients undergoing coronary angiography: a systematic review with meta-analysis of randomized, controlled trials. *J Am Coll Cardiol.* 2013;62(23):2167–2175.

76. Kelly AM, Dwamena B, Cronin P, Bernstein SJ, Carlos RC. Meta-analysis: effectiveness of drugs for preventing contrast-induced nephropathy. *Ann Intern Med.* Feb 19 2008;148(4):284–294.

77. Wang A, Holcslaw T, Bashore TM, et al. Exacerbation of radiocontrast nephrotoxicity by endothelin receptor antagonism. *Kidney Int.* 2000;57(4):1675–1680.

78. Khoury Z, Schlicht JR, Como J, et al. The effect of prophylactic nifedipine on renal function in patients administered contrast media. *Pharmacotherapy.* 1995;15(1):59–65.

26

Chemotherapeutic Agents and the Kidney

UMUT SELAMET, RAMY M. HANNA, ANJAY RASTOGI, AND ALA ABUDAYYEH

INTRODUCTION

Cancer survival has substantially improved in past decade as treatment options extended beyond conventional chemotherapy to targeted therapy and immunotherapy. Prolongation of cancer survival lead to increased prevalence of kidney failure in cancer patients. Kidney failure is partially due to nephrotoxicity of the anticancer agents. The kidney is the major site of elimination for most of the cancer drugs, and delayed clearance due to nephrotoxicity increases the risk of systemic toxicity. Conventional chemotherapeutics manifest nephrotoxicity mostly as acute kidney injury (AKI), tubulopathy, and electrolyte abnormalities. However, nephrotoxicity spectrum with targeted therapy extend to proteinuria, hypertension, and thrombotic microangiopathy (TMA) due to disruption of kidney podocyte and endothelium crosstalk. Recently, immunotherapy has revolutionized treatment options for certain cancer types, bringing along their unique nephrotoxicity profile such as immune mediated tubulointerstitial nephritis and glomerulonephritis. In this chapter, we will review nephrotoxicity of some of the conventional and newer cancer treatments.

Table 26.1 gives a broad list of cancer drugs and their nephrotoxicity profile most of which will not be discussed in this chapter.

CONVENTIONAL CHEMOTHERAPEUTICS

Cisplatin

Cisplatin is a platinum based compound. It is one of the oldest and the most-studied nephrotoxic chemotherapeutic agents used in many forms of cancer. It causes dose-dependent acute tubular necrosis (ATN) in up to one-third of the patients, and it can also cause isolated proximal tubulopathy.[1] Cisplatin-induced nephrotoxicity is mediated through several pathways including oxidative stress, inflammatory mediators, and cell apoptosis.[2] Hydrolyzation of the chloride ion on the drug releases free hydroxyl radicals that are directly toxic to cell structures.[1,3] Also, expression of proinflammatory molecules, such as tumor necrosis factor alpha, interleukin-6, interferon-gamma, and caspases increase in the kidney, which leads to kidney injury via production of cytokines.[1,4] Moreover, cisplatin may damage renal vasculature and can reduce renal blood flow, resulting in direct ischemic effects to proximal tubule.[5] Prevention of cisplatin-induced kidney injury involves volume repletion with isotonic saline. Other strategies to reduce AKI include glutathione analog amifostine and sodium thiosulfate use, which may protect kidney against free radical injury. However, use of these drugs in clinical practice is limited due to significant side effects, cost, and concern for reducing the anticancer effect of cisplatin.[6]

Ifosfamide

Ifosfamide is a nitrogen mustard alkylating agent. It produces a nephrotoxic metabolite, chlorocetaldehyde, which is directly toxic to proximal tubule cells.[7] The most common manifestation of nephrotoxicity during treatment with ifosfamide is Fanconi's syndrome or isolated proximal renal tubular acidosis. A cumulative lifetime dose >60 to 80 g/m^2 is associated with nephrotoxicity, but lower levels may also be toxic to the kidney. Pre-existing kidney disease is a risk factor for ifosfomide nephrotoxicity. Mesna binds and inactivates acrolein (the toxic metabolite of ifosfamide) to prevent hemorrhagic cystitis, but it does not protect against AKI.[8] Experts recommend close monitoring of patients with known prior kidney disease for toxicity and dose

TABLE 26.1 NEPHROTOXICITY PROFILE OF CONVENTIONAL AND NEWER CANCER
TREATMENTS

Anti-Cancer Drug	Manifestations of Nephrotoxicity
Conventional Chemotherapeutics	
Cisplatin	ATN, chronic interstitial fibrosis, renal salt and magnesium wasting, Fanconi's syndrome, nephrogenic DI, TMA
Cyclophosphamide	Hemorrhagic cystitis, hyponatremia, SIADH
Ifosfamide	Hemorrhagic cystitis, ATN, Fanconi's syndrome, proximal tubulopathy, nephrogenic DI
Methotrexate	Crystal nephropathy
Pemetrexed	ATN, AIN, tubular atrophy and interstitial fibrosis, nephrogenic DI
Gemcitabine	TMA
Mitomycin C	TMA
Melphalan	AKI, hyponatremia, SIADH
Clorafabine	AKI, proteinuria
Anthracyclines (Doxurubicin/ Daunorubicin)	Collapsing glomerulopathy, FSGS, MCD, TMA
Nitrosoureas (Carmustine/Lomustine/ Streptozocin)	Chronic tubulointerstitial nephritis, proximal tubulopathy, uric acid nephrolithiasis, nephrogenic DI
Vilka alkaloids (Vincristine/Vinblastine)	SIADH
Adrogen Deprivation Therapy	AKI
Biphosphonates	
Pamidronate	AKI, Collapsing FSGS, MCD
Zoledronate	ATN
Targeted Therapy	
VEGF/VEGFR antagonists and TKIs	
Bevacizumab	Hypertension, proteinuria, TMA
Aflibercept	Hypertension, proteinuria, TMA
Axitinib	Hypertension, proteinuria, TMA
Sunitinib	Hypertension, proteinuria, TMA
Sorafenib	Hypertension, proteinuria, TMA
Pazopanib	Hypertension, proteinuria, TMA
Vandetanib	AKI, electrolyte disorders, nephrolithiasis, proteinuria, hypertension
Imatinib	AKI, hypophosphatemia
EGFR inhibitors	
Cetuximab	AKI, hypomagnesemia
Panitumumab	Hypomagnesemia and other electrolyte disorders
Erlotinib	Electrolyte disorders
Gefitinib	Electrolyte disorders
mTOR inhibitors	
Everolimus	Proteinuria, AKI, electrolyte disorders
Temsirolimus	ATN, proteinuria, FSGS, hypophosphatemia

TABLE 26.1 CONTINUED

Anti-Cancer Drug	Manifestations of Nephrotoxicity
HER2 inhibitor	
Trastuzumab	Hypertension, cardio-renal syndrome
BRAF inhibitors	
Vemurafamib	AIN, ATN, Fanconi's syndrome, proteinuria, hyponatremia, hypokalemia
Dabrafenib	AKI, Hypophosphatemia, granulomatous AIN
MEK inhibitor	
Trametinib	Hypertension, hyponatremia, AKI
ALK-1 inhibitor	
Crizotinib	AKI, renal cysts, hypophosphatemia, hyponatremia
Proteasome inhibitors	
Bortezomib	TMA
Carfilzomib	TMA, prerenal AKI, TLS, ATN
SLAMF-7 inhibitor	
Elotuzumab	AKI
Anti-IL 6 agent	
Siltuximab	Hyperkalemia, hyperuricemia
Anti-KIR agent	
Lirilumab	AKI, hypophosphatemia
Akt inhibitor	
Perifosine	Hypophosphatemia
Immunmodulators	
Lenalidomide	AKI, AIN, Fanconi's syndrome, MCD, TMA
Pomalidomide	AKI, crystal nephropathy
Immunotherapy	
Interferon	Proteinuria, MCD, FSGS
IL-2	Prerenal AKI due to capillary leak syndrome
Ipilumumab	ATIN, immune complex GN (lupus-like)
Nivolumab	ATIN, immune complex GN (membranous nephropathy, MCD)
Pembrolizumab	ATIN, immune complex GN (membranous nephropathy, MCD)
CAR T cells	Prerenal AKI due to capillary leak syndrome, TLS, hyponatremia, hypokalemia, hypophosphatemia

AIN = acute interstitial nephritis. AKI =acute kidney injury. Akt =protein kinase B. ALK-1 =anaplastic lymphoma kinase 1. ATIN = acute tubulointerstitial nephritis. ATN =acute tubular necrosis. BRAF = v-Raf murine sarcoma viral oncogene homolog B. CAR = chimeric antigen receptor. CTLA-4 = cytotoxic T lymphocyte–associated antigen 4. EGFR =epidermal growth factor receptor. FSGS =focal segmental glomerulosclerosis. HER-2 =human epidermal growth factor receptor 2. IL6 =interleukin 6. KIR = killer IgG-like receptor. MCD = minimal change disease. MEK = mitogen-activated protein/extracellular signal-regulated kinases. mTOR, mechanistic target of rapamycin. PD-1, programmed cell death protein 1. SLAMF7 = signaling lymphocytic activation molecule F7. TKIs = tyrosine kinase inhibitors. TLS = tumor lysis syndrome. TMA = thrombotic microangiopathy. VEGF = vascular endothelial growth factor. VEGFR = vascular endothelial growth factor receptor.

reductions of ifosfomide based on creatinine clearance.

Gemcitabine

Gemcitabine is a pyrimidine antagonist. It has been shown to cause TMA by direct endothelial injury. The risk of TMA increases with a higher cumulative dose of gemcitabine. TMA is usually associated with AKI and typically develops within weeks to months of initiation of gemcitabine therapy.[9] In a retrospective analysis of 29 cases of gemcitabine-induced nephrotoxicity in a single center, all patients had AKI, anemia, thrombocytopenia, and elevated serum lactate dehydrogenase; 27 out of 29 patients had microhematuria and proteinuria.[10] Worsening or new onset hypertension was observed in 26 patients.[10] Schistocytes were present in 21 of the 24 blood smears that were reviewed.[10] The outcomes were complete or partial renal recovery in 19 patients, chronic kidney disease (CKD) in 3, and end-stage renal disease in 7 patients.[10]

It is essential to discontinue gemcitabine when TMA occurs. Plasma exchange has no or very little beneficial effect on gemcitabine-induced TMA, whereas several case reports have shown improvement in kidney function when patients are treated with eculizumab.[11]

Methotrexate

Methotrexate (MTX) is an antifolate agent that inhibits the enzymes in purine and pyrimidine synthetic pathways. High-dose MTX is associated with AKI, which can be life-threatening due to systemic toxicity of MTX as renal elimination of the drug diminishes. MTX-induced AKI is usually nonoliguric and occurs shortly after the infusion of the drug.[12] Proposed mechanisms of AKI include pH-dependent precipitation of MTX crystals in renal tubules, causing direct tubular toxicity, obstructive and inflammatory interstitial injury, and decreased renal perfusion due to afferent arteriolar vasoconstriction.[12] MTX is a weak acid molecule so it is more soluble in alkaline urine. Prevention of high-dose MTX-induced AKI include serial monitoring of serum creatinine before and after the drug infusion, monitoring of plasma MTX concentrations, alkalization of urine to keep urine pH>7, and intravenous fluid hydration for increased urinary flow. It is recommended to maintain urinary flow at least at 2500 mL/m² per day (theoretically required urinary flow 1.0–1.8 mL/min/m² at pH

7.0) prior to, during, and after high-dose MTX infusion.[13] For alkalization of urine, normal saline infusion can be supplemented with sodium bicarbonate, and for increasing urinary flow, furosemide can be added to hydration. Leucovorin is a rescue drug that prevents systemic toxicity of MTX. Leucovorin's circulating metabolite 5-methyltetrahydrofolate competes with MTX for cellular uptake and binding to target enzymes. The leucovorin dose must be adjusted to MTX concentration especially when MTX renal clearance gets delayed due to AKI and high doses of leucovorin may result in treatment failure of the cancer.[12]

Another option for prevention of high-dose MTX systemic toxicity in the setting of AKI is use of glucarpidase, a carboxypeptidase enzyme. Glucarpidase is a recombinant bacterial enzyme that inactivates MTX by hydrolyzing it into 2 nontoxic metabolites: 4-deoxy-4-amino-N10-methylpteroic acid and glutamate, which are eliminated mainly by the liver.[14] It reduces plasma MTX concentration by 95% within 15 minutes of administration.[12] The Food and Drug Administration has approved a single dose of 50 units/kg of glucarpidase for plasma MTX concentration of >1 µmol/L in patients with rising serum creatinine. It should be optimally administered within 48 to 60 hours from the start of high dose MTX infusion.[12] Glucarpidase does not rescue intracellular effects of MTX; therefore, leucovorin is still required after glucarpidase. Additionally, glucarpidase may not be readily available due to its high cost. In those situations, hemodialysis with high-flux dialyzer might be required for elimination of free plasma MTX during AKI. Large volume of distribution and high protein binding of MTX result in rebound of free MTX after discontinuation of hemodialysis.[15] Therefore, daily dialysis is required during MTX toxicity.

Pemetrexed

Pemetrexed is a structural analogue of MTX. It is excreted mostly by kidneys via the organic anion tubular pathway. Several cases of pemetrexed-associated AKI have been reported. Biopsies of kidneys in these cases showed ATN, loss of brush borders, and tubular atrophy with some interstitial fibrosis.[16] Discontinuation of the drug does not always result in renal recovery, and some patients progress to CKD. Pemetrexed has been also associated with nephrogenic diabetes insipidus and resulting hypernatremia.[17]

NEWER CANCER TREATMENTS: TARGETED THERAPY AND IMMUNOTHERAPY

Antiangiogenic Drugs

Angiogenesis is essential for cancer growth and metastatic spread. Circulating vascular endothelial growth factor (VEGF) and VEGF receptors (VEGFR) are key players in angiogenesis, and drugs that target VEGF or VEGFR are now commonly used in treatment of various cancers including lung, breast, ovarian, gastric, colorectal, and renal cell carcinoma. VEGF family consists of 5 members (VEGF-A, VEGF-B, VEGF-C, VEGF-D, and VEGF-E), which transmit signals via 3 receptors (VEGFR-1, VEGFR-2, and VEGFR-3). The most well-defined member is VEGF-A, which stimulates endothelial cell mitogenesis and cell migration leading to cancer progression and metastasis via binding to VEGFR-2. VEGF-B plays a role in the maintenance of newly formed blood vessels via VEGFR-1. VEGF-C and VEGF-D bind to VEGFR-3 and play a role in lymphogenic metastatic spread. VEGF receptors belong to tyrosine kinase family, and, therefore, the small molecule tyrosine kinase inhibitor (TKI) drugs also show antiangiogenic effects. Antiangiogenic drugs are classified according to their target molecule:

Monoclonal antibody against VEGF:
bevacizumab (VEGF-A)

Recombinant fusion protein against VEFG:
ziv-aflibercept (VEGF-A, VEGF-B)

Monoclonal antibody against VEGFR-2:
ramucirumab

VEGFR-2 specific small molecule TKIs:
cabozantinib, ponatinib, regorafenib, vandetanib, apatinib, orantinib

Pan-VEGFR small molecule TKIs:
axitinib, pazopanib, sorafenib, sunitinib, nintedanib, cediranib, lenvatinib, lucitanib

Kidney-related adverse effects of antiangiogenic drugs include proteinuria, worsening of hypertension, and, rarely, TMA. In the normal kidney, VEGF is produced by podocytes and binds to its receptor at the glomerular and peritubular endothelium to keep the integrity of the glomerular filtration membrane. In a mice model, specific knockout of the VEGF gene resulted in nephrotic range proteinuria, endotheliosis, and features of renal TMA.[18]

A recent prospective, multicenter study conducted in France to assess the safety of antiangiogenic drugs, the Management of Antiangiogenics Renovascular Safety (MARS) study,[19-21] showed de novo hypertension in 17.1%, 22.1%, and 12.9% of patients treated with bevacizumab for ovarian, lung, and breast cancers, respectively. In the same study, de novo proteinuria was seen in 36.4%, 72.1%, and 15% of patients treated with bevacizumab for ovarian, lung, and breast cancers, respectively. In the MARS study, hypertension could be effectively controlled by conventional antihypertensive therapies in most cases; however, a few cases of malignant hypertension and hypertension associated reversible refractory leukoencephalopathy syndrome were reported in patients with TKI treatment.[19-21]

Proposed mechanisms of hypertension induced by antiangiogenic drugs include inhibition of vasodilatory nitric oxide production, increased vasoconstrictor endothelin-1 secretion, and capillary rarefaction.[22-24] Highly potent TKIs such as sorafenib raise blood pressure within days whereas monoclonal antibodies such as bevacizumab raise blood pressure over weeks or months. Blood pressure typically improves with discontinuation of the antiangiogenic drug.

Hypertension has also been suggested as a potential biomarker of antitumor effect of antiangiogenic drugs. Rini et al.[25] provided evidence that hypertension could be a biomarker of sunitinib efficacy in metastatic renal cell carcinoma. However, there is a lack of evidence for other antiangiogenic agents on whether hypertension could predict the clinical response to treatment.

Multikinase Inhibitors

Imatinib is a TKI that selectively inhibits the BCR-ABL tyrosine kinase, the receptor for platelet-derived growth factor and stem cell factor c-Kit. It is used for treatment of chronic myelogenous leukemia and gastrointestinal stromal tumors. Imatinib nephrotoxicity has been reported. In 1 study of 105 chronic myelogenous leukemia patients treated with imatinib for median of 4.5 years, AKI was seen in 7% of cases and CKD in 16%.[26] AKI typically appears within the first 2 weeks of imatinib initiation, and it improves most of the time with either dose reduction or cessation of the drug; rarely it results in stable CKD. Imatinib-related AKI seems to occur either due to direct toxic effect on kidney tubules or due to tumor lysis syndrome. Additionally, electrolyte disorders, especially hypophosphatemia and rhabdomyolysis, have been reported with imatinib use.[27]

Sunitinib is a TKI with multiple binding targets approved for treatment of gastrointestinal stromal tumors and renal cell carcinoma. It has been noted to cause TMA and focal segmental glomerulosclerosis either alone or in combination therapy with sorafenib.[28] Sorafenib, another TKI with multiple binding targets, is approved for treatment of differentiated thyroid cancer, renal cell carcinoma, and hepatocellular carcinoma. It has been reported to cause TMA as well as nephrotic syndrome due to focal segmental glomerulosclerosis.[29,30] Dasatanib is a new generation TKI approved for chronic myelogenous leukemia treatment and is associated with hypertension and proteinuria[29,30]

Epidermal Growth Factor Receptor Inhibitors

The epidermal growth factor receptor inhibitors (EGFR) is overexpressed, dysregulated, or mutated in many epithelial malignancies, and EGFR activation appears important in tumor growth and progression. Two predominant classes of EGFR inhibitors include monoclonal antibodies, such as cetuximab and panitumumab, and small molecule TKIs, such as gefitinib, erlotinib, and afatinib. The most common kidney-related adverse effects of EGFR inhibitors are hypomagnesemia and secondary hypokalemia. The basolateral membrane of the distal renal tubule have EGFR, which generate signals for translocation of the transient receptor potential M6 (TRPM6) channel. This channel mediates magnesium reabsorption in the distal convoluted tubule. EGFR inhibitors disrupt EGF and EFGR binding and consequent TRPM6 translocation. As a result, renal wasting of magnesium and hypomagnesemia occur. This effect is more pronounced with monoclonal antibodies of EGFR compared to small molecule TKIs.[31]

Fig. 26.1 shows pathways of mechanism of action for anti-VEGF and TKI drugs.

Proteasome Inhibitors

Proteasome inhibitors are highly effective drugs for multiple myeloma. Bortezomib is a boronic acid dipeptide and a selective reversible inhibitor of the 26S proteasome. Several studies have evaluated the efficacy and safety of bortezomib in multiple myeloma patients with renal failure, and reversal of myeloma-related kidney injury has been observed. In a study by Dimopoulos et al.,[32] 59% of patients who received bortezomib with dexamethasone had a renal response. Nephrotoxicity due to bortezomib is uncommon, although several cases of TMA have been reported.[33,34] The International Myeloma Working Group has suggested no dose adjustments for patients with renal impairment. Bortezomib should be administered after hemodialysis in patients requiring dialysis since hemodialysis may reduce bortezomib concentrations.[35]

Carfilzomib is another proteasome inhibitor that is approved for relapsed and refractory myeloma. Compared to bortezomib, carfilzomib has more pronounced nephrotoxicity profile. A phase II study[36] of 266 patients treated with single-agent carfilzomib, demonstrated a 25% occurrence of AKI, although severe kidney injury was rare, and only 3.8% of the patients had progressive kidney disease that required cessation of the drug. Potential causes of AKI induced by carfilzomib include ATN, tumor lysis syndrome, and prerenal AKI due to hypovolemia. TMA has also been reported in patients receiving carfilzomib.[37,38] The majority of TMA cases with proteasome inhibitors resolve completely after discontinuation of the drug.

Immunomodulators

Lenalidomide is an immunomodulatory drugs that is used in multiple myeloma. Lenalidomide is predominantly metabolized by the kidney and needs to be dose adjusted in kidney disease. Patients with pre-existing kidney disease are at risk for increased systemic toxicity of lenalidomide. In 1 analysis of 72 patients with multiple myeloma who were treated with lenalidomide plus dexamethasone, individuals with creatinine clearance <40 mL/min/1.73m^2 had an 8.4-fold higher likelihood of requiring a lenalidomide dose reduction for grade 3 or worse myelosuppression.[39] Lenalidomide has been reported to cause AKI, and a few cases of biopsy-proven acute interstitial nephritis have been described. In a series of 41 patients with immunoglobulin light chain amyloidosis who were treated with lenalidomide, 66% developed ≥50% increase in serum creatinine during treatment and 32% developed severe AKI requiring dialysis.[40]

Anaplastic Lymphoma Kinase Inhibitors

Anaplastic lymphoma kinase 1 (ALK-1) is a member of the insulin receptor tyrosine kinase

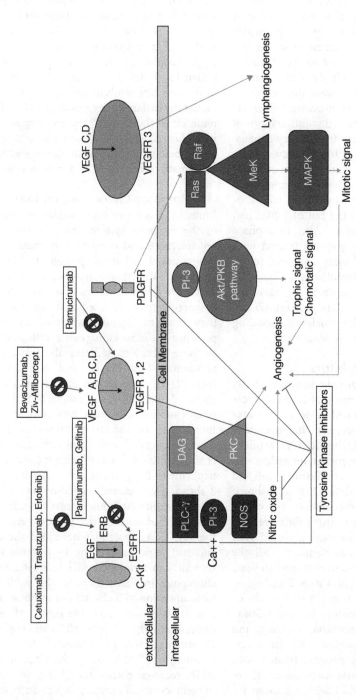

FIGURE 26.1 Pathways of targeted therapy. Akt/PKB = protein kinase B. Ca⁺⁺ = calcium. c-Kit = mast/stem cell growth factor receptor. DAG = diacyl glycerol. EGF = epidermal growth factor. EGFR = epidermal growth factor receptor. ERB = EGFR related receptor protein. MAPK = mitogen activated protein kinase. Mek = dual threonine and tyrosine recognition kinase. NOS = nitric oxide synthase. PDGFR = platelet derived growth factor receptor. PI3 = phosphatidylinositol-4,5-bisphosphate 3-kinase. PKC = Protein kinase C. PLC-ϒ = phospholipase C gamma. Raf = serine/threonine kinase/cellular homolog of viral Raf gene. Ras = rat sarcoma protein. VEGF = vascular endothelial growth factor. VEGFR = vascular endothelial growth factor receptor

family, which regulates cellular growth. Mutation of ALK-1 was first observed in anaplastic large cell lymphoma and Hodgkin lymphoma and now has been associated with rhabdomyosarcoma, neuroblastoma, and nonsmall cell lung (NSCL) cancer. Crizotinib is an oral potent inhibitor of ALK. Crizotinib has numerous nephrotoxic effects. First, it can cause increase in serum creatinine level up to 20% without an actual change in estimated glomerular filtration rate due to reduction in renal tubular creatinine secretion by inhibiting creatinine transporter.[41] This effect subsides rapidly after discontinuation of crizotinib. It can also cause true kidney damage as shown in a single case of biopsy-proven acute tubular injury.[42] Another manifestation of nephrotoxicity of crizotinib is the development and progression of renal cysts. In clinical trials[43] of crizotinib, 2% of patients (24 out of 1,205) had treatment-related renal cysts. Also, in a phase III clinical trial,[44] 7% of patients treated with crizotinib-acquired renal cysts compared to 1% patients on standard chemotherapy. The cysts that developed with crizotinib are classified as bosniak types II to IV. Rarely, crizotinib can also cause electrolyte abnormalities, including hyponatremia and hypophosphatemia.[41]

BRAF Inhibitors

The mitogen-activated protein kinase pathway includes a chain of proteins that lead to cancer development when mutated. One such mutation is v-Raf murine sarcoma viral oncogene homolog B (BRAF) V600. The BRAF V600 mutation has been identified in malignant melanoma, colorectal, and NSCL cancers. Vemurafenib and dabrafenib are BRAF inhibitors that have shown efficacy in metastatic melanomas expressing the BRAF V600 mutation. Three different case series with total of 24 patients reported AKI in patients receiving vemurafenib.[45–47] All the patients in these case series were at least 50 years old and had underlying CKD stage 2 or higher. AKI occurred at 2 peak times, 1 to 2 weeks or 1 to 2 months after initiation of vemurafenib. Nonnephrotic range proteinuria, skin rash, and photosensitivity accompanied AKI. In a retrospective study[48] of 74 patients treated with vemurafenib for metastatic melanoma, 78% of the patients developed AKI within a mean interval of 10 months of treatment. Kidney biopsy was performed in only 3 of these cases—2 of which showed ATN, and the other 1 showed focal interstitial fibrosis.

Dabrafenib is another BRAF inhibitor. The European summary of product characteristics of dabrafenib reports nephrotoxicities in <1% of patients receiving it. AKI was associated with fever and dehydration and responded well to dose interruption and general supportive measures. Dabrafenib has also been associated with granulomatous nephritis in 1 case.[49] Hypophosphatemia has been reported in 7% of patients included in clinical trials of dabrafenib. In an open-label study involving 247 patients with metastatic melanoma expressing the BRAF V600 mutation, Flaherty et al.[50] reported hyponatremia, hypophosphatemia, increased serum creatinine, and hypokalemia when dabrafenib was used in combination with the MEK inhibitor trametinib.

Immune Checkpoint Inhibitors

Immune checkpoints are inhibitory pathways of the immune system that are essential for self-tolerance and prevention of autoimmunity. Programmed cell death protein 1 (PD-1) and cytotoxic T lymphocyte–associated antigen-4 (CTLA-4) are T cell surface receptors that downregulate T cell–mediated cell death when they bind to ligands expressed by antigen-presenting cells, including cancer cells. Antibodies to these receptors, ipilimumab (anti-CTLA-4), nivolumab (anti-PD-1), and pembrolizumab (anti-PD-1), have shown efficacy in the treatment of metastatic melanoma, NSCL cancer, renal carcinoma, ovarian, and bladder cancers. Ipilimumab was the first immune checkpoint inhibitor associated with kidney disease. Izzedine et al.[51] identified 5 cases of acute tubulointerstitial nephritis (ATIN) associated with ipilimumab— 2 showing granuloma on biopsy and 1 case of lupus-like membranous glomerulopathy. All of the cases had renal recovery with corticosteroid therapy. Cortazar et al.[52] described the clinical and histologic features of 13 patients from 7 centers who developed AKI following immune checkpoint inhibitor therapy. The median time from initiation of a checkpoint inhibitor to AKI was 91 days (range, 21–245 days). All patients underwent kidney biopsy, ATIN was observed in 12 patients (3 with granulomatous features), and 1 patient had TMA. Ten of the 12 patients with ATIN received corticosteroid therapy, resulting in complete renal recovery in 2 patients and partial improvement in 7 patients. Shirali et al.[53] also recently reported 6 patients with lung cancer who developed AKI after receiving an anti–PD-1 agent. Each case showed evidence of ATIN on kidney biopsy. All of the patients were treated with other drugs such as proton pump inhibitors and nonsteroidal anti-inflammatory drugs that might have been linked to ATIN, but in most cases the use of these drugs long preceded PD-1 inhibitor therapy. Kidney functions improved in 5 of the 6 patients with corticosteroids and discontinuation of the PD-1 inhibitor as well as the potential co-offenders. AKI recurred after reexposure to the PD-1 inhibitor in 1 patient. Recently, there have been case reports of nephrotic syndrome related to immune-mediated glomerulonephritis after treatments with PD-1 inhibitors.[54,55]

Chimeric Antigen Receptor T Cells

Human T cells can be genetically modified to express chimeric antigen receptors (CAR), which are fusion proteins containing both an antigen recognition portion and a T cell activation domain, allowing the T cells to recognize a specific antigen on tumor cells. These engineered T cells are grown in the laboratory until they number in the hundreds of millions and then are infused to back into patient. CAR T cells targeting the B cell antigen CD19 have been studied extensively in acute lymphoblastic leukemia, chronic lymphocytic leukemia, and non-Hodgkin lymphoma. CAR T cell therapies are now under investigation for use in solid tumors. CAR T cell infusion can manifest toxicity mainly through cytokine release syndrome.[56] Renal toxicity includes AKI and electrolyte disturbances. Most of the time, AKI is attributed to reduced renal perfusion secondary to cytokine-mediated vasodilation, decreased cardiac output, or intravascular volume depletion due to insensible losses from high fevers. Additionally, CAR T cell infusion may lead to tumor lysis syndrome.[56] Electrolyte disturbances such as hyponatremia, hypokalemia, and hypophosphatemia have also been associated with CAR T cell therapy.[56] The mainstay of management of CAR T cell toxicity is aggressive supportive care with early intervention for hypotension. For cytokine release syndrome, pharmacologic therapy with interleukin-6 receptor blocker tocilizumab and corticosteroid may be considered in severe cases.[56]

REFERENCES

1. Arany I, Safirstein RL. Cisplatin nephrotoxicity. *Semin Nephrol.* 2003;23(5):460–464.
2. Yao X, Panichpisal K, Kurtzman N, Nugent K. Cisplatin nephrotoxicity: a review. *Am J Med Sci.* 2007;334(2);115–124.
3. Kuhlmann MK, Burkhardt G, Kohler H. Insights into potential cellular mechanisms of cisplatin nephrotoxicity and their clinical application. *Nephrol Dial Transplant.* 1997;12(12):2478–2480.
4. Ramesh G, Reeves WB. TNF-alpha mediates chemokine and cytokine expression and renal injury in cisplatin nephrotoxicity. Clin Invest. 2002;110(6):835–842.
5. Luke DR, Vadiei K, Lopez-Berestein G. Role of vascular congestion in cisplatin-induced acute renal failure in the rat. *Nephrol Dial Transplant.* 1992;7(1):1–7.
6. Ali BH, Al Moundhri MS. Agents ameliorating or augmenting the nephrotoxicity of cisplatin and other platinum compounds: a review of some recent research. *Food Chem Toxicol.* 2006 Aug;44(8):1173–1183.
7. Dubourg L, Michoudet C, Cochat P, Baverel G. Human kidney tubules detoxify chloroacetaldehyde, a presumed nephrotoxic metabolite of ifosfamide. *J Am Soc Nephrol.* 2001;12(8):1615–1623.
8. Skinner R, Sharkey IM, Pearson AD, Craft AW. Ifosfamide, mesna, and nephrotoxicity in children. *J Clin Oncol.* 1993;11:173–190.
9. Izzedine H Isnard-Bagnis C Launay-Vacher V et al. Gemcitabine-induced thrombotic microangiopathy: a systematic review. *Nephrol Dial Transplant.* 2006; 21:3038–3045.
10. Glezerman I, Kris MG, Miller V, Seshan S, Flombaum CD. Gemcitabine nephrotoxicity and hemolytic uremic syndrome: report of 29 cases from a single institution. *Clin Nephrol.* 2009;71(2):130–139.
11. Grall M, Provot F, Coindre JP, et al. Efficacy of Eculizumab in Gemcitabine-Induced Thrombotic Microangiopathy: Experience of the French Thrombotic Microangiopathies Reference Centre. *Blood.* 2016 128:136.
12. Ramsey LB, Balis FM, O'Brien MM, et al. Consensus guideline for use of glucarpidase in patients with high-dose methotrexate induced acute kidney injury and delayed methotrexate clearance. *The Oncologist.* 2018;23(1):52–61.
13. Sasaki K, Tanaka J, Fujimoto T. Theoretically required urinary flow during high-dose methotrexate infusion. *Cancer Chemother Pharmacol.* 1984;13:9–13.
14. Widemann BC, Sung E, Anderson L, et al. Pharmacokinetics and metabolism of the methotrexate metabolite 2, 4-diamino-n 10-methylpteroic acid. *J Pharmacol Exp Ther.* 2000; 294:894–901.
15. Wall SM, Johansen MJ, Molony DA, DuBose TD s, Jaffe N, Madden T. Effective

clearance of methotrexate using high-flux hemodialysis membranes. *Am J Kidney Dis.* 1996;28(6):846–854.

16. Glezerman IG, Pietanza MC, Miller V, Seshan SV. Kidney tubular toxicity of maintenance pemetrexed therapy. *Am J Kidney Dis.* 2011;58(5):817–820.

17. Vootukuru, V, Liew, Y.P, Nally, J.V. Pemetrexed-induced acute renal failure, nephrogenic diabetes insipidus, and renal tubular acidosis in a patient with non-small cell lung cancer. *Med Oncol.* 2006;23:419–422.

18. Eremina V Jefferson JA Kowalewska J et al. VEGF inhibition and renal thrombotic microangiopathy. *N Engl J Med.* 2008;13;358(11):1129–1136.

19. Launay-Vacher V, Janus N, Selle F, et al. Results of the MARS study on the management of antiangiogenics' renovascular safety in ovarian cancer: American Society of Clinical Oncology Annual Meeting. *J Clin Oncol.* 2013; 31(15 Suppl):5567–5567.

20. Goldwasser F, Janus N, Morere JF, et al. Results of the MARS study on the management of antiangiogenics' renovascular safety in lung cancer. *Eur J Cancer.* 2013; 49(Suppl 2): S819.

21. Gligorov J, Janus N, Daniel C, et al. Results of the MARS study on the management of antiangiogenics' renovascular safety in breast cancer. *Cancer Res.* 2013; 73(24 Suppl): P3–P15.

22. Facemire CS, Nixon AB, Griffiths R, Hurwitz H, Coffman TM. Vascular endothelial growth factor receptor 2 controls blood pressure by regulating nitric oxide synthase expression. *Hypertension.* 2009;54:652–658.

23. Kappers MH, van Esch JH, Sluiter W, Sleijfer S, Danser AH, van den Meiracker AH. Hypertension induced by the tyrosine kinase inhibitor sunitinib is associated with increased circulating endothelin-1 levels. *Hypertension.* 2010; 56(4):675–681.

24. Baffert F, Le T, Sennino B, Thurston G, Kuo CJ, Hu-Lowe D, McDonald DM. Cellular changes in normal blood capillaries undergoing regression after inhibition of VEGF signaling. *Am J Physiol Heart Circ Physiol.* 2006:290:H547–H559.

25. Rini BI, Cohen DP, Lu DR, et al. Hypertension as a biomarker of efficacy in patients with metastatic renal cell carcinoma treated with sunitinib. *J Natl Cancer Inst.* 2011;103(9):763–773.

26. Marcolino MS, Boesrsma E, Clementino NC, et al. Imatinib treatment duration is related to decreased estimated glomerular filtration rate in chronic myeloid leukomia patients. *Ann Oncol.* 2011;22:2073–2079.

27. Penel N, Blay JY, Adenis A. Imatinib as a possible cause of severe rhabdomyolysis. *N Engl J Med.* 2008;358(25):2746–2747.

28. Turan N, Benekli M, Ozturk SC, et al. Sunitinib- and sorafenib-induced nephrotic syndrome in a patient with gastrointestinal stromal tumor. *Ann Pharmacother.* 2012;46(10):e27.

29. Porta C, Cosmai L, Gallieni M, Pedrazzoli P, Malberti F. Renal effects of targeted anticancer therapies. *Nat Rev Nephrol.* 2015;11(6):354–370.

30. Kandula P, Agarwal R. Proteinuria and hypertension with tyrosine kinase inhibitors. *Kidney Int.* 2011;80(12):1271–1277.

31. Dimke H, van der Wijst J, Alexander TR et al. Effects of the EGFR inhibitor erlotinib on magnesium handling. *J Am Soc Nephrol.* 2010;21:1309–1316.

32. Dimopoulos MA, Roussou M, Gavriatopoulou M, et al. Reversibility of renal impairment in patients with multiple myeloma treated with bortezomib-based regimens: identification of predictive factors. *Clin Lymphoma Myelom.* 2009;9(4): 302–330.

33. Morita R, Hashino S, Shirai S, et al.: Thrombotic microangiopathy after treatment with bortezomib and dexamethasone in a patient with multiple myeloma. *Int J Hematol.* 2008;88:248–250.

34. Chan KL, Filshie R, Nandurkar H, Quach H. Thrombotic microangiopathy complicating bortezomib-based therapy for multiple myeloma. *Leuk Lymphoma.* 2015;56:2185–2186.

35. Dimopoulos MA, Sonneveld P, Leung N, et al. International Myeloma Working Group Recommendations for the Diagnosis and Management of Myeloma-Related Renal Impairment. *J Clin Oncol.* 2016;34:13,1554–1557.

36. Siegel DS, Martin T, Wang M, et al. A phase 2 study of single agent carfilzomib (PX-171-003-A1) in patients with relapsed and refractory multiple myeloma. *Blood.* 2012;120:2817–2825.

37. Sullivan MR, Danilov AV, Lansigan F, Dunbar NM. Carfilzomib associated thrombotic microangiopathy initially treated with therapeutic plasma exchange. J Clin Apher. 2015;30:308–310.

38. Hobeika L, Self SE, Velez JC. Renal thrombotic microangiopathy and podocytopathy associated with the use of carfilzomib in a patient with multiple myeloma. *BMC Nephrol.* 2014;15:156.

39. Niesvizky R, Naib T, Christos PJ, et al. Lenalidomide-induced myelosuppression is associated with renal dysfunction: adverse events evaluation of treatment-naive patients undergoing front-line lenalidomide and dexamethasone therapy. *Br J Haematol.* 2007;138 (5):640–643.

40. Specter R, Sanchorawala V, Seldin DC, et al. Kidney dysfunction during lenalidomide treatment for AL amyloidosis. *Nephrol Dial Transplant.* 2011;26 (3):881–886.

41. Perazella MA, Izzedine H. Crizitinib: renal safety evaluation. *J Onco-Nephrol.* 2017;1(1):49–56.

42. Gastaud L, Ambrosetti D, Otto J, et al. Acute kidney injury following crizotinib administration for non-small cell lung carcinoma. *Lung Cancer.* 2013;82 (2):362–364.

43. Schell P, Barlett CH, Solomon BJ, et al. Complex renal cysts associated with crizotinib treatment. *Cancer Med.* 2015; 4(6):887–896.

44. Shaw AT, Kim DW, Nakagawa K, et al. Crizotinib versus chemotherapy in advanced ALK-positive lung cancer. *N Engl J Med.* 2013;368 (25):2385–2394.

45. Uthurruague C, Thellier S, Ribes D, et al. Vemurafenib significantly decreases glomerular filtration rate. *J Eur Acad Dermatol Venerol.* 2014;28:978–979.

46. Regnier-Rosencher E, Lazareth H, Gressier L, et al. Acute kidney injury in patients with severe rash on vemurafenib treatment for metastatic melanomas. *Br J Dermatol.* 2013;169:934–938.

47. Launay-Vacher V, Zimner-Rapuch S, Poulalhon N, et al. Acute renal failure associated with the new BRAF inhibitor vemurafenib:a case series of 8 patients. *Cancer.* 2014;120:2158–2163.

48. Teuma C, Muzet CP, Pelletier S, et al. New insights in renal toxicity of BRAF inhibitor vemurafenib in patients with metastatic melanoma [abstract]. Cancer and Kidney International Network (CKIN), Annual Meeting, Brussels, Belgium, 2015.

49. Launay-Vacher V, Aapro M, De Castro G Jr, et a. Renal effects of molecular targeted therapies in oncology: a review by the Cancer and the Kidney International Network (C-KIN). *Ann Oncol.* 2015; 26:1677–1684.

50. Flaherty KT, Infante JR, Daud A, et al. Combined BRAF and MEK inhibition in melanoma with BRAF V600 mutations. *N Engl J Med.* 2012; 367: 1694–1703.

51. Izzedine H, Gueutin V, Gharbi C, et al. Kidney injuries related to ipilimumab. *Invest New Drugs.* 2014; 32:769–773.

52. Cortazar FB, Marrone KA, Troxell ML, et al. Clinicopathological features of acute kidney injury associated with immune checkpoint inhibitors. *Kidney Int.* 2016; 90:638–647.

53. Shirali AC, Perazella MA, Gettinger S. Association of acute interstitial nephritis with programmed cell death 1 inhibitor therapy in lung cancer patients. *Am J Kidney Dis.* 2016;68(2):287–229.

54. Jung K, Zeng X, Bilusic M. Nivolumab-associated acute glomerulonephritis: a case report and literature review. *BMC Nephrol.* 2016;17:188.

55. Selamet U, Ziaolhagh A, Lakhani LS et al. Nephrotoxicity of Immune Checkpoint Inhibitors: MD Anderson Cancer Center's Experience [abstract] *J Am Soc Nephrol.* 28: 2017;404.

56. Brudno JN, Kochenderfer JN. Toxicities of chimeric antigen receptor T cell: recognition and management. *Blood.* 2016;127(26):3321–3330.

27

Poisonings and Intoxications

NIKOLAS B. HARBORD AND MUHAMMAD S. AKHTER

INTRODUCTION

Nephrologists are frequently involved in the management of patients with poisoning, particularly in cases with AKI and/or electrolyte and acid-base disorders. With many intoxicants, high-quality evidence is not available. Fortunately, clinical experience and reports of therapeutic benefit (or failure) combined with careful toxicological measures are available to guide the management of poisoned patients.

This chapter will provide a clinical overview of management of poisonings and intoxications, with focus on the kidney as the organ of impact or injury. Further specific treatment within the purview of the nephrologist includes recognition and treatment of acid-base derangements, enhanced elimination, and diffusive and convective clearance.

EPIDEMIOLOGY

Poisoning is now among the leading causes of death, largely due to an epidemic of opiate overdoses. Accidental exposure remains most common particularly among children, while suicidal ingestions increase among adults.

In 2015, the American Association of Poison Control Centers[1] reported more than 2 million toxic exposures across the United States. Toxic alcohol exposures are among the most common, with 6,089 and 1,610 single-exposure cases of ethylene glycol and methanol poisoning, respectively. Reported lithium and salicylate poisoning cases were 3,597 and 10,877, respectively.

Treatment of poisonings with enteric decontamination with activated charcoal and alkalinization of the urine remain frequent at 46,030 and 11,275 treatments, respectively. Fomepizole, an inhibitor of toxic metabolites from some alcohols was used in 1,850 exposures. Extracorporeal modalities were used 2,563 times in the treatment of poisoning, of which the vast majority (2,481) were hemodialysis.[1]

MANAGEMENT CONSIDERATIONS

The initial assessment of a patient with known or suspected poisoning should include investigation of dose, timing of intoxication, measurement of levels (if available), and identification of organ dysfunction or any evident complications. Situational evidence such as from containers and the possibility of multiple ingestions should always be considered, particularly with intentional exposures and suicide attempts.

Management involves supportive care followed by more specific and directed management, as needed. Unstable patients may require an established airway, ventilation, circulatory support, and advanced cardiac life support. The route of endogenous elimination of a poison or intoxicant should be established. Further consideration should be given to improving kidney function and urine output and assessing liver function, as these may be critical determinants of the need for intervention.

Knowledge or estimation as to the timing of ingestion can facilitate enteric decontamination. Gastric lavage is not routinely recommended, with studies showing significant risk and only minimal benefit, in a small subset of recently poisoned patients.[2] Activated charcoal, administered in single[3] or multiple doses via a large lumen orogastric tube, can adsorb clinically significant quantity of the intoxicant if applied within 60 minutes of ingestion. The use of bowel irrigation or cathartics for decontamination may be of benefit if there is retained or slowly absorbed intoxicant (e.g., sustained release tablets). Induction of vomiting is contraindicated and should not be attempted.

Specific antidotes may be available and should be employed as necessary.

Enhanced elimination (through ion trapping by urinary pH modulation) and extracorporeal decontamination with hemodialysis or related procedures are potentially essential elements of treatment.[4]

Extracorporeal Therapy

The use of extracorporeal modalities in the treatment of poisoning typically involves hemodialysis (often with high-flux membranes and convective volume removal), hemofiltration, or hemoperfusion. The decision to use dialysis or other modalities for clearance is almost invariably clinical and based upon assessment of instability, organ dysfunction, or neurological deterioration despite supportive treatment. Acute kidney injury and the need for metabolic control (as with hyperkalemia or metabolic acidosis) may also influence the decision and the choice of modality. Many substances can be removed by both hemodialysis and hemoperfusion. In such cases, dialysis is preferred, as adsorption columns may be unavailable. Careful monitoring for hypotension is necessary with extracorporeal modalities, due to clearance of pressor agents, the blood circuit, and additional factors.

Hemodialysis, employing diffusive clearance down a gradient from blood across a membrane to the dialysate, is widely available and the most frequently employed modality. Solute/drug/poison removal is largely governed by molecular weight/size (in Daltons), water versus lipid solubility, protein binding, and volume of distribution (Vd), as well as blood and dialysate flow rates and dialyzer pore size and surface area. For example, small molecular weight solutes (<500 Da), with high water solubility, low protein binding, and small Vd (Vd <1 L/kg) will be cleared more than larger solutes with high lipid solubility, tight protein binding, and large Vd. Of note, with diffusive clearance, blood flow rate, drug, and dialyzer pore size are interrelated: the smallest solutes (<300 Da) are highly diffusible through conventional membranes, and clearance will increase with higher blood flow rates. Increasing blood flow rates (Qb) may, however, increase hemodynamic instability. Increases in dialysate flow rate (Qd) will increase diffusive clearance, but clearances likely plateau at Qd 1.5 times the Qb. For larger/less diffusible, small solutes (>300 Da), clearance is best increased with use of larger surface area and larger pore dialyzers. As noted, high-flux dialyzers are nearly ubiquitous and can remove substances as large as vancomycin, with a molecular weight of 1,400 Da.[5] Finally, as molecular weight increases, clearance across a hemofilter is increasingly a function of convection (the creation of an ultrafiltrate through hydrostatic pressure) and less a function of diffusion.[6] As such, extracorporeal treatment of large molecular weight intoxicants should employ convection, which can be accomplished with modern conventional dialysis machines (as convection dialysis), hemofiltration, or, in some centers, with hemodiafiltration.

Hemofiltration, in which convective clearance of solute results from hydrostatic transmembrane pressure applied to the blood against a membrane to create an ultrafiltrate (UF), is usually performed in a continuous manner (e.g., continuous veno-venous hemofiltration). Hemofiltration can clear large molecules up to a molecular weight of 50,000 Da, and convective passage is described by the sieving coefficient, a variable from 0 (negligible) to 1 (complete). Clearance is increased by increasing the ultrafiltration rate, and total clearance is equal to the sieving coefficient multiplied by UF rate. Hemofiltration is not frequently deployed in the treatment of poisoning, although continuous hemofiltration with hemodynamically tolerable low Qb and maximum UF rate with necessary replacement fluid may be of clinical utility in some exposures.

Hemoperfusion, in which solute is adsorbed from blood perfused over a large surface area column (typically charcoal) rather than through a hemofilter, is infrequently used to detoxify patients with poisoning.[7] Hemoperfusion can provide clearance but does not allow for correction of metabolic abnormalities. Furthermore, columns can become saturated with solute, while adverse effects include a flushing reaction and thrombocytopenia. Hemoperfusion is of clinical benefit and can provide superior clearance for some intoxicants such as lipid soluble drugs, barbiturates, carbemazepine, valproic acid, and theophylline.[8]

POISONINGS

Toxic Alcohols: Methanol and Ethylene Glycol

Methanol is a common solvent and cleaning agent and is typically ingested intentionally in attempted suicide or accidentally consumed during epidemic poisonings with bootleg or counterfeit alcohol. Ethylene glycol is antifreeze and is also found in many industrial solvents.

Vision impairment and severe acidosis is the classic presentation for methanol, while kidney injury with acidosis is the expectation with ethylene glycol. The metabolism of toxic alcohols produces toxic metabolites. Specifically, the hepatic enzymes alcohol dehydrogenase (ADH) and aldehyde dehydrogenase oxidize methanol to formaldehyde then formic acid whereas ethylene glycol is converted to glycoaldehyde, glycolic acid, and then oxalate (Fig. 27.1).

Formaldehyde binds to tissue proteins and can cause necrosis of retinal and optic neurons as well as the basal ganglia. Formic acid is an inhibitor of cytochrome oxidase, preventing oxidative respiration resulting in mitochondrial and organ dysfunction.

Glycoaldehyde and oxalate (which precipitates as calcium oxalate) causes hypocalcemic tetany, renal tubular injury, calcium oxalate crystalluria and stones, myocardial injury, and cerebrovascular and meningeal injury.

The clinical manifestations of intoxications depend on the route of exposure, quantity of ingestion, duration of time since ingestion, and

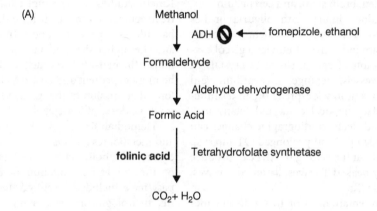

Oxidation of methanol to toxic metabolites by alcohol dehydrogenase is inhibited by fomepizole and ethanol

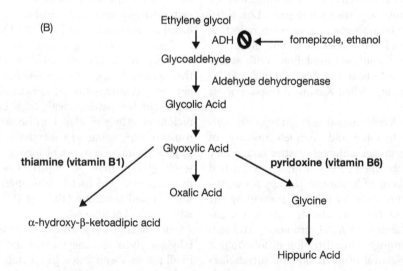

Oxidation of ethylene glycol to toxic metabolites by alcohol dehydrogenase is inhibited by fomepizole and ethanol

FIGURE 27.1 Metabolism of Toxic Alcohols

whether co-ingestion of other substances occurs. Toxic alcohols can both produce inebriation similar to ethanol, with additional early effects such as central nervous system (CNS) depression, as well as nausea and vomiting.

Methanol has been described to cause acute pancreatitis. Later findings include obtundation, seizure, and coma, as well as respiratory and cardiopulmonary failure. Methanol toxicity can present with blurry vision or visual loss; ophthalmic findings can include retinal hyperemia, papilledema, pupillary dilation, and, eventually, optic atrophy. Neurological symptoms can include rigidity, and a Parkinson's-like syndrome as well as hemorrhage and/or white matter lesions in the putamen, brain stem, and cerebellum.

Acute kidney injury with oliguria or hematuria and evidence of calcium oxalate crystalluria are indicative of ethylene glycol toxicity. Deposition of calcium oxalate crystals in the cerebral vessels, meninges, myocardium, and kidney may result in widespread organ dysfunction. Secondary hypocalcemia and tetany may be evident and electrocardiographic changes can include a wide QRS and prolonged QT interval. Hyperkalemia in the setting of AKI can produce progressively peaked T waves, flattened P waves, and widened QRS.

Initial presentation, prior to significant metabolism of the alcohol, may include an elevated serum osmolal gap, typically >25 mOsm/Kg. High anion gap metabolic acidosis is typically evident after metabolism and closure of the serum osmolal gap, with anion gap >12m to 16 mEq/L and bicarbonate consumption reflecting the magnitude of oxalate (ethylene glycol) or formate (methanol) accumulation. With severe metabolic acidosis and acidemia, rapid and labored breathing, called Kussmaul respiration, is expected.

Enteric decontamination is not typically beneficial due to rapid and complete invasion of ingested methanol, although gastric lavage may recover unabsorbed parent alcohol if performed within an hour of ingestion. Therapy for methanol exposure typically involves preventing the formation of toxic metabolites through competitive inhibition of ADH, promoting end metabolism through administration of folic/folinic acid, and removal of methanol and metabolites and correction of metabolic acidosis with dialysis. Inhibition of ADH is possible with either ethanol or fomepizole (4-methyl pyrazole or 4-MP).[9] Folic and folinic acid are cofactors for the conversion of formate to H_2O and CO_2, and 50 mg IV should be administered intravenously (IV) at intervals.

Fomepizole is the more expensive than ethanol, but because it has more predictable kinetics, longer duration of action, and fewer adverse CNS and gastrointestinal side effects, it is the preferred ADH inhibitor.[10] Dosing should follow the recommended loading dose of 15 mg/kg IV and then 10 mg/kg IV every 12 hours. Increase in dosing to 15 mg/kg IV every 12 hours after 48 hours should be used with prolonged intoxications, while the schedule should be adjusted to every 4 hours to account for dialytic removal, if used in combination with dialysis. Kinetic studies of methanol elimination during treatment with fomepizole have shown methanol half-life as high as 87 hours (mean 52 hours), and the higher the methanol concentration, the longer the half-life.[11] As such, dialysis is likely to be more expedient and cost-effective than a prolonged admission to the intensive care unit with multiple doses of fomepizole.

Hemodialysis effectively removes methanol and metabolites and delivers base/bicarbonate to correct metabolic acidosis. Accepted indications or thresholds for initiation of dialysis in the past have included levels greater than 50 mg/dL, neurologic or visual symptoms, or refractory metabolic acidosis; it should be continued until levels (which may rebound) remain below 20 mg/dL. The use of extracorporeal modalities in the treatment of methanol poisoning has been systematically reviewed, resulting in evidence-based recommendations (Table 27.1).[12]

Enteric decontamination measures provide minimal utility with ethylene glycol, other than gastric lavage within a few hours after ingestion. Administration of fomepizole has been suggested for patients with high clinical suspicion of ethylene glycol poisoning, such as osmolar gap, anion gap metabolic acidosis or oxalate crystalluria or established exposure with levels greater than 20 mg/dL. Cofactors that promote safe end metabolism, pyridoxine (50 mg IV) and thiamine (100 mg IV), should be administered at interval.

Hemodialysis also readily and rapidly clears ethylene glycol and metabolites and is indicated in all patients with anion gap metabolic acidosis and/or kidney injury. On the other hand, previous consideration of ethylene glycol levels greater than 50 mg/dL as a threshold for hemodialysis initiation has been challenged by kinetic studies

TABLE 27.1 INDICATIONS FOR DIALYSIS IN THE MANAGEMENT OF SELECTED POISONINGS

Methanol[a,]	Likely or confirmed poisoning in the setting of any of the following: a. new neurologic or vision deficit b. Metabolic acidosis or acidemia with pH ≤ 7.15 c. Elevated anion gap > 24 mmol/L d. Methanol concentration > 70 mg/dL or 21.8 mmol/L in the context of fomepizole, or > 50 mg/dL or 15.6 mmol/L in the absence of an ADH blocker
Ethylene glycol	Likely or confirmed poisoning in the setting of any of the following: a. Acute kidney injury b. Anion gap metabolic acidosis c. EG level >50mg/dL (possible management with fomepizole rather than dialysis if no AKI or acidosis)
Lithium[b]	Likely or confirmed poisoning in the setting of any of the following: a. Decreased level of consciousness, seizures, or life-threatening dysrhythmia b. level > 4.0 mEq/L while kidney function is impaired Suggested intervention: a. Level >5.0 mEq/L b. Confusion c. Expected level >1.0 mEq/L with optimal management for 36 hours
Salicylates[c]	Likely or confirmed severe salicylate poisoning in the setting of any of the following: a. Level >100 mg/dL b. Level >90 mg/dL and impaired kidney function c. Altered mental status/CNS changes d. Hypoxemia or acute respiratory distress syndrome. Suggested intervention when failure of supportive therapy and any of the following: a. Level >90 mg/dL b. Level >80 mg/dL and kidney impairment c. pH ≤ 7.20

[a]Roberts DM, Yates C, Megarbane B, et al.; EXTRIP Work Group. Recommendations for the role of extracorporeal treatments in the management of acute methanol poisoning: a systematic review and consensus statement. *Crit Care Med.* 2015;43:461–472.

[b]Decker BS, Goldfarb DS, Dargan PI, et al.; EXTRIP Workgroup. Extracorporeal treatment for lithium poisoning: systematic review and recommendations from the EXTRIP workgroup. *Clin J Am Soc Nephrol.* 2015;10:875–887.

[c] Juurlink DN, Gosselin S, Kielstein JT, Ghannoum M, Lavergne V, Nolin TD, Hoffman RS; EXTRIP Workgroup. Extracorporeal treatment for salicylate poisoning: systematic review and recommendations from the EXTRIP Workgroup. *Ann Emerg Med.* 2015;266:165–181.

CNS = central nervous system. ADH = antidiuretic hormone

involving fomepizole.[13] With fomepizole effectively inhibits the formation of toxic metabolites, renal elimination of the parent alcohol in patients with intact kidney function occurs with a mean half-life of 17 hours. In short, patients with ethylene glycol poisoning and levels greater than 50 mg/dL without kidney injury or acidosis can be managed with early administration of the antidote fomepizole, precluding hemodialysis. A systematic review of extracorporeal therapy in ethylene glycol is currently underway.

Of note, additional toxic alcohols can present with clinically important exposures or poisoning, including diethylene glycol and propylene glycol.[14]

Lithium

Lithium (Li^{3+}) salts effectively treat bipolar affective disorder but have a well-characterized toxic potential and narrow therapeutic index.[15] Toxic effects of lithium include hypothyroidism, potentially irreversible nephrogenic diabetes insipidus, symptoms of polyuria and polydipsia, and finding of impaired urinary concentrating ability and possibly hypernatremia. Additional kidney toxicity includes chronic interstitial nephritis with microcysts and nephrotic glomerulopathies. Acute toxicity can present with gastrointestinal symptoms including vomiting and diarrhea; cardiac effects include myocarditis with ST depression or lateral T wave inversions and heart block.

Lithium also causes acute neurologic effects: CNS symptoms increase with rising concentration from confusion to coma and seizures, including a characteristic fine tremor, hyperreflexia, dystonia, and cerebellar signs. The syndrome of irreversible lithium-effectuated neurotoxicity has variable clinical features including cerebellar and cognitive deficits.[16]

Immediate-release lithium is rapidly absorbed, reaching peak concentration within 2 hours, while sustained release formulations reach peak blood concentration within 5 hours. Shortly after administration, gastric lavage or bowel irrigation (for sustained release preparations) may provide enteric decontamination. Sodium polystyrene sulfonate resin binds lithium and may have a modest effect on oral bioavailabilty.[17] Absorption is followed by a rapid (alpha phase) distribution in total body water (Vd 0.5 L/kg) and then a slower (beta phase) of tissue and CNS distribution (Vd 0.7–0.9 L/kg). Lithium is not bound to blood proteins, and the delay in distribution reflects slow penetration of the blood–brain barrier.

Therapeutic steady state lithium level is 0.6 to 1.2 mEq/L, with mild toxicity noted at 1.5 to 2.5 mEq/L, moderate toxicity at 2.5 to 3.5 mEq/L, and severe toxicity at >3.5 mEq/L. Acute, chronic, or acute-on-chronic toxicity should be established due to important implications in management decisions. Of note, elderly patients and those with chronic toxicity may have symptoms at lower concentrations than with acute toxicity.

Lithium is not metabolized in the body, and the kidneys are the route of endogenous elimination. Lithium is filtered and transported like sodium in the kidneys, and any decrease in estimated glomerular filtration rate, as with volume depletion, nonsteroidal anti-inflammatory drug use, or thiazides (as it promotes more proximal tubular absorption), can decrease clearance and increase lithium concentration. Conversely, lithium concentration can be decreased with an increase in estimated glomerular filtration rate by volume expansion and natriuretic measures such as loop diuretics and amiloride or triamterene.

Like other small, unbound, water soluble solutes with low Vd, lithium is readily dialyzable. The role of extracorporeal therapy has been systematically reviewed, and evidence-based indications are available (Table 27.1).[16] Conventional intermittent hemodialysis is the optimal initial modality, whereas sustained low-efficiency dialysis and hemodiafiltration are also acceptable and are more efficient at initial Li^{3+} lowering than continuous modalities. Intervention is recommended for all patients with decreased consciousness, seizures, or severe dysrhythmia and any patient with a level >4.0 mEq/L and impaired kidney function. Extracorporeal intervention is suggested for any patient who is confused, with a level >5.0 mEq/L, or expected have a level above 1.0 mEq/L after 36 hours of supportive therapy. Treatment with dialysis should continue until clinical improvement or level <1.0 mEq/L. Repeated observation and serial measures are recommended as lithium levels may rebound after equilibration from tissue after initial lowering. Continuous treatments may have a role in subsequent treatments due to slow CNS release.

Salicylates

Salicylates are a subgroup of nonsteroidal anti-inflammatory drugs. Acetylsalicylic acid (aspirin) and methyl salicylate, in particular, are widely available without prescription and have a well-characterized acute and chronic toxicity. Ingested aspirin is the most common exposure. Oil of wintergreen (pure methyl salicylate) has lethal potential at oral doses of less than a teaspoon (5 ml), and when applied in large doses, topical analgesics containing methyl salicylate also can be toxic or even lethal.

Salicylates are rapidly absorbed from the small intestine, acetylsalicylic acid powder more rapidly than tablets or enteric-coated pills (prolonged up to 12 hours). Acetylsalicylic acid exhibits a high degree of protein binding and a small Vd (0.2–0.5 L/kg). First-pass metabolism hydrolyzes acetylsalicylic acid to salicylic acid, followed by hepatic conjugation. Salicylates are cytotoxic and uncouple oxidative phosphorylation, leading to a mitochondrial dysfunction, impaired ATP generation, and organ dysfunction with metabolic acidosis (including type B lactic acidosis).

Acute intoxication can present with tinnitus, deafness, diaphoresis and flushing; tachycardia, and hypovolemia, as well as nausea and vomiting. Acute respiratory distress syndrome (ARDS) and cerebral edema are severe complications of increased vascular permeability. Patients usually demonstrate respiratory alkalosis from hyperventilation, followed by high anion gap metabolic acidosis from accumulation of salicylates and bicarbonate consumption. Respiratory fatigue eventually results in respiratory acidosis.

Unlike adults and older children, very young children may not demonstrate hyperventilation and respiratory alkalosis. Acidemia correlates with CNS symptoms (agitation, obtundation, and coma) and facilitates entry of salicylates into the cerebrospinal fluid. Death is usually the result of cerebral edema.

Patients should receive gastrointestinal decontamination with activated charcoal and volume resuscitation. Administration of IV sodium bicarbonate should be given to treat acidemia, reduce CNS entry of salicylate, and alkalinize the urine (toward a pH of 8) to enhances elimination of salicylate through ion trapping. Bicarbonate should not be administered when there is an evident predominate alkalosis with alkalemia. The presence of ARDS and/or cerebral edema, precluding sodium chloride or bicarbonate administration, are classic indications for extracorporeal therapy.

The role of extracorporeal therapy in the treatment of salicylate poisoning has been systematically reviewed and evidence-based recommendations are available (Table 27.1).[18] Hemodialysis effectively removes salicylates, a solute with low molecular weight and low Vd, and conventional intermittent hemodialysis is preferred over sustained low-efficiency dialysis or continuous modalities. Hemoperfusion also provides clearance but does not correct acidosis. Hemodialysis is recommended for any patient with a salicylate level >100 mg/dL, a level >90 mg/dL and impaired kidney function, or any altered mental status/CNS changes, hypoxemia, or ARDS. Hemodialysis is suggested with failure of supportive therapy and any of the following: salicylate level >90 mg/dL, salicylate level >80 mg/dL and kidney impairment, or pH ≤7.20.

Toluene

Toluene is a widely available organic solvent, found in a variety of products including glue, paint thinner, lacquers, enamels, typewriter correction fluid, butane lighters, and marking pencils. Glue sniffing, the modern form of volatile substance abuse, gained popularity in the 1960s. Other names of this phenomenon are "huffing" and "bagging," based on the mode of inhalation. Toluene abuse is more common in adolescents and adults of modest socioeconomic background as it is cheap and easily accessible.

Immediate effects of toluene inhalation closely resemble acute alcohol intoxication and include euphoria and pleasant exhilaration. Diplopia, gross disorientation, vivid colorful hallucinations, delusions, stupor, respiratory depression, and even coma can result from prolonged inhalation and severe intoxication. Permanent CNS effects are also reported, including ataxia, tremors, and impaired speech, hearing, and vision. Toluene can also induce dysrhythmias, assumed to be the cause of "sudden sniffing death syndrome." Renal effects are metabolic acidosis and hypokalemia, which can also cause muscle paralysis. Repeated use can cause significant damage to the heart, liver, and kidneys.[19, 20, 21]

With glue sniffing, toluene vapor is 100 to 1,000 times more concentrated than occupational exposure limits in the solvent industry. Total dose inhaled and its effects depend upon mode, duration of inhalation, and number of exposures and is also affected by genetic factors, diet, and alcohol consumption.[22] Intoxicated patients may present with nausea and generalized weakness, and the diagnosis is usually made by history and suggestive neuropsychiatric, cardiovascular, and renal manifestations. Urinary hippuric acid is a biomarker for toluene abuse.

Inhaled toluene is available in arterial blood within 10 seconds, while T_{max} is 30 to 45 minutes. It is highly lipophilic and is deposited in adipose tissue and the CNS. The liver metabolizes toluene to benzyl alcohol via the cytochrome P450 system, followed by oxidation to benzoic acid and conjugation with glycine to form hippuric acid, which is excreted in urine.[22]

Excessive production of hippuric acid consumes bicarbonate and causes metabolic acidosis. If renal function is preserved, hippourate is actively secreted by the renal tubules and rapid excretion of this organic anion obligates urinary loss of sodium and potassium. The resulting clinical picture will be a hyperchloremic (nonanion gap) metabolic acidosis with volume depletion and hypokalemia. Toluene or its metabolites have also been noted to cause tubular injury.[21,23]

Management of toluene toxicity is supportive. IV hydration and repeated testing and replacement of serum electrolytes are the mainstay of treatment. Patients generally respond very well, although oral potassium replacement may be required even after discharge from the hospital.

Cleistanthus Collinus

Cleistanthus collinus, popularly known as oduvanthalai or garari, is a shrub found in South Asia, especially southern India. This very toxic plant is used for homicidal and suicidal purposes due to its ready availability and is favored by young women as a method of deliberate self-harm. All parts of the plant are toxic, but the leaves are most often used in poisonings or as an abortifacient. Multiple toxins have been isolated from oduvanthalai but the major constituents are cleistanthin A and B, collinusin, and diphyllin.[24]

Patients usually present with abdominal pain, vomiting, diarrhea, chest pain, palpitations, and shortness of breath. Cardiac effects include various arrhythmias including ventricular tachycardia and ventricular fibrillation. Respiratory effects include respiratory failure and ARDS. Myasthenia-like weakness has also been reported. Renal effects are common and include hypokalemia and hyperchloremic (nonanion gap) metabolic acidosis, caused by distal renal tubular acidosis from tubular toxicity.

Diagnosis is mainly clinical, but an enzyme-linked immunosorbent assay has been developed for cleistanthin A and B. High performance liquid chromatography has also been used in toxin detection. Mechanism of action is not well understood, but animal studies have implicated inhibition of renal tubular H(+)-ATPase activity.[25]

Maintenance of airway, breathing, and circulation; appropriate treatment of arrhythmias; and correction of hypokalemia and metabolic acidosis are essential in the management of *Cleistanthus collins* poisoning.

CONCLUSION

Many intoxications involve kidney injury and physiologic derangements within the purview of the nephrologist. Furthermore, the nephrologist may be central to the extracorporeal detoxification of a poisoned patient.

REFERENCES

1. Mowry JB, Spyker DA, Brooks DE, Zimmerman A, Schauben JL, 2015 Annual report of the American Association of Poison Control Centers' National Poison Data System (NPDS): 33rd annual report. *Clinical Toxicology*. 2016;54:961–1146.
2. Vale JA, Kulig K; American Academy of Clinical Toxicology, European Association of Poisons Centres and Clinical Toxicologists. Position paper: gastric lavage. *J Toxicol Clin Toxicol*. 2004;42:933–943.
3. Chyka PA, Seger D, Krenzelok EP, Vale JA; American Academy of Clinical Toxicology.; European Association of Poisons Centres and Clinical Toxicologists. Position paper: single-dose activated charcoal. *Clin Toxicol*. 2005;43:61–87.
4. Winchester JF, Harbord NB, Charen E, Ghannoum M. Use of dialysis and hemoperfusion treatment of poisoning. In Daugirdas JT, Blake PJ, Ing TS, eds. *Handbook of Dialysis*. 5th ed. Philadelphia, PA: Lippincott Willliams & Wilkins; 2015: 368–390.
5. De Bock V, Verbeelen D, Maes V, Sennesael J. Pharmacokinetics of vancomycin in patients undergoing haemodialysis and haemofiltration. *Nephrol Dial Transplant*. 1989;4:635–639.
6. Depner T, Garred L. Solute transport mechanisms in dialysis. In Horl W, Koch KM, Lindsay RM, Ronco C, Winchester JF, eds. *Replacement of Renal Function by Dialysis*. 5th ed. Dordrecht, The Netherlands; Kluwer Academic; 2004: 73–93.
7. Ghannoum M, Lavergne V, Gosselin S, et al. Practice trends in the use of extracorporeal treatments for poisoning in four countries. *Semin Dial*. 2016;29:71–80.
8. Harbord N, Winchester JF, Charen E, Sheth N, Bhansali A; Extracorporeal therapies acute intoxication and poisoning. In: Ronco C, Bellomo R, Kellum J, eds. *Critical Care Nephrology*. 3rd ed. Amsterdam, The Netherlands: Elsevier; 2017:588–594.
9. Brent J, McMartin K, Phillips S, Aaron C, Kulig K; Methylpyrazole for Toxic Alcohols Study Group. Fomepizole for the treatment of methanol poisoning. *N Engl J Med*. 2001;344:424–429.
10. Barceloux DG, Bond GR, Krenzelok EP, Cooper H, Vale JA; American Academy of Clinical Toxicology Ad Hoc Committee on the Treatment Guidelines for Methanol Poisoning. American Academy of Clinical Toxicology practice guidelines on the treatment of methanol poisoning. *J Toxicol Clin Toxicol*. 2002;40:415–447.
11. Hovda KE, Andersson KS, Urdal P, et al. Methanol and formate kinetics during treatment with fomepizole. *Clin Toxicol*. 2005;43:221–227.
12. Roberts DM, Yates C, Megarbane B, et al.; EXTRIP Work Group. Recommendations for the role of extracorporeal treatments in the management of acute methanol poisoning: a systematic review and consensus statement. *Crit Care Med*. 2015;43:461–472.
13. Sivilotti ML, Burns MJ, McMartin KE, Brent J, For the Methylpyrazole for Toxic Alcohols Study Group: Toxicokinetics of ethylene glycol during fomepizole therapy: implications for management. *Ann Emerg Med*. 2000;36:114–125.
14. Kraut JA, Kurtz I. Toxic alcohol ingestions: clinical features, diagnosis, and management. *Clin J Am Soc Nephrol*. 2008;3:208–225.
15. McKnight RF, Adida M, Budge K, Stockton S, Goodwin GM, Geddes JR. Lithium toxicity profile: a systematic review and meta-analysis. *Lancet*. 2012;379:721–728.

16. Decker B, Goldfarb DS, Dargan PI, et al.; EXTRIP Workgroup. Extracorporeal treatment for lithium poisoning: systematic review and recommendations from the EXTRIP workgroup *Clin J Am Soc Nephrol.* 10(5):875–887.

17. Belanger DR, Tierney MG, Dickinson G. Effect of sodium polystyrene sulfonate on lithium bioavailability. *Ann Emerg Med.* 1992;21:1312–1315.

18. Juurlink DN, Gosselin S, Kielstein JT, Ghannoum M, Lavergne V, Nolin TD, Hoffman RS; EXTRIP Workgroup. Extracorporeal treatment for salicylate poisoning: systematic review and recommendations from the EXTRIP Workgroup. *Ann Emerg Med.* 2015;266:165–181.

19. von Burg, R. Toluene. *J Appl Toxicol.* 1993;13: 441–446.

20. Djurendic-Brenesel M, Stojiljkovic G, Pilija V. Fatal intoxication with toluene due to inhalation of glue. *J Forensic Sci.* 2016;61:875–878.

21. Carlisle EJ, Donnelly SM, Vasuvattakul S, Kamel KS, Tobe S, Halperin ML. Glue-sniffing and distal renal tubular acidosis: sticking to the facts. *J Am Soc Nephrol.* 1991;1:1019–1027.

22. Raikhlin-Eisenkraft B, Hoffer E, Baum Y, Bentur Y. Determination of urinary hippuric acid in toluene abuse, journal of toxicology. *Clinical Toxicology.* 2001;39:73–76.

23. Tuchscherer J, Rehman H. Metabolic acidosis in toluene sniffing. *Can J. Emerg. Med.* 2013;15:249–252.

24. Das S, Hamide A, Mohanty MK, Muthusamy R. Fatal *Cleistanthus collinus* toxicity: a case report and review of literature. *J Forensic Sci.* 2014;59:1441–1447.

25. Chrispal A. *Cleistanthus collinus* poisoning. *J Emerg Trauma Shock.* 2012;5:160–166.

SECTION V

Kidney Protection in Systemic Illness

28

Diabetic Kidney Disease

JOHN CIJIANG HE

INTRODUCTION

Diabetic kidney disease (DKD) is the most common cause of end-stage renal failure (ESRD) in the world. Though the incidence rate has decreased recently with current management, the prevalence remains high. The pathogenesis of DKD is complex including genetic, hemodynamic, metabolic, and environmental factors. Histologically, DKD is characterized by thickening of glomerular basement membrane (GBM), mesangial expansion, and arteriolar hyalinosis. Clinically, patients with DKD present with glomerular hyperfiltration at the early stage and then progress to microalbuminuria, macroalbuminuria, and ESRD over several decades. However, this classic progression pattern has been changed with treatment, including tight glycemic control and renin–angiotensin system (RAS) inhibition. The diagnosis of DKD is mostly based on the clinical presentation, and kidney biopsy is required if patients have an atypical presentation, particularly in type 2 diabetic patients. The mainstay of therapy includes hyperglycemic control, blood pressure (BP) control, and angiotensin converting enzyme inhibitors (ACEIs) or angiotensin II receptor blockers (ARBs). However, both ACEIs and ARBs have only partial renal protection. Therefore, there is an urgent need to develop better therapies for DKD.

EPIDEMIOLOGY OF DKD

Diabetes affects 25.8 million people of all ages representing 8.3% of US population[1] and 347 million worldwide. DKD is the most common cause of ESRD in patients (44%) in the United States.[1,2] The epidemiology of DKD has been best studied in patients with type 1 disease, since the time of clinical onset is usually known. It has been believed that approximately 20% to 30% will have microalbuminuria after a mean duration of diabetes of 15 years.[3] Less than half of these patients will progress to overt nephropathy. It has been suggested that 25% to 45% of diabetic patients will develop clinically evident DKD during their lifetime.[3,4] The overall incidence of ESRD in diabetic patients was also substantial, with reported rates of 4% to 17% at 20 years from time of initial diagnosis and approximately 16% at 30 years.[5]

PATHOGENESIS OF DKD

The pathogenesis of DKD is very complex, including multiple factors (e.g., genetic, metabolic, hemodynamic). Considerable effort has been spent to identify genetic risk variants to account for the burden of nephropathy in patients with diabetes. However, these studies have been able to identify only some genes that confer a modest risk to DKD.[6] Glomerular hypertrophy and hyperfiltration develop in early DKD, which may lead to progression of the disease.[7] The mechanism by which high glucose causes DKD has been studied extensively in cultured cells and in animal models. It is known that high glucose increases activation of polyol (or aldose reductase) and hexosamine pathways, generation of oxidative stress, formation of advanced glycated end products, and activity of protein kinase C isoforms.[8] Several growth factors have been involved in the pathogenesis of DKD including angiotensin II, endothelin-1, transforming growth factor-beta, vascular endothelial growth factor (VEGF), and angiopoietin (Ang-1 and Ang-2). The immunologic and inflammatory elements also play an important role in initiating and orchestrating the development of DKD.[9]

PATHOLOGY OF DKD

The characteristic features of DKD with type 1 diabetes include 3 major lesions: diffuse mesangial expansion, diffuse thickened GBM, and hyalinosis of afferent and efferent arterioles.[10,11] Features that may occur relatively early (2–5 years of diabetes) are GBM thickening and mesangial matrix accumulation. Mesangial hypercellularity may be noted early but is often not a major feature in advanced disease. The classic lesion of diffuse mesangial (intercapillary) sclerosis or nodular sclerosis was described as the Kimmelstiel and Wilson nodule. Mesangiolysis and capillary microaneurysms are thought to be an important part of the development of nodular sclerosis. Hyalinosis of the arterioles results from the insudation of plasma protein with a glassy or hyaline appearance.

CLINICAL PRESENTATION
The major clinical manifestations are albuminuria, less often hematuria, and, in many patients, progressive chronic kidney disease (CKD), which usually are slow. The natural history of DKD prior to the introduction of current management is classically divided into 5 stages in type 1 diabetes mellitus. Stages 1 and 2 are preclinical stages, characterized with rise of glomerular filtration rate (GFR), normoalbuminiruia or intermittent microalbuminuria in stage 2, and normal BP. The structural changes including thickening of GBM and mild mesangial expansion can occur prior to microalbuminuria in the preclinical stages. In stage 3, which is also called the clinical stage of diabetes nephropathy is defined by persistent microalbuminuria, mild HTN, and normal or slight decline of GFR. Microalbuminuria, also referred to as moderately increased albuminuria, is defined as urinary albumin excretion between 30 and 300 mg/day or between 30 and 300 mg/g creatinine on a random urine sample. Persistent microalbuminuria is defined with 2 of 3 positive repeat measurements within 6 months. In this stage, there is more GBM thickening and mesangial expansion. Stage 4 is characterized by macroalbuminuria, also referred as severely increased albuminuria (defined as urinary albumin excretion >300 mg/day or >300 mg/g creatinine on a random urine sample). In this stage, patients have persistent HTN and further decline of GFR and subsequent slow progression to ESRD, which is stage 5. Histology reveals more glomerulosclerosis with or without Kimmelstiel-Wilson nodules, arteriolar hyalinosis, and tubular interstitial fibrosis.

However, recent studies report that microalbuminuria may revert to the normal range even without treatment with ACEIs.[12] Subsequent analysis of the Diabetes Control and Complications Trial/Epidemiology of Diabetes Interventions and Complications (DCCT/EDIC) study[13] have confirmed this finding. Regression of microalbuminuria in the DCCT/EDIC study was associated with improved glycemic, lipid, and BP control. Thus, the use of persistent microalbuminuria as a reliable risk factor for ultimate development of overt proteinuria or reduced GFR is incorrect. Furthermore, it now appears that progression of renal functional decline may occur without a transition from microalbuminuria to overt proteinuria.[14] A major factor that may contribute to the progression in these patients is acute kidney injury (AKI).[15] Nevertheless, until improved biomarkers have been identified, it is still recommended to measure urinary albumin–creatinine ratio (ACR) on repeated occasions or at least once a year to identify patients who are at increased risk of renal deterioration with diabetes. If ACR is increased on the first occasion, the clinical parameters need to be evaluated, resolved, or optimized (i.e., glycemic control, BP, volume status, intercurrent infection, etc.) before repeat testing to establish sustained albuminuria

DIAGNOSIS
When approaching any diagnosis, it is important to consider common risk factors for the disease and its progression. For DKD, these include longer duration, poor glycemic control, hypertension, and presence of proteinuria.[16] Other factors include race, genetic susceptibility (family history), and advanced age.[17] Detailed recommendations can be found in the clinical practice guidelines for DKD outlined by the Kidney Disease Outcomes Quality Initiative (KDOQI),[18] which were last updated in 2007.

Although the gold standard for the diagnosis of DKD is renal biopsy, most of the time it is still made on clinical grounds. Based on the knowledge of its natural history, it is recommended to start screening for albuminuria at 5 years in patients with type 1 diabetes and at the time of diagnosis in patients with type 2 diabetes. The type of early screening test should be an ACR with a first-morning void spot collection. Studies have confirmed the sensitivity and specificity of the ACR to be >85% compared with 24-hour collections. However, in patients with low muscle mass or obesity, the test is not as accurate.[19,20] If a positive result is obtained, the test should be confirmed for persistence with 2 of 3 positive repeat measurements within 6 months. DKD should be considered in patients with type 1 diabetics with microalbuminuria (ACR of 30–300 mg/g) and a duration of diabetes >10 years, as well as in patients with type 1 or type 2 diabetes with macroalbuminuria (ACR >300 mg/g). Albuminuria should raise concern for DKD; The KDOQI committee encourages the interpretation of albuminuria in relation to estimation of renal function to risk stratify patients.[18] Renal function should be assessed through measured serum creatinine or estimated GFR (eGFR) with knowledge of their limitations. It is important to remember that patients with early nephropathy may have evidence of hyperfiltration and may have a normal to elevated GFR. Other clues that support diabetic nephropathy aside from evidence of albuminuria and impaired renal function include large kidneys on ultrasonography and existence of diabetic retinopathy or neuropathy; however, absence of these findings in patients with type 2 diabetes does not rule out nephropathy. Because diabetes affects the microvascular circulation, the presence of retinopathy, which can be evaluated with a routine ophthalmologic exam, was thought to predict nephropathy. Studies have shown that retinopathy correlates well with overt nephropathy; however, the association is not as strong in early DKD. One study estimated that 30% of patients with type 2 diabetes with renal insufficiency had no evidence of retinopathy or albuminuria.[21]

In type 1 diabetes, most patients can be diagnosed with DKD based on clinical presentation. However, the diagnosis of DKD in type 2 diabetes often requires additional testing including kidney biopsy. Because diabetes is a common condition, coincidence with other nondiabetic CKD is relatively frequent. Patients with atypical clinical features should prompt evaluation for nondiabetic CKD by performing additional diagnostic testing. Atypical presentation of DKD include rapidly decreasing renal function, rapidly increasing proteinuria, active urinary sediment, refractory hypertension, nephrotic range of proteinuria with normal GFR, or a large reduction in GFR after start of an ACEI or ARB. Because generalized vascular disease is common in diabetes, refractory hypertension and/or a significant decrease in kidney function after RAS blockade should prompt consideration of renal artery stenosis. Patients with nephrotic syndrome but normal renal function are also inconsistent with diagnosis of DKD and require kidney biopsy to rule out membranous disease or minimal change disease. The differential diagnosis of these diseases is critical because these patients require steroid and immunosuppressive therapy while patients with DKD should not have these treatments. Differential diagnosis of DKD from other kidney diseases may require both noninvasive testing such as serological testing and imaging and invasive procedure such as kidney biopsy. Additionally, imaging studies with radiographic contrast may pose greater risks in people with diabetes and CKD than in other people.

TREATMENT

Since DKD is a complex disease with many risk factors and pathogenetic factors involved, the treatment requires multiple approaches. The current standard of treatment for DKD includes hyperglycemic control, BP control, ACEI/ARB, antilipid therapy, dietary intervention, and smoking cessation. In addition, a multiple disciplinary approach with close collaboration between nephrologist, diabetologist, nutritionist, and nurse to treat this group of patient population with complex disease is needed.

Treatment of Hyperglycemia
Tight Glycemic Control

The evidence that achieving a hemoglobin A1C (HbA1C) level of approximately 7% is able to mitigate renal complications of diabetes derives largely from the Diabetes Control and Complications Trial (DCCT)[22] and follow-up Epidemiology of Diabetes Interventions and Complications (EDIC) study.[13] Glycemic control may reduce the development of microalbuminuria in patients with type 2 diabetes as well. The Kumamoto Study,[23] the UK Prospective Diabetes Study,[24] and the Veterans Affairs Cooperative Study on Glycemic Control and Complications in Type II Diabetes Feasibility Trial[25] showed that improved glycemic control was associated with reduced incidence of microalbuminuria. However, these studies did not show benefit of tight glycemic control on the progression of DKD at the late stages. Recent studies[26-28] evaluating further tight glycemic management (A1C 6%–7%) failed to demonstrate improvement in overall cardiovascular disease or mortality (the primary endpoint), but all showed improvement in renal parameters. In the Action in Diabetes and Vascular Disease study, there was a 21% reduction in renal outcomes with tight control (HbA1C 6.5%) versus good control (HbA1C 7.3%), despite no reduction in major cardiovascular events. Similarly, the Veterans Affairs Diabetes Trial and the Action to Control Cardiovascular Risk in Diabetes.[29] Study similarly showed that more intensive control, achieving an HbA1C of 6.9% or 6.3%, respectively, compared with standard control (HbA1C of 8.4% or 7.6, respectively), resulted in a 32% reduction in the development of incident microalbuminuria and macroalbuminuria. However, these studies did not show significant benefits of more intensive glycemic control on eGFR or reduction in macrovascular complications.

Measurement of Hyperglycemic Control

In patients with diabetes and CKD, the accuracy of the HbA1c measurement in reflecting ambient glucose concentrations may be altered because of reduced red blood cell lifespan, transfusions, and hemolysis. In general, most studies find that HbA1c is lower than expected based on repeated blood glucose measurements in patients on hemodialysis (HD).[30,31] There is a poorer correlation of plasma glucose levels with HbA1c levels in patients with diabetes on HD compared with those with normal kidney function. Fructosamine (glycated albumin) has been suggested as a better marker of glycemic control in patients with CKD and dialysis; however, studies have found that the correlation of fructosamine levels with blood glucose could be better[30,32] or worse in patients with CKD[33] compared with HbA1C.

Choice of Drugs

The kidney has also been well described to play an important role in insulin metabolism; one-third of insulin degradation is carried out by the kidney proximal tubular cells,[34] and reduced kidney function is associated with a prolonged half-life of insulin. Some patients with long-standing diabetes with progressive renal dysfunction may no longer require hypoglycemic medications because of the combined effect of reduced renal gluconeogenesis and impaired insulin degradation, and it has been termed as "burnt out diabetes."[35] First-generation sulfonylureas (e.g., chlorpropamide, tolazamide, and tolbutamide) should be avoided in patients with CKD stage 3 and beyond. These drugs have increased half-lives as the parent drug and its metabolites can build up with reduced renal clearance. Since it is primarily cleared by the liver,

it does not have active metabolites, and the risk of hypoglycemia is lower, Glipizide is the preferred second-generation sulfonylurea.[35] The peroxisome proliferator-activated receptor gamma activators are primarily metabolized by the liver. This class of drugs was initially considered to reduce many of the inflammatory pathways associated with diabetes and cardiovascular disease and was also reported to reduce albuminuria to a modest extent.[36] Recently, the Food and Drug Administration restricted use of rosiglitazone because of its association with increased cardiovascular events. Metformin is cleared by the kidney, and its use in CKD is restricted. Because of its effects on impairing mitochondrial function, toxic levels have been associated with severe, life-threatening metabolic lactic acidosis.[37] The Food and Drug Administration guidelines indicate that metformin should not be used in men with a serum creatinine of >1.5 mg/dL or women with a serum creatinine of >1.4 mg/dL.[38] However, it may be preferable to consider a GFR cutoff for metformin use, because serum creatinine can translate into different eGFR levels depending on weight, race, and age. Although clearance of metformin decreases by 75% when the GFR is between 30 and 60 mL/min per 1.73 m^2, the concentrations are only 3% of the levels found in patients with metformin-induced lactic acidosis. However, all patients with metformin-induced lactic acidosis may not have elevated metformin levels. As metformin has an excellent profile to reduce hepatic gluconeogenesis, is not associated with weight gain, and is not linked to cancer, its use may need to be more liberalized.[38] Recently, the British National Formulary recommended that metformin use be reevaluated if GFR is <45 mL/min per 1.73 m^2 and be stopped if the GFR falls to <30 mL/min per 1.73 m^2. Several new hypoglycemic medications have recently been approved for diabetes. The dipeptidyl peptidase 4 inhibitors decrease the breakdown of glucagon-like peptide 1 to improve both fasting and postprandial glucose levels. Examples of this class include sitagliptin, saxagliptin, and linagliptin and can be used in CKD, although dose adjustment is required for sitagliptin and saxagliptin. A recent study[39] identified glucagon-like peptide 1 receptors in the kidney, suggesting there may be direct effects of these drugs on the kidney. As exenatide is excreted by the kidneys and its clearance is reduced when the GFR is reduced to 30 mL/min per 1.73 m^2,[40] it is not recommended for use with a GFR <30 mL/min per 1.73 m^2. There has been much interest in the class of drugs that blocks the sodium-glucose transporter (SGLT2), because it lowers glucose levels, reduces weight, and lowers insulin requirements.[41,42] Recent studies suggest that SGLT2 inhibitors also improve renal function.[43] However, inhibition of SGLT2 results in the loss of about 80 g of glucose in the urine each day,[44] and it has been associated with an increased risk of genitourinary infections.[41,44]

RAS Inhibitors
Primary Prevention
A number of clinical trials have evaluated the efficacy of ACEIs or ARBs for the primary prevention of microalbuminuria in patients with type 1 diabetes mellitus. Three randomized, placebo-controlled trials of 256 to 3,326 patients with type 1 diabetes and normoalbuminiruia (RASS, EUCLID, and DIRECT) showed no benefit from angiotensin inhibition.[45–47] We therefore do not administer these drugs for primary prevention.

Treatment for DKD
The benefit of antihypertensive therapy with an ACEIs in type 1 diabetes can be demonstrated early in the course of the disease when microalbuminuria is the only clinical manifestation. The administration of an ACEIs to normotensive type 1 diabetics with microalbuminuria decreased both albumin excretion and, at 2 years, progression to overt diabetic nephropathy when compared with patients treated with placebo.[48] A more pronounced benefit was demonstrated in the largest trial[49] to date in type 1 diabetic patients who already had overt nephropathy. There has been much less information on the effect of ACEIs in patients with nephropathy due to type 2 diabetes, although a similar benefit appears to be present. More data are currently available on the efficacy of ARBs. In the Irbesartan Diabetic Nephropathy Trial[50] (IDNT), irbesartan was associated with a reduced risk of the combined endpoint (doubling of the plasma creatinine, development of ESRD, or death from any cause). These benefits were independent of the differences in the magnitude of BP reduction among the groups. In the RENAAL trial[51], similar benefits were observed with losartan. ACEIs have been compared with placebo and with ARBs in 2 trials (ADVANCE and DETAIL)[52–53] of patients with type 2 diabetes. The results are consistent with the conclusion that ACEIs are at least as effective as ARBs in diabetic patients with

microalbuminuria. Patients with type 2 diabetes and advanced kidney disease are likely to progress relentlessly to ESRD despite treatment with ACEIs or ARBs, although more slowly. Therefore, the renal protective effect is only partial with either ACEIs or ARBs.

Combination Treatment
ONTARGET[54] and VA NEPHRON-D[55] studies confirmed that combination therapy with ACEI and ARBs does not prevent renal disease progression or death, and it increases the rate of serious adverse events. Thus, combination therapy with an ACEI plus an ARB should not be used in patients with diabetic nephropathy. The use of aliskiren in combination with either an ACEI or ARB does not appear to preserve renal function and increases the risk of adverse events as shown in the multinational Aliskiren Trial in Type 2 Diabetes Using Cardiorenal Endpoints (ALTITUDE).[56]

Potential Side Effects of RAS Inhibition
CKD patients treated with RAS blockade often develop hyperkalemia, and this is particularly common in patients with DKD due to development of type 4 renal tubular acidosis. In most cases, hyperkalemia can be controlled in these patients by giving low K diet and adding of diuretics, which increases the urinary excretion of K. However, in some patients, daily use of kayexalate is required to normalize hyperkalemia. Patients with DKD can also develop AKI with RAS blockade because of reduction of intraglomerular pressure due to relaxation of glomerular efferent artery. This occurs mostly in patients with the combination therapy with RAS inhibition and diuretics, particularly when patients have episodes of poor oral intake and diarrhea. However, these AKI episodes are usually transient and easily reversed by some hydration or discontinuation of diuretics. In severe cases, RAS blockade should be reduced or held until renal function is back to normal. When RAS blockade is initiated in DKD patients, renal function and electrolytes must be checked within 2 weeks to make sure that patients do not develop significant AKI and hyperkalemia. However, if serum creatinine rises less than 30% and remains stable, the same dose of ACEIs or ARBs may be safely continued. A reduction of glomerular filtration in these patients is expected, a sign of beneficial effects of RAS blockade. However, in stage 5 CKD patients, it is recommended to not initiate RAS blockade because of the concerns of

requiring renal replacement therapy with further reduction in GFR.

Treatment of Hypertension
Goals of BP Control in Patients with Diabetes and CKD

The target BP for patients with diabetes and CKD as recommended by the American Diabetes Association[57] and the National Kidney Foundation[58] remains a systolic BP <130 mmHg and a diastolic BP <80 mmHg. There is strong evidence that systolic BP is closely correlated with progression of kidney function in patients with diabetes. In the UK Prospective Diabetes Study,[59] for every 10 mmHg decrease in systolic BP, there was a reduction of microvascular complications by 13%. Post hoc analysis of the Irbesartan in DKD Trial (IDNT) data demonstrate that renal outcome was improved with lowering of systolic BP.[60,61] However, there remains a concern that the systolic BP should not be lowered much below 120 mmHg. In the IDNT study, there was an increase in all-cause mortality in patients who had systolic BP <120 mmHg.[61] In particular, cardiovascular events and congestive heart failure are increased with systolic BP <120 mmHg. In the Action to Control Cardiovascular Risk in Diabetes (ACCORD) study, there was not a significant reduction in the primary composite outcome, and there was a slight increase in the annual rates of death and adverse events in the group with intensive BP control.[26] Therefore, the ideal systolic BP in a patient with diabetes and CKD is thought to be between 120 and 130 mmHg. However, in a patient with diabetes and no CKD, the systolic BP that is adequate may be between 120 and 140 mmHg. A treated systolic BP <120 mmHg in a patient with DKD and underlined cardiac disease may be associated with an increase in cardiovascular events and should be avoided.

Selections of Antihypertensive Medications in DKD

Current standard therapy for patients with diabetes and kidney disease is to provide a RAS blocker as the mainstay of therapy. Initial studies evaluated various classes of calcium channel blockers (CCBs) as monotherapy for patients with diabetes and proteinuria.[62,63] Small studies showed that the dihydropyridine class of CCBs (nifedipine, amlodipine) increased proteinuria, whereas the nondihydropyridine CCBs (diltiazem, verapamil) reduced proteinuria.[62,63] A combination of an ACEI and either a dihydropyridine CCB (amlodipine) or a nondihydropyridine CCB (verapamil) was not found to reduce albuminuria in patients with nondiabetic CKD.[64] However, it is commonly accepted that a combination of an ACEI (or ARB) with a CCB is superior to placebo and equivalent or superior to ACEIs alone for progression of DKD. The benefit of this combination is likely due to an overall reduction in systemic BP with the CCB. The recent Avoiding Cardiovascular Events through Combination Therapy in Patients Living with Systolic Hypertension trial[65] suggests that a combination of an ACEI with diuretic is superior than an ACEI with amlodipine.

Antilipid Treatment for DKD Patients

The role of statins on cardiovascular outcomes in patients with DKD has been clarified somewhat with the results of the Study of Heart and Renal Protection.[66] After 5 years of follow-up, the statin plus ezetimibe therapy was associated with a significant 17% relative risk reduction of the primary clinical outcome of major atherosclerotic events compared with placebo. There was benefit for nonfatal myocardial infarction, nonhemorrhagic stroke, and any revascularization procedure. However, there was no reduction in the risk of all-cause mortality. The effect of treatment on the primary outcome was similar among the diabetic subgroup. Data from the Collaborative Atorvastatin Diabetes Study[67] supported the benefit of statins in patients with diabetes and CKD. Thus, on the basis of the existing evidence, treatment with statins or a statin/ezetimibe combination may be supported to reduce cardiovascular events alone. Reduced dosing of statins and fibric acid derivatives is generally recommended for patients with advanced CKD. The Treating to New Targets[68] trial did report a benefit for secondary prevention of major cardiovascular events from treatment with atorvastatin (80 mg/d compared with 10 mg/d) in 546 patients with diabetes and CKD and pre-existing coronary artery disease over 5 years of follow-up. There was a 32% reduction in the relative risk of major cardiovascular events in patients with CKD (with and without diabetes). Therefore, the data support the use of statins as secondary prevention in patients with diabetes and kidney disease. In the absence of a known cardiovascular event, there are data to support the use of statins as primary prevention for cardiovascular events. The lack of improvement in overall mortality is unexplained and remains a concern in these patients.

Nonmedication Intervention for DKD Patients

It remains uncertain whether dietary protein restriction slows the long-term decline in GFR in DKD. There are at least 2 explanations for the relative lack of benefit of a low-protein diet on GFR in the last study compared to the 2 previous trials. First, the difference in protein intake between the 2 groups was probably substantially less in the last trial (0.89 vs. 1.02 g/kg per day). Second, BP, albuminuria, and glycemia were aggressively and similarly controlled in both groups. Given that these factors are independent and significant risk factors for deterioration in GFR, the ability to detect subtle differences in the rate of decline due to protein restriction alone may have been masked. There are several potential problems associated with a low-protein diet. In addition to difficulty with compliance due to concurrent fat and simple carbohydrate restriction, diabetics are at increased risk for protein malnutrition because the reduction in intake may be associated with enhanced protein breakdown induced by insulin deficiency.[69] Marked decreases in proteinuria may be observed in obese diabetics who lose weight.[70] Cigarette smoking represents another important factor associated with progression of DKD, and, therefore, smoking cessation is highly recommended in these patients.

Diabetes and ESRD

Diabetic patients with ESRD are candidates for HD, peritoneal dialysis (PD), and kidney transplant. Among the prevalent US ESRD population, patients with diabetes are more likely to be maintained by HD and less likely by kidney transplant than their nondiabetic counterparts. The fraction maintained by PD is small and similar among individuals with and without diabetes. Data from the US Medicare registry indicate a 10% to 20% survival advantage for HD over PD in patients aged >45 years with diabetes. The advantage of HD over PD was most apparent among those older patients with coincident cardiovascular disease. Conversely, PD confers survival advantage over HD for diabetic individuals aged <45 years without cardiovascular comorbidity.[71] Diabetic patients on PD undergo more rapid peritoneal fibrosis, hyperpermeability, and loss of ultrafiltration than their nondiabetic counterparts; the relative risk of death associated with PD/HD only emerges after 24 months on therapy.[72] Finally, it is possible that more hemodynamically tenuous patients are disproportionately assigned to PD, based on the perception of PD as gentler therapy. The evidence also suggests that patients with residual renal function would be better to start on PD instead of HD.

Both survival and medical rehabilitation of patients with diabetes and ESRD is superior after renal transplantation, with or without pancreas transplantation (for those with type 1 diabetes mellitus).[73,74] In diabetes, preemptive living donor transplantation before initiation of dialysis is preferred, although infrequently performed.[75] Cardiovascular risk is a major concern for diabetics contemplating transplant. The cardiovascular mortality is greater in those who list diabetes as the cause of ESRD, rather than as a comorbidity.[73]

REFERENCES

1. Collins AJ, Kasiske B, Herzog C, et al. Excerpts from the United States Renal Data System 2004 annual data report: atlas of end-stage renal disease in the United States. *Am J Kidney Dis.* 2005;45 (1 Suppl 1):A5–A7, S1–S280.
2. Centers for Disease Control. Incidence of end-stage renal disease attributed to diabetes among persons with diagnosed diabetes—United States and Puerto Rico, 1996–2007. *MMWR Morb Mortal Wkly Rep.* 2010;59:1361–1366.
3. Orchard TJ, Dorman JS, Maser RE, et al. Prevalence of complications in IDDM by sex and duration. Pittsburgh Epidemiology of Diabetes Complications Study II. *Diabetes.* 1990;39:1116–1124.
4. Nathan DM, Cleary PA, Backlund JY, et al. Modern-day clinical course of type 1 diabetes mellitus after 30 years' duration: the diabetes control and complications trial/epidemiology of diabetes interventions and complications and Pittsburgh epidemiology of diabetes complications experience (1983–2005). *Arch Intern Med.* 2009;169:1307–1316.
5. Krolewski AS, Warram JH, Freire MB. Epidemiology of late diabetic complications: a basis for the development and evaluation of preventive programs. *Endocrinol Metab Clin North Am.* 1996;25:217–242.
6. Thomas MC, Groop PH, Tryggvason K. Towards understanding the inherited susceptibility for nephropathy in diabetes. *Curr Opin Nephrol Hypertens.* 2012;21:195–202.
7. Premaratne E, Macisaac RJ, Tsalamandris C, Panagiotopoulos S, Smith T, Jerums G. Renal

hyperfiltration in type 2 diabetes: effect of age-related decline in glomerular filtration rate. *Diabetologia.* 2005;48:2486–2493.

8. Brownlee, M. Biochemistry and molecular cell biology of diabetic complications. *Nature.* 2001;414:813–820.

9. You H, Gao T, Cooper TK, Brian Reeves W, Awad AS. Macrophages directly mediate diabetic renal injury. *Am J Physiol Renal Physiol.* 2013;305:F1719–F1727.

10. Najafian B, Mauer M. Progression of diabetic nephropathy in type 1 diabetic patients. *Diabetes Res Clin Pract.* 2009;83:1–8.

11. Najafian B, Alpers CE, Fogo AB. Pathology of human diabetic nephropathy. *Contrib Nephrol.* 2011;170:36–47.

12. Perkins BA, Ficociello LH, Silva KH, Finkelstein DM, Warram JH, Krolewski AS. Regression of microalbuminuria in type 1 diabetes. *N Engl J Med.* 2003;348:2285–2293.

13. de Boer IH, Rue TC, Cleary PA, et al. Intensive diabetes therapy and glomerular filtration rate in type 1 diabetes. *N Engl J Med.* 2011;365:2366–2376.

14. Perkins BA, Ficociello LH, Roshan B, Warram JH, Krolewski AS. In patients with type 1 diabetes and new-onset microalbuminuria the development of advanced chronic kidney disease may not require progression to proteinuria. *Kidney Int.* 2010;77:57–64.

15. Onuigbo MA. Can ACE inhibitors and angiotensin receptor blockers be detrimental in CKD patients? *Nephron Clin Pract.* 2011;118:407–c419.

16. Altemtam N, Russell J. El Nahas M. A study of the natural history of diabetic kidney disease (DKD). *Nephrol Dial Transplant.* 2012:27:1847–1854.

17. Ayodele OE, Alebiosu CO, Salako BL. Diabetic nephropathy—a review of the natural history, burden, risk factors and treatment. *J Natl Med Assoc.* 2004;96:1445–1454.

18. National Kidney Foundation. KDOQI clinical practice guideline for diabetes and CKD: 2012 update. *Am J Kidney Dis.* 2012;60:850–886.

19. Ellam TJ. Albumin:creatinine ratio—a flawed measure? The merits of estimated albuminuria reporting. *Nephron Clin Pract.* 2011;118:c324–c330.

20. Guidone C, Castagneto-Gissey L, Leccesi L, Arrighi E, Iaconelli A, Mingrone G. Underestimation of urinary albumin to creatinine ratio in morbidly obese subjects due to high urinary creatinine excretion. *Clin Nutr.* 2012;31:212–216.

21. Kramer HJ, Nguyen QD, Curhan G, Hsu CY. Renal insufficiency in the absence of albuminuria and retinopathy among adults with type 2 diabetes mellitus. *J Am Med Assoc.* 2003;289:3273–3277.

22. Diabetes Control and Complications Trial Research Group. The effect of intensive treatment of diabetes on the development and progression of long-term complications in insulin-dependent diabetes mellitus. *N Engl J Med.* 1993;329:977–986.

23. UK Prospective Diabetes Study Group UKPDS 28: a randomized trial of efficacy of early addition of metformin in sulfonylurea-treated type 2 diabetes. *Diabetes Care.* 1998;21:87–92.

24. Levin SR, Coburn JW, Abraira C, et al. Veterans Affairs Cooperative Study on Glycemic Control and Complications in Type 2 Diabetes Feasibility Trial Investigators. Effect of intensive glycemic control on microalbuminuria in type 2 diabetes. *Diabetes Care.* 2000;23:1478–1485.

25. Patel A, MacMahon S, Chalmers J, et al. Intensive blood glucose control and vascular outcomes in patients with type 2 diabetes. *N Engl J Med.* 2008;358:2560–2572.

26. Cushman WC, Evans GW, Byington RP, et al. Effects of intensive blood-pressure control in type 2 diabetes mellitus. *N Engl J Med.* 2010;362:1575–1585.

27. Duckworth W, Abraira C, Moritz T, et al. Glucose control and vascular complications in veterans with type 2 diabetes. *N Engl J Med.* 2009;360:129–139.

28. Kalantar-Zadeh K, Kopple JD, Regidor DL, et al. A1C and survival in maintenance hemodialysis patients. *Diabetes Care.* 2007;30:1049–1055.

29. Gerstein HC, Miller ME, Byington RP, et al. Action to control cardiovascular risk in diabetes study group. *N Engl J Med.* 2008;358(24):2545–2559.

30. Inaba M, Okuno S, Kumeda Y, et al. Glycated albumin is a better glycemic indicator than glycated hemoglobin values in hemodialysis patients with diabetes: effect of anemia and erythropoietin injection. *J Am Soc Nephrol.* 2007;18:896–903.

31. Riveline JP, Teynie J, Belmouaz S, et al. Glycaemic control in type 2 diabetic patients on chronic haemodialysis: use of a continuous glucose monitoring system. *Nephrol Dial Transplant.* 2009;24:2866–2871.

32. Freedman BI, Shihabi ZK, Andries L, et al. Relationship between assays of glycemia in diabetic subjects with advanced chronic kidney disease. *Am J Nephrol.* 2010;31:375–379.

33. Riveline JP, Hadjadj S. Assessing glycemic control in maintenance hemodialysis patients with type 2 diabetes: response to Kazempour-Ardebili. *Diabetes Care.* 2009;32:e155; author reply e156.

34. Rabkin R, Ryan MP, Duckworth WC. The renal metabolism of insulin. *Diabetologia.* 1984;27:351–357.

35. Kalantar-Zadeh K, et al. Burnt-out diabetes: impact of chronic kidney disease progression on the natural course of diabetes mellitus. *J Ren Nutr.* 2009;19:33–37.

36. Bakris G, Ruilope LM, McMorn SO, et al. Differences in glucose tolerance between fixed-dose antihypertensive drug combinations in people with metabolic syndrome. *Diabetes Care.* 2006;29:2592–2597.

37. Kovesdy CP, Sharma K, Kalantar-Zadeh K. Glycemic control in diabetic CKD patients: where do we stand? *Am J Kidney Dis.* 2008;52:766–777.

38. Lipska KJ, Bailey CJ, Inzucchi SE. Use of metformin in the setting of mild-to-moderate renal insufficiency. *Diabetes Care.* 2011;34:1431–1437.

39. Park CW, Kim HW, Ko SH, et al. Long-term treatment of glucagon-like peptide-1 analog exendin-4 ameliorates diabetic nephropathy through improving metabolic anomalies in db/db mice. *J Am Soc Nephrol.* 2007;18:1227–1238.

40. Linnebjerg H, Kothare PA, Park S, et al. Effect of renal impairment on the pharmacokinetics of exenatide. *Br J Clin Pharmacol.* 2007;64:317–327.

41. Wilding JP, Woo V, Soler NG, et al. Long-term efficacy of dapagliflozin in patients with type 2 diabetes mellitus receiving high doses of insulin: a randomized trial. *Ann Intern Med.* 2012;156:405–415.

42. Vallon V, Komers R. Pathophysiology of the diabetic kidney. *Compr Physiol.* 2011;1:1175–1232.

43. Wanner C, Inzucchi SE, Zinman B. Empagliflozin and progression of kidney disease in type 2 diabetes. *N Engl J Med.* 2016;375:1801–1802.

44. Neumiller JJ, White JR Jr., Campbell RK. Sodium-glucose co-transport inhibitors: progress and therapeutic potential in type 2 diabetes mellitus. *Drugs.* 2010;70:377–385.

45. The EUCLID Study Group. Randomised placebo-controlled trial of lisinopril in normotensive patients with insulin-dependent diabetes and normoalbuminuria or microalbuminuria. *Lancet.* 1997;349:1787–1792.

46. Mauer M, Zinman B, Gardiner R, et al. Renal and retinal effects of enalapril and losartan in type 1 diabetes. *N Engl J Med.* 2009;361:40–51.

47. Bilous R, Chaturvedi N, Sjølie AK, et al. Effect of candesartan on microalbuminuria and albumin excretion rate in diabetes: three randomized trials. *Ann Intern Med.* 2009;151:11–20, W13–W14.

48. Viberti G, Mogensen CE, Groop LC, Pauls JF. European Microalbuminuria Captopril Study Group. Effect of captopril on progression to clinical proteinuria in patients with insulin-dependent diabetes mellitus and microalbuminuria. *J Am Med Assoc.* 1994;271:275–279.

49. Lewis EJ, Hunsicker LG, Bain RP, Rohde RD. The Collaborative Study Group. The effect of angiotensin-converting-enzyme inhibition on diabetic nephropathy. *N Engl J Med.* 1993;329:1456–1462.

50. Lewis EJ, Hunsicker LG, Clarke WR, et al. Collaborative Study Group: Renoprotective effect of the angiotensin-receptor antagonist irbesartan in patients with nephropathy due to type 2 diabetes. *N Engl J Med.* 2001;345:851–860.

51. Brenner BM, Cooper ME, de Zeeuw D, et al. RENAAL Study Investigators: Effects of losartan on renal and cardiovascular outcomes in patients with type 2 diabetes and nephropathy. *N Engl J Med.* 2001;345:861–869.

52. Patel A, ADVANCE Collaborative Group, MacMahon S, et al. Effects of a fixed combination of perindopril and indapamide on macrovascular and microvascular outcomes in patients with type 2 diabetes mellitus (the ADVANCE trial): a randomised controlled trial. *Lancet.* 2007;370:829.

53. Barnett AH, Bain SC, Bouter P, et al. Angiotensin-receptor blockade versus converting-enzyme inhibition in type 2 diabetes and nephropathy. *N Engl J Med.* 2004;351:1952.

54. Cai W, He JC, Zhu L, Chen X, Striker GE, Vlassara H. AGE-receptor-1 counteracts cellular oxidant stress induced by AGEs via negative regulation of p66shc-dependent FKHRL1 phosphorylation. *Am J Physiol Cell Physiol.* 2008;294:C145–C152.

55. Fried LF, Emanuele N, Zhang JH, et al. Combined angiotensin inhibition for the treatment of diabetic nephropathy. *N Engl J Med.* 2013;369:1892–1903.

56. Parving HH, Brenner BM, McMurray JJ, et al. Cardiorenal end points in a trial of aliskiren for type 2 diabetes. *N Engl J Med.* 2012;367:2204–2213.

57. Tuttle KR, Bakris GL, Bilous RW, et al. Diabetic kidney disease: a report from an ADA Consensus Conference. *Am J Kidney Dis.* 2014;64:510–533.

58. Taler SJ, Agarwal R, Bakris GL, et al. KDOQI US commentary on the 2012 KDIGO clinical practice guideline for management of blood pressure in CKD. *Am J Kidney Dis.* 2013;62:201–213.

59. Bretzel RG, Voigt K, Schatz H. The United Kingdom Prospective Diabetes Study (UKPDS) implications for the pharmacotherapy of type 2 diabetes mellitus. *Exp Clin Endocrinol Diabetes.* 1998;106:369–372.

60. Berl T, Hunsicker LG, Lewis JB, et al. Impact of achieved blood pressure on cardiovascular outcomes in the Irbesartan Diabetic Nephropathy Trial. *J Am Soc Nephrol.* 2005;16:2170–2179.

61. Pohl MA, Blumenthal S, Cordonnier DJ, et al. Independent and additive impact of blood pressure control and angiotensin II receptor blockade on renal outcomes in the irbesartan diabetic nephropathy trial: clinical implications and limitations. *J Am Soc Nephrol.* 2005;16:3027–3037.

62. Bakris GL, Copley JB, Vicknair N, Sadler R, Leurgans S. Calcium channel blockers versus other antihypertensive therapies on progression

of NIDDM associated nephropathy. *Kidney Int.* 1996;50:1641–1650.

63. Abbott K, Smith A, Bakri, GL. Effects of dihydropyridine calcium antagonists on albuminuria in patients with diabetes. *J Clin Pharmacol.* 1996;36:274–279.

64. Boero R, Rollino C, Massara C, et al. How well are hypertension and albuminuria treated in type II diabetic patients? *J Hum Hypertens.* 2003;17:413–418.

65. Bakris GL, Sarafidis PA, Weir MR, et al. ACCOMPLISH Trial investigators: Renal outcomes with different fixed-dose combination therapies in patients with hypertension at high risk for cardiovascular events (ACCOMPLISH): a prespecified secondary analysis of a randomised controlled trial. *Lancet.* 2010;375:1173–1181.

66. Baigent C, Landray MJ, Reith C, et al. The effects of lowering LDL cholesterol with simvastatin plus ezetimibe in patients with chronic kidney disease (Study of Heart and Renal Protection): a randomised placebo-controlled trial. *Lancet.* 2011;377:2181–2192.

67. Colhoun HM, Betteridge DJ, Durrington PN, et al. Effects of atorvastatin on kidney outcomes and cardiovascular disease in patients with diabetes: an analysis from the Collaborative Atorvastatin Diabetes Study (CARDS). *Am J Kidney Dis.* 2009;54:810–819.

68. Shepherd J, Kastelein JJ, Bittner V, et al. Intensive lipid lowering with atorvastatin in patients with coronary heart disease and chronic kidney disease: the TNT (Treating to New Targets) study. *J Am Coll Cardiol.* 2008;51:1448–1454.

69. Brodsky IG, Robbins DC, Hiser E, et al. Effects of low-protein diets on protein metabolism in insulin-dependent diabetes mellitus patients with early nephropathy. *J Clin Endocrinol Metab.* 1992;75:351–357.

70. Morales E, Valero MA, Leon M, Hernandez E, Praga M. Beneficial effects of weight loss in overweight patients with chronic proteinuric nephropathies. *Am J Kidney Dis.* 2003;41:319–327.

71. Vonesh EF, Snyder JJ, Foley RN, Collins AJ. Mortality studies comparing peritoneal dialysis and hemodialysis: what do they tell us? *Kidney Int Suppl,* 2006;103:S3–11.

72. Termorshuizen F, Korevaar JC, Dekker FW, Van Manen JG, Boeschoten EW, Krediet RT. Hemodialysis and peritoneal dialysis: comparison of adjusted mortality rates according to the duration of dialysis: analysis of the Netherlands Cooperative Study on the Adequacy of Dialysis 2. *J Am Soc Nephrol.* 2003;14:2851–2860.

73. Giri M. Choice of renal replacement therapy in patients with diabetic end stage renal disease. *EDTNA ERCA J.* 2004;30:138–142.

74. Locatelli F, Pozzoni P, Del Vecchio L. Renal replacement therapy in patients with diabetes and end-stage renal disease. *J Am Soc Nephrol.* 2004;15(Suppl 1):S25–S29.

75. Locatelli F, Del Vecchio L, Pozzoni P, Manzoni C. Nephrology: main advances in the last 40 years. *J Nephrol.* 2006;19:6–11.

29

Hypertension and the Kidney

RUPINDER K. SODHI, MARIE D. PHILIPNERI, AND PAUL G. SCHMITZ

INTRODUCTION

Hypertension affects 73 million Americans (35 million men and 38 million women) and is one of the most common treatable risk factors for stroke, myocardial infarction, and progressive kidney disease.[1] Hypertension is responsible for 1 in 6 deaths in the United States and imposes an enormous economic demand on the healthcare system (>$75 billion in 2009). A specific cause of hypertension is discovered in <15% of all patients with an elevated blood pressure (e.g., secondary hypertension). In patients without a known cause, high blood pressure is referred to as primary or essential hypertension. The National Health and Nutrition Examination Survey (NHANES)[2] data estimates that 24% of individuals without chronic kidney disease (CKD) have hypertension. Approximately 36% of individuals with stage 1 CKD have hypertension, which increases to 84% in individuals with stages 4 and 5 CKD. The Kidney Early Evaluation Program (KEEP)[2] database estimates a similar prevalence of hypertension in CKD.

CLASSIFICATION AND EPIDEMIOLOGY

For 4 decades, an expert panel appointed by the National Heart, Lung and Blood Institute has prepared guidelines for the classification and management of hypertension. The Eighth Report (JNC 8) was published in 20014.[3] The JNC 8 differed considerably from previous reports, principally addressing blood pressure goals rather than the long-awaited revision of JNC 7. Despite the focused objectives of JNC 8, as of this writing, it has not been endorsed by the National Heart, Lung, and Blood Institute, American College of Cardiology, American Heart Association, American Society of Hypertension, or American Society of Nephrology. In light of the considerable controversy and fragmented support, we have chosen to use the JNC 7 as a template for this chapter, while incorporating recently published data to provide updated generally accepted approaches to the evaluation of hypertension.

The JNC 7 classifies hypertension into 4 categories, which reflect the cardiovascular risk of high blood pressure. Perhaps the most controversial issue in the classification scheme was the inclusion of the prehypertension category. The rationale for including this group was as follows:

- Patients with prehypertension usually progress to stage 1 hypertension if they live long enough.[4]
- The rate of progression to stage 1 hypertension can be relatively rapid, and, therefore, these patients should be monitored regularly for the development of stage 1 hypertension.[4]
- Patients with prehypertension are at higher risk for cardiovascular events and are more likely to exhibit cardiovascular risk factors (hyperlipidemia, diabetes, obesity) than normotensive patients.[5,6]
- Patients with prehypertension should be instructed in healthy lifestyle habits and, in some cases, be placed on drug therapy (e.g., when accompanied by additional cardiac risk factors).[7]

NHANES is designed to monitor the health and nutritional status of adults and children in the United States. In 1999, NHANES became a continuous program, which is focused on specific need-based health issues; however, data on high blood pressure are available from 1976. Trends in the awareness, treatment, and control of hypertension have been recently summarized.[8] Despite intensive efforts at physician and patient education the number of patients with controlled hypertension (defined as systolic blood pressure [SBP] <140 mmHg and diastolic blood pressure [DBP] <90 mmHg) is approximately 50% among all adults with hypertension.

PITFALLS OF BLOOD PRESSURE MEASUREMENTS

White Coat Hypertension

White coat hypertension, or hypertension only in the physician's office, is reported in up to 20% of patients diagnosed with hypertension.[9] White coat hypertension is defined as a clinic blood pressure of ≥140/90 mmHg on at least 3 occasions, with at least 2 sets of measurements of <140/90 mmHg in nonclinical settings, plus the absence of target-organ damage. Most evidence indicates that white coat hypertension is not associated with an increased incidence of cardiovascular events and should not be treated. However, the development of overt hypertension is higher in these patients; thus, regular monitoring should be employed.[10,11]

Pseudohypertension

Overestimation of the blood pressure may occur in patients with severely arteriosclerotic blood vessels because the vessel is poorly compressible with a standard cuffed sphygmomanometer. If such a condition is believed to exist, direct intraarterial measurements may be required.

Nocturnal Blood Pressure

Twenty-four-hour ambulatory blood pressure measurements reveal variations in blood pressure that follow a circadian pattern.[11] Blood pressure variability occurs throughout the daytime hours and falls to its lowest level 1 to 2 hours after sleep (referred to as "dipping").[12] Blood pressure increases sharply in the early morning hours, during the transition from sleep to wakefulness. Some patients do not exhibit dipping (e.g., "nondippers") and are at higher risk for cardiovascular events.[13] Nondipping is very common in African Americans and individuals with CKD or autonomic nervous system disease.[13] Nondipping has also been associated with increased sympathetic nervous system activity and glucocorticoid administration.[13]

Masked Hypertension

Masked hypertension is an intriguing variant of hypertension that presents as the polar opposite of white coat hypertension (i.e., hypertension at home, with normal blood pressures in the office). The prevalence of masked hypertension is believed to exceed 10% in the general population and as high as 30% in at-risk populations.[14,15] Importantly, these patients have an increased relative risk of cardiovascular events and should be treated. Since blood pressure measurements are normal in the office, at home blood pressure measurements are the only method to diagnose masked hypertension.

Blood Pressure Variability

Although some fluctuation in blood pressure invariably accompanies hypertension, dramatic, frequent variations are unusual. Anxiety and panic attacks are the most common causes of labile hypertension. Labile hypertension has been reported in pheochromocytoma. Recent studies suggest that adjusting the timing of drug administration to reduce lability (e.g., evening and split doses) may reduce cardiovascular events.[16,17]

Isolated Systolic Hypertension

Isolated systolic hypertension (ISH) is defined as SBP >160 mmHg and DBP <90 mmHg.[18,19] The predominant blood pressure variant in patients >50 is ISH. The SBP increases in a linear fashion throughout life, whereas, the DBP increases until approximately age 50 and decreases thereafter.[20] Several large population-based studies have shown that the SBP is a greater risk factor for the development of cardiovascular disease than the DBP.[20] Acknowledgement of the risk of ISH reflects an important paradigm shift in the management of hypertension. The JNC 6 amended the 2000 report to reflect these observations and further suggest that the SBP (not DBP) be the primary end point of antihypertensive therapy in patients after the age of 50.[21]

The mechanism responsible for ISH reflects a gradual increase in arterial stiffness (due to remodeling and calcification of the vessel wall).[22] The less-compliant vessel cannot stretch during systole, resulting in an augmented SBP. Conversely, the loss of elastic recoil during diastole (which augments diastolic pressure) decreases the DBP. Since arterial stiffness is governed by vascular remodeling, ISH is tantamount to a diseased blood vessel.

Several large randomized studies have shown that treatment of ISH with a diuretic, beta blocker, or calcium channel blocker produces a 25% to 50% decrease in the incidence of cardiovascular events, even in patients >80 years of age, regardless of gender.[23-25] Importantly, there was a 30% reduction in the rate of stroke and a 21% reduction in the rate of death in the treatment group of Hypertension in the Very Elderly Trial[23] ($p <$ 0.01). A reduction in death rate was observed within 6 months of initiation of therapy.

HYPERTENSIVE KIDNEY DISEASE—AN ENIGMA

Although considerable evidence indicates that hypertension accelerates kidney injury, its role in the initiation of kidney disease is surprisingly controversial.[26] There are several compelling arguments that cast doubt on the role of hypertension in promoting kidney injury, including:

- Of the 70 million Americans with hypertension, less than 1% exhibit progressive kidney injury.
- The majority of patients with a diagnosis of hypertension-associated kidney disease have not undergone kidney biopsy.
- Hypertension develops in the vast majority of patients with kidney disease, regardless of the underlying diagnosis.
- Recent studies indicate that hypertensive-associated renal disease develops in genetically susceptible patients. Specifically, African Americans with polymorphisms in the motor protein, nonmuscle myosin 2a, or MYH9 (a protein expressed in podocytes) were more likely to develop kidney failure if they were hypertensive compared to individuals without these polymorphisms.[27-29]

Hypertension is almost always characterized by pathological changes in the renal microvasculature. However, it is not possible to predict which patients will develop kidney injury based on pathological changes. Indeed, the typical vascular changes described in hypertension are so common that most refer to the pathology as "benign nephrosclerosis." Notably, malignant or severe hypertension produces severe vascular damage and acute kidney injury.

Pathology of the Kidney in Hypertension

Benign nephrosclerosis is characterized by small, atrophic kidneys that exhibit a finely granular surface (leather-like) on gross examination. Light microscopy reveals hyaline arteriolosclerosis with thickening of walls of the small arteries and arterioles, narrowed lumens, and atrophy of glomeruli and tubules with interstitial fibrosis. The larger interlobar and arcuate arteries reveal fibroelastic hyperplasia with duplication of the internal elastic lamina and fibrous thickening of the media.

Malignant nephrosclerosis is a serious clinical syndrome characterized by papilledema, encephalopathy, and acute kidney injury. The kidneys are normal to small with surface hemorrhages due to rupture of the arterioles and capillaries. The appearance is referred to as a "flea-bitten" kidney. Necrotizing arteriolitis with fibrinoid necrosis of the arterioles and small arteries with mild inflammatory infiltrates is seen microscopically. Thrombotic microangiopathy involving the glomerular capillaries, interlobular arteries, and larger arterioles is often observed. Vascular changes characterized by intimal proliferation or "onion skinning" (concentric proliferation of smooth muscle cells) is also common.

Regardless of the original cause, once the glomerular filtration rate (GFR) reaches a critical threshold (~30–60 mL/min), adaptive changes occur locally and systemically that perpetuate the injury (Fig 29.1).[29]

Recently, Griffin and colleague[30] have proposed that susceptibility to hypertension-induced renal disease (HIRD) should be quantitatively assessed in terms of blood pressure threshold for HIRD and the slope of the relationship between blood pressure and HIRD. The application of such a concept is illustrated in Figure 29.2. Moreover, this group has utilized radiotelemetry monitoring of blood pressure in several rodent models of hypertension and renal injury, revealing conceptually consistent data. An essential aspect of the "burden of blood pressure" concept is illuminated in the context of autoregulation of the preglomerular vessel. For example, in diabetes, the afferent arteriolar autoregulation is impaired, which promotes increased barotrauma to the glomerular capillaries at any given blood pressure.[31] Malignant hypertension exceeds the autoregulatory limits of the afferent arteriole resulting in transmission of pressure to the glomerular capillaries, producing hydrostatic injury. Finally, nephron loss eventually impairs renal autoregulation in the remnant nephrons, which accelerates renal injury from hypertension. Conceptually, this paradigm does not depend on blood pressure-independent effects of presumed mediators of hypertension (e.g., angiotensin II).

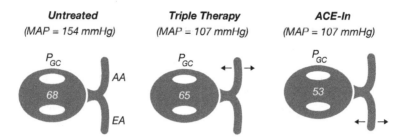

FIGURE 29.1 Experimental model of renal fibrosis illustrates the relationship between mean arterial pressure (MAP), afferent arteriolar resistance, efferent arteriolar resistance (EA), and glomerular capillary hydrostatic pressure (P_{GC}) in 3 groups of five-sixth nephrectomized rats. Untreated rats are hypertensive and have an elevated P_{GC} (normal ~45 mmHg). When the MAP is reduced with triple therapy (hydralazine/reserpine/HCTZ), renal fibrosis and proteinuria are unchanged. Since AA resistance decreased with triple therapy, the P_{GC} remained elevated. However, sustained angiotensin converting enzyme inhibitor (ACEI) use selectively reduces EA resistance and elicits a fall in P_{GC} compared to triple therapy. Since ACEIs, but not triple therapy, reduce renal fibrosis and proteinuria, it is concluded that elevated P_{GC} is responsible for progressive renal scarring. Moreover, agents that selectively reduce intraglomerular pressure confer a unique benefit in human and experimental models of progressive renal fibrosis.

Hemodynamic Manipulation

Sustained inhibition of converting-enzyme offers a selective advantage over other antihypertensive agents by engendering a reduction in glomerular pressure (P_{GC}) and protein excretion. Figure 29.1 depicts the relationship between mean arterial pressure (MAP), arteriolar resistance, and P_{GC} in 3 groups of rats with progressive renal fibrosis. Untreated rats exhibit severe systemic and glomerular hypertension and rapidly develop renal fibrosis. When the MAP was reduced with triple therapy, P_{GC} and renal fibrosis were unaffected.[32] In contrast, inhibition of converting-enzyme, reduced P_{GC}, and attenuated renal fibrosis.

Several controlled clinical studies in humans have confirmed the beneficial effects of converting-enzyme inhibition in CKD. Angiotensin receptor blocking agents have been recently shown to confer similar benefits on progressive renal fibrosis.[33–37]

CLINICAL STUDIES ASSESSING THE RENAL EFFECTS OF HYPERTENSION

Numerous clinical studies assess the renal effects of hypertension.[38] The Multiple Risk Factor Intervention Trial[39] revealed that individuals developing ESRD had higher baseline mean SBP

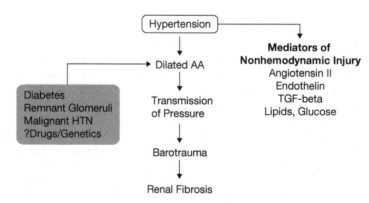

FIGURE 29.2 Model of hypertension-induced renal disease based on barotrauma to the renal microvessels with subsequent fibrosis. In this model, susceptible patients transmit more systemic pressure to the glomerular capillaries because of impaired autoregulation (i.e., dilated afferent arteriole). The pressure induces barotrauma analogous to malignant hypertension. Drugs that selectively effect the afferent arteriole may engender changes in susceptibility to systemic pressures. HTN = hypertension. AA = ascending aorta.

and DBP than individuals without ESRD (SBP 142 vs. 135 mmHg; DBP 93 vs. 91 mmHg, both $p < 0.001$).

In the Veterans Affairs hospital population, a systolic blood pressure of ≥150 mmHg carried a hazard ratio of 9.1 for progression to a renal endpoint. Furthermore, rates of progression to ESRD were a function of blood pressure control with incidence rates of 7.2%, 27.7%, and 71.4% among those with SBP of <130 mmHg, <150 mmHg, and >150 mmHg, respectively.[40] CKD progression is even more rapid among those with diabetes and uncontrolled blood pressures. The Reduction of Endpoints in Noninsulin-Dependent Diabetes Mellitus with the Angiotensin II Antagonist Losartan (RENAAL)[41] trial examined the effects of losartan on renal outcomes among those with diabetic nephropathy (albuminuria ≥300 mg/g; serum creatinine 1.3–3.0 mg/dL). Baseline SBP >160 mmHg was independently associated with progression to a doubling of serum creatinine, ESRD, or death. Additionally, the lower the blood pressure achieved, the slower the progression of CKD and ESRD. Similar results were observed in patients enrolled in the Irbesartan Diabetic Nephropathy Trial.[42]

CONTROL OF BLOOD PRESSURE AND CKD PROGRESSION

In the Modification of Diet in Renal Disease study,[43] individuals with nondiabetic CKD (mean GFR 39 mL/min; mean proteinuria 1.1 g/day) were randomized to tight or usual MAP with achieved MAP of 91 mmHg (125/75 mmHg) or 96 mmHg (130/80 mmHg), respectively. After 3 years, the rate of GFR decline was identical in both arms (11.5 mL/min). However, among those with greater than 3 g/day of proteinuria, GFR decline was 10.2 mL/min in the usual blood pressure group versus 6.7 mL/min in tight control group. After an additional 6 years of follow-up, during which no blood pressure goal was specified and blood pressures not measured, those randomized to the intensive arm were 33% less likely to require dialysis. However, this benefit was driven exclusively by lower rates of ESRD in those with at least 1 g/day of proteinuria.[43]

The African American Study of Kidney Disease trial[44] evaluated the effects of intensive blood pressure control on CKD progression. The trial found that 1,100 African Americans with a mean GFR of 46 mL/min and 600 mg of proteinuria achieved a blood pressure goal of either 128/78 mmHg (intensive therapy) or 141/85 mmHg

(usual care). Over 4 years of follow-up, the rate of GFR decline was nearly identical in both groups (2.1 mL/min/year). The Ramipril Efficacy in Nephropathy-2[45] tested a similar premise with ramipril in patients with immunoglobulin A nephropathy (mean GFR 35 mL/min; mean proteinuria 2.9 g/d). Achieved blood pressures were 130/80 mmHg (intensive group) and 134/82 mmHg (usual care). Intensive blood pressure control failed to result in further slowing of GFR decline (mean decline 2.6 mL/min in both groups) over 18 months of follow-up, an outcome noted irrespective of degree of pretreatment proteinuria. In the aggregate, these studies indicate that control of blood pressure to less than 130/80 mmHg fails to further slow progression of nondiabetic CKD; however, there may be a modest benefit among those with proteinuria in excess of 2 to 3 g/d.

The lack of prospective trials evaluating the effects of lower blood pressure targets on the progression of diabetic nephropathy has resulted in a limited understanding of optimal blood pressure goals.

The Appropriate Blood Pressure Control trial[46] has been the only attempt at prevention of CKD progression in type 2 diabetic patients. The study evaluated the effects of achieved blood pressure goals of 128/75 mmHg (intensive) versus 137/81 mmHg (usual care) among 500 normotensive individuals with type 2 diabetes, one-third of whom had diabetic nephropathy. After 5 years of follow up, no change in the rate of GFR decline was noted between groups. Moreover, the study was extended by 2.5 years, and still no difference was noted, albeit both groups had very slow decline in GFR.

FUTURE DIRECTIONS IN RESEARCH AND THERAPY

A recent subanalysis of the Systolic Blood Pressure Intervention Trial (SPRINT)[45] trial revealed that intensive blood pressure lowering (<120 mmHg) resulted in more frequent episodes of AKI (as defined and staged by modified KDIGO criteria[46]). Of the 288 participants with AKI, 179 were in the intensive arm as compared to 109 in the standard arm. Most cases were mild, and most participants had complete recovery of kidney function.

The risks of baseline DBP on outcomes in SPRINT was also recently addressed.[47] However, the effects of the intensive SBP intervention on the primary outcome were not influenced by baseline DBP level (interaction $p = 0.83$). The primary outcome hazard ratio for intensive versus standard treatment was 0.78 (95%confidence interval : 0.57–1.07) in the lowest DBP quintile (mean baseline DBP, 61±5 mmHg) and 0.74 (95% confidence interval: 0.61–0.90) in the upper 4 DBP quintiles (mean baseline DBP, 82±9 mmHg), with an interaction p value of 0.78. Although low baseline DBP was associated with increased risk of cardiovascular disease events, there was no evidence that the benefit of the intensive SBP lowering differed by baseline DBP.

Cheung et al.[48] examined outcomes in participants with baseline CKD in SPRINT. In their poststudy analysis, patients with CKD and hypertension without diabetes exhibited reduced rates of major cardiovascular events and all-cause death in the intensive arm without evidence of effect modifications by CKD or deleterious effect on the main kidney outcome.

Considerable evidence suggests that vascular wall remodeling precedes overt hypertension and progressive renal fibrosis. Therefore, employing noninvasive measurements of arterial compliance has emerged as a proxy for the hypertensive state. It is conceivable that pharmacologic therapy will be targeted at this precursor event, thus preventing the development of hypertension.[49]

REFERENCES

1. Institute of Medicine (US) Committee on Public Health Priorities to Reduce and Control Hypertension. A population-based policy and systems change approach to prevent and control hypertension. 2010;Accessed from the IOM website in 2017.
2. Saran R, Robinson B, Abbott KC, et al. US Renal Data System 2016 annual data report: epidemiology of kidney disease in the United States. *Am J Kidney Dis.* 2017;69:A7–A8.
3. Chobanian AV, Bakris GL, Black HR, et al. The Seventh Report of the Joint National Committee on Prevention, Detection, Evaluation, and Treatment of High Blood Pressure: the JNC 7 report. *J Am Med Assoc.* 2003;289:2560–2572.
4. Vasan RS, Larson MG, Leip EP, et al. Assessment of frequency of progression to hypertension in non-hypertensive participants in the Framingham Heart Study: a cohort study. *Lancet.* 2001;358:1682–1686.
5. Hsia J, Margolis KL, Eaton CB, et al. Prehypertension and cardiovascular disease risk in the Women's Health Initiative. *Circulation.* 2007;115:855–860.
6. Qureshi AI, Suri MFK, Kirmani JF, et al. Is prehypertension a risk factor for cardiovascular diseases? *Stroke.* 2005;36:1859–1863.
7. Thompson AM, Hu T, Eshelbrenner CL, et al. Antihypertensive treatment and secondary prevention of cardiovascular disease events among persons without hypertension: a meta-analysis. *J Am Med Assoc.* 2011;305:913–922.
8. Zhang Y, Moran AE. Trends in the prevalence, awareness, treatment, and control of hypertension among young adults in the United States, 1999 to 2014. *Hypertension* 2017;70:736–742.
9. Harshfield GA, Laragh JH. How common is white coat hypertension? *J Am Med Assoc.* 1988;259:225–228.
10. Pierdomenico SD, Cuccurullo F. Prognostic value of white-coat and masked hypertension diagnosed by ambulatory monitoring in initially untreated subjects: an updated meta analysis. *Am J Hypertens.* 2011;24:52–58.
11. Pickering TG, Shimbo D, Haas D. Ambulatory blood-pressure monitoring. *N Engl J Med.* 2006;354:2368–2374.
12. O'Brien E, Imai Y, Kawasaki T et al. Nocturnal blood pressure fall on ambulatory monitoring in a large international database. The "Ad Hoc" Working Group. *Hypertension.* 1997;29:30–39.
13. Bursztyn M. Predictors of all-cause mortality in clinical ambulatory monitoring: unique aspects of blood pressure during sleep. *Hypertension.* 2007;49:1235–1241.
14. Leitão CB, Canani LH, Kramer CK, et al. Masked hypertension, urinary albumin excretion rate, and echocardiographic parameters in putatively normotensive type 2 diabetic patients. *Diabetes Care.* 2007;30:1255–1260.
15. Hänninen M-RA, Niiranen TJ, Puukka PJ, et al. Target organ damage and masked hypertension in the general population: the Finn-Home study. *J Hypertens.* 2013;31:1136–1143.
16. Hermida RC, Ayala DE, Mojón A, et al. Bedtime dosing of antihypertensive medications reduces cardiovascular risk in CKD. *J Am Soc Nephrol.* 2011;22:2313–2321.
17. Orías M, Correa-Rotter R. Chronotherapy in hypertension: a pill at night makes things right? *J Am Soc Nephrol.* 2011;22:2152–2155.
18. Chobanian AV. Clinical practice. Isolated systolic hypertension in the elderly. *N Engl J Med.* 2007;357:789–796.
19. Franklin SS, Jacobs MJ, Wong ND, et al. Predominance of isolated systolic hypertension among middle-aged and elderly US hypertensives: analysis based on National Health and Nutrition Examination Survey (NHANES) III. *Hypertension.* 2001;37:869–874.

20. Franklin SS, Gustin W, Wong ND, et al. Hemodynamic patterns of age-related changes in blood pressure. The Framingham Heart Study. *Circulation.* 1997;96:308–315.

21. Izzo JL, Levy D, Black HR. Clinical advisory statement: importance of systolic blood pressure in older Americans. *Hypertension.* 2000;35:1021–1024.

22. O'Rourke MF. Aortic diameter, aortic stiffness, and wave reflection increase with age and isolated systolic hypertension. *Hypertension.* 2005;45:652–658.

23. Beckett NS, Peters R, Fletcher AE, et al. Treatment of hypertension in patients 80 years of age or older. *N Engl J Med.* 2008;358:1887–1898.

24. Staessen JA, Fagard R, Thijs L, et al. Randomised double-blind comparison of placebo and active treatment for older patients with isolated systolic hypertension. The Systolic Hypertension in Europe (Syst-Eur) Trial Investigators. *Lancet.* 1997;350:757–764.

25 Prevention of stroke by antihypertensive drug treatment in older persons with isolated systolic hypertension. Final results of the Systolic Hypertension in the Elderly Program (SHEP). SHEP Cooperative Research Group. *J Am Med Assoc.* 1991;265:3255–3264.

26. Freedman BI, Sedor JR. Hypertension-associated kidney disease: perhaps no more. *J Am Soc Nephrol* 2008;19:2047–2051.

27. Taal HR, Verwoert GC, Demirkan A et al. Genome-wide profiling of blood pressure in adults and children. *Hypertension.* 2012;59:241–247.

28. Kao WHL, Klag MJ, Meoni LA, et al. MYH9 is associated with nondiabetic end-stage renal disease in African Americans. *Nat Genet.* 2008;40:1185–1192.

29. Zhong J, Yang H-C, Fogo AB. A perspective on chronic kidney disease progression. *Am J Physiol Renal Physiol.* 2017;312:F375–F384.

30. Griffin KA. Hypertensive kidney injury and the progression of chronic kidney disease. *Hypertension.* 2017;70(4):687–694.

31. Brosius FC. New insights into the mechanisms of fibrosis and sclerosis in diabetic nephropathy. *Rev Endocr Metab Dis.* 2008;9:245–254.

32. Anderson S, Meyer TW, Rennke HG, et al. Control of glomerular hypertension limits glomerular injury in rats with reduced renal mass. *J Clin Invest.* 1985;76:612–619.

33. Remuzzi A, Gagliardini E, Sangalli F, et al. ACE inhibition reduces glomerulosclerosis and regenerates glomerular tissue in a model of progressive renal disease. *Kidney Int.* 2006;69:1124–1130.

34. Mann JFE, Schmieder RE, McQueen M, et al. Renal outcomes with telmisartan, ramipril, or both, in people at high vascular risk (the ONTARGET study): a multicentre, randomised, double-blind, controlled trial. *Lancet.* 2008;372:547–553.

35. Hou FF, Hou FF, Zhang X, et al. Efficacy and safety of benazepril for advanced chronic renal insufficiency. *N Engl J Med.* 2006;354:131–140.

36. Barnett AH, Bain SC, Bouter P, et al. Angiotensin-receptor blockade versus converting-enzyme inhibition in type 2 diabetes and nephropathy. *N Engl J Med.* 2004;351:1952–1961.

37. Lewis EJ, Hunsicker LG, Bain RP, et al.; The Collaborative Study Group. The effect of angiotensin-converting-enzyme inhibition on diabetic nephropathy. *N Engl J Med.* 1993;329:1456–1462.

38. Sternlicht H, Bakris GL. Hypertension and Chronic Kidney Disease. In Bakris GL, Sorrentino M, eds. Hyperteions: A companion to Braunwald's Heart Disease. (3rd ed.) 2017. Elsevier, Philadelphia.

39. Ishani A, Grandits GA, Grimm RH, et al. Association of single measurements of dipstick proteinuria, estimated glomerular filtration rate, and hematocrit with 25-year incidence of end-stage renal disease in the multiple risk factor intervention trial. *J Am Soc Nephrol.* 2006;17:1444–1452.

40. Agarwal R. Blood pressure components and the risk for end-stage renal disease and death in chronic kidney disease. *Clin J Am Soc Nephrol.* 2009;4:830–837.

41. Brenner BM, Cooper ME, de Zeeuw D, et al. Effects of losartan on renal and cardiovascular outcomes in patients with type 2 diabetes and nephropathy. *N Engl J Med.* 2001;345:861–869.

42. Pohl MA, Blumenthal S, Cordonnier DJ, et al. Independent and additive impact of blood pressure control and angiotensin II receptor blockade on renal outcomes in the irbesartan diabetic nephropathy trial: clinical implications and limitations. *J Am Soc Nephrol.* 2005;16:3027–3037.

43. Klahr S, Levey AS, Beck GJ, et al.; Modification of Diet in Renal Disease Study Group.The effects of dietary protein restriction and blood-pressure control on the progression of chronic renal disease. *N Engl J Med.* 1994;330:877–884.

44. Appel LJ, Wright JT, Greene T, et al. Intensive blood-pressure control in hypertensive chronic kidney disease. *N Engl J Med.* 2010;363:918–929.

45. Rocco MV, Sink KM, Lovato LC, et al. Effects of intensive blood pressure treatment on acute kidney injury events in the Systolic Blood Pressure Intervention Trial (SPRINT). *Am J Kidney Dis.* 2018;71(3):352–361.

46. National Kidney Foundation: Acute Kidney Injury Work Group. Kidney Disease: Improving Global Outcomes (KDIGO) – Clinical Practice Guideline for Acute Kidney Injury. *Kidney Int Suppl.* 2012;2:1–138.

47. Beddhu S, Chertow GM, Cheung AK, et al. Influence of baseline diastolic blood pressure on effects of intensive compared with standard blood pressure control. *Circulation.* 2018;137:134–143.

48. Cheung AK, Rahman M, Reboussin DM, et al. Effects of intensive BP control in CKD. *J Am Soc Nephrol.* 2017;28:2812–2823.

49. Dudenbostel T, Glasser SP. Effects of antihypertensive drugs on arterial stiffness. *Cardiol Rev.* 2012;20:259–263.

30

Cardiovascular Protection in Chronic Kidney Disease

JONATHAN W. WAKS, RULAN S. PAREKH, AND LARISA G. TERESHCHENKO

INTRODUCTION

Chronic kidney disease (CKD) currently affects over 15% of the United States population, and over 650,000 people (2.03 per 100,000 US population) have end-stage renal disease (ESRD) requiring dialysis.[1,2] Individuals with CKD have an increased prevalence of all forms of cardiovascular disease, including coronary artery disease (CAD), cerebrovascular disease, hypertension, dyslipidemia, diabetes, congestive heart failure, and sudden cardiac death (SCD). CKD is also an independent risk factor for developing cardiovascular disease; in the Atherosclerosis Risk in Communities (ARIC) study,[3] each 10 mL/min/1.73 m² decrease in estimated glomerular filtration rate (eGFR) was associated with a 5% increase in the risk of developing atherosclerotic cardiovascular disease, and in a large analysis[4] of over 1.1 million adults without ESRD or renal transplant, there was a graded, inverse relationship between eGFR and incident cardiovascular events (Fig. 30.1). In participants with established coronary heart disease (CHD) in the Reasons for Geographic and Racial Differences in Stroke[5] study, an eGFR <60 mL/min/1.73 m² was associated with a risk of recurrent cardiovascular events that was equivalent to other established, high-risk conditions such as smoking, diabetes, and metabolic syndrome.

Persons with ESRD have an extremely high incidence of cardiovascular disease and a high rate of cardiovascular mortality. In the Hemodialysis[6] trial, approximately 80% of participants with ESRD on dialysis had some form of cardiac disease, 40% had congestive heart failure, and 39% had CAD. CHD accounted for 43% of cardiac hospitalizations during follow-up, and approximately 1 in 4 participants died from CHD complications. Compared to the general population, those with ESRD have a rate of cardiovascular mortality that is 10- to 20-fold higher.[7]

This chapter will provide an overview of the epidemiology of cardiovascular disease in patients with CKD and will discuss strategies to diagnose cardiovascular disease and reduce cardiovascular risk, morbidity, and mortality in this high-risk population.

CORONARY HEART DISEASE

As previously noted, persons with CKD have an increased incidence of CHD, and the severity of CHD parallels the severity of CKD.[8] Those with more advanced CKD tend to present with acute myocardial infarction (MI) rather than stable angina as their initial manifestation of CHD,[9] reinforcing the importance of aggressive CHD risk factor modification and surveillance in the CKD population.

Diagnosing Coronary Heart Disease in Chronic Kidney Disease

Unfortunately, established CHD screening tools such as the Framingham Risk Score lack accuracy for predicting CHD risk in persons with advanced CKD, although modifications that improve score performance in the CKD population do exist.[10] Additionally, typical anginal symptoms are less useful in establishing the diagnosis of CHD in those with advanced CKD/ESRD; in a study of patients with ESRD or renal transplant who were undergoing coronary angiography, a history of angina had both poor sensitivity (65%) and poor specificity (66%) for discovering significant epicardial CAD during coronary angiography.[11]

Noninvasive stress testing also has limitations in advanced CKD, and stress testing in the ESRD population is less accurate overall when compared to those without ESRD.[12] In advanced CKD, the diagnostic utility of nonimaging

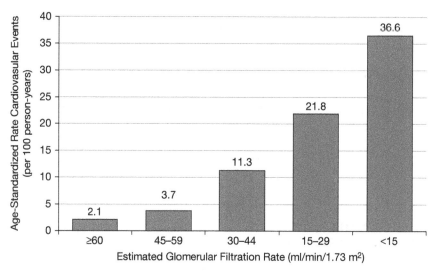

FIGURE 30.1 Relationship between adverse cardiovascular events and estimated glomerular filtration rate (GFR). Note the rapid increase in cardiovascular events once estimated GFR decreases to <44 mL/min/1.73 m². Adapted from Go AS, Chertow GM, Fan D, McCulloch CE, Hsu C-y. Chronic kidney disease and the risks of death, cardiovascular events, and hospitalization. *N Engl J Med.* 2004;351(13):1296–1305.

exercise stress testing is limited, in part due to a high prevalence of baseline electrocardiographic abnormalities such as left ventricular hypertrophy and other repolarization changes.[13,14]

In a meta-analysis of studies evaluating the utility of stress testing in renal transplant candidates, single-photon emission computed tomography (SPECT) nuclear perfusion imaging had a modest sensitivity of 74% and a specificity of 70% for obstructive CAD detected on coronary angiography. Stress test performance was slightly improved for dobutamine stress echocardiography (sensitivity 79%; specificity 89%).[15] In a study of 138 renal transplant candidates who underwent detailed cardiac evaluation with coronary artery calcium scoring, coronary computed tomography angiography, SPECT imaging, and invasive coronary angiography, 22% of patients had obstructive CAD defined as a ≥50% narrowing of a vessel lumen detected on invasive angiography. Coronary computed tomography angiography had the highest sensitivity (93%), and SPECT imaging had the highest specificity (97%) for detecting angiographically significant CAD.[16]

The most recent American College of Cardiology (ACC)/American Heart Association (AHA) guidelines[17] do not recommend any specific type of noninvasive stress testing that should be preferentially used in patients with advanced CKD. Guidelines recommend that CKD patients

be managed similarly to patients without CKD, with the decision to perform stress testing based on the presence of risk factors, symptoms, and clinical suspicion for CHD. Additionally, although supporting data are limited, the ACC/AHA guidelines give a Class IIb recommendation for noninvasive stress testing in asymptomatic men >45 years and women >55 years with CKD given the increased incidence of CHD in this population, although the evidence to support this recommendation is limited. CHD screening for patients who are undergoing evaluation for renal transplant is addressed in the following discussion in more detail.

Acute Myocardial Infarction

In patients with acute MI, poorer renal function is consistently associated with worse short- and long-term clinical outcomes. In a single center study of 3,106 patients who presented with acute MI, in-hospital mortality and postdischarge mortality increased significantly as renal function declined: in-hospital mortality was 2% for patients with normal renal function (creatine clearance [CrCl] >75 mL/min), 6% for those with mild CKD (CrCl 50–75 mL/min), 14% for those with moderate CKD (35–50 mL/min), 21% for those with severe CKD (CrCl <35 mL/min), and 30% for those with ESRD on renal replacement therapy.[18] In patients with acute ST-elevation MI, reduced CrCl was associated with significant increases in 30-day mortality, even after adjusting for multiple other risk factors: compared to patients with normal CrCl (≥90 mL/min), patients with mild CKD (CrCl 60–90 mL/min), moderate CKD (CrCl 30–60 mL/min), and severe CKD (CrCl <30 mL/min) had adjusted odds ratios (ORs) for total mortality of 1.4 (p = 0.006), 2.1 (p < 0.001), and 3.8 (p < 0.001), respectively.[19]

Poorer outcomes after acute MI may be in part related to observations that patients with more severe CKD often experience increased rates of bleeding and/or do not receive evidence-based therapies during treatment for acute MI.[20] In an analysis of >130,000 elderly patients hospitalized with acute MI, patients with CKD were less likely to receive aspirin, beta blockers, thrombolytics, or angioplasty. Mortality at 1 year was 24%, 46%, and 66% for patients with no, mild, and moderate CKD, respectively.[21] In study of greater than 40,000 participants evaluating the relationship between CKD and outcomes after non-ST-elevation MI in the era of primary percutaneous coronary intervention (PCI), those with CKD received fewer evidence-based therapies and had more comorbidities, more severe CAD, and increased rates of in-hospital mortality (OR 2.0–2.8) and major bleeding (OR 1.5–2.8).[22]

HEART FAILURE

Heart failure and CKD commonly co-exist, and the combination of CKD and heart failure is associated with poor outcomes. In the Candesartan in Heart Failure-Assessment of Reduction in Mortality and Morbidity[23] trial, approximately 35% of participants had an estimated GFR <60 mL/min/1.73 m², and impaired renal function was independently associated with an increased risk of cardiovascular death or unplanned hospital admission for heart failure management. As estimated GFR decreased, the hazard ratio for cardiovascular death or unplanned heart failure hospitalization increased (each 10 mL/min/1.73 m² decrease in GFR was associated with a 19% increase in risk in the composite endpoint).

There are a multitude of complex hemodynamic, neurohormonal, and systemic interactions that closely link impaired kidney function to impaired cardiac function and heart failure, including fluid and salt retention, low cardiac output and impaired renal perfusion, alterations in the renin–angiotensin–aldosterone system, and systemic inflammation.[24] Details of the "cardio-renal syndrome" are presented in more detail in Chapter 45.

SUDDEN CARDIAC DEATH

SCD accounts for approximately one-fourth of all deaths in patients with ESRD, and recent data suggest that the incidence of SCD in the dialysis population is 50 events per 1,000 person-years.[2] Unfortunately, the mechanisms and risk factors for SCD in the ESRD population remain poorly understood. Although SCD is often secondary to ventricular tachyarrhythmias (ventricular tachycardia and ventricular fibrillation), more recent data have suggested that bradyarrhythmias have an underappreciated role in SCD events in ESRD patients.[25] Additionally, while the presence of CAD certainly increases the risk for SCD, factors beyond CAD contribute to the extremely high risk of SCD in the ESRD population, as cardiovascular risk factor modification and coronary revascularization do not appear to reduce SCD risk.[26-28] The majority of patients with ESRD have relatively preserved left ventricular function,[29] and, therefore, left ventricular ejection fraction (LVEF) has limited utility for risk stratification of SCD and ventricular arrhythmias in ESRD patients. Other factors unique to the CKD/ESRD population, such as chronic uremia, diffuse myocardial fibrosis and hypertrophy, autonomic dysfunction, endothelial dysfunction, and cardiac calcification, likely contribute to the elevated SCD incidence observed in ESRD patients.

Studies investigating SCD risk factors specifically in the ESRD population are ongoing, and there are currently no accepted guidelines specifically for SCD risk screening or risk reduction in the CKD population. The electrocardiogram shows promise as a readily available, inexpensive, and noninvasive method of assessing SCD risk,[30,31] and cardiac imaging and serum biomarkers may also help refine SCD risk, but it remains unclear how to optimally manage patients who are found to have increased SCD risk.

REDUCING CARDIOVASCULAR RISK IN CHRONIC KIDNEY DISEASE

Given the poor outcomes associated with CHD and MI in patients with CKD, reducing cardiovascular risk is of paramount importance in the CKD population. Strategies to reduce the incidence of cardiovascular disease in patients with CKD include lifestyle modification, exercise, smoking cessation, and various medical therapies. These approaches to reduce risk are not specific to CKD patients, but their beneficial effects may be modified by the presence of advanced CKD. A summary of interventions to reduce cardiovascular risk in persons with CKD is presented in Table 30.1.

Lifestyle Interventions

Although high-quality randomized control trials evaluating cardiovascular endpoints are not available, lifestyle education, dietary modification, and exercise training appear to improve cardio-pulmonary function and quality of life across the spectrum of CKD.[32,33] Kidney Disease Outcomes Quality Initiative (KDOQI)[34] guidelines support use of lifestyle interventions in all patients with CKD.

HMG-coA Reductase Inhibitors (Statins)

HMG-coA reductase inhibitors (statins) primarily act by lowering lipid levels, although they have other important pleotropic effects as well. Multiple studies have demonstrated that statins reduce cardiovascular events and improve survival in patients with known cardiovascular disease[35-37] and are beneficial in select patients being treated for primary prevention of cardiovascular disease.[38-40] In addition to their beneficial lipid-lowering effects, limited data suggest that statins might also benefit CKD patients by improving vascular stiffness[41-43] and reducing inflammation.[44,45]

In general, the benefits of statins appear to extend to the majority with CKD. In a meta-analysis of 37,274 participants in 38 studies that evaluated the effects of statins in CKD patients not requiring dialysis, statin therapy was associated with a 28% reduction in major cardiovascular events, a 21% reduction in all-cause mortality, a 23% reduction in cardiovascular mortality, and a 45% reduction in incident MI.[46]

The beneficial effects of statins in those with ESRD on dialysis, however, are less clear. The Study to Evaluate the Use of Rosuvastatin in Subjects on Regular Hemodialysis: An Assessment of Survival and Cardiovascular Events[27] randomized 2,776 patients aged 50 to 80 years on maintenance hemodialysis to treatment with rosuvastatin or placebo. Participants in the rosuvastatin arm had a 43% reduction in low-density lipoprotein (LDL) cholesterol levels, but despite this, rosuvastatin treatment had no effect on the composite outcome of death from cardiovascular causes, nonfatal MI, or stroke (9.2 vs. 9.5 events per 100 patient-years, $p = 0.59$), total mortality (13.5 vs. 14.0 events per 100 patient-years, $p = 0.51$), or the individual outcomes

of cardiovascular death (7.2 vs. 7.3 events per 100 patient years, $p = 0.97$ for rosuvastatin and placebo groups, respectively), nonfatal MI ($p = 0.23$), or nonfatal stroke ($p = 0.42$). Similar results were seen in the German Diabetes and Dialysis study,[28] a randomized controlled trial comparing atorvastatin to placebo in 1,255 diabetics on maintenance hemodialysis: despite a 42% reduction in LDL in atorvastatin treated patients, there was no difference in the composite outcome of cardiac death, nonfatal MI, and stroke (38 vs. 37%, $p = 0.37$), or the individual outcomes of cardiac death (23 vs. 20%, $p = 0.08$), all-cause mortality ($p = 0.33$), nonfatal MI ($p = 0.42$), or sudden death ($p = $ n.s.).

The Study of Heart and Renal Protection[47] randomized 9,270 participants with various levels of CKD (33% on dialysis) and without a history of CAD to treatment with simvastatin plus ezetimibe or placebo. During a mean follow-up period of 4.9 years, simvastatin and ezetimibe treatment reduced major atherosclerotic events by 17% (11.3 vs. 13.4%, $p = 0.002$, for treatment and placebo groups, respectively). When subgroups were analyzed, however, a reduction in major atherosclerotic events due to treatment with simvastatin plus ezetimibe was seen only in patients who were not on dialysis (risk ratio [RR] 0.78; 95% confidence interval [CI]: 0.67–0.91). No benefit to simvastatin plus ezetimibe use was seen in dialysis patients (RR 0.90; 95% CI: 0.75–1.08). Similarly, in a meta-analysis[48] of 8,289 participants with ESRD in 25 studies, statins did not reduce major cardiovascular events, all-cause mortality, cardiovascular mortality, MI, or stroke, despite being associated with significant reductions in cholesterol levels.

The 2013 National Kidney Foundation's KDOQI and Kidney Disease: Improving Global Outcomes (KDIGO) clinical practice guidelines recommend treatment of dyslipidemia in patients with CKD based on the presence or absence of cardiovascular risk factors rather than serum cholesterol levels.[49] These guidelines mirror the most recent ACC/AHA lipid management guidelines[50] in that both recommend against using specific LDL cholesterol targets when initiating lipid-lowering therapy and deciding on treatment goals.

The KDIGO guidelines recommend that all adults with CKD who are ≥50 years old be treated with a statin and/or ezetimibe based on the observation that most of these patients are at high-risk for CHD with an estimated 10-year

TABLE 30.1 INTERVENTIONS FOR CARDIOVASCULAR PROTECTION IN CHRONIC KIDNEY DISEASE—SUMMARY

Intervention	Persons with CKD	Persons on Dialysis	Persons with Renal Transplant
Lifestyle interventions[a]	Recommended for all persons regardless of renal function		
Statins[b]	• Guidelines recommend use of statins in adults with CKD who are ≥50 year old be treated with a statin (or ezetimibe) given that most of these persons will have a high risk of CHD. • In adults 18–49 years old, statins are recommended in persons with known CAD, diabetes, stroke, or estimated 10-year CHD incidence of >10%	• Multiple high quality randomized control trials have revealed no significant benefit in CV outcomes associated with statin use in dialysis patients regardless of effects on cholesterol lowering.	• Transplant patients have a high rate of cardiovascular disease, and statin therapy is therefore indicated in renal transplant patients.
Aspirin/antiplatelet agents[c]	• Aspirin recommended for secondary prevention of CAD regardless of renal function. • Data supporting use for primary prevention of CAD specifically in the CKD population are more limited. Reasonable to consider aspirin based on patient CV risk factors.	• No specific data for use of aspirin in dialysis patients—follow general guidelines regarding secondary prevention of CAD. • Decision to use aspirin for primary prevention of CV events based on patient risk factors.	• Although rates of CV events post renal transplant are high, there are no high-quality data supporting use of antiplatelet therapy for primary prevention of CV events specifically in renal transplant patients. • Follow general guidelines. Reasonable to consider aspirin based on patient CV risk factors.
BP control[d]	• KDIGO guidelines recommend goal BP ≤140/90 mmHg (no proteinuria), and ≤130/80 mmHg (significant proteinuria), although other guidelines have slightly different goals	• Optimal BP targets for dialysis patients remains controversial.	• Goal BP ≤130/80 mmHg
Coronary revascularization[e]	• In general, more severe CKD is associated with increased complications after CABG or PCI. ESRD is associated with even higher procedural risks. Optimal method of revascularizing patients with severe CKD and multivessel CAD remains controversial. • Guidelines recommend against routine coronary revascularization prior to renal transplant in the absence of CV symptoms or high-risk coronary anatomy.		

(continued)

TABLE 30.1 CONTINUED

Intervention	Persons with CKD	Persons on Dialysis	Persons with Renal Transplant
Implantable cardioverter-defibrillators for primary prevention of sudden cardiac death[f]	• Recommendations for primary prevention ICD implantation are based on current guidelines which focus on LVEF and functional class. CKD attenuates the efficacy of primary prevention ICD implantation.	• Data for primary prevention ICD use in the dialysis population are lacking, although trials are ongoing. Dialysis patients were excluded from the major ICD trials. • Risks of ICD implantation (such as bleeding and device infection) are also increased in patients on dialysis.	• No specific data in this population, and the decision to implant a primary prevention ICD in a renal transplant patient should be based on current guidelines focusing on LVEF and functional class. • There is an increased risk of infectious complications in patients who are on immunosuppression.

[a]Howden EJ, Leano R, Petchey W, Coombes JS, Isbel NM, Marwick TH. Effects of exercise and lifestyle intervention on cardiovascular function in CKD. *Clin J Am Soc Nephrol.* 2013;8(9):1494–1501; Barcellos FC, Santos IS, Umpierre D, Bohlke M, Hallal PC. Effects of exercise in the whole spectrum of chronic kidney disease: a systematic review. *Clin Kidney J.* 2015;8(6):753–765; K/DOQI Workgroup. K/DOQI clinical practice guidelines for cardiovascular disease in dialysis patients. *Am J Kidney Dis.* 2005;45(Suppl):S1–S153.

[b]Wanner C, Krane V, Marz W, et al. Atorvastatin in patients with type 2 diabetes mellitus undergoing hemodialysis. *N Engl J Med.* 2005;353(3):238–248; Palmer SC, Navaneethan SD, Craig JC, et al. HMG CoA reductase inhibitors (statins) for people with chronic kidney disease not requiring dialysis. *Cochrane Db Sys Rev.* 2014(5):Cd007784; Baigent C, Landray MJ, Reith C, et al. The effects of lowering LDL cholesterol with simvastatin plus ezetimibe in patients with chronic kidney disease (Study of Heart and Renal Protection): a randomised placebo-controlled trial. *Lancet.* 2011;377(9784):2181–2192; Palmer SC, Navaneethan SD, Craig JC, et al. HMG CoA reductase inhibitors (statins) for dialysis patients. *Cochrane Db Sys Rev.* 2013(9):Cd004289; Kidney Disease Improving Global Outcomes. KDIGO clinical practice guideline for lipid management in chronic kidney disease. *Kidney Intern Suppl.* 2013;3(3):259–305. http://www.kdigo.org/clinical_practice_guidelines/Lipids/KDIGO%20Lipid%20Management%20Guideline%202013.pdf; Stone NJ, Robinson J, Lichtenstein AH, et al.; American College of Cardiology/American Heart Association Task Force on Practice Guidelines. 2013 ACC/AHA guideline on the treatment of blood cholesterol to reduce atherosclerotic cardiovascular risk in adults: a report of the American College of Cardiology/American Heart Association Task Force on Practice Guidelines. *Circulation.* 2014;129(25 Suppl 2):S1–45; Bibbins-Domingo K, on behalf of the USPSTF. Aspirin use for the primary prevention of cardiovascular disease and colorectal cancer: U.s. preventive services task force recommendation statement. *Ann Intern Med.* 2016;164(12):836–845; Fellstrom BC, Jardine AG, Schmieder RE, et al. Rosuvastatin and cardiovascular events in patients undergoing hemodialysis. *N Engl J Med.* 2009;360(14):1395–1407.

[c]Palmer SC, Di Micco L, Razavian M, et al. Antiplatelet agents for chronic kidney disease. *Cochrane Db Sys Rev.* 2013(2):Cd008834; Kidney Disease Improving Global Outcomes. KDIGO 2012 clinical practice guideline for the evaluation and management of chronic kidney disease. *Kidney Int Suppl.* 2013;3:1–150; Kasiske BL, Zeier MG, Chapman JR, et al. KDIGO clinical practice guideline for the care of kidney transplant recipients: a summary. *Kidney Int.* 2010;77(4):299–311.

[d]Kidney Disease Improving Global Outcomes. KDIGO clinical practice guideline for the management of blood pressure in chronic kidney disease. *Kidney Int Suppl.* 2012;2(5):337–414; Kasiske BL, Zeier MG, Chapman JR, et al. KDIGO clinical practice guideline for the care of kidney transplant recipients: a summary. *Kidney Int.* 2010;77(4):299–311.

[e]Cooper WA, O'Brien SM, Thourani VH, et al. Impact of renal dysfunction on outcomes of coronary artery bypass surgery: results from the Society of Thoracic Surgeons National Adult Cardiac Database. *Circulation.* 2006;113(8):1063–1070; Latif F, Kleiman NS, Cohen DJ, et al. In-hospital and 1-year outcomes among percutaneous coronary intervention patients with chronic kidney disease in the era of drug-eluting stents: a report from the EVENT (Evaluation of Drug Eluting Stents and Ischemic Events) Registry. *JACC-Cardiovasc Interv.* 2009;2(1):37–45; McFalls EO, Ward HB, Moritz TE, et al. Coronary-artery revascularization before elective major vascular surgery. *N Engl J Med.* 2004;351(27):2795–2804.

[f]Goldenberg I, Vyas AK, Hall WJ, et al. Risk stratification for primary implantation of a cardioverter-defibrillator in patients with ischemic left ventricular dysfunction. *J Am Coll Cardiol.* 2008;51(3):288–296; Singh SM, Wang X, Austin PC, Parekh RS, Lee DS. Prophylactic defibrillators in patients with severe chronic kidney disease. *JAMA-Intern Med.* 2014;174(6):995–996; Tompkins C, McLean R, Cheng A, et al. End-stage renal disease predicts complications in pacemaker and ICD implants. *J Cardiovasc Electrophysiol.* 2011;22(10):1099–1104; de Bie MK, Lekkerkerker JC, van Dam B, et al. Prevention of sudden cardiac death: rationale and design of the Implantable Cardioverter Defibrillators in Dialysis patients (ICD2) Trial—a prospective pilot study. *Curr Med Res Opin.* 2008;24(8):2151–2157; Tracy CM, Epstein AE, Darbar D, et al. 2012 ACCF/AHA/HRS focused update of the 2008 guidelines for device-based therapy of cardiac rhythm abnormalities: a report of the American College of Cardiology Foundation/American Heart Association Task Force on Practice Guidelines. *J Am Coll Cardiol.* 2012;60(14):1297–1313.

BP = blood pressure. CV = cardiovascular. CAD = coronary artery disease. CKD = chronic kidney disease. ICD = implantable cardioverter-defibrillator. LVEF = left ventricular ejection fraction. CABG = coronary artery bypass grafting. PCI = percutaneous coronary intervention. CHD = coronary heart disease. KDIGO = kidney disease: improving global outcomes

CHD risk of >10%. For patients who have CKD but are between the ages of 18 and 49 years, statins are recommended in patients who have known CAD, diabetes, prior ischemic stroke, or an estimated 10-year CHD incidence of >10%. Additionally, despite a very high incidence of cardiovascular disease in ESRD patients on dialysis, due to lack of cardiovascular benefit in multiple studies as previously noted, guidelines recommend against the routine use of statins in the ESRD population. Unlike the ACC/AHA guidelines, the KDIGO guidelines[49] recommend avoiding high doses of statins in patients with eGFR <60 mL/min/1.73 m².

Although KDIGO guidelines recommend against initiating statins in patients on dialysis, statins are recommended in kidney transplant recipients due to the high rate of dyslipidemia in this population (often secondary to immunosuppression drugs), because data suggest that dyslipidemia is strongly related to future cardiovascular events in this population.[49]

Aspirin/Antiplatelet Agents

Aspirin has been shown to reduce the incidence of cardiovascular events in a wide variety of patient populations.[51-53] Data specifically evaluating the efficacy of aspirin for primary or secondary prevention of cardiovascular events in the CKD population are more limited. In a subanalysis of the Hypertension Optimal Treatment study[54] in which 18,597 participants (the vast majority of whom were being treated for primary prevention of cardiovascular disease) were randomized to low-dose aspirin (75 mg/d) or placebo, 3,619 participants (19.5%) had a baseline estimated GFR <60 mL/min/1.73 m². Aspirin therapy resulted in a greater absolute reduction in major cardiovascular events and total mortality and a nonsignificant increase in major bleeding among patients with CKD as compared to those with preserved renal function.

However, in a meta-analysis of over 27,000 participants evaluating multiple antiplatelet agents in patients with CKD in both primary and secondary prevention studies, antiplatelet agents reduced the risk of MI (RR 0.87; 95% CI: 0.76–0.99) but had no effect on total mortality, cardiovascular mortality, or stroke. Antiplatelet agents also increased the risk of major bleeding by 33%. Results did not change based on the degree of renal impairment.[55] KDIGO guidelines suggest that aspirin is useful for secondary prevention of cardiovascular disease in patients with CKD

but that data supporting its use for primary prevention are lacking.[56] Data supporting use of antiplatelet agents other than aspirin for primary prevention of cardiovascular disease are even less robust.

Blood Pressure Control

Good control of blood pressure is of critical importance for both preservation of renal function and for reducing cardiovascular risk in patients with and without CKD.[57-60] The target blood pressure for persons with CKD remains controversial. The most recent KDIGO guidelines[61] recommend that patients with CKD and without significant proteinuria be treated to reach a target blood pressure of ≤140/90 mmHg and those with significant proteinuria (>30 mg/24 h) be treated to reach a target blood pressure of ≤130/80 mmHg. These guidelines are similar to the most recent guidelines proposed by the European Society of Hypertension/European Society of Cardiology.[62] Notably, the 2014 guidelines from the Eighth Joint National Committee (JNC 8)[63] recommend a blood pressure goal of ≤140/90 mmHg regardless of proteinuria. In general, angiotensin converting enzyme inhibitors and angiotensin receptor blockers are considered the first-line agents in patients with CKD.[61-63] Further information on the important link between CKD and hypertension and the relative benefit of different medications, can be found in Chapter 32. Even more controversial are the blood pressure targets for those on dialysis. The optimal blood pressure measurement such as before dialysis, after dialysis, or between dialysis is not known.

Coronary Artery Revascularization

In general, accepted indications for coronary revascularization (acute coronary syndrome, angina, and high risk stress test results) do not consider the presence or severity of CKD. The risk associated with revascularization, however, is strongly influenced by CKD severity. Patients with CKD have poorer outcomes after coronary artery bypass grafting (CABG) surgery compared to those with preserved renal function, and the majority of cardiac surgery risk scoring systems include renal function as a predictor for surgical risk.[64-66] Although ESRD has been long recognized as an independent risk factor for post-CABG mortality (persons on dialysis have a 3-fold increase in the odds of in-hospital mortality compared to those not on dialysis),[67] even moderate CKD increases complications associated with CABG. In an analysis of >483,000 patients who had isolated CABG between 2000 and 2003, 22% of patients had no renal dysfunction (eGFR >90 mL/min/1.73 m²), 51% of patients had mild CKD (eGFR 60–90 mL/min/1.73 m²), 24% had moderate CKD (eGFR 30–59 mL/min/1.73 m²), 2% had severe CKD (eGFR <30 mL/min/1.73 m² but not on dialysis), and 1.5% had ESRD requiring dialysis. Preoperative eGFR was a strong predictor of operative mortality and other postoperative complications, and there was a sharp increase in operative mortality as soon as eGFR decreased to <60 mL/min/1.73 m². Compared to patients with no CKD, the relative risk of operative mortality increased by 55% in patients with moderate CKD, 2.9-fold in patients with severe CKD not requiring dialysis, and 3.8-fold in dialysis patients. Among patients with mild CKD, there was a nonsignificant increase in operative mortality.[68] Other studies have corroborated the significant risk associated with CABG as the eGFR decreases below approximately 60 mL/min/1.73 m².[69]

Long-term survival post-CABG is also strongly linked to preoperative renal function.[70] Interventions such as performing CABG "off-pump" without placing the patient on cardiopulmonary bypass seem to reduce the risk of acute renal injury but had no impact on long-term renal function.[71] Other potential strategies that are being investigated to reduce kidney injury associated with CABG are discussed elsewhere.[72]

CKD is also a strong predictor of adverse outcomes after PCI. In an older series of 5,327 patients who underwent PCI (approximately 25% of patients treated with balloon angioplasty and approximately 66% of patients treated with bare-metal stenting) at a single center between 1994 and 1999, patients with more severe CKD tended to have more complex CAD involving multiple vessels. Despite a high rate of procedural success, there was a dose-dependent increase in total mortality, cardiovascular mortality, and other adverse events including post-procedure acute kidney injury, as renal function declined.[73]

In a more recent study of 4,791 patients in the Evaluation of Drug Eluting Stents and Ischemic Events Registry, there was a graded increase in peri-procedural bleeding complications as eGFR decreased (3.3%, 5.0%, 8.8%, and 14.3% for patients with CrCl >75 mL/min, 50–75 mL/min, 30–49 mL/min, and <30 mL/min, respectively, $p < 0.0001$). There was also a graded increase in death or MI during the index hospitalization (5.8%, 7.4%, 8.4%, and 10% for patients with CrCl >75 mL/min, 50–75 mL/min, 30–49 mL/min, and <30 mL/min, respectively, $p = 0.0016$) and at 1 year (8.5%, 12.3%, 15.1%, 22.1% for patients with CrCl >75 mL/min, 50–75 mL/min, 30–49 ml/min, and <30 mL/min, respectively, $p < 0.0001$).[74] Limited data suggest that drug-eluting stents are likely more beneficial than bare-metal stents in patients with ESRD who are undergoing PCI.[75,76]

The optimal method of coronary revascularization in patients with severe CKD and multivessel CAD remains controversial. In an analysis of the Future Revascularization Evaluation in Patients with Diabetes Mellitus: Optimal Management of Multivessel Disease trial[77] comparing CABG to PCI in diabetics with multivessel CAD, patients with eGFR <60 mL/min/1.73 m² derived similar benefit to CABG as compared to those with eGFR ≥60 mL/min/1.73 m², with a significant reduction in rates of MI and need for revascularization but no difference in time to all-cause mortality. In a meta-analysis[78] of 38,740 patients in 28 studies assessing outcomes related to CABG and PCI for treatment of multivessel CAD in patients with CKD (defined as eGFR <60 mL/min/1.73 m²), CKD patients treated with PCI had a 45% reduction in the odds of short term mortality but a 29% increase in the odds of long-term mortality, a 78% increase in the odds of incidence of MI, and a 2.9-fold increase in the odds of needing additional revascularization procedures compared to CABG-treated patients. In a separate meta-analysis[79] of 32,350 ESRD patients in 16 studies comparing PCI and CABG for treatment for multivessel CAD, CABG (as compared to PCI) was associated with a significant increase in early mortality but a 10% reduction in late mortality risk, a 56% reduction in the risk of recurrent MI, and a 78% reduction in the risk of the need for recurrent revascularization.

In general, the decision to perform CABG or PCI in CKD patients with multivessel CAD should be based on evaluation of patient comorbidities (especially diabetes, for which benefit from CABG over PCI has been demonstrated in multiple studies), coronary anatomy, and cardiac function. In patients who are renal transplant candidates with multivessel CAD, CABG likely provides a more durable result and decreases the risk of needing additional procedures with the need to administer intravenous contrast.[80]

Therapy to Reduce the Incidence of SCD in ESRD

Despite the high incidence of both cardiovascular disease and SCD in the ESRD population, no interventions have been shown to reduce the risk of SCD. Randomized control trials have demonstrated that statins and other cholesterol lowering medications do not reduce the incidence of SCD in ESRD patients.[28] Additionally, coronary revascularization has not been shown to significantly reduce SCD events in dialysis patients. The reasons for the disconnect between cardiovascular risk factors and SCD events are not entirely clear, but they likely reflect a limited understanding of SCD mechanisms unique to the ESRD population.

Given the high rates of SCD in ESRD patients, it would seem plausible that implantable cardioverter-defibrillator (ICD) therapy would reduce the incidence of SCD in this population. However, patients with ESRD or severe CKD were not well represented in large ICD trials. Additionally, retrospective data have repeatedly demonstrated that CKD significantly attenuates the benefit associated with ICD utilization,[81,82] likely due to competing causes of mortality, increasing complications related to ICD implantation,[83] and mechanisms of SCD events that are distinct from ventricular arrhythmias in the advanced CKD population. Studies specifically investigating the use of ICDs for the primary prevention of SCD in patients with ESRD are currently enrolling patients.[84]

There are no guidelines specifically for implantation of ICDs in patients with CKD/ESRD, and clinicians should follow the standard ACC/AHA/Heart Rhythm Society guidelines[85] while understanding that persons with severe CKD were underrepresented in clinical trials that form the basis for the current guidelines, that device-related complications are more common, and that the overall benefit to survival is attenuated in patients with severe CKD.

CARDIOVASCULAR CONSIDERATIONS IN THE SETTING OF KIDNEY TRANSPLANTATION

Cardiovascular disease is the leading cause of death after successful kidney transplantation, accounting for 30% to 50% of all deaths in renal transplant recipients with functioning allografts.[80,86,87] Unfortunately, there remains a lack of consensus for how to optimally screen patients for CHD prior to renal transplant. Although ACC/AHA guidelines for preoperative cardiac evaluation state that stress testing should only be performed on patients who have symptoms and/or a functional capacity below 4 metabolic equivalents,[88] a 2012 ACC/AHA consensus statement[80] specifically on cardiac evaluation prior to renal transplantation recommends (Class IIb, level of evidence C) that among kidney transplant candidates without active cardiac conductions (acute coronary syndrome, severe angina, decompensated heart failure, unstable arrhythmias, or severe valvular disease), noninvasive stress testing may be considered regardless of functional status based on CAD risk factors, which include diabetes, >1 year on dialysis, prior cardiovascular disease, age >60 years, left ventricular hypertrophy, smoking, hypertension, and dyslipidemia. The number of these risk factors that should prompt testing remains unclear and controversial.

The 2005 KDOQI guidelines[34] recommend performing annual stress testing in patients awaiting kidney transplant, although the utility of this approach remains unclear with limited supportive data. ACC/AHA guidelines[80] also note that it is reasonable to perform an assessment of left ventricular function with echocardiography (Class IIa, level of evidence B) based on data suggesting poorer outcomes among ESRD patients with reduced left ventricular function or severe pulmonary hypertension. Patients with valvular disease may also require more frequent echocardiographic surveillance.

The utility of prophylactic coronary revascularization in ESRD patients awaiting kidney transplant is unclear, although older, small studies have suggested that revascularization might improve outcomes in a subset with significant CAD. Large randomized control trials evaluating coronary revascularization prior to noncardiac surgery (not transplants) have not shown a benefit to routine pretransplant revascularization in the absence of severe angina or high risk coronary anatomy.[89,90] ACC/AHA guidelines recommend that revascularization should be considered in kidney transplant candidates who meet criteria for revascularization independent of their ESRD/transplant status. CABG is considered the preferred method of revascularization in ESRD patients with high-risk of multivessel CAD. Notably, guidelines recommend against prophylactic coronary revascularization in patients with stable CAD without symptoms or high-risk lesions prior to renal transplant.[90]

After transplantation, aggressive cardiovascular risk factor reduction is critical, as cardiovascular disease remains the leading cause of death despite improved kidney function. Transplanted patients should be treated with a statin.[49] Although much effort has been put forth to better understand cardiovascular risk in renal transplant candidates, guidelines for follow-up cardiovascular testing after successful transplant are limited at this point in time.

CONCLUSION

Persons with CKD, and especially ESRD, have a high incidence of cardiovascular disease and poor cardiovascular outcomes. The benefit of interventions that have shown efficacy in non-CKD populations, such as aspirin, statins, and ICDs, appear to be attenuated in patients with severe CKD. Unfortunately, patients with significant CKD have been excluded from the majority of large cardiovascular trials, and for this reason, it remains unclear how to optimally treat these patients to reduce the incidence of cardiovascular events. Future, high-quality randomized controlled studies designed to assess interventions and cardiovascular outcomes specifically in the advanced CKD population will be required to identify high-yield risk-reduction strategies and to reduce the incidence of cardiovascular disease, adverse cardiovascular complications, and cardiovascular mortality in this high-risk population.

REFERENCES

1. Coresh J, Selvin E, Stevens LA, et al. Prevalence of chronic kidney disease in the United States. *J Am Med Assoc.* 2007;298(17):2038–2047.
2. Parikh NI, Gona P, Larson MG, et al. Long-term trends in myocardial infarction incidence and case fatality in the National Heart, Lung, and Blood Institute's Framingham Heart study. *Circulation.* 2009;119(9):1203–1210.
3. Manjunath G, Tighiouart H, Ibrahim H, et al. Level of kidney function as a risk factor for atherosclerotic cardiovascular outcomes in the community. *J Am Coll Cardiol.* 2003;41(1):47–55.
4. Go AS, Chertow GM, Fan D, McCulloch CE, Hsu C-y. Chronic kidney disease and the risks of death, cardiovascular events, and hospitalization. *N Engl J Med.* 2004;351(13):1296–1305.
5. Baber U, Gutierrez OM, Levitan EB, et al. Risk for recurrent coronary heart disease and all-cause mortality among individuals with chronic kidney disease compared with diabetes mellitus, metabolic syndrome, and cigarette smokers. *Am Heart J.* 2013;166(2):373–380.e372.
6. Cheung AK, Sarnak MJ, Yan G, et al. Cardiac diseases in maintenance hemodialysis patients: results of the HEMO Study. *Kidney Int.* 2004;65(6):2380–2389.
7. Foley RN, Parfrey PS, Sarnak MJ. Clinical epidemiology of cardiovascular disease in chronic renal disease. *Am J Kidney Dis.* 1998;32(5 Suppl 3):S112–S119.
8. Ix JH, Shlipak MG, Liu HH, Schiller NB, Whooley MA. Association between renal insufficiency and inducible ischemia in patients with coronary artery disease: the heart and soul study. *J AmSoc Nephrol.* 2003;14(12):3233–3238.
9. Go AS, Bansal N, Chandra M, et al. Chronic kidney disease and risk for presenting with acute myocardial infarction versus stable exertional angina in adults with coronary heart disease. *J Am Coll Cardiol.* 2011;58(15):1600–1607.
10. Weiner DE, Tighiouart H, Elsayed EF, et al. The Framingham predictive instrument in chronic kidney disease. *J Am Coll Cardiol.* 2007;50(3):217–224.
11. Schmidt A, Stefenelli T, Schuster E, Mayer G. Informational contribution of noninvasive screening tests for coronary artery disease in patients on chronic renal replacement therapy. *Am J Kidney Dis.* 2001;37(1):56–63.
12. Marwick TH, Steinmuller DR, Underwood DA, et al. Ineffectiveness of dipyridamole SPECT thallium imaging as a screening technique for coronary artery disease in patients with end-stage renal failure. *Transplantation.* 1990;49(1):100–103.
13. Bangalore S. Stress testing in patients with chronic kidney disease: The need for ancillary markers for effective risk stratification and prognosis. *Journal Nucl Cardiol.* 2016;23(3):570–574.
14. Sharma R, Pellerin D, Gaze DC, et al. Dobutamine stress echocardiography and the resting but not exercise electrocardiograph predict severe coronary artery disease in renal transplant candidates. *Nephrol Dial Transplant.* 2005;20(10):2207–2214.
15. Wang LW, Fahim MA, Hayen A, et al. Cardiac testing for coronary artery disease in potential kidney transplant recipients. *Cochrane Db Sys Rev.* 2011(12):Cd008691.
16. Winther S, Svensson M, Jorgensen HS, et al. Diagnostic performance of coronary CT angiography and myocardial perfusion imaging in kidney transplantation candidates. *JACC-Cardiovasc Imagi.* 2015;8(5):553–562.
17. Gibbons RJ, Balady GJ, Timothy Bricker J, et al. ACC/AHA 2002 guideline update for exercise testing: summary article: A report of the American

college of cardiology/American heart association task force on practice guidelines (committee to update the 1997 exercise testing guidelines) 12345. *J Am Coll Cardiol.* 2002;40(8):1531–1540.

18. Wright RS, Reeder GS, Herzog CA, et al. Acute myocardial infarction and renal dysfunction: a high-risk combination. *Ann Intern Medi.* 2002;137(7):563–570.

19. Gibson CM, Pinto DS, Murphy SA, et al. Association of creatinine and creatinine clearance on presentation in acute myocardial infarction with subsequent mortality. *J Am Coll Cardiol.* 2003;42(9):1535–1543.

20. Fox CS, Muntner P, Chen AY, et al. Use of evidence-based therapies in short-term outcomes of ST-segment elevation myocardial infarction and non-ST-segment elevation myocardial infarction in patients with chronic kidney disease: a report from the National Cardiovascular Data Acute Coronary Treatment and Intervention Outcomes Network registry. *Circulation.* 2010;121(3):357–365.

21. Shlipak MG, Heidenreich PA, Noguchi H, Chertow GM, Browner WS, McClellan MB. Association of renal insufficiency with treatment and outcomes after myocardial infarction in elderly patients. *Ann Intern Med.* 2002;137(7):555–562.

22. Hanna EB, Chen AY, Roe MT, Wiviott SD, Fox CS, Saucedo JF. Characteristics and in-hospital outcomes of patients with non-ST-segment elevation myocardial infarction and chronic kidney disease undergoing percutaneous coronary intervention. *JACC-Cardiovasc Interv.* 2011;4(9):1002–1008.

23. Hillege HL, Nitsch D, Pfeffer MA, et al. Renal function as a predictor of outcome in a broad spectrum of patients with heart failure. *Circulation.* 2006;113(5):671–678.

24. Schefold JC, Filippatos G, Hasenfuss G, Anker SD, von Haehling S. Heart failure and kidney dysfunction: epidemiology, mechanisms and management. *Nat Rev Nephrol.* 2016;12(10):610–623.

25. Wong MC, Kalman JM, Pedagogos E, et al. Bradycardia and asystole is the predominant mechanism of sudden cardiac death in patients with chronic kidney disease. *J Am Coll Cardiol.* 2015;65(12):1263–1265.

26. Herzog CA, Strief JW, Collins AJ, Gilbertson DT. Cause-specific mortality of dialysis patients after coronary revascularization: why don't dialysis patients have better survival after coronary intervention? *Nephrol Dial Transplant.* 2008;23(8):2629–2633.

27. Fellström BC, Jardine AG, Schmieder RE, et al. Rosuvastatin and cardiovascular events in patients undergoing hemodialysis. *N Engl J Med.* 2009;360(14):1395–1407.

28. Wanner C, Krane V, Marz W, et al. Atorvastatin in patients with type 2 diabetes mellitus undergoing hemodialysis. *N Engl J Med.* 2005;353(3):238–248.

29. Parfrey PS, Foley RN, Harnett JD, Kent GM, Murray DC, Barre PE. Outcome and risk factors for left ventricular disorders in chronic uraemia. *Nephrol Dial Transplant.* 1996;11(7):1277–1285.

30. Waks JW, Tereshchenko LG, Parekh RS. Electrocardiographic predictors of mortality and sudden cardiac death in patients with end stage renal disease on hemodialysis. *J Electrocardiol.* 2016;49(6):848–854.

31. Tereshchenko LG, Kim ED, Oehler A, et al. Electrophysiologic substrate and risk of mortality in incident hemodialysis. *J Am Soc Nephrol.* 2016;27(11):3413–3420.

32. Howden EJ, Leano R, Petchey W, Coombes JS, Isbel NM, Marwick TH. Effects of exercise and lifestyle intervention on cardiovascular function in CKD. *Clin J Am Soc Nephrol.* 2013;8(9):1494–1501.

33. Barcellos FC, Santos IS, Umpierre D, Bohlke M, Hallal PC. Effects of exercise in the whole spectrum of chronic kidney disease: a systematic review. *Clin Kidney J.* 2015;8(6):753–765.

34. Workgroup K. KDOQI clinical practice guidelines for cardiovascular disease in dialysis patients. *Am J Kidney Dis.* 2005;45(Suppl):S1–S153.

35. Scandinavian Simvastatin Survival Study Group. Randomised trial of cholesterol lowering in 4444 patients with coronary heart disease: the Scandinavian Simvastatin Survival Study (4S). *Lancet.* 344(8934):1383–1389.

36. Cannon CP, Braunwald E, McCabe CH, et al. Intensive versus moderate lipid lowering with statins after acute coronary syndromes. *N Engl J Med.* 2004;350(15):1495–1504.

37. Long-Term Intervention with Pravastatin in Ischaemic Disease (LIPID) Study Group. Prevention of cardiovascular events and death with pravastatin in patients with coronary heart disease and a broad range of initial cholesterol levels. *N Engl J Med.* 1998;339(19):1349–1357.

38. Ridker PM. Rosuvastatin in the primary prevention of cardiovascular disease among patients with low levels of low-density lipoprotein cholesterol and elevated high-sensitivity C-reactive protein: rationale and design of the JUPITER trial. *Circulation.* 2003;108(19):2292–2297.

39. Taylor F, Huffman MD, Macedo AF, et al. Statins for the primary prevention of cardiovascular disease. *Cochrane Db Sys Rev.* 2013(1):Cd004816.

40. Ford I, Murray H, McCowan C, Packard CJ. Long term safety and efficacy of lowering ldl cholesterol with statin therapy: 20-year follow-up of West of Scotland Coronary Prevention Study. *Circulation.* 2016;133(11):1073–1080.

41. Dogra G, Irish A, Chan D, Watts G. A randomized trial of the effect of statin and fibrate therapy on arterial function in CKD. *Am J Kidney Dis.* 2007;49(6):776–785.

42. Ichihara A, Hayashi M, Ryuzaki M, Handa M, Furukawa T, Saruta T. Fluvastatin prevents development of arterial stiffness in haemodialysis patients with type 2 diabetes mellitus. *Nephrol Dial Transplant.* 2002;17(8):1513–1517.

43. Veringa SJ, Nanayakkara PW, van Ittersum FJ, et al. Effect of a treatment strategy consisting of pravastatin, vitamin E, and homocysteine lowering on arterial compliance and distensibility in patients with mild-to-moderate chronic kidney disease. *Clin Nephrol.* 2012;78(4):263–272.

44. Panichi V, Paoletti S, Mantuano E, et al. In vivo and in vitro effects of simvastatin on inflammatory markers in pre-dialysis patients. *Nephrol Dial Transplant.* 2006;21(2):337–344.

45. Fassett RG, Robertson IK, Ball MJ, Geraghty DP, Coombes JS. Effects of atorvastatin on biomarkers of inflammation in chronic kidney disease. *Clin Nephrol.* 2014;81(2):75–85.

46. Palmer SC, Navaneethan SD, Craig JC, et al. HMG CoA reductase inhibitors (statins) for people with chronic kidney disease not requiring dialysis. *Cochrane Db Sys Rev.* 2014(5):Cd007784.

47. Baigent C, Landray MJ, Reith C, et al. The effects of lowering LDL cholesterol with simvastatin plus ezetimibe in patients with chronic kidney disease (Study of Heart and Renal Protection): a randomised placebo-controlled trial. *Lancet.* 2011;377(9784):2181–2192.

48. Palmer SC, Navaneethan SD, Craig JC, et al. HMG CoA reductase inhibitors (statins) for dialysis patients. *Cochrane Db Sys Rev.* 2013(9):Cd004289.

49. Kidney Disease Improving Global Outcomes. KDIGO clinical practice guideline for lipid management in chronic kidney disease. *Kidney Intern Suppl.* 2013;3(3):259–305. http://www.kdigo.org/clinical_practice_guidelines/Lipids/KDIGO%20Lipid%20Management%20Guideline%202013.pdf

50. Stone NJ, Robinson J, Lichtenstein AH, et al.; American College of Cardiology/American Heart Association Task Force on Practice Guidelines. 2013 ACC/AHA guideline on the treatment of blood cholesterol to reduce atherosclerotic cardiovascular risk in adults: a report of the American College of Cardiology/American Heart Association Task Force on Practice Guidelines. *Circulation.* 2014;129(25 Suppl 2):S1–45.

51. Bibbins-Domingo K, on behalf of the USPSTF. Aspirin use for the primary prevention of cardiovascular disease and colorectal cancer: U.s. preventive services task force recommendation statement. *Ann Intern Med.* 2016;164(12):836–845.

52. Berger JS, Brown DL, Becker RC. Low-dose aspirin in patients with stable cardiovascular disease: a meta-analysis. *The American journal of medicine.* 2008;121(1):43–49.

53. Baigent C, Blackwell L, Collins R, et al.; Antithrombotic Trialists Collaboration. Aspirin in the primary and secondary prevention of vascular disease: collaborative meta-analysis of individual participant data from randomised trials. *Lancet.*373(9678):1849–1860.

54. Jardine MJ, Ninomiya T, Perkovic V, et al. Aspirin is beneficial in hypertensive patients with chronic kidney disease: a post-hoc subgroup analysis of a randomized controlled trial. *J Am Coll Cardiol.* 2010;56(12):956–965.

55. Palmer SC, Di Micco L, Razavian M, et al. Antiplatelet agents for chronic kidney disease. *Cochrane Db Sys Rev.* 2013(2):Cd008834.

56. Kidney Disease Improving Global Outcomes. KDIGO 2012 clinical practice guideline for the evaluation and management of chronic kidney disease. *Kidney Int Suppl.* 2013;3:1–150.

57. Buxton AE, Sweeney MO, Wathen MS, et al. QRS duration does not predict occurrence of ventricular tachyarrhythmias in patients with implanted cardioverter-defibrillators. *J Am Coll Cardiol.* 2005;46(2):310–316.

58. Mann JF, Gerstein HC, Pogue J, Bosch J, Yusuf S. Renal insufficiency as a predictor of cardiovascular outcomes and the impact of ramipril: the HOPE randomized trial. *Ann Intern Med.* 2001;134(8):629–636.

59. Berl T, Hunsicker LG, Lewis JB, et al. Impact of achieved blood pressure on cardiovascular outcomes in the Irbesartan Diabetic Nephropathy trial. *J Am Soc Nephrol.* 2005;16(7):2170–2179.

60. Pohl MA, Blumenthal S, Cordonnier DJ, et al. Independent and Additive Impact of Blood Pressure Control and Angiotensin II Receptor Blockade on Renal Outcomes in the Irbesartan Diabetic Nephropathy Trial: Clinical Implications and Limitations. *J Am Soc Nephrol.* 2005;16(10):3027–3037.

61. Kidney Disease Improving Global Outcomes. KDIGO clinical practice guideline for the management of blood pressure in chronic kidney disease. *Kidney Int Suppl.* 2012;2(5):337–414.

62. Mancia G, Fagard R, Narkiewicz K, et al. 2013 ESH/ESC guidelines for the management of arterial hypertension: the Task Force for the Management of Arterial Hypertension of the European Society of Hypertension (ESH) and of the European Society of Cardiology (ESC). *Eur Heart J.* 2013;34(28):2159–2219.

63. James PA, Oparil S, Carter BL, et al. 2014 evidence-based guideline for the management

of high blood pressure in adults: Report from the panel members appointed to the eighth joint national committee (JNC 8). *J Am Med Assoc.* 2014;311(5):507–520.

64. Wu C, Camacho FT, Wechsler AS, et al. Risk score for predicting long-term mortality after coronary artery bypass graft surgery. *Circulation.* 2012;125(20):2423.

65. Nashef SA, Roques F, Sharples LD, et al. EuroSCORE II. *Eur J Cardio Thorac Surg.* 2012;41(4):734–744; discussion 744–735.

66. Shahian DM, O'Brien SM, Filardo G, et al. The Society of Thoracic Surgeons 2008 cardiac surgery risk models: part 1—coronary artery bypass grafting surgery. *Ann Thorac Surg.* 2009;88(1 Suppl):S2–S22.

67. Liu JY, Birkmeyer NJO, Sanders JH, et al. Risks of morbidity and mortality in dialysis patients undergoing coronary artery bypass surgery. *Circulation.* 2000;102(24):2973–2977.

68. Cooper WA, O'Brien SM, Thourani VH, et al. Impact of renal dysfunction on outcomes of coronary artery bypass surgery: results from the Society of Thoracic Surgeons National Adult Cardiac Database. *Circulation.* 2006;113(8):1063–1070.

69. Zakeri R, Freemantle N, Barnett V, et al. Relation between mild renal dysfunction and outcomes after coronary artery bypass grafting. *Circulation.* 2005;112(9 Suppl):I270–I275.

70. Dacey LJ, Liu JY, Braxton JH, et al. Long-term survival of dialysis patients after coronary bypass grafting. *Ann Thorac Surg.* 2002;74(2):458–462; discussion 462–453.

71. Garg AX, Devereaux PJ, Yusuf S, et al. Kidney function after off-pump or on-pump coronary artery bypass graft surgery: a randomized clinical trial. *J Am Med Assoc.* 2014;311(21):2191–2198.

72. Rosner MH, Okusa MD. Acute kidney injury associated with cardiac surgery. *Clinical J Am Soc Nephrol.* 2006;1(1):19–32.

73. Best PJ, Lennon R, Ting HH, et al. The impact of renal insufficiency on clinical outcomes in patients undergoing percutaneous coronary interventions. *J Am Coll Cardiol.* 2002;39(7):1113–1119.

74. Latif F, Kleiman NS, Cohen DJ, et al. In-hospital and 1-year outcomes among percutaneous coronary intervention patients with chronic kidney disease in the era of drug-eluting stents: a report from the EVENT (Evaluation of Drug Eluting Stents and Ischemic Events) Registry. *JACC-Cardiovasc Interv.* 2009;2(1):37–45.

75. Chang TI, Montez-Rath ME, Tsai TT, Hlatky MA, Winkelmayer WC. Drug-eluting versus bare-metal stents during PCI in patients with end-stage renal disease on dialysis. *J Am Coll Cardiol.* 2016;67(12):1459–1469.

76. Tsai TT, Messenger JC, Brennan JM, et al. Safety and efficacy of drug-eluting stents in older patients with chronic kidney diseasea report from the Linked CathPCI Registry–CMS Claims Database. *J Am Coll Cardiol.* 2011;58(18):1859–1869.

77. Baber U, Farkouh ME, Arbel Y, et al. Comparative efficacy of coronary artery bypass surgery vs. percutaneous coronary intervention in patients with diabetes and multivessel coronary artery disease with or without chronic kidney disease. *Eur Heart J.* 2018;9(30):21201–21210.

78. Chen Y-Y, Wang J-F, Zhang Y-J, Xie S-L, Nie R-Q. Optimal strategy of coronary revascularization in chronic kidney disease patients: A meta-analysis. *Eur J Intern Med.* 2013;24(4):354–361.

79. Zheng H, Xue S, Lian F, Huang RT, Hu ZL, Wang YY. Meta-analysis of clinical studies comparing coronary artery bypass grafting with percutaneous coronary intervention in patients with end-stage renal disease. *Eur J Cardio Thorac Surg.* 2013;43(3):459–467.

80. Lentine KL, Costa SP, Weir MR, et al. Cardiac disease evaluation and management among kidney and liver transplantation candidates: a scientific statement From the American Heart Association and the American College of Cardiology Foundation. *J Am Coll Cardiol.* 2012;60(5):434–480.

81. Goldenberg I, Vyas AK, Hall WJ, et al. Risk stratification for primary implantation of a cardioverter-defibrillator in patients with ischemic left ventricular dysfunction. *J Am Coll Cardiol.* 2008;51(3):288–296.

82. Singh SM, Wang X, Austin PC, Parekh RS, Lee DS. Prophylactic defibrillators in patients with severe chronic kidney disease. *JAMA-Intern Med.* 2014;174(6):995–996.

83. Tompkins C, McLean R, Cheng A, et al. End-stage renal disease predicts complications in pacemaker and ICD implants. *J Cardiovasc Electrophysiol.* 2011;22(10):1099–1104.

84. de Bie MK, Lekkerkerker JC, van Dam B, et al. Prevention of sudden cardiac death: rationale and design of the Implantable Cardioverter Defibrillators in Dialysis patients (ICD2) Trial— a prospective pilot study. *Curr Med Res Opin.* 2008;24(8):2151–2157.

85. Tracy CM, Epstein AE, Darbar D, et al. 2012 ACCF/AHA/HRS focused update of the 2008 guidelines for device-based therapy of cardiac rhythm abnormalities: a report of the American College of Cardiology Foundation/American Heart Association Task Force on Practice Guidelines. *J Am Coll Cardiol.* 2012;60(14):1297–1313.

86. Ojo AO, Hanson JA, Wolfe RA, Leichtman AB, Agodoa LY, Port FK. Long-term survival in renal

transcript recipients with graft function. *Kidney Int.* 2000;57(1):307–313.

87. Briggs JD. Causes of death after renal transplantation. *Nephrol Dial Transpl.* 2001;16(8): 1545–1549.

88. Fleisher LA, Fleischmann KE, Auerbach AD, et al. 2014 ACC/AHA guideline on perioperative cardiovascular evaluation and management of patients undergoing noncardiac surgery: a report of the American College of Cardiology/American Heart Association Task Force on Practice Guidelines. *J Am Coll Cardiol.* 2014;64(22):e77–e137.

89. McFalls EO, Ward HB, Moritz TE, et al. Coronary-artery revascularization before elective major vascular surgery. *N Engl J Med.* 2004;351(27):2795–2804.

90. Poldermans D, Schouten O, Vidakovic R, et al. A clinical randomized trial to evaluate the safety of a noninvasive approach in high-risk patients undergoing major vascular surgery: the DECREASE-V Pilot Study. *J Am Coll Cardiol.* 2007;49(17):1763–1769.

31

Lupus Nephritis

AISHA SHAIKH AND KIRK N. CAMPBELL

INTRODUCTION

Systemic lupus erythematosus (SLE) is a chronic inflammatory disease that can affect multiple organ systems. Lupus nephritis (LN) occurs in approximately 40% to 60% of all patients with SLE, leading to end-stage renal disease (ESRD) in 5% to 10% of patients at 10 years.[1] Renal involvement in lupus results in significant morbidity and mortality.[2,3]

LN refers to inflammation of the kidney that encompasses a wide array of renal histologic patterns. Renal biopsy is essential for its diagnosis and classification. The International Society of Nephrology/Renal Pathology Society classification of LN is based on a number of factors, including the location of immune complex deposition, presence of endocapillary or mesangial proliferation, degree of glomerular involvement, and the extent of inflammation and scarring as outlined in Table 31.1.[4] This classification system is limited by the fact that it does not include the entire spectrum of lupus-related renal diseases, such as thrombotic microangiopathy, tubulointerstitial nephritis, and lupus podocytopathy.[5] It nonetheless serves as a useful prognostic and therapeutic guide.

Renal outcomes in LN vary considerably among different histological classes, with prognosis being worse for proliferative LN (class III and class IV). The risk of progression to ESRD with proliferative LN, approaches 44% over 15 years.[6] Class IV is the most aggressive form of LN, and without immunosuppressive therapy, the 5-year patient survival has been reported to be 17%.[7]

TREATMENT OF LUPUS NEPHRITIS

Treatment of Classes I and II Lupus Nephritis

Classes I and II LN generally carry a good prognosis; however, close monitoring of disease activity and optimal blood pressure control are essential.

Class I Lupus Nephritis (Minimal Mesangial Lupus Nephritis)

Class I is the mildest form of LN. There are no abnormalities present on light microscopy (LM), and mesangial immune deposits are observed with immunofluorescence (IF) alone or by both IF and electron microscopy (EM). Patients typically have normal renal function and minimal to no proteinuria. No immunosuppressive therapy is needed for class I LN.

Class II Lupus Nephritis (Mesangial Proliferative Lupus Nephritis)

In class II LN, there is mesangial hypercellularity and/or mesangial matrix expansion on LM (Fig 31.1). A few isolated subepithelial or subendothelial deposits may be present on IF or EM.[8]

Clinical manifestations include microscopic hematuria and/or proteinuria. However, nephrotic-range proteinuria or renal insufficiency is not usually present in this class of LN. Treatment involves renin–angiotensin system (RAS) blockade with the use of angiotensin converting enzyme inhibitors or angiotensin receptor blockers to not only reduce proteinuria but to also maintain blood pressure of <130/80 mmHg.[7,9] Immunosuppressive therapy is generally not indicated for this class of LN; however, if nephrotic-range proteinuria is present or if proteinuria cannot be controlled with RAS blockade, then it is reasonable to treat with glucocorticoids or calcineurin inhibitors (CNIs), as used in the treatment of minimal change disease or focal segmental glomerulosclerosis.[10]

Treatment of Proliferative Lupus Nephritis (Classes III and IV)

In class III LN (focal LN), less than 50% of the glomeruli are affected by LM. Endocapillary

TABLE 31.1 INTERNATIONAL SOCIETY OF NEPHROLOGY/RENAL PATHOLOGY SOCIETY 2003 CLASSIFICATION OF LUPUS NEPHRITIS

Class	Description
Class I	**Minimal mesangial lupus nephritis**
	Normal glomeruli by light microscopy. but mesangial immune deposits by immunofluorescence
Class II	**Mesangial proliferative lupus nephritis**
	Purely mesangial hypercellularity of any degree or mesangial matrix expansion by light microscopy. with mesangial immune deposits
	A few isolated subepithelial or subendothelial deposits may be visible by immunofluorescence or electron microscopy, but not by light microscopy
Class III	**Focal lupus nephritis[a]**
	Active or inactive focal, segmental or global endo- or extracapillary glomerulonephritis involving <50% of all glomeruli. typically with focal subendothelial immune deposits, with or without mesangial alterations
Class III (A)	Active lesions: focal proliferative lupus nephritis
Class III (A/C)	Active and chronic lesions: focal proliferative and sclerosing lupus nephritis
Class III (C)	Chronic inactive lesions with glomerular scars: focal sclerosing lupus nephritis
Class IV	**Diffuse lupus nephritis[b]**
	Active or inactive diffuse, segmental or global endo- or extracapillary glomerulonephritis involving 50% of all glomeruli, typically with diffuse subendothelial immune deposits, with or without mesangial alterations. This class is divided into diffuse segmental (IV-S) lupus nephritis when ≥50% of the involved glomeruli have segmental lesions, and diffuse global (IV-G) lupus nephritis when ≥50% of the involved glomeruli have global lesions. Segmental is defined as a glomerular lesion that involves less than half of the glomerular tuft. This class includes cases with diffuse wire loop deposits but with little or no glomerular proliferation.
Class IV-S (A)	Active lesions: diffuse segmental proliferative lupus nephritis
Class IV-G (A)	Active lesions: diffuse global proliferative lupus nephritis
Class IV-S (A/C)	Active and chronic lesions: diffuse segmental proliferative and sclerosing lupus nephritis
Class IV-G (A/C)	Active and chronic lesions: diffuse global proliferative and sclerosing lupus nephritis
Class IV-S (C)	Chronic inactive lesions with scars: diffuse segmental sclerosing lupus nephritis
Class IV-G (C)	Chronic inactive lesions with scars: diffuse global sclerosing lupus nephritis
Class V	**Membranous lupus nephritis**
	Global or segmental subepithelial immune deposits or their morphologic sequelae by light microscopy and by immunofluorescence or electron microscopy, with or without mesangial alterations
	Class V lupus nephritis may occur in combination with class III or IV in which case both will be diagnosed
	Class V lupus nephritis may show advanced sclerosis
Class VI	**Advanced sclerotic lupus nephritis**
	≥90% of glomeruli globally sclerosed without residual activity

[a]Indicate the proportion of glomeruli with active and with sclerotic lesions.

[b] Indicate the proportion of glomeruli with fibrinoid necrosis and/or cellular crescents.

Reprinted with permission from Weening JJ, D'Agati VD, Schwartz MM, et al. The classification of glomerulonephritis in systemic lupus erythematosus revisited. *Kidney Int.* 2004;65(2):521–530.

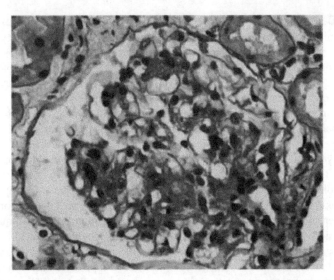

FIGURE 31.1 Periodic acid Schiff staining of lupus nephritis class II, demonstrating mild mesangial hypercellularity. Reprinted with permission from Houssiau FA, Vasconcelos C, D'Cruz D, et al. The 10-year follow-up data of the Euro-Lupus Nephritis Trial comparing low-dose and high-dose intravenous cyclophosphamide. *Ann Rheum Dis.* 2010;69(1):61–64.

or extracapillary proliferation is segmental (involving >50% of the glomerular tuft). In class IV LN (diffuse LN), <50% of the glomeruli are affected on LM, and the endocapillary or extracapillary proliferation is diffuse (involving <50% of the glomerular tuft; Fig. 31.2). EM usually reveals subendothelial immune deposits, and occasionally mesangial immune deposits are also observed. The histological lesions are classified further as active or chronic (Table 31.2).

Clinical manifestations of classes III and IV LN include hematuria, proteinuria, hypertension, and renal insufficiency. Proliferative LN is the most aggressive form of LN and requires immunosuppressive therapy

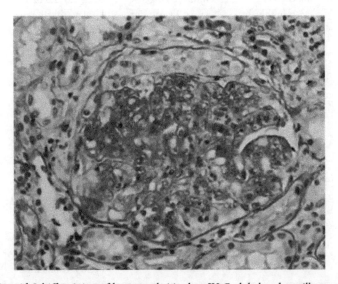

FIGURE 31.2 Periodic acid Schiff staining of lupus nephritis class IV-G global endocapillary proliferation, crescent formation, and disruption of Bowman's capsule Reprinted with permission from Houssiau FA, Vasconcelos C, D'cruz D, et al. The 10-year follow-up data of the Euro-Lupus Nephritis Trial comparing low-dose and high-dose intravenous cyclophosphamide. *Ann Rheum Dis.* 2010;69(1):61–64.

Background

In the 1950s, use of steroids for the treatment of proliferative LN resulted in an improvement in patient survival from a dismal 17% at 5 years to 55% at 5 years.[11,12]

In the 1970s, the addition of cytotoxic therapy to the steroid regimen resulted in further improvement in patient survival, which went up to 80% at 5 years.[13,14]

After several years following the introduction of cytotoxic therapy for proliferative LN, mycophenolate mofetil (MMF) emerged as an alternative to cytotoxic therapy.[15,16]

The goal of therapy is to achieve clinical and histological remission and avoid progression to chronic kidney disease. Remission of LN not only improves renal outcomes but also results in significant improvement in overall patient mortality.

Treatment of proliferative LN includes induction therapy and maintenance therapy.

Induction Therapy

The goal of induction therapy is to rapidly halt the acute inflammatory process in the kidney and to disrupt the autoimmune pathways to achieve remission, reduce renal disease progression, and prevent relapses.

Induction therapy for diffuse or moderate to severe focal proliferative LN consists of potent immunosuppressive therapy. The induction regimen should include glucocorticoids with either cyclophosphamide or MMF.[10,17]

The induction therapy is typically administered for 3 to 6 months. During this time, close monitoring is required, and if signs of disease progression such as worsening of creatinine and/or proteinuria are observed, then the immunosuppressive agents can be switched (cyclophosphamide to MMF, or vice versa).

Glucocorticoids should not be used as monotherapy for proliferative LN. Long-term renal outcomes are better when glucocorticoids are combined with an immunomodulatory

---

TABLE 31.2 REGIMEN FOR INITIAL THERAPY FOR CLASSES III AND IV LUPUS NEPHRITIS

Regimen	NIH	Euro-Lupus	Oral Cyclophosphamide	MMF
Cyclophosphamide	IV cyclophosphamide 0.5–1 g/ m²; monthly for 6 months	IV cyclophosphamide 500 mg; every 2 weeks for 3 months	Oral cyclophosphamide 1.0–1.5 mg/ kg/day (maximum dose 150 mg/d) for 2–4 months	—
MMF	—	—	—	MMF up to 3 g/day for 6 months
Benefit shown by RCT in proliferative LN	Yes	Yes	Yes	Yes
Benefit shown by RCT in severe proliferative LN	Yes	Untested	Untested	Untested
Comments	Effective in whites, blacks, Hispanics, Chinese	Effective in whites. Untested in blacks, Hispanics, Chinese	Effective in whites, blacks, Chinese; easy to administer and lower cost than IV cyclophosphamide	Effective in whites, blacks, Hispanics, Chinese; high cost

IV = intravenous. LN =lupus nephritis. MMF =mycophenolate mofetil. RCT = randomized controlled trial. All regimens include corticosteroids:
  • Oral prednisone, initial dose up to 0.5–1 mg/kg/day, tapering over 6–12 months according to clinical response.
  • IV methylprednisolone is sometimes added initially for severe disease.

agent.[13] The initial oral prednisone dose used is 1 mg/kg/day (maximum 80 mg/day). In severe proliferative disease, intravenous (IV) methylprednisolone 500 to 1,000 mg for 1 to 3 days is administered before switching to oral prednisone. The prednisone is tapered over several weeks to a maintenance dose of 5 to 10 mg/day.[17]

Cyclophosphamide may be administered as a high-dose regimen (National Institutes of Health [NIH] protocol) or as a low-dose regimen (Euro-lupus protocol). The NIH regimen includes IV cyclophosphamide 0.5 to 1 gram/m[2] monthly for 6 to 7 months.[18] The Euro-lupus regimen consists of IV cyclophosphamide 500 mg every 2 weeks for a total of 6 doses. It is important to note that the cumulative dose of cyclophosphamide in the Euro-lupus regimen is 3 grams, which is at least 50% lower than the NIH regimen. It is equally important to note that the Euro-lupus regimen has been found to be equivalent to the NIH regimen for remission induction and preservation of renal function at 5 and 10 years and has fewer side effects.[2,19] The Euro-lupus regimen was originally studied in a predominantly white cohort with mild to moderate LN; however, more recently the short-term efficacy of this regimen was verified in a more diverse cohort of patients with LN.[20]

Oral cyclophosphamide can also be used as induction therapy at 1 to 1.5 mg/kg/day (maximum 150 mg/day) for 2 to 4 months. This regimen of oral cyclophosphamide provides a cumulative dose of cyclophosphamide that is similar to the NIH regimen.

The use of cyclophosphamide is associated with significant adverse effects including leucopenia, gonadal failure, malignancies, infections, and hemorrhagic cystitis.[21]

MMF has been found to be equivalent to cyclophosphamide as induction therapy for LN.[22] Recently some concerns have been raised regarding the long-term renal outcomes with MMF being equivalent to cyclophosphamide, as the risk of developing ESRD from LN has risen slightly since the introduction of MMF as induction therapy.[6] However, as of now, MMF along with cyclophosphamide remains an agent of choice for LN induction therapy.

MMF dose used for induction therapy is 2 to 3 g/day for 6 months.[22] To assure better tolerability, MMF is started at a dose of 0.5 g twice daily in week 1, 1 g twice daily in week 2, with a target of 1.5 g 2× daily or 1 gram 3× daily thereafter. The adverse event rate with MMF has been found to be similar to that of cyclophosphamide; however, the types of adverse events with these agents are different. MMF has a lower incidence of ovarian failure and alopecia.[22]

Even though the treatment guidelines for proliferative LN recommend that either cyclophosphamide or MMF can be used as induction therapy, one agent may preferable to the other in certain clinical situations:

- MMF is associated with a better response rate in black and Hispanic patients.[23]
- Asian patients are more likely to be intolerant of higher doses of MMF but have similar response rates even at a lower dose.[23]
- MMF may be preferable in women of childbearing age due to the risk of ovarian failure associated with cyclophosphamide.
- Cyclophosphamide (NIH) protocol is recommended for severe and/or crescentic proliferative LN.[10]

Maintenance Therapy

Following the induction therapy, patients are switched to a maintenance therapy. The goal of maintenance therapy is to sustain clinical and histological remission achieved by induction therapy and to prevent renal relapses.

The maintenance therapy for LN is essential, as studies have shown that up to 50% patients may suffer from a relapse after completion of induction therapy.[2,10,24] MMF has emerged as the agent of choice for maintenance therapy. It has been shown to be more effective than azathioprine and less toxic than cyclophosphamide.[24,25] MMF dose during the maintenance therapy is 1 to 2 g/day, and it is used in conjunction with low dose prednisone 5 to 10 mg/day.

If a patient is unable to tolerate MMF, then azathioprine (2 mg/kg/day) along with low dose prednisone can be used. Azathioprine is also the agent of choice in women who are in remission and planning to become pregnant. MMF is contraindicated in pregnancy.

The duration of maintenance therapy is not well defined but can last for several months to years depending on disease severity, presence of clinical and histological remission, and the risk of relapse.

TREATMENT OF MEMBRANOUS LUPUS NEPHROPATHY (CLASS V)

In class V LN, there is diffuse thickening of the glomerular capillary wall on LM (Fig 31.3), and subepithelial deposits are present on IF and EM. Presence of subendothelial deposits may indicate presence of coexisting class III or class IV LN.

Patients with combined class III + class V or class IV + class V carry a worse prognosis than pure class V.[26] These patients should be treated according to proliferative LN treatment guidelines as previously noted.

Patients with pure class V LN typically present with proteinuria; however, hematuria, hypertension, and renal insufficiency may accompany proteinuria. Proteinuria can be in the subnephrotic or nephrotic range.

There is no consensus for the management of pure class V LN due to lack of randomized clinical trials. All patients are treated with RAS blockade to lower proteinuria, anti-hypertensive therapy with a target blood pressure of <130/80 mmHg, lipid-lowering agents, and anticoagulation therapy if risk factors for thromboembolism are present.[27-29]

Use of immunosuppressive therapy in patients with class V LN associated with subnephrotic range proteinuria and normal renal function remains controversial. Most experts recommend not using immunosuppressive therapy unless poor prognostic signs (such as worsening proteinuria or renal insufficiency) develop, while some have made a case for using immunosuppression due to the fact that, unlike idiopathic membranous nephropathy, membranous lupus nephropathy rarely remits spontaneously.

Patients with class V LN associated with nephrotic range proteinuria and/or renal insufficiency are treated with immunosuppressive therapy. The induction therapy typically involves use of use of glucocorticoids along with an immunosuppressive agent. Monotherapy with glucocorticoids is not recommended for treatment of class V LN.

The choice of the immunosuppressive therapy for class V LN is not guided by robust clinical trials. The potential treatment options are addressed in the following discussion.

MMF plus Prednisone

MMF has been shown to be as effective as IV cyclophosphamide for induction therapy for lupus membranous nephropathy.[30] During induction therapy MMF is administered at 1.5 g 2× daily for 6 months. The dose is lowered to 1 g 2× daily during the maintenance phase. In patients who are unable to tolerate MMF or have a contraindication to MMF use, CNIs or cyclophosphamide in combination with glucocorticoids can be used.

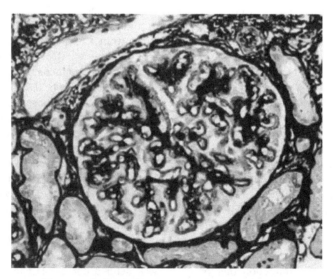

FIGURE 31.3 Silver staining of lupus nephritis class V showing subepithelial immune deposits and interdigitating spike formation. Reprinted with permission from Houssiau FA, Vasconcelos C, D'Cruz D, et al. The 10-year follow-up data of the Euro-Lupus Nephritis Trial comparing low-dose and high-dose intravenous cyclophosphamide. Ann Rheum Dis. 2010;69(1):61–64.

Calcineurin Inhibitors plus Prednisone

Cyclosporine is typically initiated at a dose of 200 mg/m² body surface area (approximately 5 mg/kg body weight) per day and given in 2 equal doses at 12-hour intervals (adjustment in the dose is required if the glomerular filtration rate [GFR] declines). The antiproteinuric effect is more rapid with cyclosporine compared to cyclophosphamide; however, the relapse rate with cyclosporine is also higher.[31] Due to the high relapse rate, once remission is achieved on cyclosporine therapy, cyclosporine is typically continued for 12 to 24 months.

Cyclosporine has been more extensively studied than tacrolimus in class V LN; however, tacrolimus can be used as an alternative as it is associated with fewer cosmetic side effects.

Calcineurin inhibitors may be the preferred agent in women of childbearing age as cyclophosphamide may result in ovarian failure and infertility. Calcineurin inhibitors may also be preferable to cyclophosphamide and MMF in women who are planning to become pregnant as both these agents can cause congenital malformations.

CNIs should be used with caution in patients with a low GFR due to the potential of nephrotoxicity associated with these agents.

Cyclophosphamide plus Prednisone

IV or oral cyclophosphamide can be used by to treat class V LN. In the study for membranous LN, intravenous cyclophosphamide was used every other month for 6 doses (ranging from 0.5–1.0 g/m² body surface area per month.[31] Once remission is achieved, patients are generally switched to MMF-based maintenance therapy. However, if the patient has failed MMF therapy in the past or is unable to tolerate MMF, CNIs can be used for maintenance therapy.[31]

Glucocorticoids

Glucocorticoids should not be used as monotherapy for class V LN as renal remission rates are significantly higher when they are used in combination with another agent.[31]

Dosing of prednisone (for treatment of lupus membranous nephropathy) with the previously mentioned regimens is not based on robust clinical data. Prednisone can be initiated at an oral dose of 1 mg/kg/day (maximum 60 mg/day) and gradually tapered every 2 weeks till a dose of 5 to 10 mg/day is reached.[32] Another option is alternate-day oral prednisone initiated at 40 mg/m² body surface area (approximately 1 mg/kg body weight) every other day for 8 weeks, followed by gradual tapered (5 mg/week) to 10 mg/m² body surface area.[31]

TREATMENT OF CLASS VI (ADVANCED SCLEROSIS LUPUS NEPHRITIS)

The renal biopsy in class VI LN shows sclerosis of at least 90% of the glomeruli, along with significant interstitial fibrosis and tubular atrophy. It usually results from chronic injury and without signs of acute immunologic activity. Therefore, immunosuppressive therapy for class VI LN is only indicated for extrarenal manifestations of lupus.[10]

HYDROXYCHLOROQUINE

All patients with LN of any class should be treated with hydroxychloroquine (maximum daily dose of 6–6.5 mg/kg ideal body weight) unless a contraindication exists for its use. There is some evidence to suggest that hydroxychloroquine increases likelihood of renal remission and decreases occurrence of renal relapses.[33,34]

However, due to its association with retinal toxicity, patients on hydroxychloroquine should receive annual eye exams.

TREATMENT OF RELAPSING LUPUS NEPHRITIS

The relapse rates in LN are high. Typically, patients present with worsening proteinuria and/or worsening GFR. A repeat renal biopsy should always be considered in relapsing LN as patients can spontaneously transform from one class of LN to another. If the class of LN diagnosed on the repeat biopsy is similar to the previous biopsy findings, it is reasonable to retreat the patient with the same agent that was successful in achieving remission in the past. However, the cumulative exposure to cyclophosphamide should not exceed the lifetime allowable dose of 36 g due to increased risk of malignancy.[21]

TREATMENT OF REFRACTORY/RESISTANT LUPUS NEPHRITIS

In patients who fail to respond to more than one of the initial recommended treatment regimens, treatment with Rituximab, IV immunoglobulins, or CNIs can be considered. These recommendations are not based on robust clinical trials but rather on small observational studies.[10,35–38]

SOME OTHER RENAL MANIFESTATIONS OF LUPUS

Thrombotic Microangiopathies

Thrombotic microangiopathies in lupus can occur alone or in combination with immune-complex LN. Thrombotic microangiopathies are not a singular entity and can occur in association with a variety of clinical conditions such as accelerated hypertension, systemic sclerosis, anti-phospholipid antibody syndrome, and thrombotic thrombocytopenic purpura. Treatment is directed toward the underlying condition.

Lupus Podocytopathy

Diffuse epithelial foot process effacement without immune-complex deposition has been described in patients with lupus. These patients are treated with glucocorticoids (like patients with minimal change disease).

Collapsing Focal Segmental Glomerulosclerosis

Collapsing focal segmental glomerulosclerosis has been described in patient with lupus. Treatment is not well studied. Glucocorticoids are used as first line therapy. CNIs and MMF can be used in combination with glucocorticoids, but these recommendations are not based on robust clinical data.

Lupus in Pregnancy

Pregnancy should be delayed until LN is in complete remission as evidence suggests that active LN is associated with increased fetal loss and increase renal relapses during pregnancy.[39,40] MMF, cyclophosphamide, angiotensin converting enzyme inhibitors, and angiotensin receptor blockers are teratogenic. Hydroxychloroquine, azathioprine, CNIs, and glucocorticoids can be used during pregnancy.

EMERGING THERAPIES

The current induction and maintenance therapies have improved patient survival with LN to 80% in 10 years; however, the renal response rates remain poor with complete remission seen in only 10% to 40% patients. Furthermore, the rate of progression to ESRD in patients with LN remains unacceptably high.[14,19,22,41] These statistics have compelled scientists and clinicians to search for better therapeutic options for LN.

Several therapeutic targets for LN have been studied recently including those targeting CD20, CLTA4-B7, IL-6, calcineurin, C5a, and other targets. These and other therapies have been well reviewed recently by Parikh et al.[42]

LUPUS NEPHRITIS AND END-STAGE RENAL DISEASE

Patients who develop ESRD due to LN may experience partial or complete resolution of their extrarenal lupus manifestations.[43] However, some studies have shown that such a remission is not observed in all LN patients.[44] The long-term prognosis of LN patients on dialysis is similar to the general population with ESRD.[41]

LUPUS NEPHRITIS AND RENAL TRANSPLANTATION

Most studies have shown that the outcome of renal transplantation in LN patients is similar to patients with other diseases.[43,45,46] However, the timing of renal transplant in LN patients has been a subject of debate. The general consensus is that LN patients who have a rapid progression to ESRD may benefit from being on dialysis for 3 to 6 months on minimal immunosuppression, allowing for reduction in lupus activity and potential for recovery of renal function. However, LN patients who have a slow and progressive decline in renal function associated with findings of chronic fibrotic changes on renal biopsy may not need to wait before transplantation and may even undergo preemptive kidney transplantation. The immunosuppression used in LN patients is similar to that used in other renal transplant patients. The recurrence rate of LN postrenal transplant varies from 2% to 11%, and graft loss due to recurrence is low, between 2 to 4%.[43,47]

CONCLUSION

The goal of LN treatment is to achieve complete remission and to prevent renal relapses to halt progression of chronic kidney disease. Though much progress has been made in this arena, there is still a need for therapeutic agents that are less toxic and more effective than the currently available therapies. Future studies may shed light on the new agents for LN.

REFERENCES

1. Houssiau FA, Vasconcelos C, D'Cruz D, et al. The 10-year follow-up data of the Euro-Lupus Nephritis Trial comparing low-dose and

high-dose intravenous cyclophosphamide. *Ann Rheum Dis.* 2010;69(1):61–64.

2. Yap DY, Tang CS, Ma MK, Lam MF, Chan TM. Survival analysis and causes of mortality in patients with lupus nephritis. *Nephrol Dial Transplant.* 2012;27(8):3248–3254.

3. Bernatsky S, Boivin JF, Joseph L, et al. Mortality in systemic lupus erythematosus. *Arthritis Rheum.* 2006;54(8):2550–2557.

4. Weening JJ, D'Agati VD, Schwartz MM, et al. The classification of glomerulonephritis in systemic lupus erythematosus revisited. *J Am Soc Nephrol.* 2004;15(2):241–250.

5. Wilhelmus S, Alpers CE, Cook HT, et al. The revisited classification of GN in SLE at 10 years: time to re-evaluate histopathologic lesions. *J Am Soc Nephrol.* 2015;26(12):2938–2946.

6. Tektonidou MG, Dasgupta A, Ward MM. Risk of end-stage renal disease in patients with lupus nephritis, 1971–2015: a systematic review and bayesian meta-analysis. *Arthritis Rheumatol.* 2016;68(6):1432–1441.

7. Jafar TH, Stark PC, Schmid CH, et al. Progression of chronic kidney disease: the role of blood pressure control, proteinuria, and angiotensin-converting enzyme inhibition: a patient-level meta-analysis. *Ann Intern Med.* 2003;139(4):244–252.

8. Weening JJ, D'Agati VD, Schwartz MM, et al. The classification of glomerulonephritis in systemic lupus erythematosus revisited. *Kidney Int.* 2004;65(2):521–530.

9. Duran-Barragan S, McGwin G, Jr., Vila LM, Reveille JD, Alarcon GS, cohort LamU. Angiotensin-converting enzyme inhibitors delay the occurrence of renal involvement and are associated with a decreased risk of disease activity in patients with systemic lupus erythematosus—results from LUMINA (LIX): a multiethnic US cohort. *Rheumatology (Oxford).* 2008;47(7):1093–1096.

10. Radhakrishnan J, Cattran DC. The KDIGO practice guideline on glomerulonephritis: reading between the (guide)lines—application to the individual patient. *Kidney Int.* 2012;82(8):840–856.

11. Heller BI, Jacobson WE, Hammarsten JF. The effect of cortisone in glomerulonephritis and the nephropathy of disseminated lupus erythematosus. *J Lab Clin Med.* 1951;37(1):133–142.

12. Cameron JS. Lupus nephritis: an historical perspective 1968-1998. *J Nephrol.* 1999;12(Suppl 2):S29–S41.

13. Austin HA, 3rd, Klippel JH, Balow JE, et al. Therapy of lupus nephritis: controlled trial of prednisone and cytotoxic drugs. *N Engl J Med.* 1986;314(10):614–619.

14. Ginzler EM, Bollet AJ, Friedman EA. The natural history and response to therapy of lupus nephritis. *Annu Rev Med.* 1980;31:463–487.

15. Chan TM, Li FK, Tang CS, et al. Efficacy of mycophenolate mofetil in patients with diffuse proliferative lupus nephritis. *N Engl J Med.* 2000;343(16):1156–1162.

16. Ginzler EM, Dooley MA, Aranow C, et al. Mycophenolate mofetil or intravenous cyclophosphamide for lupus nephritis. *N Engl J Med.* 2005;353(21):2219–2228.

17. Bertsias GK, Tektonidou M, Amoura Z, et al. Joint European League against Rheumatism and European Renal Association–European Dialysis and Transplant Association (EULAR/ERA-EDTA) recommendations for the management of adult and paediatric lupus nephritis. *Ann Rheum Dis.* 2012;71(11):1771–1782.

18. Boumpas DT, Austin HA, 3rd, Vaughn EM, et al. Controlled trial of pulse methylprednisolone versus two regimens of pulse cyclophosphamide in severe lupus nephritis. *Lancet.* 1992;340(8822):741–745.

19. Houssiau FA, Vasconcelos C, D'Cruz D, et al. Immunosuppressive therapy in lupus nephritis: the Euro-Lupus Nephritis Trial, a randomized trial of low-dose versus high-dose intravenous cyclophosphamide. *Arthritis Rheum.* 2002;46(8):2121–2131.

20. Access Trial Group. Treatment of lupus nephritis with abatacept: the Abatacept and Cyclophosphamide Combination Efficacy and Safety study. *Arthritis Rheumatol.* 2014;66(11):3096–3104.

21. Faurschou M, Sorensen IJ, Mellemkjaer L, et al. Malignancies in Wegener's granulomatosis: incidence and relation to cyclophosphamide therapy in a cohort of 293 patients. *J Rheumatol.* 2008;35(1):100–105.

22. Appel GB, Contreras G, Dooley MA, et al. Mycophenolate mofetil versus cyclophosphamide for induction treatment of lupus nephritis. *J Am Soc Nephrol.* 2009;20(5):1103–1112.

23. Isenberg D, Appel GB, Contreras G, et al. Influence of race/ethnicity on response to lupus nephritis treatment: the ALMS study. *Rheumatology (Oxford).* 2010;49(1):128–140.

24. Dooley MA, Jayne D, Ginzler EM, et al. Mycophenolate versus azathioprine as maintenance therapy for lupus nephritis. *N Engl J Med.* 2011;365(20):1886–1895.

25. Contreras G, Pardo V, Leclercq B, et al. Sequential therapies for proliferative lupus nephritis. *N Engl J Med.* 2004;350(10):971–980.

26. Sloan RP, Schwartz MM, Korbet SM, Borok RZ. Lupus Nephritis Collaborative Study Group.

Long-term outcome in systemic lupus erythematosus membranous glomerulonephritis. *J Am Soc Nephrol.* 1996;7(2):299–305.

27. Bomback AS, Appel GB. Updates on the treatment of lupus nephritis. *J Am Soc Nephrol.* 2010;21(12):2028–2035.

28. Mercadal L, Montcel ST, Nochy D, et al. Factors affecting outcome and prognosis in membranous lupus nephropathy. *Nephrol Dial Transplant.* 2002;17(10):1771–1778.

29. Lionaki S, Derebail VK, Hogan SL, et al. Venous thromboembolism in patients with membranous nephropathy. *Clin J Am Soc Nephrol.* 2012;7(1):43–51.

30. Radhakrishnan J, Moutzouris DA, Ginzler EM, Solomons N, Siempos, II, Appel GB. Mycophenolate mofetil and intravenous cyclophosphamide are similar as induction therapy for class V lupus nephritis. *Kidney Int.* 2010;77(2):152–160.

31. Austin HA, 3rd, Illei GG, Braun MJ, Balow JE. Randomized, controlled trial of prednisone, cyclophosphamide, and cyclosporine in lupus membranous nephropathy. *J Am Soc Nephrol.* 2009;20(4):901–911.

32. Sinclair A, Appel G, Dooley MA, et al. Mycophenolate mofetil as induction and maintenance therapy for lupus nephritis: rationale and protocol for the randomized, controlled Aspreva Lupus Management Study (ALMS). *Lupus.* 2007;16(12):972–980.

33. Fangtham M, Petri M. 2013 update: Hopkins lupus cohort. *Curr Rheumatol Rep.* 2013;15(9):360.

34. Ruiz-Irastorza G, Ramos-Casals M, Brito-Zeron P, Khamashta MA. Clinical efficacy and side effects of antimalarials in systemic lupus erythematosus: a systematic review. *Ann Rheum Dis.* 2010;69(1):20–28.

35. Melander C, Sallee M, Trolliet P, et al. Rituximab in severe lupus nephritis: early B-cell depletion affects long-term renal outcome. *Clin J Am Soc Nephrol.* 2009;4(3):579–587.

36. Rauova L, Lukac J, Levy Y, Rovensky J, Shoenfeld Y. High-dose intravenous immunoglobulins for lupus nephritis—a salvage immunomodulation. *Lupus.* 2001;10(3):209–213.

37. Ogawa H, Kameda H, Amano K, Takeuchi T. Efficacy and safety of cyclosporine A in patients with refractory systemic lupus erythematosus in a daily clinical practice. *Lupus.* 2010;19(2):162–169.

38. Miyasaka N, Kawai S, Hashimoto H. Efficacy and safety of tacrolimus for lupus nephritis: a placebo-controlled double-blind multicenter study. *Mod Rheumatol.* 2009;19(6):606–615.

39. Carvalheiras G, Vita P, Marta S, et al. Pregnancy and systemic lupus erythematosus: review of clinical features and outcome of 51 pregnancies at a single institution. *Clin Rev Allergy Immunol.* 2010;38(2–3):302–306.

40. Wagner SJ, Craici I, Reed D, et al. Maternal and foetal outcomes in pregnant patients with active lupus nephritis. *Lupus.* 2009;18(4):342–347.

41. Costenbader KH, Desai A, Alarcon GS, et al. Trends in the incidence, demographics, and outcomes of end-stage renal disease due to lupus nephritis in the US from 1995 to 2006. *Arthritis Rheum.* 2011;63(6):1681–1688.

42. Parikh SV, Rovin BH. Current and emerging therapies for lupus nephritis. *J Am Soc Nephrol.* 2016;27(10):2929–2939.

43. Mojcik CF, Klippel JH. End-stage renal disease and systemic lupus erythematosus. *Am J Med.* 1996;101(1):100–107.

44. Krane NK, Burjak K, Archie M, O'Donovan R. Persistent lupus activity in end-stage renal disease. *Am J Kidney Dis.* 1999;33(5):872–879.

45. Ponticelli C, Moroni G. Renal transplantation in lupus nephritis. *Lupus.* 2005;14(1):95–98.

46. Bumgardner GL, Mauer SM, Payne W, et al. Single-center 1-15-year results of renal transplantation in patients with systemic lupus erythematosus. *Transplantation.* 1988;46(5):703–709.

47. Contreras G, Mattiazzi A, Guerra G, et al. Recurrence of lupus nephritis after kidney transplantation. *J Am Soc Nephrol.* 2010;21(7): 1200–1207.

32

Thrombotic Microangiopathies

LEWIS KAUFMAN

INTRODUCTION

Thrombotic microangiopathies syndromes include a heterogeneous group of disorders that are unified by their clinical and pathological features.[1] They all include the clinical characteristics of microangiopathic hemolytic anemia (MAHA), thrombocytopenia, and end-organ dysfunction. All forms of TMA have common blood vessel wall pathology that includes widespread endothelial injury with the formation of diffuse microvascular thrombosis (Fig. 32.1). Over the last few decades, the specific causes of the primary TMA syndromes have in many cases been elucidated, and their nomenclature has been changing to reflect their underlying cause: thrombotic thrombocytopenic purpura (TTP; or TMA resulting from severe ADAMTS13 deficiency), hemolytic uremic syndrome (HUS; or Shiga-toxin mediated TMA), complement-mediated TMA, drug-induced TMA, metabolism-mediated TMA, and coagulation-mediated TMA. Of these, the older term "atypical HUS," which was originally meant to differentiate a previously poorly characterized TMA syndrome from HUS with diarrhea, has been completely replaced by the specific term "complement-mediated TMA." This chapter will review these primary causes of TMA with a specific focus on how the underlying cause effects treatment, management, and the development of novel therapeutic approaches (Table 32.1).

Importantly, many systemic disorders are also associated with MAHA and thrombocytopenia including pregnancy complications, severe hypertension, systemic infections (including bacterial, viral, rickettsial, and fungal), malignancy, systemic rheumatological disorders, hematopoietic stem cell transplant, and disseminated intravascular coagulation. The treatment of these patients is focused entirely on the underlying disorder. Although primary TMA syndromes can often be unmasked by an acute event such as surgery or pregnancy, the treatment here is entirely focused on the underlying causal abnormality (such as ADAMTS13 deficiency or complement mutation) and not on the precipitating events. The rapid evolution of treatments and outcomes of TMA syndromes over the last decade correlates with our accelerated understanding of the pathogenesis of these disorders.

THROMBOTIC THROMBOCYTOPENIC PURPURA

Cause

TTP is a thrombotic microangiopathy caused by severe reductions in activity of the von Willebrand factor-cleaving protein ADAMTS13.[2] ADAMTS13 functions to cleave von Willebrand multimers that are secreted by vascular endothelial cells.[1] When ADAMTS13 is deficient, von Willebrand multimers become unusually large, which leads directly to the development of small vessel platelet thrombi and subsequent end-organ dysfunction.[3] TTP can be acquired, due to an autoantibody inhibitor, or it can be inherited, caused by inherited homozygous or compound heterozygous mutations in ADAMTS13.[2] The acquired form of TTP is mediated by autoantibodies that block ADAMTS13 protease function or nonneutralizing antibodies that cause clearance of ADAMTS13 protease.[4]

Clinical Manifestations and Diagnosis

The presence of MAHA and thrombocytopenia without an apparent alternative clinical explanation should raise the diagnostic possibility of TTP. The presentation of acquired TTP is quite variable, ranging from minimal organ involvement to critical multiorgan failure.[5] Importantly,

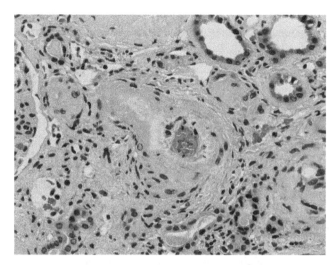

FIGURE 32.1 Common pathological features of primary thrombotic microangiopathy (TMA). All type of primary TMA include common vascular pathological findings, including renal arteriole occlusion with endotheliosis, mucoid intimal degeneration, and fibrin deposition. Courtesy of Fadi Salem, Department of Pathology, Icahn School of Medicine at Mount Sanai.

TTP is distinctive among all causes of TMA as only rarely causing acute kidney injury. The reasons for this are not known. Transient focal neurological abnormalities are common but are absent in up to one-third of patients. Other presenting clinical features are varied and include weakness, gastrointestinal symptoms such as abdominal pain or gastrointestinal bleeding, purpuric skin lesions, or cardiac ischemia or failure.[6]

TABLE 32.1 PRIMARY THROMBOTIC MICROANGIOPATHY SYNDROMES

Thrombotic thrombocytopenic purpura	Deficiency of ADAMTS13, the von Willebrand factor cleaving metalloprotease. Acquired due to autoimmune antibody to ADAMTS13, or hereditary due to mutation in ADAMTS13. Acute kidney injury uncommon. Treatment is plasma infusion.
Complement-mediated TMA	Uncontrolled activation of alternate complement pathway. Mediated by loss of function mutations in complement regulatory proteins (CFH, CFI, CD46) or gain of function in an effector gene (CFB or C3). Can also be caused by autoimmune antibodies to CFH or CFI. Treatment is the anti-complement agent eculizumab, or if autoantibody is cause plasma exchange and immunosuppression.
Hemolytic uremic syndrome	Enteric infection with a Shiga-toxin secreting strain of *Escherichia Coli* or *Shigella dysenteriae*. Toxin causes direct damage to renal cells. Most common in children less than 5 years old. Treatment is mainly supportive.
Drug-induced TMA	Immune-mediated caused by drug-dependent antibodies that directly damage cells (quinine is best described). Toxic-dose related reaction cause by direct cellular toxicity of drug (calcineurin inhibitors such as cyclosporine and tacrolimus, VEGF inhibitors, oxymorphone)
Metabolism-mediated TMA	Disorders of intracellular vitamin B12 metabolism due to mutations in MMACHC gene. Treated with parenteral vitamin B12 administration.
Coagulation-mediated TMA	Caused by mutations in DGKE, most commonly. Mutations in PLC and THBD also implicated. Treatment usually plasma infusion.

TMA = thrombotic microangioapathy.

A presumptive diagnosis of TTP is usually made based on clinical and laboratory parameters, even without fully excluding other forms of TMA first. Making an early diagnosis is of paramount importance to allow for early initiation of therapy, most notably plasma exchange. ADAMTS13 activity testing levels are an important adjunct to the initial clinical diagnosis. A level of less than 10% of normal activity supports a diagnosis of acquired TTP. However, some individuals with acquired TTP may have higher ADAMTS13 levels, and, therefore, this test must not be used as the sole diagnostic determinant and plasma exchange not withheld based on this criteria alone. In most clinical laboratories, severe deficiency of ADAMTS13 reflexively triggers testing for the presence of an autoantibody inhibitor. These autoantibodies are present in the great majority of acquired TTP cases, and their absence raises the possibility of late-onset hereditary TTP, which is caused by a genetic mutation in ADAMTS13 and not an autoantibody. ADAMTS13 levels and autoantibody titers are routinely followed during treatment and remission although they do not always correlate with clinical response or overall patient outcome.

Treatment and Outcomes

The cornerstone of TTP therapy is plasma exchange, which results in ADAMTS13 replacement. Prior to routine use of plasma exchange, survival rates from TTP were dismal, typically less than 10% overall.[7] After the advent of routine treatment of TTP with plasma exchange, the survival rates have improved to 78%. This dramatic survival benefit adds clear urgency for early initiation of plasma exchange, even when other causes of thrombotic microangiopathy are still being considered. Our new in-depth understanding of the root causes of acquired TTP has led to several novel therapeutic strategies that either inhibit the production of autoantibodies against ADAMTS13 or prevent the accumulation of von Willebrand factor-platelet complexes that are the cause of end-organ dysfunction.[8] In congenital TTP, our understanding of the basic genetic cause of this entity has led to the development of recombinant ADAMTS13 protease for therapeutic use. Overall, these exciting therapeutic approaches describe a new highly targeted strategy to TTP therapy that will be evaluated in clinical trials over the coming years.

Using first-line approaches, more than 80% of newly diagnosed TTP patients will achieve clinical remission. However, many of these patients will relapse, particularly those who keep an undetectable ADAMTS13 activity or continue to show detectable anti-ADAMTS13 antibodies. TTP patients are at increased risk for many other co-morbid conditions including cognitive impairment, depression, hypertension, cardiovascular disease, and death.[9] Newer, yet untested, therapies include administration of recombinant ADAMTS13 or inhibitors of von Willebrand factor complex formation. Such novel targeted approaches would make attractive, safe, and simple candidates for prophylactic and/or maintenance therapy.

COMPLEMENT-MEDIATED TMA

Cause

Complement-mediated TMA is mediated by dysregulation of the alternative complement pathway. The alternative complement pathway, unlike the classical or lectin pathways, is always active with the continuous formation of small amounts of C3b on the cell surface. To prevent continuous and unopposed activation, this complement system is tightly regulated. Disruption of this network of complement regulatory proteins can lead to unopposed activation of the alternative pathway, resulting in the formation of the membrane attack complex and cellular injury. Endothelial cell injury, in particular to renal endothelial cells, results in the complement-mediated TMA phenotype. Unlike for TTP, acute kidney injury and hypertension are prominent features of complement-mediated TMA.

Many cases of complement-mediated TMA can be linked directly to mutations in the complement regulatory network: either loss of function mutations in regulatory genes (complement factor H [CFH], complement factor I [CFI], CD46) or gain of function mutations in effector genes (complement factor B [CFB] or C3).[1,10] The most frequently identified genetic abnormality is in CFH. CFH with CFI compete with CFB for binding to C3b and accelerates C3 convertase decay.[11] Over 100 different mutations in CFH have been described, with the great majority of these being heterozygous. As such, these patients have normal, or near normal, CFH and/or C3 levels. Unfortunately, patients with CFH mutations have the worst outcomes of all patients with atypical HUS: two thirds of all patients progress to ESRD or death within 1 year of diagnosis.[12] Interestingly, complement mutations that cause atypical HUS are usually heterozygous and are often carried by related family members who remain completely asymptomatic. This suggests the existence of additional genetic and/or environmental modifiers. CFH antibodies have also been implicated in approximately 10% of patients with complement-mediated TMA. These antibodies interfere with binding of CFH to the C3 convertase and prevent CFH-mediated complement regulation.

Clinical Manifestations and Diagnosis

Clinical features of complement-mediated TMA include MAHA, thrombocytopenia, and acute kidney injury with hypertension. Typically, levels of ADAMTS13 are greater than 5%, and stool cultures are negative for Shiga-toxin producing bacteria. The criteria are not specific and can occur in other forms of primary and secondary TMA syndromes. Measurements of plasma levels of C3, C4, CFB, CFH, or CFI are indicated, but normal results do not exclude the diagnosis of complement-mediated TMA. In approximately 25% of patients, a family history of TMA is evident. In the majority of patients (>75%), there is an antecedent trigger event such as an upper respiratory infection, a diarrheal infection, or pregnancy.

Genetic studies of major causative mutations are possible and can add invaluable diagnostic and prognostic information. Unfortunately, such testing is still not widely available and needs to be arranged through special laboratories that can be found on the National Center for Biotechnology Information website.[1] Such screening should be strongly considered in those patients with a clear family history, recurrent disease, and presentation within the first year of life or during pregnancy or in those who have a poor or unexpected clinical course.

Treatment and Outcomes

Besides supportive care, all patients with a diagnosis of complement-mediated TMA should receive anticomplement therapy, for which eculizumab is currently the only approved agent. Eculizumab is a humanized monoclonal antibody to C5. In multiple large case series, its administration has shown to be an effective treatment for patients with a variety of genetic mutations in complement proteins, in those with autoantibodies to CFH, and in kidney transplant recipients.[13,14] This included improvement in kidney function and hematological parameters as

well as the ability to discontinue plasma therapy. As a result of these studies, the US Food and Drug Administration granted accelerated approval for the use of eculizumab for complement-mediated TMA in 2011. The benefit of the drug was limited, however, in complement-mediated TMA patients who carry mutations in C5.

The main issues with eculizumab therapy continues to be the high cost, estimated to be in excess of $400,000 per year per patient. Because the diagnostic criteria are relatively nonspecific and even patients without a complement abnormality may show a beneficial response to eculizumab, the decision to start and continue the drug can at times be difficult. In addition, it remains unknown whether patients who have had a favorable response to eculizumab can ever be taken safely off of the drug. Small case series suggest high risk of relapse with eculizumab withdrawal. This implication is problematic given the huge associated cost. Certainly, all patients being treated with eculizumab should be tested for anti-CFH antibodies, where more conventional immunosuppression and/or plasma exchange may be equally beneficial. In those with severe disease, where eculizumab is not available because of cost, plasma exchange is recommended. Combined liver–kidney transplantation provides a potentially definitive cure for complement-mediated TMA caused by CFH, CFI, CFB, or C3 mutations, in particular for children with severe disease.

The main adverse event with eculizumab therapy is life-threatening and fatal meningococcal infections with a reported annual rate of 0.5%.[1] All patient should be vaccinated again *neisseria meningitis* as well as to *strep pneumoniae* and *haemophilus influenza* type B.

HEMOLYTIC UREMIC SYNDROME

Cause

HUS is the major systemic complication of enterohemorrhagic infection. Specifically, in North America and Europe, the most common cause of HUS in is Shiga toxin-producing *Escherichia coli* (*E. coli*; STEC). *Shigella dysenteriae* is another important cause worldwide, particularly in South Asia and parts of Africa.[15] It is much more common in children under the age of 5, where it is a major cause of acute kidney injury with a mortality rate of 3%. In adults, it is much less common, but when it occurs, it is more severe with higher mortality rates. Many different

E. coli stains can produce Shiga toxin, with *E. coli* O157:H7 the most common. Healthy cattle are the main source of STEC, which are commonly present in their intestine and stool. Human infection occurs after ingestion of contaminated food products including undercooked meat, unpasteurized milk, water, or fruit and vegetables. Human-to-human transmission is also possible, particularly among children in daycare-type settings. Although outbreaks of this illness do occur and are often publicized,[16] sporadic cases happen more commonly. Endemic HUS happens more often in rural versus urban settings and in the summer months, which is consistent with exposure to cattle being the primary infectious source. Cellular damage is the direct result of Shiga toxin binding to ceramide trihexoside on the cell surface.[1] Effected cells include endothelial cells as well as many cells within the kidney including podocytes, mesangial, and tubular cell types.

Clinical Manifestations and Diagnosis

Typically, severe abdominal pain, vomiting, and diarrhea begin soon after the contaminated food is ingested, but this prodromal illness typically precedes the development of HUS by approximately 5 to 10 days. The HUS syndrome includes MAHA, thrombocytopenia, and acute kidney injury. Acute kidney injury is often severe, more than half the time requiring dialysis therapy. Other organs can be involves as well, in particular the central nervous system, which occurs in approximately 25% of all cases. Severe neurological involvement such as seizures or somnolence portends a bad outcome with higher mortality.

Diagnostic evaluation for STEC infection should be done, including stool cultures, Shiga toxin stool enzyme-linked immunosorbent assay, as well as testing for STEC specific serum immunoglobulin M levels. Because the STEC may only be present in the stool during the prodromal period, stool culture results may be negative and not reliable as evidence of recent infection.

Treatment and Outcomes

Management of HUS is aggressive supportive care to include intravenous fluids to maintain intravascular volume, transfusion of blood products as needed, and hemodialysis initiation where appropriate. In general, approximately 25% of patients with HUS will develop long-term sequela with death or ESRD occurring in about 10%. In general, the acuity of the initial illness including the need for dialysis or presence of neurological symptoms was strongly associated with worse long-term outcomes.[17] Improvements in food safety via continued public health improvement measures should help to reduce its incidence.[18]

DRUG-INDUCED TMA

Cause

Drug-induced TMA is an acquired condition caused by exposure to a drug. It can be difficult to diagnose because specific laboratory tests to identify a specific drug are not generally available, and the role of the implicated drug may not be entirely clear. Overall, there are 2 specific types of drug-induced TMA: immune-mediated and toxicity-mediated.[1] Both induce classic findings of TMA including MAHA, thrombocytopenia, and acute kidney injury. The immune-mediated form of drug-induced TMA is caused by exposure to any amount of the drug, even in very small amounts, and is caused by an idiosyncratic, antibody-dependent mechanism. The toxicity-mediated form of drug-induced TMA is caused by a dose and time-dependent mechanism of the offending agent. Each of these 2 mechanisms involves differences in prognosis, presentation, and management.

In the immune-mediated mechanism, the drug itself induces antibody formation, and the antibodies react with multiple cell types including endothelial cells, platelets, and neutrophils. The binding of antibodies to these multiple targets induces cellular damage and subsequently TMA. The antibody generation requires previous or ongoing exposure to the drug, and the severity of the reaction is independent of dose. Even very small doses may produce a severe reaction. Quinine is the most common and well-characterized cause of this syndrome.[19] The existence of drug-dependent quinine antibodies has been definitively established. Other implicated drugs include quetiapine and gemcitabine and, to lesser extent, trimethoprim-sulfomethaxazole, proteasome inhibitors such as bortezomib and immunomodulatory agents such as OKT3 or adalimumab.

In the toxicity-mediated mechanism, TMA may develop by a variety of mechanisms, in general, due to direct tissue injury from the implicated agent. These reactions are often mediated by dose and time-dependent toxicity. There are 3 major categories of drugs causing toxicity-mediated drug-induced TMA: (i) cancer therapies such as gemcitabine (causes both immune and toxic-mediated TMA) mitomycin, vascular endothelial growth factor inhibitors, and hematopoietic cell transplantation; (ii) immunosuppressive agents such as calcineurin inhibitors (both cyclosporine and tacrolimus) and sirolimus; and (iii) drugs of abuse such as inappropriate intravenous administration of extended release oxymorphone, ecstasy, or cocaine. The reaction to vascular endothelial growth factor inhibitors has been well described and appears to be mediated by direct action of the drug on glomerular endothelial and podocyte function.[20] Calcineurin inhibitor reactions seem to be mediated by direct effects of the drug on glomerular endothelial cell signaling pathways.

Clinical Manifestations and Diagnosis

Immune-mediated drug induced TMA typically involves the sudden onset of severe systemic symptoms including anuric kidney failure beginning within hours of drug exposure. This is most classically illustrated by our experience with quinine. Exposure to quinine is often missed unless specifically asked for by the healthcare team. Exposure may be from quinine tablets or quinine-containing drinks such as tonic water. Patients may report nonspecific illnesses with previous exposures to the drug that were previously unrecognized.

Toxicity-mediated drug-induced TMA usually involves gradual or subacute decline in kidney function, usually with hypertension and, at times, neurological findings such as headache or confusion. The exception to this is with drugs of abuse, where sudden onset, severe TMA may occur.

Treatment and Outcomes

Primary management of all drug-induced TMAs is drug discontinuation or avoidance and supportive care. Recovery from immune-mediated drug-induced TMA is very gradual and often incomplete. Chronic kidney disease is common. Recovery from toxicity-mediated drug-induced TMA is highly variable, and although hematological findings often normalize, chronic kidney disease often persists.

METABOLISM-MEDIATED AND COAGULATION-MEDIATED TMA

A rare cause of TMA is from a hereditary defect in vitamin B12 metabolism, called cobalamin

C disease.[21] It usually presents in infancy with multiple organ dysfunction including TMA. It is caused by mutations in methylmalonic aciduria and homocystinuria type C protein. It is associated with elevated homocysteine and low methionine levels in plasma, with methylmalonic aciduria. Treatment is parenteral administration of vitamin B12.

Once considered part of the spectrum of atypical HUS, rare mutations in coagulation-associated proteins are now classified as coagulation-mediated TMA.[22] These include mutations in thrombomodulin, protein kinase C-associated protein, and diacylglycerol kinase ε (DGKE). Most patients present in early childhood and are found to have acute kidney injury requiring dialysis. The pathophysiology of these disorders is uncertain, but in the case of DGKE, mutations seems to involve activation of protein kinase C and upregulation of prothrombotic factors.[23]

CONCLUSION

Over the last decade, there has been a dramatic growth in our understanding of the underlying causes of the primary TMA syndromes. These discoveries have opened up entire new avenues for specific disease-targeted treatments. As these therapies come into use, it is clear that there are still many unmet therapeutic needs for TMA both at time of initial presentation as well as for maintenance therapy to prevent disease recurrence and other long-term morbidities.

REFERENCES

1. George JN, Nester CM. Syndromes of thrombotic microangiopathy. *N Engl J Med.* 2014;371(19):1847–1848.
2. Levy GG, Nichols WC, Lian EC, et al. Mutations in a member of the ADAMTS gene family cause thrombotic thrombocytopenic purpura. *Nature.* 2001;413(6855):488–494.
3. Moake JL, Rudy CK, Troll JH, et al. Unusually large plasma factor VIII: von Willebrand factor multimers in chronic relapsing thrombotic thrombocytopenic purpura. *N Engl J Med.* 1982;307(23):1432–1435.
4. Froehlich-Zahnd R, George JN, Vesely SK, et al. Evidence for a role of anti-ADAMTS13 autoantibodies despite normal ADAMTS13 activity in recurrent thrombotic thrombocytopenic purpura. *Haematologica.* 2012;97(2):297–303.
5. George JN, Chen Q, Deford CC, Al-Nouri Z. Ten patient stories illustrating the extraordinarily

diverse clinical features of patients with thrombotic thrombocytopenic purpura and severe ADAMTS13 deficiency. *J Clin Apher.* 2012;27(6):302–311.

6. Reese JA, Muthurajah DS, Kremer Hovinga JA, Vesely SK, Terrell DR, George JN. Children and adults with thrombotic thrombocytopenic purpura associated with severe, acquired Adamts13 deficiency: comparison of incidence, demographic and clinical features. *Pediatr Blood Cancer.* 2013;60(10):1676–1682.

7. Kremer Hovinga JA, Vesely SK, Terrell DR, Lammle B, George JN. Survival and relapse in patients with thrombotic thrombocytopenic purpura. *Blood.* 2010;115(8):1500–1511; quiz 1662.

8. Cataland SR, Wu HM. Acquired thrombotic thrombocytopenic purpura: new therapeutic options and their optimal use. *J Thromb Haemost.* 2015;13(Suppl 1):S223–S229.

9. Deford CC, Reese JA, Schwartz LH, et al. Multiple major morbidities and increased mortality during long-term follow-up after recovery from thrombotic thrombocytopenic purpura. *Blood.* 2013;122(12):2023–2029; quiz 2142.

10. Bu F, Maga T, Meyer NC, et al. Comprehensive genetic analysis of complement and coagulation genes in atypical hemolytic uremic syndrome. *J Am Soc Nephrol.* 2014;25(1):55–64.

11. Stahl AL, Vaziri-Sani F, Heinen S, et al. Factor H dysfunction in patients with atypical hemolytic uremic syndrome contributes to complement deposition on platelets and their activation. *Blood.* 2008;111(11):5307–5315.

12. Noris M, Caprioli J, Bresin E, et al. Relative role of genetic complement abnormalities in sporadic and familial aHUS and their impact on clinical phenotype. *Clin J Am Soc Nephrol.* 2010;5(10):1844–1859.

13. Legendre CM, Licht C, Loirat C. Eculizumab in atypical hemolytic-uremic syndrome. *N Engl J Med.* 2013;369(14):1379–1380.

14. Palma LM, Langman CB. Critical appraisal of eculizumab for atypical hemolytic uremic syndrome. *J Blood Med.* 2016;7:39–72.

15. Tarr PI, Gordon CA, Chandler WL. Shigatoxin-producing *Escherichia coli* and haemolytic uraemic syndrome. *Lancet.* 2005;365(9464):1073–1086.

16. Bell BP, Goldoft M, Griffin PM, et al. A multistate outbreak of *Escherichia coli* O157:H7-associated bloody diarrhea and hemolytic uremic syndrome from hamburgers. The Washington experience. *J Am Med Assoc.* 1994;272(17):1349–1353.

17. Garg AX, Suri RS, Barrowman N, et al. Long-term renal prognosis of diarrhea-associated hemolytic uremic syndrome: a systematic review, meta-analysis, and meta-regression. *J Am Med Assoc.* 2003;290(10):1360–1370.

18. Maki DG. Don't eat the spinach—controlling foodborne infectious disease. *N Engl J Med.* 2006;355(19):1952–1955.

19. Kojouri K, Vesely SK, George JN. Quinine-associated thrombotic thrombocytopenic purpura-hemolytic uremic syndrome: frequency, clinical features, and long-term outcomes. *Ann Intern Med.* 2001;135(12):1047–1051.

20. Eremina V, Jefferson JA, Kowalewska J, et al. VEGF inhibition and renal thrombotic microangiopathy. *N Engl J Med.* 2008;358(11):1129–1136.

21. Geraghty MT, Perlman EJ, Martin LS, et al. Cobalamin C defect associated with hemolytic-uremic syndrome. *J Pediatr.* 1992;120(6):934–937.

22. Lemaire M, Fremeaux-Bacchi V, Schaefer F, et al. Recessive mutations in DGKE cause atypical hemolytic-uremic syndrome. *Nat Genet.* 2013;45(5):531–536.

23. Bruneau S, Neel M, Roumenina LT, et al. Loss of DGKepsilon induces endothelial cell activation and death independently of complement activation. *Blood.* 2015;125(6):1038–1046.

33

Systemic Inflammatory Diseases and the Kidney

JOSE MANUEL MONROY-TRUJILLO AND DUVURU GEETHA

INTRODUCTION

The antineutrophil cytoplasmic antibodies (ANCA) associated vasculitis (AAV) are rare multisystem autoimmune diseases, which is common in older individuals. AAV should be considered in the differential diagnosis of rapidly progressive glomerulonephritis (GN) and pulmonary renal syndrome.

Combination of glucocorticoids with cyclophosphamide or rituximab is effective in inducing disease remission.

AAV is a relapsing disease, and maintenance immunosuppression is needed to prevent disease relapses, but the duration of maintenance immunosuppression remains to be defined.

Definition

AAV are autoimmune diseases characterized by the presence of circulating ANCA and inflammatory cell infiltration causing necrosis of small blood vessels. The AAV comprise granulomatosis with polyangiitis (GPA), microscopic polyangiitis (MPA) and eosinophilic GPA (EGPA).

Epidemiology

AAV is more common in patients over the age of 60 and is disproportionately more common in whites compared to African Americans.[1] AAV are not genetic or inheritable diseases. Genome-wide association studies have identified reproducible genetic association of HLA-DPB1*0401 for patients with ANCA and allele deficiency of alpha-1 antitrypsin for patients with GPA. More important, these studies have shown that the strongest genetic associations are with ANCA specificity rather than with clinical syndrome (GPA vs. MPA). Proteinase 3 AAV is associated with HLA-DP whereas myeloperoxidase AAV is associated with HLA-DQ.[2]

The estimated annual incidence of GPA and MPA in Europeans vary from 2 to 12 cases per million population with prevalence of 23 to 160 cases per million population. EGPA is much less common than GPA or MPA with incidence of 1 to 4 cases per million population and prevalence of 10 to 20 cases per million population.[2]

Pathogenesis

The pathogenesis of AAV remains incompletely understood and involves interaction between the immune system and nonimmune factors. Neutrophils play a central role in AAV by being targets of ANCA as well as effectors cells mediating endothelial damage. Imbalances in T cell subtypes and cytokines play role by breaking tolerance, cause oxidative burst targeting endothelial cells, and trigger autoimmunity. B cells are thought to play a major role since they produce ANCA, which have been shown to be pathogenic in animal models of AAV. More recent data have strengthened the role of alternate complement pathway activation in the pathogenesis of AAV.[3] Certain drugs have been implicated in the etiology of AAV, the most common being propylthiouracil, hydralazine, and levamisole-adulterated cocaine.

Clinical Manifestations

Most patients with AAV often trace the onset of vasculitis to a flu-like illness and have constitutional symptoms of fever, sweats, anorexia, and weight loss. GPA and EGPA have granulomatous manifestations while GPA, MPA, and EGPA have vasculitic manifestations. The granulomatous manifestations include sinusitis, nasal collapse, ocular inflammation, otitis media, subglottic stenosis, lung nodules, and cavities. Vasculitic manifestations include pauci-immune GN, leucocytoclastic skin vasculitis, scleritis, alveolar hemorrhage, and mononeuritis multiplex. Patients with EGPA have asthma and eosinophilia.[1] Renal involvement is more common in GPA and MPA than in EGPA and presents clinically as rise in serum creatinine, proteinuria, and hematuria. Cardiac involvement occurs more commonly in EGPA and GPA and can range from cardiomyopathy and conduction abnormalities to life-threatening myocarditis. Other rare manifestations include hepatitis and pancreatitis.

Laboratory Findings/Renal Histopathology

Majority of patients have elevated levels of erythrocyte sedimentation rate and C-reactive protein. A positive ANCA serology has a high diagnostic predictive value in the right clinical setting. It is recommended that the laboratory testing for ANCA include immunofluorescence and enzyme-linked immunosorbent assay. About 90% of GPA and MPA patients are ANCA positive compared to 45% of patients with EGPA. GPA patients are more often c-ANCA/proteinase 3 ANCA positive while MPA patients are often p-ANCA/myeloperoxidase ANCA positive. The hallmark of renal vasculitis histologically is a pauci-immune GN, but granulomatous interstitial nephritis and evidence of immune complex GN can be also be seen in some patients. A new ANCA GN classification proposed by the international working group of renal pathologists categorizing ANCA GN to focal, crescentic, mixed, and sclerotic classes has been shown to have predictive value with focal class having the best renal outcome and sclerotic class having the worst renal outcome.

Treatment

The treatment of AAV involves a 2-staged approach of remission induction and maintenance phases.[1,2] Remission is defined clinically by stabilization or improvement in serum creatinine, resolution of hematuria, and absence of signs of extrarenal disease. Treatment advances have transformed these uniformly fatal diseases to chronic illness with a relapsing course with a 5-year survival of 75%. Induction therapy involves using glucocorticoids with either cyclophosphamide or rituximab. Plasma exchange is recommended in the setting of alveolar hemorrhage or severe renal disease requiring dialysis at presentation. The glucocorticoid regimen typically consists of pulse methyl prednisone 1000 mg/day for 3 days followed by oral prednisone 1 mg/kg/day, which is tapered over 6 months. Cyclophosphamide can be given intravenously or orally for 3 to 6 months until disease remission is achieved. The dose of cyclophosphamide is adjusted for renal function and older age. The recommended dose of rituximab for remission induction is 375 mg/m^2 once a week for 4 weeks. Rituximab is preferred for remission induction in patients with relapsing disease and young patients who wish to preserve fertility. During the induction phase, it is recommended that patients receive *Pneumocystis jiroveci* pneumonia prophylaxis. Following remission induction, either azathioprine, mycophenolate mofetil, or rituximab is used for remission maintenance up to 18 to 24 months with close clinical monitoring after that. The value of ANCA serology monitoring for prediction of relapses remains controversial.

Considerations in Management of End-Stage Renal Disease Patients

About 20% to 25% of AAV patients reach end-stage renal disease (ESRD) within a few years of diagnosis, with ESRD being more common in MPA than GPA patients. Patients with AAV are more likely to be on hemodialysis than peritoneal dialysis due to concern for increased infection risk in immunosuppressed patients. The 10-year probability of survival for AAV patients on dialysis is similar to patients with nondiabetic nephropathies on dialysis. The risk of vasculitis relapse is less in dialysis patients. Renal transplantation is the preferred renal replacement therapy option with a 10-year patient and allograft survival of 75% and 64%, respectively. Relapses following transplant are rare with current immunosuppressive regimens. It is recommended that AAV patients are transplanted after being in remission for at least 6 months on dialysis to minimize the risk of recurrent disease.

ANTIGLOMERULAR BASEMENT MEMBRANE DISEASE

Antiglomerular basement membrane disease (anti-GBM) should be considered in the differential diagnosis of rapidly progressive GN and should be considered when in patients presenting with hemoptysis and increased serum creatinine with an active urine sediment.

The standard therapy is plasmapheresis combined with glucocorticoids and cyclophosphamide in all patients except those with dialysis dependent renal failure.

Definition
Anti-GBM disease is a small vessel vasculitis affecting glomerular capillaries and/or lung capillaries with GBM deposition of anti-GBM antibodies causing alveolar hemorrhage and necrotizing and crescentic GN.

Epidemiology
Anti-GBM disease is rare, with an annual incidence of 0.5 to 1 cases per million in Europe. There are 2 age-dependent peaks of incidence, in the third decade of life where presentation with both lung and renal disease is observed and in the seventh decade of life where isolated renal involvement is more common.[4] There is a slight male predominance in the younger age group and female predominance in the older age group.

Pathogenesis
Anti-GBM disease is caused by autoimmunity to the non-collagenous domain 1 of the α3-chain of type intravenous collagen in response to an unknown inciting stimulus. The pathogenicity of these antibodies has been demonstrated in animal models. There is strong association between anti-GBM disease and HLA class II alleles including DRB1*1501 and DR4 alleles.[4] Interestingly, hydrocarbon exposure has been linked in several case reports. Smoking can precipitate lung hemorrhage in patients with circulating anti-GBM antibodies. Additional reported predisposing factors include presence of small vessel renal vasculitis, membranous nephropathy, lithotripsy for renal calculi, and alemtuzumab treatment for multiple sclerosis.

Clinical Manifestations
The classic presentation is a pulmonary–renal syndrome with alveolar hemorrhage and rapidly progressive renal failure. Rapidly progressive GN occurs in 80% to 90% of patients, and 40% to 50% present with isolated alveolar hemorrhage. About 70% to 90% of patients can experience fatigue, malaise, and weight loss. All patients will have microscopic hematuria and moderate proteinuria, and it is common to see rapid progression of renal failure. When the lungs are involved, patients present with cough, hemoptysis, and hypoxemia. The anemia resulting from alveolar hemorrhage can be out of proportion

to renal failure and can be a clue to the disease presentation.

Laboratory/Renal Histopathology
Circulating anti-GBM antibodies detected by commercially available enzyme immunoassays or bead-based fluorescence assays are universally present and diagnostic.[5] About one-third of patients can have circulating ANCA, especially in the setting of severe renal disease. Renal biopsy should be performed in patients with renal involvement unless there is a contraindication. Light microscopy reveals widespread crescent formation involving more than 80% of glomeruli. The crescents are of uniform age compared to ANCA-associated GN where one might see combination of cellular, fibro-cellular, and fibrous crescents. Interstitial fibrosis and tubular atrophy are uncommon given the acuity of the disease. The pathognomonic finding is a linear staining of IgG along the glomerular capillaries on immunofluorescence (Fig. 33.1).

Treatment
The standard of therapy is combination of plasmapheresis to remove circulating anti-GBM antibodies, glucocorticoids to halt neutrophil driven inflammation, and cyclophosphamide to stop formation of new antibodies. The treatment outcome depends on the severity of renal disease due to poor renal prognosis in patients with dialysis dependent renal failure and in those who have 100% crescents on renal biopsy.[6] In these patients, the risk of immunosuppression outweighs any potential benefit. Treatment with plasmapheresis and immunosuppressive therapy is recommended in patients with alveolar hemorrhage regardless of severity of renal disease, in patients who are serologically positive for both ANCA and anti-GBM antibody, and in patients with renal involvement who do not require dialysis at presentation. Plasmapheresis is performed daily for 14 days or until the antibody level is undetectable.[4] The optimal duration of therapy is not clear. In general, therapy is continued until anti-GBM antibody is negative. If anti-GBM antibody remains positive after 4 months of therapy, cyclophosphamide is replaced with azathioprine for 6 to 9 months.

Considerations in ESRD Patients Undergoing Renal Transplantation
Renal transplant is recommended for ESRD patients when the anti-GBM antibody has been

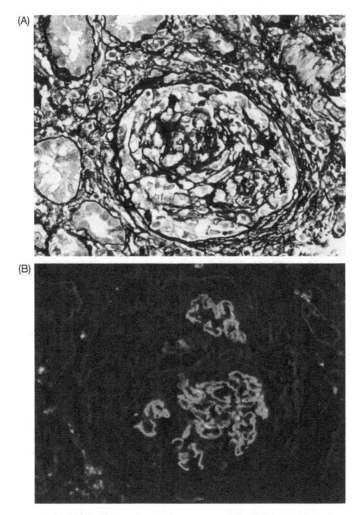

FIGURE 33.1 (A) Glomerulus with cellular crescent and disruption of the glomerular basement membrane, (Periodic acid Schiff- methenamine silver stain 200×). (B) Strong linear immunoglobin G staining by immunofluorescence along the glomerular basement membrane.

negative for 12 months and the disease has been quiescent for 6 months post treatment in the absence of immunosuppressive therapy. Up to 50% of transplanted patients will have positive linear IgG staining on immunofluorescence, but clinical recurrence of disease is low when transplant is performed during disease quiescence.

IGA VASCULITIS

IgA vasculitis is common in children and typically affects skin, joints, kidneys, and gastrointestinal system. In older adults, renal disease is common and carries a worse prognosis. IgA renal disease should be differentiated from IgA-dominant postinfectious GN.

Renal biopsy is indicated in IgA vasculitis when there is high grade proteinuria or renal insufficiency.

Definition

IgA vasculitis, previously known as Henoch-Schonlein purpura is a small-vessel vasculitis affecting skin, kidney, joints, and gastrointestinal tract and characterized by tissue deposition of IgA. The hallmark of renal disease is mesangial IgA deposition and is indistinguishable from IgA nephropathy.

Epidemiology

IgA vasculitis is a childhood disease and occurs between ages 3 and 5. The annual incidence is

20 cases per 100,000 in children under the age of 17 and 5 per 100,000 in adults.[7] The disease is less frequent in African Americans compared to whites and Asians with a male preponderance. IgA vasculitis peaks in spring, summer, and fall and is less common in winter.

Pathogenesis

The underlying cause of IgA vasculitis is not known. It is an immune complex-mediated vasculitis characterized by IgA deposition. A multihit hypothesis has been proposed in the pathogenesis of IgA vasculitis. Overproduction of galactose deficient IgA1 (Gd-IgA1) and autoantibodies against Gd-IgA1 is followed by formation of immune complexes and deposition of those immune complexes in glomeruli.[8] Genetic factors and secondary immune dysregulation might be involved in the production of Gd-IgA1. Additionally, mucosal immune dysregulation may contribute to the production of Gd-IgA1 and Gd-IgA1 immune complexes.

Clinical Manifestations

The classic tetrad of IgA vasculitis includes a palpable purpura with lower limb predominance, arthritis/arthralgias, abdominal pain, and renal disease. These can develop in any order and at any time over a period of few days to few weeks. The frequency of renal involvement ranges from 25% to 50% and is common in older children and adults. The renal disease usually occurs within a month of onset of systemic symptoms and is not related in a predictable fashion to development of extrarenal disease. The most common renal manifestation is microscopic hematuria with or without red blood cell casts. In severe cases, these result in moderate to severe proteinuria and a rise in serum creatinine.

Laboratory Findings/Renal Histopathology

The renal biopsy is indistinguishable from IgA nephropathy and demonstrates focal mesangial proliferation in mild disease and more cellular proliferation with crescent formation in those with severe proteinuria or renal insufficiency. Immunofluorescence reveals classic finding of diffuse mesangial IgA staining (Fig. 33.2). Co-staining with C3 is seen in 90% of patients. Electron microscopy demonstrates electron dense deposits in mesangial and paramesangial areas. It is important to differentiate IgA vasculitis from IgA dominant post infectious GN, the findings of which are supported by findings of subepithelial deposits on microscopy.

Treatment

Patients with microscopic hematuria or low-grade proteinuria with preserved renal function require only supportive therapy and do not need to undergo renal biopsy. Renal biopsy is performed when there is high-grade proteinuria or rise in serum creatinine. If there is evidence of crescentic GN with >50% glomeruli involved by crescents, a course of glucocorticoids is

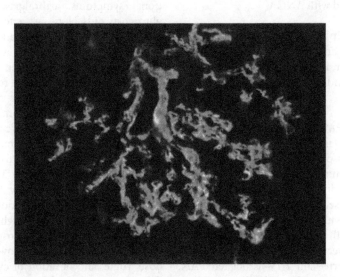

FIGURE 33.2 Immunofluorescence stain for immunoglobin A. Intense granular glomerular staining in the mesangium of an affected glomerulus.

recommended.[9] Addition of cyclophosphamide was not beneficial to steroids alone in severe Henoch-Schonlein nephritis in a French trial.[10]

Considerations in Management of ESRD Patients

The rates of ESRD ranges from 10 % to 30% at 10 years. Renal transplantation can be performed for ESRD due to IgA vasculitis. The deposition of IgA in allograft is common, although most cases remain subclinical. The incidence of recurrent disease is higher in live donors and in patients who have had an aggressive course with rapid progression of their renal disease.

POLYARTERITIS NODOSA

Polyarteritis nodosa (PAN) is a medium vessel vasculitis. It can involve almost any medium vessel, causing a wide variety of symptoms. It usually spares pulmonary arteries. Renal arteries are affected in 50% to 60% of cases causing hypertension and renal failure.

As PAN does not affect capillaries, it does not cause GN. It can also affect gastrointestinal tract, heart, skin, muscle, and central nervous system.

Prognosis is very poor without treatment. Main treatment is extrapolated from literature on AAV.

Definition

PAN was defined in the 2012 Chapel Hill Consensus Conference[11] as necrotizing arteritis of medium- and small-sized arteries without GN or vasculitis of arterioles, capillaries, or venules and not associated with ANCA.

Epidemiology

PAN is rare with an annual incidence in Europe of 4.4 to 9.7 per million. PAN affects middle aged or older individuals with a slight male preponderance.

Pathogenesis

Most cases of polyarteritis nodosa are idiopathic. PAN has been associated with hepatitis B virus infection in a minority of cases. PAN occurring in the setting of infections and hairy cell leukemia are called secondary PAN. In 1970, up to 36% of patients with PAN were related to hepatitis B virus.[12] With the advent of hepatitis B vaccine, this has decreased to 7.3%. There are reports of hepatitis C virus and HIV-associated PAN. In other instances, monogenetic diseases with loss of function mutation can lead to deficiency of adenosine deaminase-2 and cause PAN-like syndrome.

Clinical Manifestations

The clinical manifestations are mainly related to affected organs.[13] For unclear reasons, it does not usually affect pulmonary artery vessels. Kidneys are involved in up to 60% of cases producing hypertension, infarction, or hematoma secondary to rupture of microaneurysms. Nonspecific symptoms are common including weight loss, abdominal pain, malaise, and myalgias. Gastrointestinal involvement can lead to ischemia, perforation, or infarction.

There are no serologic markers for diagnosis of PAN. Arteriogram may reveal microaneurysms that tend to occur in bifurcation vessels. They occur more commonly in renal, mesenteric, and hepatic arteries.

Treatment

Without any treatment, a 5-year survival has been reported between 10% and 20%. Main treatment consist of cyclophosphamide and steroids. Prognosis in treated PAN improves to a 5-year survival of almost 80%.[14] Most of the literature about treatment of PAN is obtained from AAV. The Factor-Five Score and Birmingham Vasculitis Activity Score have been used to evaluate therapeutic response. The Factor-Five Score consist of 4 variables: renal insufficiency (creatine >1.7 mg/dL), gastrointestinal involvement, cardiac involvement, and age >65. For patients with mild disease manifesting with constitutional symptoms, arthralgias, and skin rash, glucocorticoids alone are effective in inducing remission. For resistant cases with mild disease, azathioprine 2 mg/kg/day or methotrexate 20 to 25 mg once weekly may need to be added. For severe cases manifesting with renal, cardiac, gastrointestinal, and neurologic manifestations, it is recommended to use a combination of high-dose steroids followed by cyclophosphamide. In organ or life-threatening manifestations, it is recommended to give pulse therapy with intravenous methylprednisone for 3 days followed by oral prednisone 1 mg/kg/day, tapered over 6 to 8 months. There are no randomized controlled trials comparing pulse and high-dose glucocorticoid therapy in PAN. Cyclophosphamide has been used extensively in PAN.[15] However, the optimal dose, route, and duration of cyclophosphamide is uncertain. Cyclophosphamide can be given as pulse therapy or as oral cyclophosphamide until remission is achieved but no more than 12 months.

Patients with hepatitis B or C virus-related PAN should be treated with antivirals rather than immunosuppressant therapy.

SCLERODERMA RENAL CRISIS

Scleroderma is an autoimmune disorder affecting multiple organs. It causes excessive fibrosis and vascular damage. Renal disease involvement is common in scleroderma with scleroderma renal crisis (SRC) being the most serious manifestation.

SRC is characterized by abrupt onset of hypertension, acute kidney injury, and a benign urinalysis. However up to 10% of SRC patients can be normotensive. The main stay of treatment is angiotensin converting enzyme inhibitors.

Definition

Scleroderma is a multisystem disease of unknown origin affecting predominantly the skin, gastrointestinal tract, lungs, and kidneys. It is classified as diffuse cutaneous systemic sclerosis and limited cutaneous systemic sclerosis. SRC occurs predominantly in diffuse scleroderma and is an early complication of scleroderma. SRC is characterized by acute onset of renal failure in the absence of prior renal disease and abrupt onset of moderate to severe hypertension, though it is important to remember that 10% of cases are normotensive.

Epidemiology

SRC is more common in women. Main risk factors include diffuse scleroderma, high-dose steroid use in the recent month, use of cyclosporine and presence of positive anti-RNA polymerase III antibodies.[16] SRC affects about 18% of patients with diffuse systemic sclerosis and about 2% of limited cutaneous sclerosis.

Pathologic Findings

The pathologic findings on renal biopsy are localized in the small arcuate and interlobular arteries. The histologic hallmark is intimal proliferation and thickening with concentric "onion-skin thickening" and edema that leads to narrowing and occlusion of vascular lumen (Fig. 33.3). Pathologic changes in SRC are similar to those observed in malignant hypertension.

Clinical Manifestations

SRC is characterized by abrupt onset of accelerated hypertension or rapidly progressive oliguric renal failure.[17] Hypertension is seen in 90% of cases (>150/85 mmHg). It usually occurs early in the course of the disease. Seventy-five percent of them occur in the first 4 years of diagnosis. Laboratory findings include elevated creatinine and proteinuria (53%). Microangiopathy hemolytic anemia is only seen in 33% to 46% of cases. The risk of SRC is increased in patients with antibodies against RNA polymerase III and decreased in patients with, anticentromere antibodies.[16] Hyperreninemia has been reported in 96% of cases, but there is limited clinical relevance.

Treatment

The main treatment is angiotensin converting enzyme inhibitors (ACEIs), and a number of studies have confirmed their role in better

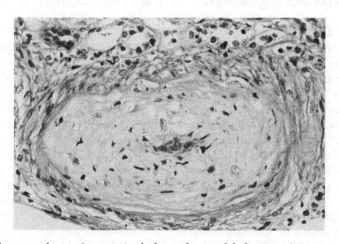

FIGURE 33.3 Scleroderma renal crisis: Severe intimal edema of an interlobular artery (Masson trichrome).

control of hypertension and preservation of renal function.[16,18] The most experience has been with captopril. Although, the data on other ACE inhibitors like lisinopril are limited, they are equally efficacious. ACEIs, however, have not been shown to prevent SRC when given prophylactically. Addition of calcium channel blockers may be beneficial to improve blood pressure control.

Considerations in Management of ESRD Patients

Renal recovery from dialysis can occur as late as 18 months after onset of SRC and because of this, decision regarding transplant should not be made immediately following dialysis initiation for SRC. Renal allograft survival is reduced in SRC patients compared to renal transplant recipients for other causes of ESRD; however, the overall outcomes are better in transplanted SRC patients compared to those remaining on dialysis.[19] Following transplant, it is important to continue ACEI and avoid using high-dose glucocorticoids and cyclosporine to minimize the risk of SRC.

IGG4-RELATED DISEASE

IgG4-related disease (IgG4-RD) is an emerging disorder that is characterized by tumor-like swelling of involved organs and infiltration of plasma cells (IgG4+) with a variable degree of fibrosis that has a "storiform" pattern and elevated IgG4.

The kidney is one of the main affected organs (23% of cases in a series of 235 patients). The most common renal finding is tubulointerstitial nephritis.[20]

Majority of patients with early disease respond to glucocorticoid therapy; 30% of patients can experience relapse after stopping steroids.

Definition

IgG4-RD has been recently defined by the following criteria: (i) presence of kidney damage (abnormal urinalysis, elevated creatinine with either elevated serum IgG levels, hypocomplementemia, or elevated IgE levels), (ii) abnormal renal imaging, (iii) elevated IgG4 levels (>135 mg/dL), and (iv) histologic findings (dense lymphoplasmacytic infiltration IgG4-positive plasma cells >10/high power field and/or IgG4/IgG-positive plasma cells >40%).[21]

Epidemiology

IgG4-RD mostly affects middle-aged men as most of patients are >50 years old. Male to female

ratio 4:1. When present in females, the salivary glands are predominantly affected. IgG4-RD has been associated with malignancies, mainly of the gastrointestinal tract. The pancreas is the main organ involved (60% of the cases).

Pathogenesis

IgG4 immunoglobulin is the least abundant in the body. It binds weakly to both C1q and FcγR (fragment crystallizable-gamma receptors). IgG4-RD typically has low serum complement levels. It is regulated by type 2 helper T cells. Pathologic diagnosis of IgG4-RD requires immunohistochemical confirmation with IgG4 immunostaining. Elevated serum IgG4 levels alone are not enough to establish the diagnosis.[22]

Clinical Manifestations

The most common lesion is tubulointerstitial nephritis. This can lead to progressive increase in serum creatinine. About 50% of patients have mild proteinuria or microscopic hematuria. The glomeruli can also be affected in cases of membranous nephropathy. Hypocomplementemia (both C3 and C4) is another common feature. IgG4-RD can be seen in other conditions such as Mikulicz syndrome (salivary and lacrimal glands), thyroiditis, retroperitoneal fibrosis, autoimmune pancreatitis, and periaortitis.[23]

Renal Histopathology

The histologic hallmark is a lymphoplasmacytic infiltration of the renal interstitium and the presence of storiform pattern of interstitial fibrosis. Immunohistochemistry of renal biopsy tissue demonstrates increased numbers of IgG4-positive plasma cells (Fig. 33.4).

Treatment

One of the characteristics of IgG4-related kidney disease is rapid improvement with glucocorticoids therapy. Glucocorticoids are therefore the first-line therapy. One regimen described is to start 40 mg orally daily for 4 weeks and then taper over the next 7 weeks by decreasing 5 mg per week.[24] In patients, not responding or having intolerance to glucocorticoids, rituximab 1 gm administered every 2 weeks for 2 doses is used. Azathioprine and mycophenolate mofetil are other second-line agents. Patients need close monitoring after induction of remission as relapses are common. About 30% of patients can experience relapses after stopping steroids.

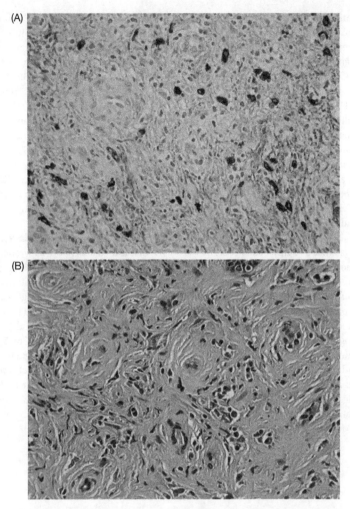

FIGURE 33.4 Immunoglobin G4 (IgG4) related nephropathy. (A) Immunostain for IgG4 shows many positive plasma cells in the interstitial inflammatory infiltrate (400×). (B) Typical storiform pattern of interstitial fibrosis (hematoxylin and eosin 400×).

REFERENCES

1. Yates M, Watts R. ANCA associated vasculitis. *Clin Med (Lond)*. 2017;17(1):60–64.

2. Pagnoux C. Updates in ANCA associated vasculitis. *Eur J Rheumatol*. 2016;3(3):122–133.

3. Xiao H, Hu P, Falk RJ, Jennette JC. Overview of the pathogenesis of ANCA associated vasculitis. *Kidney Dis (Basel)*. 2016;1(4):205–215.

4. McAdoo SP, Pusey CD. Anti glomerular basement membrane disease. *Clin J Am Soc Nephrol*. .12;2017: 1–11.

5. Bolton WK. Goodpasture's syndrome. *Kidney Int*. 1996;50:1753–1766.

6. Levy JB, Turner AN, Rees AJ, Pusey CD. Long-term outcome of anti–glomerular basement membrane antibody disease treated with plasma exchange and immunosuppression. *Ann Intern Med*. 2001;134:1033–1042.

7. Yang YH, Yu HH, Chiang BL. The diagnosis and classification of Henoch-Schönlein purpura: an updated review. *Autoimmun Rev*. 2014;13(4–5):355–358.

8. Suzuki H, Yasutake J, Makita Y, et al. IgA nephropathy and IgA vasculitis with nephritis have a shared feature involving galactose-deficient IgA1-oriented pathogenesis. *Kidney Int*. 2018;93(3):700–705.

9. Pillebout E, Thervet E, Hill G, et al. Henoch-Schönlein purpura in adults: outcome and prognostic factors. *J Am Soc Nephrol*. 2002;13:1271–1278.

10. Pillebout E, Alberti C, Guillevin L, et al. Addition of cyclophosphamide to steroids provides no

benefit compared with steroids alone in treating adult patients with severe Henoch Schönlein Purpura. *Kidney Int.* 2010;78:495–502.

11. Jennette JC, Falk RJ, Bacon PA, et al. 2012 revised International Chapel Hill Consensus Conference Nomenclature of Vasculitides. *Arthritis Rheum.* 2013;65(1):1–11.

12. Trepo C, Guillevin L. Polyarteritis nodosa and extrahepatic manifestations of HBV infection: the case against autoimmune intervention in pathogenesis. *J Autoimmun.* 2001; 16(30) 269–274.

13. Forbess L, Bannykh S. Polyarteritis nodosa. *Rheum Dis Clin N Am.* 2015;(41):33–46.

14. Pagnoux C, Seror R, Henegar C, et al.; French Vasculitis Study Group. Clinical features and outcomes in 348 patients with polyarteritis nodosa: a systematic retrospective study of patients diagnosed between 1963 and 2005 and entered into the French Vasculitis Study Group Database. *Arthritis Rheum.* 2010;62(2):616–626.

15. Guillevin L, Cohen P, Mahr A, et al. Treatment of polyarteritis nodosa and microscopic polyangiitis with poor prognosis factors: a prospective trial comparing glucocorticoids and six or twelve cyclophosphamide pulses in sixty-five patients. *Arthritis Rheum.* 2003;49(1):93–100.

16. Penn H, Howie AJ, Kingdon EJ, et al. Scleroderma renal crisis: patient characteristics and long-term outcomes. *QJM.* 2007;100(8):485–494.

17. Traub YM, Shapiro AP, Rodnan GP, et al. Hypertension and renal failure (scleroderma renal crisis) in progressive systemic sclerosis. Review of a 25-year experience with 68 cases. *Medicine (Baltimore).* 1983; 62(6):335–352.

18. Steen VD, Costantino JP, Shapiro AP, Medsger TA Jr. Outcome of renal crisis in systemic sclerosis: relation to availability of angiotensin converting enzyme (ACE) inhibitors. *Ann Intern Med.* 1990; 113(5):352–357.

19. Gibney EM, Parikh CR, Jani A, Fischer MJ, Collier D, Wiseman AC. Kidney transplantation for systemic sclerosis improves survival and may modulate disease activity. *Am J Transplant.* 2004;4(12):2027–2031.

20. Inoue D, Yoshida K, Yoneda N, et al. IgG4-Related disease: dataset of 235 consecutive patients. *Medicine (Baltimore).* 2015 Apr;94(15):e680.

21. Kawano M, Saeki T, Nakashima H, et al. Proposal for diagnostic criteria for IgG4-related kidney disease. *Clin Exp Nephrol.* 2011 Oct;15(5):615–626.

22. Stone JH, Zen Y, Deshpande V. IgG4-related disease. *N Engl J Med.* 2012;366:539–551.

23. Kawano M, Yamada K. IgG4-related kidney disease and IgG4-related retroperitoneal fibrosis. *Semin Liver Dis.* 2016;36:283–290.

24. Khosroshahi A, Stone JH. Treatment approaches to IgG4-related systemic disease. *Curr Opin Rheumatol.* 2011, 23:67–71.

34

The Kidney in Patients with Cancer

RAMNIKA GUMBER, AKASH SETHI, AND JONATHAN J. HOGAN

INTRODUCTION

The kidney-associated complications in patients with cancer are diverse and common. In select large cohort studies, the risk of developing acute kidney injury (AKI; defined as a 50% increase in serum creatinine) in incident cancer patients was 17.5% and 27% at 1 and 5 years, respectively,[1] and 52.9% of patients with solid tumors had an abnormal estimated glomerular filtration rate (eGFR).[2] Further, an analysis of 1998–2002 United States Renal Database System, End Stage Renal Disease found that approximately one-third of end stage renal disease (ESRD) patients had cancer when beginning renal replacement therapy.[3] Importantly, renal disease in the setting of cancer can be associated with significant morbidity, mortality, and treatment interruption.

The etiology of kidney injury can be multi-factorial as shown in Table 34.1. In this chapter, we will focus on etiopathologies that are unique to this group—specifically, direct tumor involvement of the kidney, paraneoplastic renal diseases, treatment-associated kidney disease, tumor lysis syndrome (TLS), and kidney disease after hematopoietic stem cell transplantation (HCT).

DIRECT TUMOR INVOLVEMENT OF THE KIDNEY

Renal Cell Carcinoma

The management of primary renal tumors can affect long-term renal function. Nephron-sparing procedures may be recommended for patients with localized (T1 and T2) renal tumors to minimize surgical complications and improve long-term renal outcomes versus radical nephrectomy. The European Organization for Research and Treatment of Cancer randomized trial[4] found that partial nephrectomy was noninferior to radical nephrectomy in patients with T1 or T2 with no spread to lymph nodes or distant organs renal cell carcinomas <5.0 cm for overall survival and oncologic outcomes. At a median follow-up of 6.7 years, radical nephrectomy was associated with higher rates of moderate renal dysfunction (<60 mL/min/1.73m^2) but not more severe stages (eGFR <30 or <15 mL/min/1.73m^2) of kidney disease.[5] A recent meta-analysis comparing the treatment of localized tumors with radical nephrectomy, partial nephrectomy, or thermal ablation found that radical nephrectomy was associated with a larger decline in eGFR (–10.5 mL/min/1.73m^2) versus partial nephrectomy and that partial nephrectomy and thermal ablation were both associated with lower risk of stage 3 or worse chronic kidney disease (CKD) and ESRD compared to radical nephrectomy.[6] Rates of AKI were not different between groups.

Metastatic Disease to the Kidney

Solid tumor metastases to the kidney are rare. Past autopsy series found that the kidney was an uncommon site for metastases, occurring in 2% to 12% of patients with cancer. One recent retrospective study[7] described 151 patients diagnosed with renal metastases from primary nonrenal malignancies by nephrectomy, fine-needle aspiration, or biopsy. Flank pain (30%), hematuria (16%), and weight loss (12%) were the most common symptoms. The majority of tumors were solitary (75%) and carcinomas (80.8%), and the most common primary site was lung (43.7%). Patients treated with surgery had improved overall survival in this study.

Lymphomatous Infiltration of the Kidney

The literature describing lymphomatous infiltration of the kidney is composed of older autopsy series and more recent epidemiologic and kidney biopsy series. The autopsy series in patients with

TABLE 34.1 CAUSES OF KIDNEY INJURY IN THE SETTING OF CANCER

Mechanism of Injury	Examples
Related to tumor infiltration or burden	Lymphomatous infiltration of the kidney
	Metastatic disease to the kidney (usually carcinomas)
	In setting of primary renal cancer and/or its surgical management
Paraneoplastic renal disease	Paraprotein-associated kidney disease
	Light chain cast nephropathy
	Monoclonal immunoglobulin (AL, AH, AHL) amyloidosis
	Monoclonal immunoglobulin deposition disease (LCDD, HCDD, LHCDD)
	Type I (monoclonal) cryoglobulinemic glomerulonephritis
	Monoclonal gammopathies of renal Significance
	Additional glomerular diseases
	Cancer-associated membranous nephropathy
	Minimal change disease
Treatment-associated kidney disease	Various, see Table 34.2
Tumor lysis syndrome	Common in hematologic malignancies with rapid cell turnover, high tumor burden, and that are more sensitive to treatment (i.e. Burkitt lymphoma, acute lymphoblastic leukemia)
Kidney disease after HCT	Acute kidney injury
	Chronic kidney disease
	Glomerular disease/nephrotic syndrome
	Thrombotic microangiopathy

AL = light chain amyloidosis. AH = heavy chain amyloidosis. AHL = heavy and light chain amyloidosis. LCDD = light chain deposition disease. HCDD = heavy chain deposition disease. HLCDD = light and heavy chain deposition disease. HCT = hematopoetic cell transplantation.

various types of lymphomas found that most patients did not have clinical evidence or suspicion for renal involvement and that the prevalence of renal involvement differed by lymphoma type.[8] Using chronic lymphocytic leukemia (CLL) as an example, 59% to 90% of patients were found to have renal infiltration on autopsy.[9] More recent studies have found that the incidence of renal insufficiency (serum creatinine >1.5 mg/dL) was 7.5% at baseline in patients with CLL,[10] that 12% of patients with CLL who underwent a kidney biopsy were found to have significant infiltration,[10] and that as of 2013, only 17 cases were reported where a kidney biopsy found renal CLL infiltration.[11] Reports exist of patients with lymphomatous infiltration of the kidney whose renal function improved with antilymphoma treatment.[10] Taken together, these data indicate that clinically relevant renal lymphomatous infiltration can occur but that the majority of cases are likely to be subclinical.

Paraneoplastic Conditions Affecting the Kidney

Paraneoplastic kidney diseases occur due to the secretion of tumor products, rather than through direct tumor involvement of renal tissue or extrarenal obstruction. Ideally, diagnosing paraneoplastic kidney disease establishes a direct mechanistic link between the cancer and kidney disease with the use of biomarkers. This is the case with myeloma cast nephropathy and light chain (AL) amyloidosis, where malignant plasma cells secrete pathogenic monoclonal immunoglobulins that cause kidney damage. However, since few specific biomarkers exist in nephrology, evidence for paraneoplastic renal disease is often limited to a temporal correlation between the diagnosis, activity, remission, and relapse of both the cancer and the renal disease.

Paraprotein-Mediated Kidney Disease

AL amyloidosis is a prototypical paraneoplastic disease where within malignant plasma cells produce amyloidogenic monoclonal immunoglobulin light chains that deposit in the kidney (among other organs) and cause renal damage. Until the 1990s, the prognosis for patients with AL amyloidosis was dismal, with median survival after diagnosis of 7 months. Since then, the use of high-dose melphalan followed by autologous stem cell transplant or bortezomib-based chemotherapies has dramatically improved patient outcomes. Baseline renal parameters and response to therapy are predictive of renal survival in AL amyloidosis, with baseline proteinuria >5 grams/24 h and eGFR $\leq$50 mL/min associated with 3-year ESRD rates of 4%, 30%, and 85% for patients meeting 0, 1, or both criteria, respectively.[12] Renal progression ($\geq$25% decrease in eGFR) is associated with worse renal prognosis, while renal response (>30% decrease in proteinuria to <0.5 gm/day and nonprogression of eGFR) is associated with improved renal outcomes. Light chain cast nephropathy in the setting of multiple myeloma is also an important paraneoplastic renal disease and is discussed elsewhere (see Chapter 38).

The monoclonal gammopathies of renal significance are a collection of paraprotein-mediated kidney diseases in patients who do not meet criteria for multiple myeloma or systemic lymphoma.[13] These disorders include the monoclonal immunoglobulin deposition diseases (light chain deposition disease, heavy chain deposition disease, and light and heavy chain deposition disease), proliferative glomerulonephritis with monoclonal immunoglobulin deposits, type I (monoclonal) cryoglobulinemia, and paraprotein-associated C3 glomerulonephritis. In these patients, treatment is directed against the pathogenic underlying plasma or B cell clone.

Other Paraneoplastic Glomerular Diseases

Malignancy-associated membranous nephropathy has mostly been reported in the setting of solid tumors. Clinical evidence for this association includes a higher incidence of cancer in patients with membranous nephropathy versus age- and sex-adjusted general population, the close temporal proximity of diagnosing both conditions, and multiple reported cases of improvement in proteinuria with anti-neoplastic treatment.[14] The recent discovery of 2 important biomarkers have led a reevaluation of relating membranous nephropathy and malignancy. Patients who are positive for anti-M-type phospholipase A2 receptor (PLA2R) antibodies have been shown to have decreased incidences of malignancy versus those who are anti-PLA2R negative,[15] and tumor production of thrombospondin type-1 domain-containing 7A may be the cause of malignancy-associated membranous nephropathy in some patients,[16] However, while these associations are still being validated, age-appropriate cancer screening is still prudent in older patients given the historical link between membranous nephropathy and cancer.

Minimal change disease has been classically associated with Hodgkin disease but has also been reported in the setting of non-Hodgkin lymphomas. Unlike with membranous nephropathy, there are no biomarkers for minimal change disease, and so the evidence for these associations is mostly observed temporal clinical correlations.

TREATMENT-ASSOCIATED KIDNEY DISEASE

Anti-neoplastic agents can cause a wide variety of renal-relevant adverse effects (Table 34.2). Here, we highlight important kidney-associated side effects of 5 classes of agents: platinum therapies, antifolate agents, vascular endothelial growth factor (VEGF) inhibitors, immune checkpoint inhibitors, and proteasome inhibitors.

Platinum-Based Chemotherapies (Cisplatin, Carboplatin, Oxaliplatin)

Cisplatin is a cytotoxic agent that inhibits DNA synthesis by crosslinking with DNA purine bases and is commonly used to treat pulmonary, gastrointestinal, urogenital, head, neck, and skin cancers.[17] It has been shown to cause a variety of renal adverse events, including direct proximal tubular injury and impairment of renal vascular autoregulation resulting in AKI, CKD, renal sodium wasting, and magnesium wasting. Typically, the urinalysis exhibits minimal or tubular proteinuria and no microscopic hematuria. Kidney biopsy in cisplatin-treated patients may show acute tubular necrosis, interstitial fibrosis with tubular atrophy, and, rarely, thrombotic microangiopathy (TMA), especially if administered with bleomycin.[18]

Cisplatin-associated kidney damage is dose-dependent. One study showed that high-dose cisplatin at 40 mg/m^2 daily for 5 days for 3 cycles decreased GFR from 109 mL/min/1.73m^2 to 68 mL/min/1.73m^2, and all patients developed tubular proteinuria.[19] A 23% reduction in GFR has been observed with a cumulative dose of 180 to 900 mg of cisplatin.[20] Hypomagnesemia is common with a study showing that it affected 100% patients receiving a cumulative dose of 300 mg/m^2 over 6 cycles with mean resultant serum magnesium level of 1.2 mg/dL.[21] The average time for recovery from hypomagnesemia after stopping the drug ranges from few months to several years. Recovery of renal function may not

TABLE 34.2 RENAL ADVERSE EVENTS ASSOCIATED WITH ANTINEOPLASTIC AGENTS

Drug	Renal Adverse Effect	Note
Platinum based (cisplatin>carboplatin> oxaliplatin	AKI CKD Hypomagnesemia	AKI is dose-dependent and may not be reversible[a]
Aklylating agents (Ifosfamide, cyclophosphamide)	Fanconi syndrome—more common with prior cisplatin use Hypomagnesemia Hyponatremia (SIADH)- observed with cyclophosphamide AKI	Adverse events are dose-dependent and may progress despite drug discontinuation[b]
Mitomycin-C	TMA	Dose-dependent; may occur after treatment is completed. Conventional treatment of hemolytic uremic syndrome is not effective[c]
Antifolate agents (methotrexate, pemetrexate)	AKI	Dose-dependent and reversible
Ipilimumab	Granulomatous AIN Lupus-like glomerulonephritis (case reports)	Reversible; consider corticosteroids after drug discontinuation
Pyrimidine analogue (gemcitabine 5-fluorouracile, cytarabine)	TMA	Not dose-dependent; full or partial recovery of renal function may occur after drug discontinuation[d]
VEGF inhibitors, TK inhibitors (sunitinib, sorafenib, axitinib, ramacirumab, bevacizumab)	AKI, proteinuria, hypertension, TMA, hypophosphatemia with imatinib	Dose-dependent
Anti-EGFR monoclonal antibodies (cetuximab, panitumumab)	Hypomagnesemia	Reversible after drug discontinuation
Checkpoint Inhibitors (pembrolizumab, nivolumab, atezolizumab, ipililumab)	AIN	May improve with steroids and discontinuing the agent

[a]Duagaard G, Rossing N, Rorth M. Effects of cisplatin on different measures of glomerular function in the human kidney with special emphasis on high dose. *Cancer Chemothr Pharmacol.* 1988;21(2):163–167; Macleod PM, Tyrell CJ, Keeling DH. The effect of cisplatin on renal function in patients with testicular tumors. *Clin Radiol.* 1988;39(2):190–192; Labaye J, Sarret D, Duvic C et al. Renal toxicity of oxaliplatin. *Nephrol Dial Transplant.* 2005;20(6):1275–1276.

[b]Rossi R, Pleyer J, Schäfers P, et al. Development of ifosfamide-induced nephrotoxicity: prospective follow-up in 75 patients. *Med Pediatr Oncol.* 1999;32(3):177–182.

[c]Lesesne JB, Rothschild N, Erickson B, et al. Cancer-associated hemolytic-uremic syndrome: analysis of 85 cases from a national registry. *J Clin Oncol.* 1989;7(6):781–789.

[d]Glezerman I, Kris MG, Miller V, Seshan S, Flombaum CD. Gemcitabine nephrotoxicity and hemolytic uremic syndrome: report of 29 cases from a single institution. *Clin Nephrol.* 2009;71(2):130–139.

AKI = acute kidney injury. CKD = chronic kidney disease. SIADH = syndrome of inappropriate antidiuretic hormone. TMA = thrombotic microangiopathy. AIN = acute intertitial nephritis. VEGF = vascular endothelial growth facgtor. TK = tyrosine kinase. EGFR = epidermal growth factor receptor.

occur after drug withdrawal.[20] The renal-relevant side effects of carboplatin are similar to those of cisplatin but are less common. Oxaliplatin has a more favorable side-effect profile, with only a few case reports describing an association with acute tubular necrosis.[22]

Prevention of AKI in cisplatin-treated patients involves volume expansion along with drug infusion.[23] Amifostine is approved by the Food and Drug Administration for protecting against nephrotoxicity induced by both single and repeated doses of cisplatin in ovarian and nonsmall-cell lung cancer patients receiving cisplatin, likely without interfering with antitumor activity. Its use, however, is limited by side effects and cost.[24]

Antifolate Agents (Methotrexate)

Methotrexate is used in the treatment of non-Hodgkin's lymphoma and leukemia.[17] Methotrexate enters the cell through a reduced folate carrier using an endocytic pathway activated by a folate receptor. After entering the cell, methotrexate is polyglutamated. Methotrexate and its polyglutamates inhibit the enzyme dihydrofolate reductase, ultimately inhibiting DNA synthesis.[25,26] Both methotrexate and its metabolite 7-hydroxymethotrexate are poorly soluble in acidic urine. Hence, they are susceptible to direct intratubular precipitation, which can cause acute tubular necrosis. Urine microscopy may show characteristic methotrexate crystals, and kidney biopsy may show tubular deposits of methotrexate crystal deposits.

Methotrexate nephrotoxicity is dose-dependent but usually moderate and reversible.[27] In a study[28] of 102 patients treated with high-dose methotrexate, 3.9% of patients developed AKI, though none required dialysis, and AKI resolved in all of the affected patients. AKI may also occur in the absence of toxic plasma methotrexate levels 24 to 48 hours after infusion.[29] Methotrexate-associated AKI is treated with leucovorin rescue therapy, which concurrently decreases the antitumor effect, with or without glucarpidase, which results in >88% decrease in methotrexate levels within 15 minutes. Drug removal with hemodialysis or hemoperfusion is an option for patients with severe AKI, but rebound of plasma methotrexate levels should be expected and leucovorin redosed.[30,31] To prevent AKI, patients are treated with alkali therapy to urinary pH ≥7.0 and volume expansion 12 hours prior to and up to 48 to 72 hours post methotrexate administration,[32] and drugs interfering with methotrexate excretion (probenecid, penicillin, salicylate, nonsteroidal anti-inflammatory drugs, sulfisoxazole, weak organic acids) are avoided.

Vascular Endothelial Growth Factor Targeting Agents (Sunitinib, Sorafenib, Axitinib, Ramucirumab, Bevacizumab)

Bevacizumab, the first drug approved by the Food and Drug Administration in this class, is a recombinant humanized VEGFA-specific monoclonal antibody, which has been used in the treatment of metastatic colon cancer, metastatic renal cell carcinoma, nonsmall-cell lung cancer, and gynecological and breast cancers. Sunitinib and sorafenib have been used in metastatic renal cell carcinoma, and cabozantinib, vandetanib, and lenvantinib have been used in thyroid cancer. VEGFA secreted by tumor cells and surrounding stroma stimulates the proliferation and survival of endothelial cells, leading to the formation of new blood vessels, which may be structurally abnormal and leaky. The VEGF ligands bind to and activates 3 structurally similar type 3 receptor tyrosine kinases, designated VEGFR1 (also known as FLT1), VEGFR2 (also known as KDR), and VEGFR3 (also known as FLT4). In response to ligand binding, the VEGFR tyrosine kinases activate a network of distinct downstream signaling pathways. Accordingly, several strategies to inhibit the VEGFA–VEGFR signaling pathway for the treatment of cancer have been employed.[33,34]

Anti-VEGF therapy, leading to low free VEGF levels, causes endothelial dysfunction and glomerular epithelial cell (podocyte) dysregulation, leading to hypertension and proteinuria.[35] A systematic review of patients treated for renal cell carcinoma with any VEGF inhibitor reported an incidence of mild asymptomatic proteinuria of 21% up to 63%, but heavy proteinuria (more than 4+ proteinuria on urinalysis or >3.5 gm/24 h) in up to 6.5%.[36] Incidence of bevacizumab-associated hypertension and proteinuria was shown to increase with higher doses (relative risk of developing proteinuria of 2.2 with 10 or 15 mg/kg per dose vs. 1.4 with 3, 5, or 7.5 mg/kg per dose.[37]

Thrombotic microangiopathy is the most common finding in patients taking VEGF inhibitors who undergo kidney biopsy,[38] with many of these cases being renal-limited (i.e., not systemic). Other described kidney biopsy findings include minimal change disease, collapsing focal segmental glomerulosclerosis, and acute interstitial nephritis.[39]

While discontinuation of anti-VEGF agents can lead to a significant reduction in proteinuria, persistence of some proteinuria is common.[40] Drug continuation or reintroduction can result in a more severe recurrence of TMA. There are no strong data to guide management of hypertension secondary to VEGF inhibitors. Expert opinion recommends the use of angiotensin converting enzyme inhibitors and dihydropyridine calcium channel blockers for antiproteinuric and vasodilatory effects, respectively. Nondihydropyridine calcium channel blockers should be avoided in patients on sunitinib and sorafenib as there is interference with CYP3A4 system. Dose reduction or interruption may need to be considered in the case of severe, refractory hypertension or in the case of hypertensive crisis.[41,42]

Immune Checkpoint Inhibitors

Immune check point inhibitors (CPI) are a relatively new class of monoclonal antibodies against inhibitory receptors on a variety of cells, including tumors and T cells. The most commonly used CPIs target programmed death 1 protein (pembrolizumab, nivolumab), programmed death ligand-1 (atezolizumab), and cytotoxic T lymphocyte associated antigen 4 (ipilimumab). These agents are being used in a variety of hematologic and solid malignancies. Since CPIs target signaling pathways that normally inhibit T cells, they are associated with a variety of immune-mediated adverse events.[43,44] The incidence of

AKI with CPI use has been estimated at 2% to 29%.[45] Patients with CPI-associated AKI have most often exhibited acute interstitial nephritis on kidney biopsy.[46] Acute cellular rejection in the allograft has also been reported in patients with kidney transplants treated with CPIs.[47] The management of patients with CPI-associated AKI includes consideration of kidney biopsy to determine the pattern of injury and corticosteroid treatment in cases of interstitial nephritis.

Proteasome Inhibitors (Bortezomib and Carfilzomib)

The proteasome inhibitors, bortezomib and carfilzomib, have been approved for use in multiple myeloma, and bortezomib has also been approved in mantle cell lymphoma. The primary mechanism of action of these agents is to inhibit the removal of misfolded proteins in the endoplasmic reticulum, resulting in induction of the terminal unfolded protein response and cellular apoptosis.[13]

Recent case reports and case series describe patients who develop renal insufficiency during protease inhibitor (PI) therapy, with TMA found on kidney biopsy (Fig. 34.1). Previous reports have postulated a link between PI's action on the VEGF pathway via NFκB inhibition, causing microvascular injury to the glomerular capillaries, similar to other medications with anti-VEGF

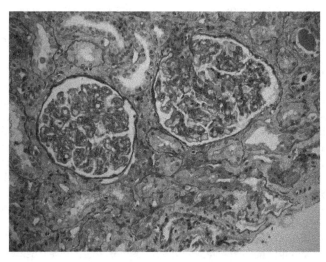

FIGURE 34.1 Thrombotic microangiopathy in a patient treated with carfilzomib (periodic acid Schiff, 400×). Glomerular basement membranes show diffuse duplication and focal wrinkling. There is swelling of endothelial cells and occasional marginating leukocytes. There is segmental rarefaction of mesangium consistent with mesangiolysis. Image courtesy of Dr. Matthew Palmer, Department of Pathology and Laboratory Medicine, University of Pennsylvania, Philadelphia, PA.

activity. Carfilzomib may be associated with a higher risk of TMA compared to bortezomib, which may be due to the irreversible inhibition of the ubiquitin–proteasome pathway with carfilzomib, in contrast with the reversible inhibition that bortezomib provides.[48] A recent case series of 11 patients (8 of whom were using carfilzomib) who developed TMA during PI reported a median time from medication initiation to TMA diagnosis of 21 days (range 5 days to 17 months). At diagnosis, patients were found have evidence of hemolytic anemia and AKI (median serum creatinine 3.12 mg/dL), with 4 patients requiring dialysis. No patient had another identifiable etiology for TMA. Four patients were treated with plasma exchange, and 3 patients received eculizumab. Nine patients had resolution of TMA without evidence of hemolysis after withdrawal of PI. Two patients had stabilization of laboratory values but persistent evidence of hemolysis despite medication withdrawal. One patient had recurrence of TMA with rechallenge of PI.[48]

TUMOR LYSIS SYNDROME

TLS is a potentially life-threatening complication that occurs when intracellular components (specifically potassium, phosphorus, and nucleic acids) are released into the systemic circulation by massive cell turnover and cell lysis. The nucleic acids are catabolized into uric acid, which can precipitate in the kidney and cause vasoconstriction, inflammation, oxidative injury and impaired autoregulation. Acute deposition of calcium and phosphorus into the renal tubules also causes AKI in TLS.

TLS may occur spontaneously (primary) or in response to therapy (secondary). TLS is more common in acute hematologic malignancies as well as those with rapid cell turnover, higher tumor burdens, and that are more chemosensitive. These include Burkitt lymphoma and T-cell acute lymphoblastic leukemia.[49] However, an increased incidence of TLS has been observed in the setting of more indolent malignancies with the development of targeted anti-neoplastic agents.[49]

TLS is diagnosed using the Cairo-Bishop classification system, which requires 2 or more laboratory (hyperuricemia, hyperkalemia, hyperphosphatemia, or hypocalcemia) and clinical (AKI, cardiac arrhythmia, seizure, or death) features to occur 3 days before to 7 days after initiation of treatment.[50,51] The risk of TLS

is increased in the setting of pre-existing CKD, volume depletion, and hyperuricemia.

The treatment and prophylaxis of TLS involve optimizing intravascular volume status, using hypouricemic agents, and managing electrolyte abnormalities. A 2008 International Expert Panel recommended that adults at risk for TLS receive 2 to 3 L/m^2/day of intravenous fluids. While sodium bicarbonate or acetazolamide increase urine pH, thus decreasing the risk of uric acid precipitation, they also increased the risk of calcium phosphorus deposition. Since similar outcomes have been observed with normal saline, the consensus was to avoid urine alkalinization unless needed to correct a metabolic acidosis. Allopurinol and rasburicase are hypouricemic agents used in TLS. Allopurinol, a xanthine oxidase inhibitor, prevents uric acid formation and carries the risk of acute uric acid crystal deposition if used in the setting of hyperuricemia. Rasburicase is a recombinant urate oxidase that is used to rapidly lower serum uric acid concentrations. The remainder of TLS treatment focuses on management of electrolyte abnormalities (hyperkalemia, hypocalcemia, hyperphosphatemia) and renal replacement therapy (intermittent hemodialysis, continuous renal replacement therapy, or peritoneal dialysis), if needed.[50]

KIDNEY DISEASE AFTER HEMATOPOIETIC CELL TRANSPLANTATION

HCT includes allogeneic and autologous bone marrow and stem cell transplants (SCT) and is used in the treatment of numerous benign and malignant hematologic disorders. The number of patients undergoing HCT has increased dramatically over time. Over 50,000 patients/year worldwide undergo HCT; up to 2014, over 340,000 patients had undergone HCT in the United States alone.[52] Kidney injury after HCT is more common after allogeneic transplants than autologous transplants.

Up to 70% of adults experience AKI in the first 100 days after allogeneic stem cell transplants in association with various conditioning regimens, medication exposures, and posttransplant complications (e.g., sepsis, acute graft-versus host disease, and hepatic sinusoidal obstructive disease). AKI after HCT is associated with decreased survival and increased risk of developing CKD. CKD also develops in up to 70% of HCT survivors and may occur due to TMA (systemic or renal-limited) in the setting of conditioning regimens, medication exposure (e.g., calcineurin inhibitors), BK virus nephropathy, and development of nephrotic syndrome, the latter of which is hypothesized to be a renal manifestation of chronic graft versus host disease.[53]

REFERENCES

1. Christiansen CF, Johansen MB, Langeberg WJ, Fryzek JP, Sørensen HT. Incidence of acute kidney injury in cancer patients: a Danish population-based cohort study. *Eur J Intern Med.* 2011;22:399-40.

2. Launay-Vacher V, Oudard S, Janus N et al. Prevalence of renal insufficiency in cancer patients and implications for anticancer drug management: the Renal Insufficiency and Anticancer Medications (IRMA) study. *Cancer.* 2007;110(6):1376-1384.

3. Jay L Xue DVM, Fred Dalleska, Anne M Murray, Allan J Collins. Cancer prevalence in patients with end-stage renal disease. Paper presented at: American Society of Nephrology Kidney Week; 2005; Philadelphia, PA.

4. Van Poppel H, Da Pozzo L, Albrecht W et al. A prospective, randomised EORTC intergroup phase 3 study comparing the oncologic outcome of elective nephron-sparing surgery and radical nephrectomy for low-stage renal cell carcinoma. *Yearb Urol.* 2011; 59(4):543-552.

5. Scosyrev E, Messing EM, Sylvester R, Campbell S, Poppel HV. Renal function after nephron-sparing surgery versus radical nephrectomy: results from EORTC randomized trial 30904. *Eur Urol.* 2014;65(2):372-377.

6. Patel HD, Pierorazio PM, Johnson MH, et al. renal functional outcomes after surgery, ablation, and active surveillance of localized renal tumors: a systematic review and meta-analysis. *Clin J Am Soc Nephrol.* 2017;12(7):1057-1069.

7. Zhou C, Urbauer DL, Fellman BM, et al. Metastases to the kidney: a comprehensive analysis of 151 patients from a tertiary referral centre. *BJU Int.* 2015;117(5):775-782.

8. Richmond J, Sherman RS, Diamond HD, Craver LF. Renal lesions associated with malignant lymphomas. *Am J Med.* 1962;32(2):184-207.

9. Schwartz JB, Shamsuddin AM. The effects of leukemic infiltrates in various organs in chronic lymphocytic leukemia. *Human Pathol.* 1981;12(5):432-440.

10. Strati P, Nasr SH, Leung N, et al. Renal complications in chronic lymphocytic leukemia and monoclonal B-cell lymphocytosis: the Mayo Clinic experience. *Haematologica.* 2015;100(9):1180-1188.

11. Uprety D, Peterson A, Shah BK. Renal failure secondary to leukemic infiltration of kidneys in CLL-a case report and review of literature. *Ann Hematol.* 2012;92(2):271-273.

12. Palladini G, Hegenbart U, Milani P. A staging system for renal outcome and early markers of renal response to chemotherapy in AL amyloidosis. *Blood.* 2014;Oct 9;124(15):2325-2332.

13. Hogan JJ, Weiss BM. Bridging the divide: an onco-nephrologic approach to the monoclonal gammopathies of renal significance. *Clin J Am Soc Nephrol.* 2016;11:1681-1691.

14. Cambier JF, Ronco P. Onco-nephrology: glomerular diseases with cancer. *Clin J Am Soc Nephrol.* 2012;7(10):1701-1712.

15. Timmermans SA, Ayalon R, van Paassen P. Anti-phospholipase A2 receptor antibodies and malignancy in membranous nephropathy. *Am J Kidney Dis.* 2013;62(6):1223-1225.

16. Hoxha E, Wiech T, Stahl PR. A Mechanism for cancer-associated membranous nephropathy. *N Engl J Med.* 2016;19;374(20):1995-1996.

17. SACT report. National Cancer Intelligence Network; March 18, 2015. http://www.chemodataset.nhs.uk/reports/

18. Jackson AM, Rose BD, Graff LG et al. Thrombotic microangiopathy and renal failure associated with antineoplastic chemotherapy. *Ann Intern Med.* 1984:101(1):41-44.

19. Duagaard G, Rossing N, Rorth M. Effects of cisplatin on different measures of glomerular function in the human kidney with special emphasis on high dose. *Cancer Chemothr Pharmacol.* 1988;21(2):163-167.

20. Macleod PM, Tyrell CJ, Keeling DH. The effect of cisplatin on renal function in patients with testicular tumors. *Clin Radiol.* 1988;39(2):190-192.

21. Buckley JE, Clark VL, Meyer TJ, Pearlman NW. Hypomagnesemia after cisplatin combination chemotherapy. *Arch Intern Med.* 1984;144(12):2347-2348.

22. Labaye J, Sarret D, Duvic C et al. Renal toxicity of oxaliplatin. *Nephrol Dial Transplant.* 2005;20(6):1275-1276.

23. Cornelison TL, Reed E. Nephrotoxicity and hydration management for cisplatin, carboplatin, and ormaplatin. *Gynecol Oncol.* 1993;50(2):147-158.

24. Capizzi RL. Amifostine reduces the incidence of cumulative nephrotoxicity from cisplatin: laboratory and clinical aspects. *Semin Oncol.* 1999;26(2 Suppl 7):72-81.

25. Gorlick R, Goker E, Trippett T, Waltham M, Banerjee D, Bertino JR. Intrinsic and acquired resistance to methotrexate in acute leukemia. *New Engl J Med.* 1996;335,1041-1048.

26. Chabner BA, Roberts TG Jr. Chemotherapy and the war on cancer. *Nat Rev Cancer.* 2005;5:65–72.

27. Frei E III, Jaffe N, Tattersall MH, Pitman S, Parker L. New approaches to cancer chemotherapy with methotrexate. *N Engl J Med.*1975;17;292(16):846–851.

28. Mashhadi MA, Kaykhaei MA, Sanadgol H. Low prevalence of high-dose methotrexate nephropathy in patients with malignancy. *Iran J Kidney Dis.* 2012;6(2):105–109.

29. Garneau AP, Riopel J, Isenring P. Acute methotrexate-induced crystal nephropathy. *N Engl J Med.* 2015;373:2691–2693.

30. Howard SC, McCormick J, Pui CH, Buddington RK, Harvey RD. Preventing and managing toxicities of high-dose methotrexate. *Oncologist.* 2016;21(12):1471–1482.

31. Fermiano M, Bergsbaken J, Kolesar JM. Glucarpidase for the management of elevated methotrexate levels in patients with impaired renal function. *Am J Health Syst Pharm.* 2014;71(10):793–798.

32. Relling MV, Fairclough D, Ayers D. Patient characteristics associated with high-risk methotrexate concentrations and toxicity. *J Clin Oncol.*1994;12(8):1667–1672.

33. Napoleone F, Anthony PA. Ten years of anti-vascular endothelial growth factor therapy. *Nat Rev Drug Discov.* 2016;15:385–403.

34. Kerbel RS. Tumor angiogenesis. *N Engl J Med.* 2008;358:2039–2049.

35. Hayman SR, Leung N, Grande JP, Garovic VD. VEGF inhibition, hypertension, and renal toxicity. *Curr Oncol Rep.* 2012;14(4): 285–294.

36. Izzedine H, Massard C, Spano JP, Goldwasser F, Khayat D, Soria JC. VEGF signalling inhibition-induced proteinuria: Mechanisms, significance and management. *Eur J Cancer.* 2010;46(2):439–448.

37. Zhu X, Wu S, Dahut WL, Parikh CR. Risks of proteinuria and hypertension with bevacizumab, an antibody against vascular endothelial growth factor: systematic review and meta-analysis. *Am J Kidney Dis.* 2007;49(2):186–193.

38. Vigneau C, Lorcy N, Dolley-Hitze T, et al. All anti-vascular endothelial growth factor drugs can induce "pre-eclampsia-like syndrome": a RARe study. *Nephrol Dial Transplant.* 2014;29(2):325–332.

39. Izzedine H, Escudier B, Lhomme C, et al. Kidney diseases associated with anti-vascular endothelial growth factor (VEGF): an 8-year observational study at a single center. *Medicine.* 2014;93(24):333–339.

40. Nazer B, Humphreys BD, Moslehi J. Effects of novel angiogenesis inhibitors for the treatment of cancer on the cardiovascular system focus on hypertension. *Circulation.* 2011;124:1687–1691.

41. Kalaitzidis RG, Elisaf MS. Uncontrolled hypertension and oncology: clinical tips. *Curr Vasc Pharmacol.* 2017;16(1):23–29.

42. Derosa L, Izzedine H, Albiges L, Escudier B. Hypertension and angiotensin system inhibitors in patients with metastatic renal cell carcinoma. *Oncol Rev.* 2016; 10(2): 298.

43. Lievense LA, Hegmans JP, Aerts JG. Biomarkers for immune checkpoint inhibitors. *Lancet Oncol.* 2014;15(1):e1.

44. Ribas A. Tumor immunotherapy directed at PD-1. *N Engl J Med.* 2012;366(26):2517–2519.

45. Wanchoo R, Karam S, Uppal NN, et al. Adverse renal effects of immune checkpoint inhibitors: a narrative review on behalf of Cancer and Kidney International Network Workgroup on Immune Checkpoint Inhibitors. *Am J Nephrol.* 2017;45:160–169.

46. Cortazar FB, Marrone KA, Troxell ML, et al. Clinicopathological features of acute kidney injury associated with immune checkpoint inhibitors. *Kidney Int.* 2016;90(3):638–647.

47. Alhamad T, Venkatachalam K, Linette GP, Brennan DC. Checkpoint inhibitors in kidney transplant recipients and the potential risk of rejection. *Am J Transplant.* 2016;16(4):1332–1333.

48. Yui JC, Van Keer J, Weiss BM, et al. Proteasome inhibitor associated thrombotic microangiopathy. *Am. J. Hematol.* 2016;91:E348–E352.

49. Senbanjo IO. Tumor lysis and acute renal failure in Burkitt's lymphoma: a review on pathophysiology and management. *Indian J Nephrol.* 2009;19(3):83–86.

50. Howard SC, Jones DP, Pui CH. The tumor lysis syndrome. *N Engl J Med.* 2011;364(19):1844–1854.

51. Cairo MS, Coiffier B, Reiter A, Younes A. Recommendations for the evaluation of risk and prophylaxis of tumour lysis syndrome (TLS) in adults and children with malignant diseases: an expert TLS panel consensus. *Brit J Haematol.* 2010;149(4):578–586.

52. D'Souza A, Fretham C. Current uses and outcomes of hematopoietic cell transplantation (HCT). CIBMTR Summary Slides; 2017. https://www.cibmtr.org/ReferenceCenter/SlidesReports/pages/index.aspx

53. Hingorani S. Renal complications of hematopoietic-cell transplantation. *N Engl J Med.* 2016;374:2256–2267.

35

Cast Nephropathy in Plasma Cell Dyscrasias

SANDHYA MANOHAR AND NELSON LEUNG

INTRODUCTION

Plasma cell dyscrasias represent a group of diseases that are characterized by the clonal expansion of abnormal plasma cells. These cells, in turn, produce increased amounts of monoclonal protein either in whole or its fragments (light or heavy chain). The most common of the plasma cell dyscrasias are represented in Table 35.1 and include monoclonal gammopathy of undetermined significance (MGUS), smoldering multiple myeloma, multiple myeloma, and Waldenström's macroglobulinemia, among others. Studies have shown that nearly all patients evolve from the premalignant disease state of MGUS to a malignant condition like multiple myeloma.[1,2] The malignant state is defined by clonal mass and end-organ damage, which necessitate the initiation of treatment. However, a number of kidney diseases can occur even in the premalignant conditions. Despite their premalignant state, these diseases may require chemotherapy for treatment, and, hence, the new term "monoclonal gammopathy of renal significance" (MGRS) was created to distinguish these conditions from the benign MGUS.[3]

Plasma cell dyscrasias are associated with a wide spectrum of renal lesions (Table 35.2). This is related to the differential handling of the monoclonal proteins at various segments of the nephron and the molecular diversity of these proteins. Large intact immunoglobulins (Ig) are generally not filtered at the glomerulus but the smaller free light chains (FLC) are readily filtered.[4] Under normal conditions, at the level of the proximal tubule, the FLC undergo reabsorption via the megalin–cubulin receptors,[5] such that there is minimal detectable FLC in the urine.[4] In the setting of a plasma cell dyscrasia, the megalin–cubulin pathways are saturated by the overwhelming load of FLCs causing FLC to appear in the urine in large quantities as Bence Jones protein. In certain situations, these FLCs aggregate with the naturally occurring Tamm-Horsfall protein (THP) in the distal tubules to form intraluminal proteinaceous cast. The resulting tubular obstruction and inflammatory reaction manifest as deterioration in kidney function. This condition is termed "light chain cast nephropathy."

Light chain cast nephropathy is one of the most common renal manifestations in multiple myeloma. The updated criteria of the International Myeloma Working Group[6] from 2014, considers renal failure by light chain cast nephropathy as a myeloma-defining event. The diagnosis of light chain cast nephropathy should be made by a kidney biopsy. However, this is not always feasible in clinical setting, and a presumptive diagnosis can be made in the setting of severe renal failure based on the presence of high levels of the involved FLC (>500 mg/L) and low urinary albumin excretion.[6] In patients with a plasma cell dyscrasia and kidney disease, cast nephropathy is noted in about 20% to 30% of the cases.[7,8] It is most commonly seen in patients with multiple myeloma; hence, the name "myeloma kidney" has been used, but it has also been rarely reported in patients with Waldenström macroglobulinemia,[9] lymphoma,[10] and chronic lymphocytic leukemia.[11] Therefore, the term "myeloma cast nephropathy" should be reserved for patients with multiple myeloma and "light chain cast nephropathy" for patients with other hematologic conditions. Another renal lesion, although rare, associated with plasma cell dyscrasia is infiltration of renal parenchyma by plasma cells.

HISTORY OF THE TERMINOLOGY

One of the first recognitions of plasma cell disorder dates back to the 1840s. It started with the

TABLE 35.1 SUMMARY OF SELECTED MONOCLONAL PLASMA CELL DISORDERS WITH RENAL MANIFESTATIONS BASED ON 2014 INTERNATIONAL MYELOMA WORKING GROUP DIAGNOSTIC CRITERIA FOR MULTIPLE MYELOMA AND RELATED PLASMA CELL DISORDERS

Disease	Diagnostic Criteria
MGRS	All criteria are required: • Evidence of monoclonal protein either in circulation or in the kidney seen on kidney biopsy • Not meeting criteria for symptomatic multiple myeloma or lymphoma—absence of end-organ damage such as lytic bone lesions, anemia, hypercalcemia, or renal failure from cast nephropathy
Smoldering multiple myeloma	All criteria are required: • Serum monoclonal protein (IgG or IgA) ≥3 g/dL or urinary monoclonal protein ≥500 mg per 24 hours and/or clonal bone marrow plasma cells 10%–60% • Absence of myeloma defining events or amyloidosis
Multiple myeloma	• meet criteria for smoldering multiple myeloma AND at least one of the following: • Presence of biomarker associated with near inevitable progression to end-organ damage: clonal bone marrow plasma cells ≥60% or involved FLC of >100 mg/L with ratio of involved/uninvolved of 100 or more or MRI with more than one focal lesion. • Presence of end-organ damage (CRAB): hypercalcemia, Renal failure from cast nephropathy, Anemia, lytic Bone lesions
Waldenström macroglobulinemia	All criteria are required: • IgM monoclonal gammopathy • >10% bone marrow lymphoplasmacytic infiltration (usually intertrabecular) by small lymphocytes that exhibit plasmacytoid or plasma cell differentiation and a typical immunophenotype
AL amyloidosis	All criteria are required: • Positive amyloid staining by Congo red in any tissue • Amyloid is composed of one of the immunoglobulin light chains • Amyloid-related systemic syndrome (such as renal, liver, heart, • Gastrointestinal tract, or autonomic or peripheral nerve involvement)

FLC = free light chain; Ig = immunoglobulin; MGRS = monoclonal gammopathy of renal significance; MRI = magnetic resonance imaging. CRAB = hypercalcemia, renal insufficiency, anemia, and bony lesions. AL = immunoglobulin light chain

observation of a single patient, an English grocer named Mr. Thomas McBean who complained to his physician, Dr. William Macintyre that "his body linen was stiffened by his urine." He also had been suffering with back pains, and his physicians had diagnosed him with an unusual variant of "mollities and fragilitas ossium," a terminology used for referring to a condition of bone fragility.[12] The quest for this mysterious substance in the urine finally ended in the lab of a chemical pathologist named Henry Bence Jones. He performed an exhaustive series of experiments and concluded that this was probably a new form of protein that he believed was a "hydrated deutoxide of albumen." In the meanwhile, the index patient passed away, and his autopsy revealed kidneys that were normal, both grossly and microscopically.[12] Mistakenly, the Bence Jones protein was deemed to be nonpathological at that time. It was not until the middle of the 20th century that the true origin and pathogenic potential was elucidated from the work of numerous researchers. It was later discovered that there were 2 subtypes of the Bence Jones protein. These were the 2 immunoglobulin light chains, kappa and lambda, identified by New York biochemists Leonhard Korngold and his assistant Rosa Lipari. In honor of their

TABLE 35.2 SUMMARY OF RENAL MANIFESTATIONS IN MONOCLONAL PLASMA CELL DISORDERS

Plasma Cell Disease		Common Renal Manifestations
MGRS	MGUS Smoldering multiple myeloma	Organized: • Type I and type II cryoglobulinemic GN • AL/AHL/AH amyloidosis • Immunotactoid Glomerulopathy • Light chain proximal tubulopathy (with or without Fanconi syndrome) • Crystal-storing histiocytosis[a] Nonorganized: • MIDD • Proliferative GN with monoclonal Ig deposits • Monoclonal gammopathy-associated C3 glomerulopathy
Malignancies	Multiple myeloma Waldenström's macroglobulinemia	Organized: • Type I and type II cryoglobulinemic GN • AL/AHL/AH amyloidosis • Crystal-storing histiocytosis • Light chain proximal tubulopathy (with or without Fanconi syndrome) • Immunotactoid Glomerulopathy[a] Non-Organized: • Myeloma cast nephropathy • MIDD • Proliferative GN with monoclonal Ig deposits[a]

[a]Meyer E, Carss KJ, Rankin J, et al. Mutations in the histone methyltransferase gene KMT2B cause complex early-onset dystonia. *Nat Genet.* 2017;49(2):223–237.
AL = immunoglobulin light chain. AHL = immunoglobulin heavy and light chain. AH = immunoglobulin heavy chain. GN = glomerulonephritis. Ig = Immunoglobulin. MIDD = monoclonal immunoglobulin deposition disease. MGRS = monoclonal gammopathy or renal significance.

work, the immunoglobulin light chains were hence named after them. The terminology "cast nephropathy" has been credited to Dr. Oliver who in his microdissection studies found large amounts of casts in patients with multiple myeloma that died from renal failure.[13]

MECHANISM OF LIGHT CHAIN CAST FORMATION

Light chains are unique in that they are capable of producing many different kinds of renal lesions. They have been associated with glomerular diseases like type 1 and type 2 cryoglobulinemic glomerulonephritis (GN), immunoglobulin light chain (AL) amyloidosis, immunotactoid GN, fibrillary GN, monoclonal immunoglobulin deposition disease (MIDD), and proliferative GN with monoclonal Ig deposits.[14] In the tubulointerstitial compartment, paraprotein-related kidney injury can present as light chain

proximal tubulopathy (with or without Fanconi syndrome), crystal-storing histiocytosis, and light chain cast nephropathy. Vascular involvement is also common in these diseases.[14] Patients can sometimes have a combination of glomerular, tubulointerstitial, and vascular lesions. This is due to the complex interactions between the light chains, host, and kidney-related factors. Light chain cast nephropathy is a major renal lesion associated with Bence Jones proteinuria, and this will be discussed in detail in this chapter.

Light chain casts are intraluminal proteinaceous aggregations and are made up of FLCs and THP (Fig. 35.1). Rat studies have reproduced the phenomenon of cast nephropathy by intravenous and/or intratubular infusion of purified Bence Jones proteins.[15] THP, also known as uromodulin, is a tubular protein that is exclusively generated by the cells of the thick ascending limb of the loop of Henle. This is also the initial site of light chain

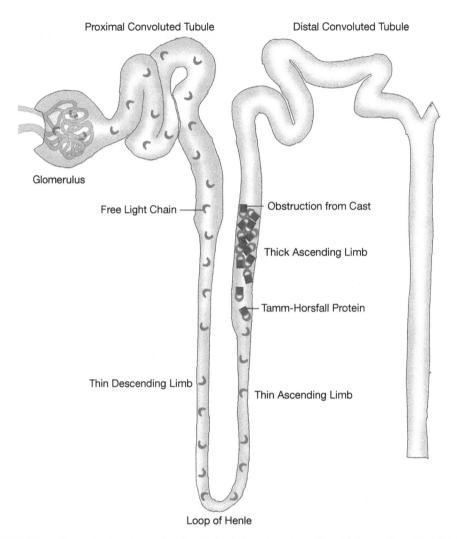

Proximal Convoluted Tubule

Distal Convoluted Tubule

Glomerulus

Free Light Chain

Obstruction from Cast

Thick Ascending Limb

Tamm-Horsfall Protein

Thin Descending Limb

Thin Ascending Limb

Loop of Henle

FIGURE 35.1 Figure demonstrating obstruction from light chain cast nephropathy with interaction of free light chain and Tamm-Horsfall protein in the ascending limb of the loop of Henle.

cast formation. The function of THP is not well understood, but it has been noted to be associated with many kidney diseases like kidney stones[16] and Balkan nephropathy.[17] THP is a glycoprotein with a peptide backbone. Work by Sanders et al.[18] has shown evidence of a common binding site on the kappa and lambda light chains, which interacts in a noncovalent fashion with the carbohydrate moiety on the THP. Patients with light chains of a particular amino acid sequence will have a higher affinity to THP and, hence, higher propensity to cause cast nephropathy.

Not all patients with multiple myeloma develop cast nephropathy, and a unique combination of factors is required. The distal nephron milieu is an important factor in cast formation.

Any prerenal event that decreases the tubular fluid flow rate increases the interaction time in the distal tubule between the 2 culprit proteins.[19] The tubular fluid pH is another important factor: the more acidic the pH, the more the interaction between the light chains and THP.[20] THP has an isoelectric point of about 3.5, making it a highly polyanionic (negatively charged) molecule even in the most acidic urine. The light chains, on the other hand, have a isoelectric point that is quite variable, ranging between 4.7 to 7.4. So an interaction between THP and an appropriately charged light chain at a suitable pH can result in precipitation of the 2 proteins.[20] In vitro studies have shown evidence that a higher urinary concentration of sodium, chloride, and calcium augment cast formation. This is presumed to be related to promotion of THP self-aggregation, which, in turn, serves as a nidus for light chain cast formation. Some of the light chains themselves cause loop segment dysfunction, resulting in increased tubular chloride concentration.[21] This, in turn, affects the sodium and calcium concentration of the tubular fluid to favor precipitation of the proteins. The increased chloride concentration can also result in afferent arteriolar constriction via a feedback mechanism, which causes a drop in glomerular filtration rate (GFR) and, hence, tubular fluid rate, thus further exacerbating the protein precipitation. Hypercalcemia and loop diuretics also alter the intratubular fluid ion concentration by increasing the sodium, chloride, and calcium concentration.[21]

Light chain cast nephropathy is associated with inflammatory reaction in the interstitium. It is believed that once the THP–FLC interaction has resulted in a cast formation and tubular obstruction, there is a secondary leaking of FLC into the interstitium, and this triggers an intense inflammatory reaction, though direct evidence is lacking. However, there is evidence of FLC initiating an intracellular signaling cascade that results in a proinflammatory state by elaboration of monocyte chemoattractant protein-1, interleukin-6, and hydrogen peroxide, and increased nuclear factor kappa B pathway has been discovered in the tubular cells.[22,23] This is mostly in the proximal convoluted tubule where the FLC are likely triggering it during the process of reclamation. Such tubulointerstitial damage eventually leads to tubulointerstitial fibrosis and irreversible kidney injury.

CLINICAL PICTURE

Renal failure is a major cause of early mortality in patients with multiple myeloma, being second only to infection. Patients with light chain cast nephropathy typically present with severe acute kidney injury (AKI). This is acute in nature in about 50% of the patients with average serum creatinine of 7 mg/dL or more.[24] There is usually a precipitating factor like dehydration, contrast exposure, nonsteroidal anti-inflammatory drugs (NSAIDs), infection, or hypercalcemia (Table 35.3).

TABLE 35.3 SUMMARY OF KNOWN PRECIPITATING FACTORS FOR LIGHT CHAIN CAST NEPHROPATHY

Factor	Mechanism
Immunoglobulin light chain concentration	Clonal free light chains concentration of 500 mg/L or greater increases the likelihood of cast nephropathy.
Immunoglobulin light chain type	Light chains with higher isoelectric point (polycationic) would have a more favorable charge to interact with the polyanionic THP.
THP concentration	Higher the THP concentration, greater than risk of cast formation.
Prerenal events like intravascular volume depletion, diuretics, NSAIDs use, contrast drug use	Afferent arteriolar vasoconstriction leads to decrease in glomerular filtration rate and hence a decrease in tubular fluid rate. This increases the interaction time between the culprit proteins.
Chloride concentration in distal nephron	Light chains can cause loop segment dysfunction and increase the intratubular chloride concentration. This can in turn lead to an increase in sodium and calcium concentration. Chlorides can also via a feedback mechanism cause afferent arteriolar constriction and hence decrease the tubular fluid rate. Together they increase the THP aggregation.
Sodium concentration in distal nephron	The higher concentration of sodium and calcium augment cast formation presumably due to an increase in self-aggregation which in turn serves as a nidus for cast formation.
Calcium concentration in distal nephron	
Tubular fluid pH	The more acidic the tubular fluid pH, the more the interaction between the light chains and THP.

NSAIDs = nonsteroidal anti-inflammatory drugs; THP = Tamm-Horsfall protein

Urinalysis would show evidence of proteinuria of at least 2 g/day, though less than 10% are in the nephrotic range.[24] These urinary proteins are typically low molecular weight in nature, consisting predominantly of Bence Jones proteins, though other tubular proteins from tubular injury can also be present and can range from 0.1 to 19.7 g/day.[25] Larger molecular weight proteins like albumin are less commonly seen. A study from a large referral center[25] noted that the percentage of urinary albumin excretion in patients with a histological diagnosis of light chain cast nephropathy was consistently less than 25% with a median of 7%. This is important as routine urine dipstick detects only albumin, and low molecular weight proteins like Bence Jones proteins can be easily missed.[26] Quantification of individual types of protein by urine protein electrophoresis can add valuable information, especially in those who are at a high risk for kidney biopsy.

A urine protein electrophoresis though requires an early morning urine sample or a 24-hour urine sample for optimal results, which can be challenging clinically.[27] The alternative test to assess for FLC is the serum FLC assay. Serum FLC assay is a nephelometric assay that uses sheep-derived polyclonal antibodies to kappa and lambda FLCs. It accurately measures even low levels of FLC quantitatively, and the monoclonality can be identified by the presence of an abnormal kappa–lambda ratio.[28] Patients who present with cast nephropathy have a high tumor burden as would be in multiple myeloma and would have a highly abnormal FLC ratio. The normal FLC ratio of kappa-to-lambda is 0.26 to 1.65,[28] and in the context of renal failure the threshold is raised with the accepted normal range being 0.37 to 3.17.[29] Patients who present with AKI and have a clonal FLCs of 500 mg/L or greater must be strongly suspected to have cast nephropathy.[30] Patients with monoclonal kappa FLC tend to present with more severe renal failure.[31]

The role of kidney biopsy in patients with light chain cast nephropathy is debated. This is mainly due to concerns of high bleeding risk in these patients. But this theoretical concern has not been seen in practice. Ecotière et al.[32] noted in their study that none of their patients had any serious bleeding after a kidney biopsy. Fish et al.[33] noted that hemorrhagic complications were seen in 4.1% of patients with monoclonal gammopathy as compared to 3.9% in patients without any monoclonal gammopathy. Six of the 92 patients with cast nephropathy had significant bleeding complications defined as presence of hematoma or macroscopic hematuria, none of which required surgical intervention.

A school of thought believes that kidney biopsy is not required to prove the diagnosis of cast nephropathy if patients have a bland urine sediment, serum FLC >1,500 mg/L, and minimal albuminuria.[25] In fact, the 2014 International Myeloma Working Group updated criteria[6] for the diagnosis of multiple myeloma in its definition of light chain cast nephropathy as a myeloma-defining event calls for either a histological diagnosis or a presumed diagnosis based on the presence of high involved FLC levels, typically >1,500 mg/L. However, in addition to the diagnostic value, the role of kidney biopsy in prognostication is also important. Leung et al.[34] found in their study that only patients with biopsy-proven cast nephropathy showed renal function recovery with FLC reduction. Ecotière et al[32] had noted in their study that on multivariate analysis looking at treated patients who responded hematologically, the median number of casts and tubular atrophy were independent predictors of renal response. Knowledge of other plasma dyscrasia-associated renal lesions is important as well. Coexistence of 2 forms of paraprotein-associated lesions was seen in 6% of the biopsies in a study at Mayo clinic with light chain cast nephropathy seen in conjunction with light chain deposition disease, AL amyloidosis and fibrillary GN. Ecotière et al. found that even in a highly selected group of myeloma patients, there was significant heterogeneity in the noted renal lesions. This information can further dictate the presence of other end-organ involvement as well.[14] For instance, cardiac involvement is common in AL amyloidosis and an important factor when considering future bone marrow transplantation.

PRECIPITATING FACTORS

One of the major precipitating factors of cast nephropathy is dehydration. In a study of patients with AKI and myeloma cast nephropathy,[35] this risk factor was seen in 65% of the patients. NSAIDs and intravenous contrast use also precipitated myeloma cast nephropathy, most likely due to vasoconstriction of the afferent arterioles with decrease in GFR. Pathophysiologically, all these factors cause a decrease in the tubular fluid flow rate. This results in an increase in the interaction time between THP and light chains. See Table 35.3 for more detailed list of precipitating factors.

PATHOLOGY

The characteristic finding seen on histology is the presence of multiple intraluminal proteinaceous casts.[14] These are acellular and homogenous and have characteristic fracture lines. They stain eosinophilic on hematoxylin and eosin stain and pale or negative on periodic acid–Schiff stain and are polychromatic (red and blue) on the trichrome stain. They are accompanied by varying degrees of interstitial inflammation and a typical giant cell reaction in the interstitium that surrounds the cast. Casts are also associated with acute tubular injury. This may be as part of cast nephropathy or from inherent nephrotoxic potential of light chains. Immunofluorescence staining shows the casts as being restricted for either kappa or lambda light chain. The light chain in the cast would be the same as in the serum and urine. Typically kappa is more commonly seen than lambda chains. Theoretically, lambda chains have a greater tendency to polymerize into covalently bond dimers as compared to kappa.[36] Hence, the slightly larger sized lambda may not necessarily filter into the tubular lumen as easily as kappa chains, but studies have shown no significant difference in the light chain predominance in cast nephropathy.[31] On electron microscopy, the cast's ultrastructural evaluation would have a varied appearance with no specific substructure formation. Other light chain–related renal lesions like amyloidosis and MIDD can also be expected to be seen in the same patient.[37]

TREATMENT

Treatment of AKI in light chain cast nephropathy is a medical urgency. Patients who present with AKI as their myeloma-defining event had worse outcomes than patients who met criteria for multiple myeloma via other criteria. Even with modern chemotherapy, there is a higher early death compared with patients without AKI, although the overall prognosis is no longer significantly different.[38] Most patients require hospitalization for symptom control, initiation of chemotherapy, and accelerated removal of circulating FLCs. See Table 35.4 for an overview of the treatment strategies.

SYMPTOMATIC MEASURES

Patients presenting with cast nephropathy may be volume depleted, and it is important to correct their volume status by infusion of fluids and/or blood if with significant symptomatic anemia.

TABLE 35.4 TREATMENT OVERVIEW IN PATIENTS WITH LIGHT CHAIN CAST NEPHROPATHY FROM MULTIPLE MYELOMA

Supportive Measures	Extracorporeal Light Chain Removal	Antimyeloma Therapy
Stop NSAIDs, ACEI, and ARB	Plasma exchange	CyBorD or VCD
Optimize volume status with goal 2–3 L of urine output per day, if possible		VTD
Assess for ongoing infection and treat		
Pain control	High cut-off dialysis (not available in United States)	Lenalidomide—avoided in AKI, given in refractory cases
Hemodialysis—if with symptoms of uremia, significant electrolyte disturbances		
Hypercalcemia—optimize volume status, pamidronate		Hematopoietic cell transplantation, when stabilized and if eligible
Avoid loop diuretics, unless with symptoms of volume overload		
Avoid contrast exposure, if possible		

ACEI = angiotensin converting enzyme inhibitor. ARB = angiotensin receptor blocker. AKI = acute kidney injury; CyBorD = cyclophosphamide-bortezomib–dexamethasone; NSAIDs = nonsteroidal anti-inflammatory drugs; US, United State; VCD = Velcade[R]-cyclophosphamide-dexamethasone. VTD = bortezomib, thalidomide, and dexamethasone

Hypotonic saline solution is preferred to reduce the amount of salt intake. This will also help in the correction of their hypercalcemia. Patients with mild hypercalcemia (<12 mg/dL) can be managed with hydration and dexamethasone (part of antimyeloma therapy), but those with moderate to severe hypercalcemia (12–18 mg/dL) or who are symptomatic will require the use of calcitonin in conjunction with a bisphosphonate like pamidronate for rapid reduction of calcium levels. Infection is another common complication as these patients are significantly immunocompromised, and this would need to be appropriately worked up and antibiotic regimen initiated. Appropriate prevention such as minimizing the use of catheters is also important. Pain control would also need to be addressed as fractures are common in patients with multiple myeloma. They could potentially already be using NSAIDs for pain control, and this would have to be discontinued and switched to a less nephrotoxic regimen. Other nephrotoxic agents like angiotensin converting enzyme inhibitors or angiotensin receptor blockers should be stopped. Use of contrast agent should be avoided if possible.[39] In patients who have severe AKI with symptoms or signs of uremia then dialysis should be considered. Conventional dialysis does not remove FLCs and must not be initiated for this reason. But in those patients who need both dialysis and plasmapheresis, typically dialysis will follow plasmapheresis to correct the electrolyte disturbances caused by the citrate anticoagulation.

ANTIMYELOMA THERAPY

The decision for the type of treatment regimen for multiple myeloma is based on the individual patient's tumor cytogenetics. But in patients with renal failure from cast nephropathy, regimens that can rapidly decrease light chain production are preferred. Bortezomib, cyclophosphamide, and high-dose dexamethasone (cyclophosphamide–bortezomib–dexamethasone or Velcade'–cyclophosphamide–dexamethasone) is a preferred regimen in these patients.[40] Bortezomib is a novel proteasome inhibitor that works by inducing unfolded protein response resulting in cell death.[41] It also inhibits NF-κB pathway by affecting its degradation by proteasomes.[42] Light chains are known to cause tissue injury by activating the same NF-κB pathway.[43] The drug is metabolized through the liver mainly and so can be given in patients with renal failure with no dose adjustment.[38]

Neurotoxicity is its major dose-limiting side effect, and the neuropathy can be debilitating for the patients.[44] Lenalidomide is typically avoided in patients with renal insufficiency unless the patient is refractory to a bortezomib-based therapy. Lenalidomide also seems to affect a later stem cell mobilization.[45] Thalidomide-based regimen, a combination of bortezomib, thalidomide, and dexamethasone, is used in Europe and has been reported to be superior to Velcade'–cyclophosphamide–dexamethasone.[46]

Once the patient is more stabilized, an autologous stem cell transplantation can be considered, if eligible. Patients on dialysis can undergo autologous stem cell transplantation without excessive risk.[47,48] Melphalan dose will need to be reduced by 30% to 140 mg/m^2. Transfusion needs may be higher than patients without renal failure. Platelet transfusion may also be required for dialysis in patients using a fistula during the thrombocytopenic phase.

EXTRACORPOREAL LIGHT CHAIN REMOVAL

The concept of extracorporeal light chain removal in conjunction with chemotherapy stems from the evidence that early reduction in serum light chains is associated with recovery of renal function. It is now recommended to aim for a 60% to 80% reduction in FLCs by day 21 as it was found to be associated with recovery of renal function in 80% of the patients.[49] Despite the halting of production of the FLC with effective chemotherapy, patients with renal dysfunction will have difficulty clearing the high levels of FLC that are responsible for acute ongoing kidney injury.[29] Extracorporeal light chain removal by the use of plasmapheresis or high cut-off (HCO) dialyzer has been theorized to assist in the removal and enhance recovery.

Plasmapheresis is performed while guided by the measurement of serum FLCs daily. The goal is for a minimum of 60% reduction of the serum FLC. Typically patients with light chain cast nephropathy require 5 to 7 exchanges performed once a day to achieve this. This must be performed in conjunction with antimyeloma therapy. High cut-off dialysis is performed by utilizing dialyzers with larger pore size as compared to the currently available high-flux dialyzers and so more efficiently removes proteins. This is currently not available in United States. A recent randomized clinical trial, the European Trial of FLC Removal by

Extended Hemodialysis in Cast Nephropathy[50] had randomized patients to a standard dialysis with a high flux dialyzer versus extended dialysis using a HCO dialyzer in addition to bortezomib-based chemotherapy. Ninety patients were recruited and dialysis with HCO dialyzer failed to improve renal recovery. On the other hand, another multicenter phase 3 randomized clinical trial from France, Studies in Patients with Multiple Myeloma and Renal Failure due to Myeloma Cast Nephropathy,[51] found that patients with multiple myeloma and severe renal failure from biopsy-proven myeloma cast nephropathy requiring hemodialysis showed a positive result with the HCO dialyzer. Here 98 patients were randomized to either an intensive hemodialysis regimen (8 sessions over the first 10 days, then 3× a week) using either a dialyzer with very high permeability to proteins (Theralite™ HCO) or a conventional high-flux dialyzer, while receiving bortezomib-based chemotherapy. Independence from hemodialysis was achieved in 37.5% and 60% ($p = 0.03$) of patients at 6 months in the control and HCO arms, respectively. The role of HCO dialysis remains uncertain and at this point cannot be recommended.

PROGNOSIS

When looking at multiple myeloma patients, those with renal failure have a significantly lower overall survival when compared to those who do not have renal failure. However, patients who recover their renal function have a longer median survival (28 months vs. 4 months) as compared to those who do not recover.[52] In fact, their survival is similar to those myeloma patients with no renal impairment. This makes recovery from renal failure a critical prognostic indicator in myeloma patients.[31] The presence of numerous casts on kidney biopsy and diffuse tubular atrophy is associated with poor renal prognosis.[53] The percentage of FLC reduction at day 21 has been found to be a strong predictor of renal response in multiple studies,[49,53] and Hutchinson et al.[49] have established that a 60% reduction of FLC by day21 would enable about 80% of renal function recovery. Scheid et al.,[38] in their elegantly done randomized phase 3 study, showed that the use of bortezomib-based therapy before and after autologous stem cell transplant in newly diagnosed myeloma patients with renal insufficiency overcame the known negative effect of renal failure with an overall 3-year survival of 74%.

Prior to the introduction of bortezomib, Blade et al.[52] had noted about 26% of patients had renal recovery, and the factors associated with it were serum creatinine <4 mg/dL, serum calcium ≥11.5 mg/dL, and amount of proteinuria <1 g/day. This has significantly improved with the newer chemotherapies that can be used safely in patients with renal failure and has an ability to cause rapid reduction in FLC. Ludwig et al.[54] noted in their study involving patients whose presenting feature of multiple myeloma was AKI, bortezomib was quite well tolerated with 72% having complete remission of myeloma. They measured renal response based on the updated criteria to measure renal response based on improvement in GFR and not creatinine values. An improvement of GFR to >60 mL/min/body surface area was defined as a complete response, and this was seen in 58% of patients. The median time to such a complete renal response though was long at 111 days though hematological response was seen in 25.5 days.

FUTURE RESEARCH IN CAST NEPHROPATHY

A cyclized peptide was recently designed to successfully interfere with the binding of FLC with THP in animal models.[55] Cyclized peptides are also more stable, and hence further studies would be needed to determine its oral bioavailability. This can certainly be a potential therapeutic modality in the future for patients who are known to have a high tumor burden and are at risk for developing cast nephropathy.

CONCLUSION

Light chain cast nephropathy is one of the most common renal lesions in patients with multiple myeloma. It is rarely seen in other plasma cell dyscrasias like Waldenström macroglobulinemia, lymphoma, and chronic lymphocytic leukemia. The FLC bind with THP in the distal tubule forming casts and inciting a inflammatory response in the kidney. They typically present with severe AKI precipitated by volume depletion or use of nephrotoxic agent. Management involves a combination of antimyeloma therapy with bortezomib-based chemotherapy to kill FLC-producing plasma myeloma cells and extracorporeal FLC removal for management of ongoing AKI in conjunction with supportive measures.

REFERENCES

1. Kyle RA, Therneau TM, Rajkumar SV, et al. A long-term study of prognosis in monoclonal

gammopathy of undetermined significance. *N Engl J Med*. 2002;346(8):564–569.

2. Weiss BM, Abadie J, Verma P, Howard RS, Kuehl WM. A monoclonal gammopathy precedes multiple myeloma in most patients. *Blood*. 2009;113(22):5418–5422.

3. Leung N, Bridoux F, Hutchison CA, et al. Monoclonal gammopathy of renal significance: when MGUS is no longer undetermined or insignificant. *Blood*. 2012;120(22):4292–4295.

4. Wochner RD, Strober W, Waldmann TA. The role of the kidney in the catabolism of Bence Jones proteins and immunoglobulin fragments. *J Exp Med*. 1967;126(2):207–221.

5. Klassen RB, Allen PL, Batuman V, Crenshaw K, Hammond TG. Light chains are a ligand for megalin. *J Appl Physiol (1985)*. 2005;98(1):257–263.

6. Rajkumar SV, Dimopoulos MA, Palumbo A, et al. International Myeloma Working Group updated criteria for the diagnosis of multiple myeloma. *Lancet Oncol*. 2014;15(12):e538–e548.

7. Herrera GA, Joseph L, Gu X, Hough A, Barlogie B. Renal pathologic spectrum in an autopsy series of patients with plasma cell dyscrasia. *Arch Pathol Lab Med*. 2004;128(8):875–879.

8. Paueksakon P, Revelo MP, Horn RG, Shappell S, Fogo AB. Monoclonal gammopathy: significance and possible causality in renal disease. *Am J Kidney Dis*. 2003;42(1):87–95.

9. Isaac J, Herrera GA. Cast nephropathy in a case of Waldenstrom's macroglobulinemia. *Nephron*. 2002;91(3):512–515.

10. Burke JR, Jr., Flis R, Lasker N, Simenhoff M. Malignant lymphoma with "myeloma kidney" acute renal failure. *Am J Med*. 1976;60(7):1055–1060.

11. Strati P, Nasr SH, Leung N, et al. Renal complications in chronic lymphocytic leukemia and monoclonal B-cell lymphocytosis: the Mayo Clinic experience. *Haematologica*. 2015;100(9):1180–1188.

12. Steensma DP, Kyle RA. A history of the kidney in plasma cell disorders. *Contrib Nephrol*. 2007;153:5–24.

13. Oliver J. New directions in renal morphology. *Harvey Lectures*. 1944–1945;40:102–155.

14. Nasr SH, Valeri AM, Sethi S, et al. Clinicopathologic correlations in multiple myeloma: a case series of 190 patients with kidney biopsies. *Am J Kidney Dis*. 2012;59(6):786–794.

15. Sanders PW, Herrera GA, Galla JH. Human Bence Jones protein toxicity in rat proximal tubule epithelium in vivo. *Kidney Int*. 1987;32(6):851–861.

16. Mo L, Huang HY, Zhu XH, Shapiro E, Hasty DL, Wu XR. Tamm-Horsfall protein is a critical renal defense factor protecting against calcium oxalate crystal formation. *Kidney Int*. 2004;66(3):1159–1166.

17. Cvoriscec D, Stavljenic A, Radonic M. Tamm-Horsfall protein in Balkan endemic nephropathy. *J Clin Chem Clin Biochem*. 1985;23(4):177–181.

18. Huang ZQ, Sanders PW. Localization of a single binding site for immunoglobulin light chains on human Tamm-Horsfall glycoprotein. *J Clin Invest*. 1997;99(4):732–736.

19. Sanders PW. Pathogenesis and treatment of myeloma kidney. *J Lab Clin Med*. 1994;124(4):484–488.

20. Pesce AJ, Clyne DH, Pollak VE, Kant SK, Foulkes EC, Selenke WM. Renal tubular interactions of proteins. *Clin Biochem*. 1980;13(5):209–215.

21. Sanders PW, Booker BB, Bishop JB, Cheung HC. Mechanisms of intranephronal proteinaceous cast formation by low molecular weight proteins. *J Clin Invest*. 1990;85(2):570–576.

22. Ying WZ, Wang PX, Aaron KJ, Basnayake K, Sanders PW. Immunoglobulin light chains activate nuclear factor-kappaB in renal epithelial cells through a Src-dependent mechanism. *Blood*. 2011;117(4):1301–1307.

23. Wang PX, Sanders PW. Immunoglobulin light chains generate hydrogen peroxide. *J Am Soc Nephrol*. 2007;18(4):1239–1245.

24. Montseny JJ, Kleinknecht D, Meyrier A, et al. Long-term outcome according to renal histological lesions in 118 patients with monoclonal gammopathies. *Nephrol Dial Transplant*. 1998;13(6):1438–1445.

25. Leung N, Gertz M, Kyle RA, et al. Urinary albumin excretion patterns of patients with cast nephropathy and other monoclonal gammopathy-related kidney diseases. *Clin J Am Soc Nephrol*. 2012;7(12):1964–1968.

26. Caring for Australians with Renal I. The CARI guidelines: urine protein as diagnostic test: performance characteristics of tests used in the initial evaluation of patients at risk of renal disease. *Nephrology (Carlton)*. 2004;9(Suppl 3):S8–S14.

27. Brigden ML, Neal ED, McNeely MD, Hoag GN. The optimum urine collections for the detection and monitoring of Bence Jones proteinuria. *Am J Clin Pathol*. 1990;93(5):689–693.

28. Katzmann JA, Clark RJ, Abraham RS, et al. Serum reference intervals and diagnostic ranges for free kappa and free lambda immunoglobulin light chains: relative sensitivity for detection of monoclonal light chains. *Clin Chem*. 2002;48(9):1437–1444.

29. Hutchison CA, Harding S, Hewins P, et al. Quantitative assessment of serum and urinary polyclonal free light chains in patients with

chronic kidney disease. *Clin J Am Soc Nephrol.* 2008;3(6):1684–1690.

30. Yadav P, Leung N, Sanders PW, Cockwell P. The use of immunoglobulin light chain assays in the diagnosis of paraprotein-related kidney disease. *Kidney Int.* 2015;87(4):692–697.

31. Knudsen LM, Hjorth M, Hippe E; Nordic Myeloma Study Group. Renal failure in multiple myeloma: reversibility and impact on the prognosis. *Eur J Haematol.* 2000;65(3):175–181.

32. Ecotiere L, Thierry A, Debiais-Delpech C, et al. Prognostic value of kidney biopsy in myeloma cast nephropathy: a retrospective study of 70 patients. *Nephrol Dial Transplant.* 2016;31(5):850.

33. Fish R, Pinney J, Jain P, et al. The incidence of major hemorrhagic complications after renal biopsies in patients with monoclonal gammopathies. *Clin J Am Soc Nephrol.* 2010;5(11):1977–1980.

34. Leung N, Gertz MA, Zeldenrust SR, et al. Improvement of cast nephropathy with plasma exchange depends on the diagnosis and on reduction of serum free light chains. *Kidney Int.* 2008;73(11):1282–1288.

35. Rota S, Mougenot B, Baudouin B, et al. Multiple myeloma and severe renal failure: a clinicopathologic study of outcome and prognosis in 34 patients. *Medicine (Baltimore).* 1987;66(2):126–137.

36. Solling K. Light chain polymerism in normal individuals in patients with severe proteinuria and in normals with inhibited tubular protein reabsorption by lysine. *Scand J Clin Lab Invest.* 1980;40(2):129–134.

37. Lorenz EC, Sethi S, Poshusta TL, et al. Renal failure due to combined cast nephropathy, amyloidosis and light-chain deposition disease. *Nephrol Dial Transplant.* 2010;25(4):1340–1343.

38. Scheid C, Sonneveld P, Schmidt-Wolf IG, et al. Bortezomib before and after autologous stem cell transplantation overcomes the negative prognostic impact of renal impairment in newly diagnosed multiple myeloma: a subgroup analysis from the HOVON-65/GMMG-HD4 trial. *Haematologica.* 2014;99(1):148–154.

39. Kumar SK, Callander NS, Alsina M, et al. Multiple myeloma, version 3.2017, NCCN clinical practice guidelines in oncology. *J Natl Compr Canc Netw.* 2017;15(2):230–269.

40. Rajkumar SV. Multiple myeloma: 2016 update on diagnosis, risk-stratification, and management. *Am J Hematol.* 2016;91(7):719–734.

41. Adams J. The proteasome: a suitable antineoplastic target. *Nat Rev Cancer.* 2004;4(5):349–360.

42. Hideshima T, Ikeda H, Chauhan D, et al. Bortezomib induces canonical nuclear factor-kappaB activation in multiple myeloma cells. *Blood.* 2009;114(5):1046–1052.

43. Sanders PW. Mechanisms of light chain injury along the tubular nephron. *J Am Soc Nephrol.* 2012;23(11):1777–1781.

44. Mohty B, El-Cheikh J, Yakoub-Agha I, Moreau P, Harousseau JL, Mohty M. Peripheral neuropathy and new treatments for multiple myeloma: background and practical recommendations. *Haematologica.* 2010;95(2):311–319.

45. Moreau P, Hulin C, Marit G, et al. Stem cell collection in patients with de novo multiple myeloma treated with the combination of bortezomib and dexamethasone before autologous stem cell transplantation according to IFM 2005-01 trial. *Leukemia.* 2010;24(6):1233–1235.

46. Rosinol L, Oriol A, Teruel AI, et al. Superiority of bortezomib, thalidomide, and dexamethasone (VTD) as induction pretransplantation therapy in multiple myeloma: a randomized phase 3 PETHEMA/GEM study. *Blood.* 2012;120(8):1589–1596.

47. Glavey SV, Gertz MA, Dispenzieri A, et al. Long-term outcome of patients with multiple [corrected] myeloma-related advanced renal failure following auto-SCT. *Bone Marrow Transplant.* 2013;48(12):1543–1547.

48. Lee CK, Zangari M, Barlogie B, et al. Dialysis-dependent renal failure in patients with myeloma can be reversed by high-dose myeloablative therapy and autotransplant. *Bone Marrow Transplant.* 2004;33(8):823–828.

49. Hutchison CA, Cockwell P, Stringer S, et al. Early reduction of serum-free light chains associates with renal recovery in myeloma kidney. *J Am Soc Nephrol.* 2011;22(6):1129–1136.

50. Hutchison CA, Cook M, Heyne N, et al. European trial of free light chain removal by extended haemodialysis in cast nephropathy (EuLITE): A randomised control trial. *Trials.* 2008;9.

51. Frank Bridoux BP, Augeul-Meunier K, Royer B, et al. Treatment of myeloma cast nephropathy (MCN): A randomized trial comparing intensive haemodialysis (HD) with high cut-off (HCO) or standard high-flux dialyzer in patients receiving a bortezomib-based regimen (the MYRE Study, by the Intergroupe Francophone du Myélome [IFM] and the French Society of Nephrology [SFNDT]). 58th ASH Annual Meeting; 2016; San Diego, CA.

52. Blade J, Fernandez-Llama P, Bosch F, et al. Renal failure in multiple myeloma: presenting features and predictors of outcome in 94 patients from a single institution. *Arch Intern Med.* 1998;158(17):1889–1893.

53. Ecotiere L, Thierry A, Debiais-Delpech C, et al. Prognostic value of kidney biopsy in myeloma cast nephropathy: a retrospective study of 70 patients. *Nephrol Dial Transplant.* 2016;31(1):64–72.

54. Ludwig H, Adam Z, Hajek R, et al. Light chain-induced acute renal failure can be reversed by bortezomib-doxorubicin-dexamethasone in multiple myeloma: results of a phase II study. *J Clin Oncol.* 2010;28(30):4635–4641.

55. Ying WZ, Allen CE, Curtis LM, Aaron KJ, Sanders PW. Mechanism and prevention of acute kidney injury from cast nephropathy in a rodent model. *J Clin Invest.* 2012;122(5):1777–1785.

36

Sickle Cell Nephropathy

KATIA LÓPEZ REVUELTA AND MARÍA PILAR RICARD ANDRES

INTRODUCTION

Hemoglobin S (HbS) is the most common and well-known structural hemoglobinopathy in the world. This abnormality causes sickle cell disease (SCD), which is a group of disorders that includes the most severe homozygote state (HbSS) and the compound heterozygote states HbSC and HbS/β-thalassemia. SCD is characterized by vaso-occlusive episodes due to erythrocyte sickling and hemolysis, which cause a multiorgan systemic disease associated with acute and chronic continuous ischemia-reperfusion injury and inflammation (Fig. 36.1).[1] Recent estimates consider the overall prevalence of the problem is increasing because of improved survival in SCD and immigration to higher income countries,[2] emphasizing the need to develop specific national public health policies particularly in low- and middle-income countries. On this basis, SCD has been recognized as a public health priority by United Nations Educational, Scientific and Cultural Organization (UNESCO), the African Union, and World Health Organization (WHO).

The dramatic improvement in life expectancy of SCD patients, with more than half of affected people surviving to their mid-60s,[3,4] has allowed the kidney abnormalities in SCD to emerge and been better studied, which will undoubtedly help their control.

At the moment, renal disease in SCD and its causes and complications are being inadequately and inconsistently addressed in adults, in part because of our limited awareness of its clinical presentation.

In this review, we will address kidney structural and functional abnormalities associated with SCD, known as sickle cell nephropathy (SCN); the mechanisms of kidney injury and its manifestations; and prevention strategies.

EPIDEMIOLOGY

The global prevalence of the S gene in the world is estimated at 30 million people. It especially affects individuals from tropical and subtropical Africa, the Arabian Peninsula, India, the Mediterranean basin, and Central and North America.

The annual birth rate estimated between 300,000 to 400,000 infants with hereditary hemoglobin diseases (83% SCD) is increasing.[1] The sickle cell trait is 40 to 50 times more common than SCD with a prevalence of 2% to 30% in African populations.[1]

Migration movements and mosaicism with other races are responsible for the high rates of hemoglobinopathies that are observed in Central and North America and for the increased burden of sickle cell trait in Europe around 1%.

Longitudinal and large cohort studies estimate that chronic kidney disease (CKD) is the second most common chronic complication (75%), after chronic lung disease in SCD patients over a period of 40 years of follow-up.[5,6]

CKD is responsible for one-third of the deaths in SCD patients, being the main cause of death in the long term.[5-7] The median survival for patients with SCD estimated to be 51 years declines to 29 years in those with CKD.[8] SCN accounts for 1% of all new cases of end-stage renal disease in the world.

The presence of CKD in SCD is a predictor of the detrimental outcome of other systemic complications of SCD such as cardiac dysfunction, tricuspid valve insufficiency, and even stroke.

PATHOGENESIS

The central fact of the pathophysiology of SCD is the abnormal polymerization of deoxygenated HbS, which deforms the erythrocyte to its typical sickle shape, of greater fragility, less deformability,

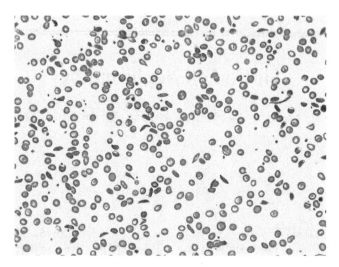

FIGURE 36.1 Peripheral blood smear (Wright stain, 250×). Red cell picture of a hemoglobin SS untreated adult patient.

and increased adherence to endothelium (see Fig. 36.1). Whereas the vascular lesions of SCD can affect the entire kidney, the inner renal medulla is especially prone to polymerization of HbS because of its hypertonicity, hypoxia, and relative acidotic state. Moreover, the relatively slow blood flow in the vasa recta lengthens red cell transit through the medulla, thereby promoting further HbS polymerization and sickled red cell adhesion to the endothelium. There is also abnormal adhesion of leukocytes, reticulocytes, and platelets to an activated endothelium, with a procoagulant state, all of which lead to tissue ischemia and organ damage.[9,10] Additional pathobiological pathways include hemolysis and increased free plasma hemoglobin.[1,11,12]

Thereby, SCN largely reflects an underlying renal vasculopathy that leads to a perfusion paradox, wherein medullary hypoperfusion occurs in conjunction with kidney and/or cortical hyperperfusion. The renal vasculopathy also leads to aberrant renal vascular responses to stress that occur systemically or in distant organs and tissues. This response is characterized by enhanced renal vasoconstriction and resultant vaso-occlusion. Recurrent cycles of ischemia and ischemia–reperfusion injury thus occur, thereby leading to subclinical and clinical acute kidney injury. These processes summate in the initiation and progression of SCN.[13] Genetic and nongenetic factors modulate the heterogeneity of SCN phenotypic expression.

CLINICAL SYNDROMES

Very few diseases have as varied a spectrum of kidney complications as SCD has. All the structures along the nephron can be damaged. Changes are most marked in patients with homozygous hemoglobin SS (HbSS) but are also seen in those with compound heterozygous states and the sickle cell trait.

Some of the manifestations occur early in life and are directly dependent on alterations in renal hemodynamics, hypoperfusion at the renal medulla (hematuria, hyposthenuria, distal tubular dysfunction), and parallel kidney/cortical hyperperfusion (hyperfiltration, glomerular hypertrophy, proximal tubular hyperfunction).

Other SCN manifestations need more time to develop, and the whole vasculopathic renal complex with the repetitive ischemia reperfusion injury, inflammation, and epithelial cell injury, probably interacting with genetic factors, can result in irreversible CKD (interstitial nephritis, proteinuria, and glomerular disease).

Hematuria

Hematuria is considered to be the most prevalent clinical feature of SCN, being usually macroscopic, asymptomatic, and self-limited. It can develop at any age, and it is much more frequent in patients with sickle cell trait (HbAS) than in the homozygous form. Hematuria is probably a consequence of cell sickling in the renal medulla combined with vascular obstruction and red cell extravasation into the tubular lumen.

Renal Papillary Necrosis

The papillae are dependent on the vasa recta; therefore, when vasa recta are destroyed, small repeated focal infarctions of the papillae occurs. The subsequent papillary infarcts are focal and localized to the core of the papilla, not at the tip, resulting in characteristic fistula formation that predisposes patients to recurrent infections.[8] The clinical presentation of this condition varies from asymptomatic macroscopic hematuria, not always present, to an acute condition involving pain, fever, and even obstructive acute kidney injury. Renal infarction has been estimated in 30% to 40% of homozygous HbSS patients.

Interstitial Nephritis

The principal pathologic lesion of the kidney in SCD is interstitial nephritis. There are variable clinical and laboratory manifestations depending on predominant and combinations of the tubular segments affected.

Hyposthenuria is a universal finding in patients with SCD. It can be manifested by enuresis very early in life and in patients older than 15 years by polyuria and polydipsia. The juxtamedullary nephrons (circulation supplied by vasa recta) are implicated in urine concentration mechanisms. Obstruction and congestion of vasa recta by the mechanisms previously discussed impair the ability to concentrate urine, alter countercurrent medullary mechanisms, and impede the reabsorption of free water and sodium, which can become a vasopressin-resistant nephrogenic diabetes insipidus when permanent damage befalls.

The most incipient abnormality that accompanies hyposthenuria is an incomplete distal tubular acidosis, usually normokalemic, which has been observed in 40% of patients with SCD and arises from diminished availability of ammonium.[14] Impaired potassium excretion in SCD likely reflects resistance of the distal nephron to aldosterone.[15] Hyperkalemic hyperchloremic metabolic acidosis is also recognized in patients with SCD that usually reflect a type 4 renal tubular acidosis defect.[16]

The increased loss of sodium and water in association with hyperfiltration that occurs in SCN leads to a reactive increased reabsorption by the proximal tubule to maintain glomerulotubular balance. This drives supranormal proximal tubular reabsorption of sodium, phosphate, and $\beta 2$-microglobuline and increased secretion of uric acid and creatinine. Hence, methods based on creatinine overestimate glomerular filtration rate (GFR) in patients with SCD.

Hyperfiltration

Increased GFR is one of the earliest signs of SCN, along with the increase of total renal blood flow.[17] With growth, the GFR rises further and can often range above 200 mL/min/1.73 m[2]. This may be partially accounted for by an increased cardiac output driven by anemia, but several mechanisms are suspected to interact, mainly an increase in vasodilatation hormones (prostaglandins, kallikreins). Essentially, the oxidative stress and inflammation secondary to vaso-occlusion activates the heme oxygenase–carbon monoxide system, which leads to increased levels of carbon monoxide and thus contributes to hyperperfusion.[13]

Glomerulopathy

Glomerular enlargement is an early finding reported in SCD children as young as 2 years (Fig. 36.2). The natural history of SCN is not known, but it has been suggested that hyperfiltration would be the early step of a sequence of events leading from albuminuria to proteinuria and ultimately CKD by development of a glomerulopathy.

Albuminuria is detected in 20% of SCD children,[18] increasing with age, and it is more prevalent in HbSS patients than in those with other hemoglobinopathies.[19] The prevalence of albuminuria continues to increase with age, being detectable in approximately 30% in the 15 to 23 age group, 40% in the 24 to 35 age range, and >60% over 35 years of age.[19] Pathophysiology of microalbuminuria is likely multifactorial, with contributions from hyperfiltration, glomerular hypertension, ischemia reperfusion injury, oxidative stress, decreased nitric oxide bioavailability, and endothelial dysfunction.

Proteinuria is also age-dependent in SCD and is seen in 20% of SCD patients (HbSS or HbSC).[20]

SCN is now felt to be a spectrum of different patterns of glomerular lesions that may coexist. In a biopsy review of patients with SCD and proteinuria and/or renal failure,[21] focal segmental glomerulosclerosis (FSGS; Fig. 36.3) was the most frequent glomerulopathy (39%), followed by membranoproliferative glomerulonephritis (28%) and thrombotic microangiopathy glomerulopathy (17%).

FSGS found in SCD is a secondary form of FSGS included in the group called the adaptive types, which are thought to result from

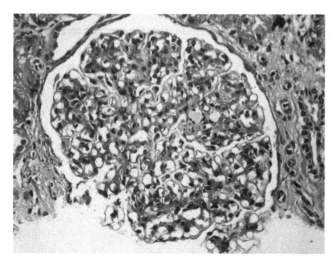

FIGURE 36.2 Kidney biopsy (Masson's trichrome stain, 400×). Glomerulomegaly in a 29-year-old patient with sickle cell disease and arterial hypertension, chronic kidney disease, and nephrotic range proteinuria. With permission of Luis F. Arias, MD, PhD. Departamento de Patología, Facultad de Medicina, Universidad de Antioquia. Medellín, Colombia. luisfer_uda@yahoo.com. http://www.kidneypathology.com/

structural and functional adaptations mediated by intrarenal vasodilatation, increased glomerular capillary pressures, and plasma flow rates. Unlike primary FSGS, adaptive disease is often associated with normal serum albumin levels, despite nephrotic-range proteinuria.

Irrespective of the initiating insult in the kidneys of Hb SS patients, the renal disease will progress to CKD. The exact role of environmental and co-inherited genetic factors for the development of CKD in SCD is not completely understood, although mechanisms common to most types of progressive renal diseases are likely to occur. The gene APOL1 has been implicated in the propensity to proteinuria and glomerulosclerosis in SCD.[22]

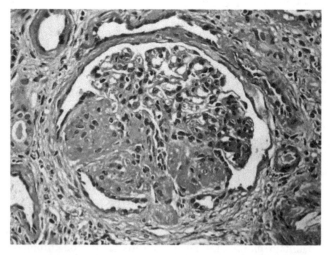

FIGURE 36.3 Kidney biopsy (Masson's trichrome stain, 400×). Segmental sclerosis in a 29-year-old patient with sickle cell disease, arterial hypertension, chronic kidney disease, and nephrotic range proteinuria. With permission of Luis F. Arias, MD, PhD. Departamento de Patología, Facultad de Medicina, Universidad de Antioquia. Medellín, Colombia. luisfer_uda@yahoo.com. http://www.kidneypathology.com/

Blood Pressure Effects

Patients with SCD tend to have a lower systemic blood pressure (BP) than age- and ethnicity-matched controls.[23] Lower BP may reflect a hemodynamic response to anemia caused by excessive systemic vasodilatation (nitric oxide and prostacyclin mediated) and endothelial dysfunction. Although unproven, it is possible that moderate and even high-normal BP (systolic BP 120–139 mmHg; diastolic BP 70–89 mmHg) are damaging from a renal perspective in patients with SCD than without SCD as they have been associated with higher creatinine levels when compared with SCD patients with lower pressures.[24,25]

Renal Medullary Carcinoma

Renal medullary carcinoma is a universally fatal tumor almost always metastatic at presentation, is considered to be specific to sickle cell hemoglobinopathies, and is associated with sickle cell trait and, to a lesser degree, with SCD. Renal medullary carcinoma is rare; it appears in most cases before 20 years of age with a higher incidence in males. A genetic predisposition is suggested and is distinguished from collecting tube carcinoma by certain markers, including a hypoxia-inducible factor. Medullary hypoxia in SCD can promote its development. The typical clinical presentation is macroscopic hematuria, lumbar pain, and abdominal mass and/ or constitutional syndrome. The appearance of macroscopic hematuria should alert its diagnostic possibility in the child with sickle cell trait or SCD, and it should be excluded by computed tomography in these situations. The existence of metastasis is common at the time of diagnosis so that the removal of the tumor is not curative. Survival after diagnosis does not exceed 6 to 12 months.[26,27]

PREVENTION STRATEGIES

Before addressing both general and more specific measures on the treatment of SCN, there are some aspects of concern on these patients. SCD is a chronic disease that in many cases is asymptomatic or subclinical. Early diagnosis, treatment, and monitoring are pivotal goals to prevent patients from developing acute problems and chronic end-organ damage. The adult patient with SCD usually has a complex psychosocial context, that results in a pattern of erratic and inconstant healthcare that threatens the effectiveness of any treatment.[23]

The lack of scientific evidence in the clinical management of adult SCD patients hinders high-quality care outside specialized centers.

Screening

Early diagnosis of SCD significantly reduces mortality and improves patient status by allowing necessary preventive measures (antibiotic prophylaxis and vaccination) and multidisciplinary care to reduce morbidity and mortality.[11]

The data are limited for early intervention through screening for renal disease in people with SCD. Therefore, clinical guidelines[28,29] consider indirect evidence from non-SCD populations in which pharmacological interventions are beneficial in people with proteinuria. They recommend annual screening of persons with SCD for microalbuminuria and proteinuria with spot urine testing by 10 years of age and refer cases with proteinuria (> 300 mg/24 h) to a nephrologist for further evaluation.[28,29]

Having in mind that spot urine albumin–creatinine ratio has not been validated in SCD because creatinine is hypersecreted and microalbuminuria quantification by 24-hour urine collection is not practical in patients with enuresis, in our opinion, we would recommend based on our opinion to be on alert and refer to a specialist when albumin–creatinine is positive below the limit of 30 mg/g.

Attention should to be paid to urinary density at the urinalysis, which along with the anamnesis can make us suspect the existence of hyposthenuria.

Identification of renal disease in people with SCD is also complicated by creatinine hypersecretion by masking significant renal impairment before serum creatinine rises.

Determination of serum cystatin C provides a more accurate estimation of GFR to detect early deterioration of renal function in patients with SCD in the clinical setting.[30,31] Nevertheless it has not yet fully validated, and it is not always available.

The pattern and rate of change of serum creatinine and creatinine-based GFR equations can be a useful manner to monitor renal function in SCD patients, meaning a modest increase in creatinine at high levels of estimated GFR, represents a significant decline in renal function.

Once CKD is diagnosed, other causes of kidney disease should be screened for.

General Measures

Care of SCD patients, especially of those who require hospitalization, should involve maneuvers to prevent acute kidney injury. Particularly, SCD patients are prone to volume depletion and drugs such as nonsteroidal anti-inflammatory drugs, which inhibit renal compensatory mechanisms mediated by prostaglandins, are harmful for these patients.

Because of hyposthenia and the risk to hypovolemia, we recommend avoiding diuretics in SCD patients.

We recommend supplementing bicarbonate when acidosis is present as this may be deleterious in HbSS patients, because it favors sickling.

Angiotensin converting enzyme inhibitors (ACEIs) have been in use for a long time to reduce proteinuria and delay the progression of CKD in patients with SCD.[32] Although this approach has not been vigorously tested in patients with SCD,[33] a panel of experts in 2014[28] recommends initiating ACEI inhibitor therapy for SCD adults with microalbuminuria or proteinuria without other apparent cause of kidney disease, even in the presence of normal blood pressure.

Though presumably angiotensin receptor blockers should have the same benefit, given the different mechanism of action and side-effect profile compared to ACEIs, losartan efficacy is being evaluated with promising results.[34] A phase 3 randomized, placebo-controlled trial is being designed to determine the efficacy of losartan for individuals with SCN and micro- or macroalbuminuria.

For the same reason, inhibitors of the renin-angiotensin system are the treatment of choice for hypertensive SCD patients. It would be advisable to recommended to treat relative hypertension in SCN to a target pressure below normal (<130/80 mmHg). These drugs must be introduced cautiously for the risk on developing hypotension and potential hyperkalemia.

Long-term studies using randomized controlled design are warranted to prove the efficacy of these drugs in slowing the progression of CKD in SCD.

Specific SCD Therapies
Hydroxyurea

There is uncertainty if hydroxyurea (HU) reduces or prevents progression of kidney disease.[35] The BABY HUG multicenter study[17] was designed to ascertain whether HU therapy is safe in infants and whether it influences renal function. Although there was no impact on this primary endpoint, those children treated with HU improved the ability to concentrate urine compared with placebo-treated children.

Although there is not conclusive evidence that HU treatment prevents the progression of SCN to CKD directly, overall, HU should have a beneficial effect through reduction of frequency of vaso-occlusive crises that can precipitate acute kidney injury and can limit some of the early symptoms and signs of renal involvement and should be considered in all patients with SCN, unless indicated otherwise.

A recent Cochrane review[35] did not identify trials that looked at red cell transfusions nor any combination of interventions to prevent or reduce kidney complications.

Promising Therapies

New therapeutic targets are focused on the vasculopathic mechanism previously discussed.

Statins have been shown to improve vascular function independently of its lipid-lowering properties, suppressing the inflammatory response to endothelial damage and restoring nitric oxide bioavailability, representing a new way of preventing vaso-occlusion. Pilot studies on simvastatin have observed reductions in pain rate and markers of inflammation that were greatest in patients receiving HU, suggesting a synergistic effect of simvastatin.[36] These results provide preliminary clinical data to support larger trials of statins in SCD and SCN. An ongoing study is evaluating the effect of atorvastatin on endothelial dysfunction and albuminuria in SCD (Clinicaltrials.gov identifier: NCT01732718).

New antiadhesive therapies include rivipansel, crizanlizumab, and blocking P-selectins, which promote adhesion to vascular endothelium and other intercellular interactions that are overexpressed in the inflammatory response.[1,37]

Chronically reducing plasma adenosine levels could reduce renal vascular congestion. In this line, the effects of adenosine A2AR receptor agonist regadenoson are under evaluation.

Another therapeutic target are drugs avoiding the polymerization of HbS, such as the GBT440 molecule, which in vitro and in vivo has shown its potent anti-sickling effect by increasing hemoglobin oxygen affinity.

Antiplatelet agents such as prasugrel and ticagrelor are also worthy of research.[1]

Hemopoietic stem cell transplantation is the only curative therapy for SCD.

Human leukocyte antigen–compatible sibling transplants with bone marrow or cord blood as progenitor sources offer 90% event-free survival, unlike using peripheral blood hemopoietic progenitors, which is associated with increased mortality. The good results are tempered by the limited availability of donors and concern about their safety.[1] It is worth remembering than hemopoietic stem cell transplantation itself carries a significant risk of long-term renal disease, even in patients without other risk factors.[38,39]

CONCLUSION

SCD is an increasing chronic disease of significant economic and psychosocial burden. Kidney disease (SCN) is one of the most frequent and severe complications of SCD. An early diagnosis and treatment with HU with broader criteria of SCD patients and SCN screening with early referral to a specialist are needed to improve patient survival and quality of life.

REFERENCES

1. Ware RE, Montalembert M, Thisiolo L, Abboud MR. Sickle cell disease. *Lancet.* 2017; 90: 311–323
2. Piel FB, Hay SI, Gupta S, Weatherall DJ, Williams TN. Global burden of sickle cell anaemia in children under five, 2010–2050: modelling based on demographics, excess mortality, and interventions. *PLoS Med.* 2013; 10(7): e1001484.
3. Prabhakar H, Haywood C Jr, Molokie R. Sickle cell disease in the United States: looking back and forward at 100 years of progress in management and survival. *Am J Hematol.* 2010; 85(5):346–353.
4. Chakravorty S, Williams TN. Sickle cell disease: a neglected chronic disease of increasing global health importance. *Arch Dis Child.* 2015; 100(1):48–53.
5. Powars DR, Elliott-Mills DD, Chan L, et al. Chronic renal failure in sickle cell disease: risk factors, clinical course, and mortality. *Ann Intern Med.* 1991;115(8):614–620.
6. Powars DR, Chan LS, Hiti A, Ramicone E, Johnson C. Outcome of sickle cell anemia: a 4-decade observational study of 1056 patients. *Medicine (Baltimore).* 2005; 84(6):363–376.
7. Platt OS, Brambilla DJ, Rosse WF, et al. Mortality in sickle cell disease. Life expectancy and risk factors for early death. *N Engl J Med.* 1994; 330(23):1639–1644.
8. Gargiulo R, Pandya M, Seba A, Haddad RY, Lerma EV. Sickle cell nephropathy. *Dis Mon.* 2014;60(10):494–499.
9. Hebbel RP. Ischemia-reperfusion injury in sickle cell anemia: relationship to acute chest syndrome, endothelial dysfunction, arterial vasculopathy, and inflammatory pain. *Hematol Oncol Clin North Am* 2014; 28(2):181–198.
10. Nath KA, Katusic ZS. Vasculature and kidney complications in sickle cell disease. *J Am Soc Nephrol.* 2012; 23(5):781–784.
11. Azar S, Wong TE. Sickle cell disease: a brief update. *Med Clin North Am.* 2017; 101(2):375–393.
12. Piel FB, Steinberg MH, Rees DC. Sickle cell disease. *N Eng J Med.* 2017; 377(3):305.
13. Nath KA, Hebbel RP. Sickle cell disease: renal manifestations and mechanisms. *Nat Rev Nephrol.* 2015; 11(3):161–171.
14. Maurel S, Stankovic Stojanovic K, Avellino V, et al. Prevalence and correlates of metabolic acidosis among patients with homozygous sickle cell disease. *Clin J Am Soc Nephrol.* 2014; 9(4):648–653.
15. DeFronzo RA, Taufield PA, Black H, McPhedran P, Cooke CR. Impaired renal tubular potassium secretion in sickle cell disease. *Ann Intern Med.* 1979; 90(3):310–316.
16. Batlle D, Itsarayoungyuen K, Arruda JA, Kurtzman NA. Hyperkalemic hyperchloremic metabolic acidosis in sickle cell hemoglobinopathies. *Am J Med.* 1982; 72(2):188–192.
17. Alvarez O, Miller ST, Wang WC, et al.; BABY HUG Investigators. Effect of hydroxyurea treatment on renal function parameters: results from the multi-center placebo-controlled BABY HUG clinical trial for infants with sickle cell anemia. *Pediatr Blood Cancer.* 2012;59(4):668–674.
18. McPherson Yee M, Jabbar SF, Osunkwo I, et al. Chronic kidney disease and albuminuria in children with sickle cell disease. *Clin J Am Soc Nephrol.* 2011;6(11):2628–2633.
19. Day TG, Drasar ER, Fulford T, Sharpe CC, Thein SL. Association between hemolysis and albuminuria in adults with sickle cell anemia. *Haematologica.* 2012;97(2):201–205.
20. Drawz P, Ayyappan S, Nouraie M, et al. Kidney disease among patients with sickle cell disease, hemoglobin SS and SC. *Clin J Am Soc Nephrol.* 2016;11(2):207–215.
21. Maigne G, Ferlicot S, Galacteros F, et al. Glomerular lesions in patients with sickle cell disease. *Medicine.* 2010;89:18–27.
22. Ashley-Koch AE, Okocha EC, Garrett ME, et al. MYH9 and APOL1 are both associated with sickle cell disease nephropathy. *Br J Haematol.* 2011;155(3):386–394.
23. Lanzkron S, Haywood C. The five key things you need to know to manage adult patients with sickle cell disease. *Hematology.* 2015;2015:420–425.

24. Thompson J, Reid M, Hambleton I, Serjeant GR. Albuminuria and renal function in homozygous sickle cell disease: observations from a cohort study. *Arch Intern Med*. 2007;167(7):701–708.

25. Novelli EM, Hildesheim M, Rosano C, et al. Elevated pulse pressure is associated with hemolysis, proteinuria and chronic kidney disease in sickle cell disease. *PLoS One*. 2014;9(12):e114309.

26. Key NS, Connes P, Derebail VK. Negative health implications of sickle cell trait in high income countries: from the football field to the laboratory. *Br J Haematol*. 2015;170:5–14.

27. Tsaras G, Owusu-Ansah A, Boateng FO, Amoateng-Adjepong Y. Complications associated with sickle cell trait: a brief narrative review. *Am J Med*. 2009;122:507–512.

28. Yawn BP, Buchanan GR, Afenyi-Annan AN, et al: Management of sickle cell disease summary of the 2014 evidence-based report by expert panel members. *J Am Med Assoc*. 2014;312(10):1033–1048.

29. Yawn BP, John-Sowah J: Management of sickle cell disease: recommendations from the 2014 expert panel report. *Am Fam Physician*. 2015;92(12):1069–1076.

30. Alvarez O, Zilleruelo G, Wright D, Montane B, Lopez-Mitnik G. Serum cystatin C levels in children with sickle cell disease. *Pediatr Nephrol*. 2006;21(4):533–537.

31. Voskaridou E, Terpos E, Michail S, et al. Early markers of renal dysfunction in patients with sickle cell/beta-thalassemia. *Kidney Int*. 2006;69(11):2037–2042

32. Falk RJ, Scheinman J, Phillips G, Orringer E, Johnson A, Jennette JC. Prevalence and pathologic features of sickle cell nephropathy and response to inhibition of angiotensin-converting enzyme. *N Eng J Med*. 1992;326:910–915.

33. Sasongko TH, Nagalla S, Ballas SK. Angiotensin-converting enzyme (ACE) inhibitors for proteinuria and microalbuminuria in people with sickle cell disease. *Cochrane Db Sys Rev*. 2015;6:CD009191.

34. Quinn CT, Saraf SL, Gordeuk VR, et al. Losartan for the nephropathy of sickle cell anemia: A phase-2, multicenter trial. *Am J Hematol*. 2017;92(9):E520–E528.

35. Roy NB, Fortin PM, Bull KR, et al. Interventions for chronic kidney disease in people with sickle cell disease. *Cochrane Db Sys Rev*. 2017;7:CD012380.

36. Hoppe C, Jacob E, Styles L, Kuypers F, Larkin S, Vichinsky E. Simvastatin reduces vaso-occlusive pain in sickle cell anaemia: a pilot efficacy trial. *Br J Haematol*. 2017;177(4):620–629.

37. Field JJ. Can selectin and iNKT cell therapies meet the needs of people with sickle cell disease? *Hematology*. 2015;2015:426–432.

38. Singh N, McNeely J, Parikh S, Bhinder A, Rovin BH, Shidham G. Kidney complications of hematopoietic stem cell transplantation. *Am J Kidney Dis*. 2013;61(5):809–821.

39. Upadhyay K, Fine RN. Solid organ transplantation following end-organ failure in recipients of hematopoietic stem cell transplantation in children. *Pediatric Nephrol*. 2014;29(8):1337–1347.

37

Kidney Disease in HIV Infection and Treatment

CHRISTINA M. WYATT

INTRODUCTION

Based on estimates from the Joint United Nations Programme on HIV/AIDS (UNAIDS), nearly 37 million people worldwide were living with HIV infection or acquired immunodeficiency syndrome (AIDS) at the end of 2015, and approximately 2 million people become newly infected each year. HIV-positive individuals are at increased risk of kidney injury, including intrinsic kidney disease that has been linked to HIV infection itself, acute or chronic kidney injury secondary to antiretroviral therapy and concomitant medications, and accelerated progression of comorbid kidney disease.[1] This chapter will focus on common manifestations of kidney disease that nephrologists are likely to encounter in clinical practice and where there is potential to intervene and improve the clinical course of disease.

HIV-ASSOCIATED NEPHROPATHY

Epidemiology of HIV-Associated Nephropathy

Kidney disease was first recognized as a rare but clinically significant complication of HIV infection early in the AIDS epidemic, when physicians reported a unique form of collapsing focal segmental glomerulosclerosis in patients with AIDS. HIV-associated nephropathy (HIVAN) was first reported in individuals of African descent and has since been strongly associated with single nucleotide polymorphisms in the *APOL1* gene.[2] The incidence of classic HIVAN and related end-stage renal disease (ESRD) has declined substantially since the introduction of effective antiretroviral therapy, with most cases now occurring in antiretroviral-naive individuals or in the setting of treatment interruption or nonadherence.

Clinical Presentation of HIVAN

In individuals who are not taking antiretroviral therapy, HIVAN typically presents with heavy proteinuria and rapid deterioration of kidney function, although it is likely that many cases of early HIVAN go unrecognized. Kidney biopsy in patients with a fulminant clinical presentation typically demonstrates collapsing focal segmental glomerulosclerosis with proliferation of glomerular epithelial cells, tubular dilatation, and interstitial inflammation (Fig 37.1). The initiation of antiretroviral therapy with suppression of HIV viremia can improve the clinical course and histology, although relapse may occur if antiretroviral therapy is interrupted.

Pathogenesis of HIVAN

Consistent with the observed improvements in the clinical course and epidemiology of HIVAN with the introduction of antiretroviral therapy, the pathogenesis is directly linked to HIV infection. Viral sequences can be detected in both tubular and glomerular epithelial cells in human kidney biopsies, and reciprocal transplantation of kidneys between wild type and HIV-transgenic mice confirmed that HIV gene expression in the kidney is required for the development of HIVAN. More recent studies have focused on the mechanisms of infection and the potential for kidney to serve as a reservoir for HIV infection.[3]

IMMUNE COMPLEX KIDNEY DISEASE IN THE SETTING OF HIV INFECTION

In addition to HIVAN, investigators have hypothesized a link between HIV infection or HIV-related immune dysregulation and a variety of immune complex kidney diseases. The term "HIV immune complex kidney disease," or HIVICK, has been used in the past to

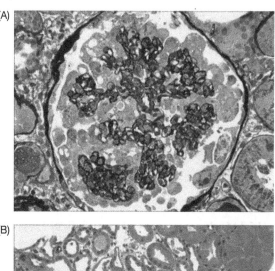

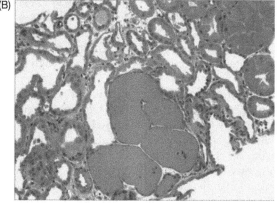

FIGURE 37.1 Pathology of HIV-associated nephropathy. Kidney biopsy in individuals with HIV-associated nephropathy demonstrates collapsing focal segmental glomerulosclerosis with proliferation of glomerular epithelial cells and accompanying tubulointerstitial lesions. (A) The glomerular capillary lumina are obliterated globally by collapse of glomerular basement membranes with hypertrophy and hyperplasia of overlying glomerular epithelial cells (Jones methenamine silver, 400×). (B) There are focally distended tubules forming microcysts that contain proteinaceous casts. Adjacent cortical tubules display degenerative changes (hematoxylin and eosin, 200×). Reproduced with permission from Wyatt CM, Klotman PE, D'Agati VDD. HIV-associated nephropathy: clinical presentation, pathology, and epidemiology in the era of antiretroviral therapy. *Semin Nephrol.* 2008;28:513–522.

describe this spectrum of disease. In several well-characterized cases, identification of HIV antigens suggests a causal relationship between HIV infection and immune complex kidney disease,[4] but overall the relationship has been difficult to investigate because of the heterogeneity of pathology and lack of an animal model. The role of antiretroviral therapy in the treatment of HIVICK is also unclear,[5] although this distinction has become less important with current guidelines recommending the initiation of antiretroviral therapy in all HIV-positive individuals.

Individuals with viral hepatitis co-infection may also be at risk for membranous nephropathy or membranoproliferative glomerulonephritis related to hepatitis B virus or hepatitis C virus (HCV) infection, respectively. Of note, the treatment of HCV with direct acting antivirals may be associated with nephrotoxicity secondary to drug–drug interactions, as discussed in the next section.

ANTIRETROVIRAL NEPHROTOXICITY

Current guidelines recommend the immediate initiation of antiretroviral therapy in all HIV-positive individuals, regardless of CD4 cell count. At the end of 2015, UNAIDS estimated that approximately 18 million people worldwide were receiving antiretroviral therapy for the treatment of HIV infection. Although early initiation of antiretroviral therapy is associated with a clear

TABLE 37.1 ANTIRETROVIRAL AGENTS WITH EFFECTS ON KIDNEY FUNCTION OR GFR ESTIMATES

Antiretroviral Agent	Relevant Effect	Risk Factors
Tenofovir disoproxil fumarate (Nucleotide reverse transcriptase inhibitor)	Proximal tubulopathy Acute kidney injury Chronic kidney disease[a]	High plasma tenofovir concentration; low body weight; decreased kidney function; drug-drug interactions; concomitant nephrotoxins
Indinavir (Protease inhibitor)	Nephrolithiasis/ urolithiasis Obstructive nephropathy Interstitial nephritis Chronic kidney disease[a]	Volume depletion; history of nephrolithiasis
Atazanavir (Protease inhibitor)	Nephrolithiasis/ urolithiasis Chronic kidney disease[a]	Volume depletion; history of nephrolithiasis
Other protease inhibitors	Rare cases of nephrolithiasis	Volume depletion; history of nephrolithiasis
Dolutegravir (Integrase inhibitor)	Inhibits tubular creatine secretion	Greater increase in creatinine may occur with low eGFR
Cobicistat (Pharmacoenhancer)	Inhibits tubular creatine secretion	Greater increase in creatinine may occur with low eGFR
Ritonavir (Pharmacoenhancer)	Inhibits tubular creatine secretion	Greater increase in creatinine may occur with low eGFR
Rilpivirine (Nonnucleoside reverse transcriptase inhibitor)	Inhibits tubular creatine secretion	Greater increase in creatinine may occur with low eGFR

[a]Tenofovir disoproxil fumarate, indinavir, and atazanavir have been associated with decreased eGFR in multiple cohort studies.
GFR = glomerular filtration rate.

mortality benefit, several commonly used antiretroviral agents have been linked to acute or chronic kidney injury (Table 37.1).

Tenofovir

The commonly used nucleotide reverse transcriptase inhibitor tenofovir is currently available as either of 2 prodrugs, tenofovir disoproxil fumarate (TDF) and tenofovir alafenamide (TAF). TDF was first approved and marketed for the treatment of HIV and hepatitis B virus infections and was more recently approved as a component of pre-exposure prophylaxis in individuals at high risk for HIV acquisition. Although no significant kidney toxicity was observed in premarketing clinical trials, TDF has been linked to rare cases of overt proximal tubular injury and has been more commonly associated with mild proximal tubular dysfunction and with declines in bone mineral density. Cumulative use of TDF for HIV treatment or prevention has also been associated with declines in creatinine clearance (CrCl) or estimated glomerular filtration rate (eGFR).[6–10] Expert guidelines recommend consideration of alternative antiretroviral therapy in individuals with eGFR <60 mL/min/1.73m^2,[11] and observational data suggest that TDF is often discontinued in clinical practice when the eGFR declines to <70 mL/min/1.73m^2.[12]

The kidney and bone toxicity of TDF have been correlated with higher plasma concentrations of tenofovir and with factors that increase plasma concentration, such as lower baseline kidney function, lower body weight, and drug–drug interactions.[13] The most common drug–drug interactions involve the boosted protease inhibitors, several of which have been shown to increase the absorption of TDF. More recently, the direct acting antiviral agent ledipasvir, which is approved in combination with sofosbuvir for the treatment of HCV infection, has been shown to increase tenofovir plasma concentrations in individuals taking TDF. Because this effect may be magnified by concomitant use of a boosted protease inhibitor or the pharmacoenhancer cobicistat, the prescribing information recommends consideration of alternative antiretroviral therapy in individuals planning to initiate treatment with ledipasvir or sofosbuvir.

The alternative prodrug TAF was approved in late 2016 based on evidence of noninferiority for viral suppression and the potential for improved safety. TAF has a longer plasma half-life as the prodrug, resulting in lower plasma concentrations of tenofovir, which is anticipated to translate into lower risk of kidney and bone toxicity. Premarketing clinical trials of TAF demonstrated improvements in biomarkers of proximal tubular function compared to TDF, but the studies were not designed to demonstrate an improvement in hard clinical outcomes. TAF is approved for use in individuals with CrCl >30 mL/min, but tenofovir concentrations and the related risk of nephrotoxicity are likely to be higher as this dosing threshold is approached.[14]

Protease Inhibitors

The older protease inhibitor indinavir has been strongly linked to nephrolithiasis, obstruction, and interstitial nephritis and is now rarely used in high-income countries. Other protease inhibitors have also been implicated in rare cases of nephrolithiasis, secondary to poor solubility of these drugs at urine pH, and the prescribing information for atazanavir includes a warning about reported cases of nephrolithiasis.

Protease inhibitors, in particular, indinavir and atazanavir, have also been associated with declines in CrCl and/or eGFR.[7,8] Some of the ritonavir-boosted protease inhibitors are known to increase tenofovir concentrations, but the association with decreased kidney function appears to be independent of TDF use. As addressed in the following discussion, there is also some impact of the pharmacoenhancer ritonavir on tubular secretion of creatinine, making it difficult to determine the true risk of nephrotoxicity with the boosted protease inhibitors.

Interference with Creatinine-Based GFR Estimates

In addition to the potential for kidney injury, several antiretroviral agents have been shown to inhibit tubular creatinine secretion, causing an increase in serum creatinine and a decline in estimated, but not true, GFR.[15] The agents with the strongest clinical effect appear to be the novel pharmacoenhancer cobicistat and the integrase inhibitor dolutegravir, but ritonavir and rilpivirine also appear to interfere with creatinine secretion. Some experts recommend the use of an alternative marker of GFR, such as cystatin C, in this setting. Elevated levels of cystatin C should be interpreted with caution, because cystatin C also reflects systemic inflammation and may provide a biased estimate of kidney function in HIV-positive individuals.[16,17] Nonetheless, a normal cystatin C result or a stable result before and after the initiation of a new antiretroviral regimen therapy can be reassuring in some cases.

COMORBID CKD IN HIV-POSITIVE INDIVIDUALS

In addition to kidney disease related to HIV infection or its treatment, HIV-positive individuals are also at risk for comorbid kidney disease. With improved survival and aging of the HIV population, traditional CKD risk factors such as diabetes and hypertension are increasingly prevalent. Studies in humans and in animal models have suggested an additive effect of HIV infection and diabetes on the development and progression of CKD.[18,19] In the animal model, the additive effect of HIV appears to be related to upregulation of inflammatory pathways that lead to downstream kidney injury,[19] suggesting a potential mechanism for the increased risk of CKD that is observed even in individuals with early HIV infection and no exposure to antiretroviral therapy.[20]

ACUTE KIDNEY INJURY IN HIV-POSITIVE INDIVIDUALS

The risk of acute kidney injury (AKI) is also higher in HIV-positive individuals. Older studies suggested that sepsis and medication toxicity were the leading causes of AKI in the years immediately following the introduction of effective antiretroviral therapy, and more recent data suggest that sepsis remains an important cause of AKI in hospitalized patients with HIV.[21] As in the general population, AKI is strongly associated with increased morbidity and mortality in HIV-positive individuals.[21,22]

CONSIDERATIONS IN ADVANCED CKD AND ESRD

HIV-positive individuals with progressive CKD should be educated about ESRD and prepared for renal replacement therapy according to clinical practice guidelines for the general population. Additional guidance is available in expert guidelines developed for the diagnosis and management of CKD in HIV-positive individuals.[11] The limited available evidence suggests that both hemodialysis and peritoneal dialysis should be considered in HIV-positive individuals, with the decision based on personal preference and other medical considerations. As in the general population, early planning is important to avoid the risks associated with central venous catheters.

CONSIDERATIONS IN KIDNEY TRANSPLANTATION

HIV-positive individuals with ESRD may also be candidates for kidney transplantation. Observational studies have demonstrated the safety of solid organ transplantation in individuals with well-controlled HIV infection, although there does appear to be an increased risk of acute allograft rejection.[23] Significant drug–drug interactions can complicate the care of HIV-positive transplant recipients; in particular, "boosted" protease inhibitors increase calcineurin inhibitor levels, often requiring a dramatic decrease in the dose and dosing frequency of the calcineurin inhibitor to achieve target trough levels.[23] This interaction is observed with both ritonavir and cobicistat, although it has not been as well studied with the latter. Many experts would recommend avoiding protease inhibitors in potential transplant recipients when possible.[11]

Based on promising results from South Africa,[24] several centers across the United States began an observational study of transplantation from HIV-positive donors to HIV-positive recipients in 2016. This study will evaluate the safety of using HIV-positive donors to expand the donor pool and decrease waiting times for HIV-positive transplant candidates.

CONCLUSION

HIV-positive individuals are at increased risk of AKI and CKD as a result of HIV-related kidney disease, medication toxicity, and accelerated progression of comorbid kidney disease. Because of the broad spectrum of disease that can occur in individuals with HIV infection, kidney biopsy should be considered in all HIV-positive individuals who present with newly diagnosed kidney disease. While the management of kidney disease in this population largely mirrors that

in the general population, nephrologists should be aware of unique drug–drug interactions and drug effects on creatinine-based GFR estimates.

REFERENCES

1. Mallipattu S, Salem F, Wyatt C. The changing epidemiology of HIV-related chronic kidney disease in the era of antiretroviral therapy. *Kidney Int.* 2014;86:259–265.
2. Kopp JB, Nelson GW, Sampath K, et al. APOL1 genetic variants in focal segmental glomerulosclerosis and HIV-associated nephropathy. *J Am Soc Nephrol.* 2011;22:2129–2137.
3. Blasi M, Balakumaran B, Chen P, et al. Renal epithelial cells produce and spread HIV-1 via T-cell contact. *AIDS.* 2014;28:2345–2353.
4. Kimmel PL, Phillips TM, Ferreira-Centeno A, Farkas-Szallasi T, Abraham AA, Garrett CT. HIV-associated immune-mediated renal disease. *Kidney Int.* 1993;44:1327–1340.
5. Foy MC, Estrella MM, Lucas GM, et al. Comparison of risk factors and outcomes in HIV immune complex kidney disease and HIV-associated nephropathy. *Clin J Am Soc Nephrol.* 2013;8:1524–1532.
6. Cooper RD, Wiebe N, Smith N, Keiser P, Naicker S, Tonelli M. Systematic review and meta-analysis: renal safety of tenofovir disoproxil fumarate in HIV-infected patients. *Clin Infect Dis.* 2010;51:496–505.
7. Mocroft A, Kirk O, Reiss P, et al. Estimated glomerular filtration rate, chronic kidney disease and antiretroviral drug use in HIV-positive patients. *AIDS.* 2010;24:1667–1678.
8. Mocroft A, Lundgren JD, Ross M, et al. Cumulative and current exposure to potentially nephrotoxic antiretrovirals and development of chronic kidney disease in HIV-positive individuals with a normal baseline estimated glomerular filtration rate: a prospective international cohort study. *Lancet HIV.* 2016;3:e23–e32.
9. Mugwanya KK, Wyatt C, Celum C, et al. Changes in glomerular kidney function among HIV-1-uninfected men and women receiving emtricitabine-tenofovir disoproxil fumarate pre-exposure prophylaxis: a randomized clinical trial. *JAMA Intern Med.* 2015;175:246–254.
10. Solomon MM, Lama JR, Glidden DV, et al. Changes in renal function associated with oral emtricitabine/tenofovir disoproxil fumarate use for HIV pre-exposure prophylaxis. *AIDS.* 2014;28:851–859.
11. Lucas GM, Ross MJ, Stock PG, et al. Clinical practice guideline for the management of chronic kidney disease in patients infected with HIV: 2014 update by the HIV Medicine Association of the

Infectious Diseases Society of America. *Clin Infect Dis*. 2014;59:e96–e138.

12. Ryom L, Mocroft A, Kirk O, et al. Predictors of advanced chronic kidney disease and end-stage renal disease in HIV-positive persons. *AIDS*. 2014;28:187–199.

13. Gupta SK, Anderson AM, Ebrahimi R et al. Fanconi syndrome accompanied by renal function decline with tenofovir disoproxil fumarate: a prospective, case-control study of predictors and resolution in HIV-infected patients. *PLoS One*. 2014;9:e92717.

14. Wyatt C. Will a new tenofovir prodrug for the treatment of HIV reduce the risk of nephrotoxicity? *Kidney Int*. 2016;89:5–6.

15. Lepist EI, Zhang X, Hao J, et al. Contribution of the organic anion transporter OAT2 to the renal active tubular secretion of creatinine and mechanism for serum creatinine elevations caused by cobicistat. *Kidney Int*. 2014;86:350–357.

16. Inker LA, Wyatt C, Creamer R, et al. Performance of creatinine and cystatin C GFR estimating equations in an HIV-positive population on antiretrovirals. *J Acquir Immune Defic Syndr*. 2012;61:302–309.

17. Gagneux-Brunon A, Delanaye P, Maillard N, et al. Performance of creatinine and cystatin C-based glomerular filtration rate estimating equations in a European HIV-positive cohort. *AIDS*. 2013;27(10):1573–1581.

18. R M, Parikh C, Gordon K, et al. Comorbid diabetes and the risk of progressive chronic kidney disease in HIV-infected adults. *J Acquir Immune Defic Syndr*. 2012;60(4):393–399.

19. Mallipattu SK, Liu R, Zhong Y, et al. Expression of HIV transgene aggravates kidney injury in diabetic mice. *Kidney Int*. 2013;83:626–634.

20. Achhra A, Mocroft A, Ross M, et al. Kidney disease in antiretroviral-naive HIV-positive adults with high CD4 counts: prevalence and predictors of kidney disease at enrolment in the INSIGHT Strategic Timing of AntiRetroviral Treatment (START) trial. *HIV Med*. 2015;16(Suppl 1):55–63.

21. Nadkarni GN, Patel AA, Yacoub R, et al. The burden of dialysis-requiring acute kidney injury among hospitalized adults with HIV infection: a nationwide inpatient sample analysis. *AIDS*. 2015;29:1061–1066.

22. Choi AI, Li Y, Parikh C, Volberding PA, Shlipak MG. Long-term clinical consequences of acute kidney injury in the HIV-infected. *Kidney Int*. 2010;78:478–485.

23. Stock PG, Barin B, Murphy B, et al. Outcomes of kidney transplantation in HIV-infected recipients. *N Engl J Med*. 2010;363:2004–2014.

24. Muller E, Barday Z, Mendelson M, Kahn D. HIV-positive-to-positive kidney transplantation--results at 3 to 5 years. *N Engl J Med*. 2015;372:613–620.

38

Cystic Kidney Diseases

FOUAD T. CHEBIB AND VICENTE E. TORRES

INTRODUCTION

Autosomal dominant polycystic kidney disease (ADPKD) is the most common monogenic kidney disease. It is characterized by relentless development of kidney cysts, hypertension, and eventually end-stage renal disease (ESRD). It is responsible for 5% to 10% of cases of ESRD globally; making it the fourth leading cause for kidney failure.[1-3] ADPKD affects 1 in 400 to 1,000 live births, or 12.5 million people worldwide. It affects both sexes equally and occurs in all ethnicities. ADPKD is a Mendelian autosomal dominant disorder. It is genetically heterogeneous, with 2 major causative genes identified: *PKD1*, which encodes polycystin 1 (PC-1) and accounts for 85%[4]; *PKD2*, which encodes polycystin 2 (PC-2) and accounts for ~15% of resolved cases.[5] More recently, mutations in *GANAB*, encoding the glucosidase IIα subunit were found to cause mild cases of ADPKD.[6]

ADPKD has strikingly high phenotypic variability.[7,8] Mutations in *PKD2* versus *PKD1* lead to much milder disease, with average ages at ESRD of 58.1 and 79.7 years for *PKD1* and *PDK2*, respectively.[9] Cysts start forming in utero and originate from the epithelia of only 1% to 5% of nephrons. Typically, the enlargement of the bilateral kidney cysts is gradual throughout the lifetime of the patient until little renal parenchyma is recognizable. At that stage, the average rate of GFR decline is 4.4 to 5.9 mL/min per year.[10] Eventually, ESRD ensues after the fourth decade of life. Over the past few years, several advancements in the genetic and radiologic diagnosis have been made. Total kidney volume (TKV) has been recognized as a biomarker for monitoring disease progression. An imaging classification of ADPKD has been developed as a tool to predict the progression of renal decline in ADPKD patients. The natural course of ADPKD makes it an ideal disease

to be targeted for renal protection. This chapter will discuss various aspects of pathophysiology, molecular pathways and targets, and pharmaceutical and nonpharmaceutical interventions in the journey of prevention of clinical complications of ADPKD.

PATHOGENESIS OF ADPKD

Despite the large advancement in understanding ADPKD pathogenesis and the discovery of *PKD1* and *PKD2* genes over 2 decades ago, the function of the polycystins (particularly PC-1) remain poorly understood. The polycystins constitute a subfamily of protein channels and are thought to regulate intracellular calcium signaling. PC-1 is localized to the primary cilium and structures involved in cell–cell contacts such as tight junctions. PC-1 likely functions as a receptor and/or adhesion molecule, whereas PC-2, a calcium-permeable nonselective cation channel, is found on the primary cilium, endoplasmic reticulum, and possibly the plasma membrane. These polycystins interact to form the PC complex, which localizes to the primary cilia and plays a role in intracellular calcium regulation.[11,12] Mutations in *PKD1* or *PKD2* lead to a reduction in intracellular calcium, an increase in cyclic adenosine monophosphate (cAMP), activation of protein kinase A, and an increase in sensitivity of collecting duct principal cells to the constant tonic effect of vasopressin.[12] The reduction in intracellular calcium determines a striking switch in the cellular response to cAMP from suppression to stimulation of proliferation. The enhanced cAMP signaling activates downstream signaling pathways responsible for impaired tubulogenesis, cell proliferation, increased fluid secretion, and interstitial inflammation. Abnormal epithelial chloride secretion occurs through the cAMP-dependent transporter encoded by the *CFTR* gene and plays an important role in generating and maintaining fluid-filled cysts in ADPKD. Other pathogenic pathways may include activation of mammalian target of rapamycin (mTOR) signaling, direct effects of PC-1 fragments on gene transcription, and increased aerobic glycolysis. Increased vasopressin concentrations have been associated with disease severity and progression in ADPKD. Blocking vasopressin effects on the kidney via the vasopressin V2 receptor has shown to inhibit disease progression in experimental studies as well large randomized clinical trials, which are addressed in the following discussion.

DIAGNOSIS

The diagnosis of ADPKD relies primarily on imaging although some cases require genetic testing. Typical imaging findings from patients with ADPKD reveal large kidneys with multiple bilateral cysts. Age-dependent diagnostic criteria have been established for patients with positive family history. The presence of a total of 3 or more kidney cysts for at-risk individuals aged 15 to 39 years and 2 or more cysts in each kidney for at-risk individuals aged 40 to 59 years are sufficient for a diagnosis of ADPKD.[13] If ultrasonography results are equivocal, magnetic resonance imaging (MRI) or computed tomography (CT) may clarify the diagnosis. Excluding the disease in at-risk individuals also depends on their age, which, in turn, dictates the imaging modality. For individuals >40 years, the absence of kidney cysts on ultrasound excludes ADPKD; in younger individuals (<40 years), MRI is superior to ultrasonography for excluding ADPKD. In the absence of a family history, these imaging based criteria do not apply. In such situations, multiple factors should be considered, including the age of the patient, the presence of associated manifestations (e.g., liver cysts), and findings or family history suggestive of other genetic disorders. ADPKD is the most likely diagnosis in the presence of bilaterally enlarged kidneys and innumerable (>10) cysts in each kidney. Of note, other genetic diseases (e.g., tuberous sclerosis, von Hippel-Lindau disease, and autosomal dominant tubulointerstitial kidney disease) can be associated with kidney cysts. When suggestive findings are noted, the differential diagnosis should be broadened. A practical algorithm for diagnostic evaluation of patients ≥18 years with kidney cysts is shown in Figure 38.1.

CLINICAL MANIFESTATIONS

ADPKD is a systemic disease. The renal manifestations include early onset hypertension, flank pain, hematuria, proteinuria, and decreased glomerular filtration rate. Most patients with ADPKD reach ESRD, although its onset varies between individuals even in the same family. Mean age of ESRD onset is 58.1 years for *PKD1*-associated ADPKD and 79.7 years for *PKD2*-associated ADPKD. Several extrarenal manifestations are associated with ADPKD including hepatic cysts, intracranial aneurysms, mitral valve prolapse, dilated and hypertrophic cardiomyopathies, diverticulosis, and bronchiectasis.

MARKERS FOR DISEASE PROGRESSION AND CLASSIFICATION

ADPKD is characterized by the gradual formation and enlargement of bilateral kidney cysts during the lifetime of the patient. Typically, renal function remains within normal range until destruction of normal renal parenchyma by enlarging cysts. The decline in GFR occurs at later stages at an average rate of 4.4 to 5.9 mL/min per year. This makes GFR a poor marker for monitoring disease progression in early to mid-stages of the disease. TKV has been established as a better tool for monitoring and prognosticating in early stages of ADPKD. TKV, measured by CT or MRI, increases exponentially in all patients with ADPKD but at variable rates (5%–6% per year on average).[10] A classification of ADPKD has been developed based on age- and height-adjusted TKV. This classification stratifies patients into different classes (class 1A–1E), which translate into varying rates of decline in GFR.[14] This tool is useful in identifying individuals who are at higher risk for disease progression and for estimating the age at which the patient will reach ESRD. For instance, comparing subclass 1E to 1A, the frequency of reaching ESRD within 10 years is substantially greater (66.9% vs. 2.4%). Knowing the patient's classification would be helpful in clinical practice for counseling and treatment planning. Class 1C to 1E would benefit from aggressive nephroprotection strategies.

CONVENTIONAL STRATEGIES FOR NEPHROPROTECTION

Until recently, there was little to offer to families with ADPKD except implementing a healthy lifestyle for all family members, early detection

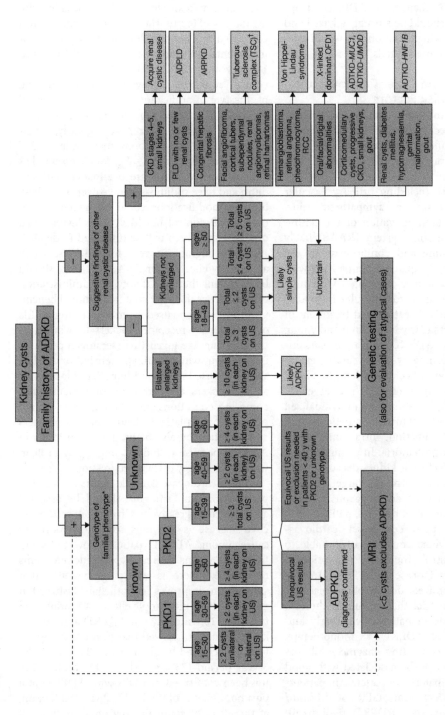

FIGURE 38.1 Practical algorithm for diagnostic evaluation of patients 18 years or older with kidney cysts. At least 1 affected member with ESRD ≤50 years old strongly suggests *PKD1* mutation; at least 1 affected family member without ESRD ≥70 years old suggests *PKD2* mutation. Polycystic kidneys with multiple angiomyolipomas (contiguous PKD1–TSC2 syndrome). ADPLD = autosomal dominant polycystic kidney disease. ADPLD = autosomal dominant polycystic liver disease. ADTKD-MUC1 = autosomal dominant tubulointerstitial kidney disease–tumor-associated mucin (previously known as medullary cystic kidney disease type 1). ADTKDUMOD = autosomal dominant tubulointerstitial kidney disease–uromodulin (previously known as medullary cystic kidney disease type 2). ARPKD = autosomal recessive polycystic kidney disease. CKD = chronic kidney disease. ESRD = end-stage renal disease. MRI = magnetic resonance imaging. OFD1 = oral–facial–digital syndrome type 1. PKD1 = polycystic kidney disease 1. PKD2 = polycystic kidney disease 2. RCC = renal cell carcinoma. US = ultrasound.

and strict control of hypertension, and assessment for cardiovascular risk factors including hyperlipidemia and aggressive treatment. Other interventions include dietary changes based on pathophysiological changes in ADPKD. If applicable, patients should be strongly advised and counseled for smoking cessation. We will discuss few of these strategies in details.

Hypertension and Other Cardiovascular Risk Factors

Hypertension is the most common manifestation of ADPKD occurring in 50% to 70% of cases prior to any significant decline in kidney function, with an average onset of 30 years. Several factors contribute to blood pressure (BP) elevation in ADPKD, including primary vascular dysfunction, increase in sympathetic tone, and, more important, activation of the renin–angiotensin–aldosterone system (RAAS) likely caused by stretching and compression of the vascular tree by cyst expansion. In patients with ADPKD, hypertension is associated with progression to ESRD and cardiovascular morbidity and mortality. Early detection and treatment of hypertension, particularly in children and young adults, is indicated. ADPKD from age 5 years onward, with rescreening every 3 years when no hypertension is found, seems prudent. In adults, home BP monitoring is advised. The target BP is ≤140/90 mmHg but should be individualized and lowered to ≤130/80 mmHg in patients with left ventricular dysfunction, intracranial aneurysm, diabetes, or proteinuria. In young patients with ADPKD with chronic kidney disease (CKD) stages 1 to 2, tight BP control (BP target, 95–110/60–75 mmHg) may be advantageous. Studies have shown that in recent decades, patients with ADPKD have experienced lower cardiovascular mortality, which could be attributable to improved BP control. The Halt Progression of Polycystic Kidney Disease (HALT-PKD) study is a recent randomized, double-blind, placebo-controlled clinical trial that examined the role of RAAS blockade in patients with early and advanced stages of ADPKD.[15,16] Monotherapy with angiotensin converting enzyme inhibitors (ACEIs) was found to be associated with good BP control in the majority of patients. In patients with early (aged 15–49 years; GFR >60 mL/min/1.73 m^2) versus later stage ADPKD, rigorous BP control (BP target range, 95–110/60–75 mmHg) was associated with a slower increase in TKV; more rapid decline in estimated GFR (eGFR)

during the first 4 months of treatment, with a slower decline thereafter (an overall eGFR effect was absent); a smaller increase in renal vascular resistance; and a greater decline in left ventricular mass index. Dual RAAS blockade with lisinopril and telmisartan had no beneficial effect compared to lisinopril alone in these patients or in patients with more advanced ADPKD (aged 18–64 years; GFR 25–60 mL/min/1.73 m^2). BP control could be achieved by a combination of lifestyle modifications and pharmaceutical therapies. It is important to encourage patients and their families to exercise regularly, maintain a healthy weight (body mass index, 2,025 Kg/m^2). Salt restriction (≤2 g/day) is essential as patients with ADPKD are overloaded with sodium and have sodium-sensitive overload. These lifestyle modifications could be beneficial not only in BP control but likely in delaying renal cyst growth (which will be discussed in details). ACEIs or angiotensin receptor blockers, which are equally effective for RAAS blockade, should be a first-line therapy. Of note, co-administration of these drugs does not confer additional benefit. Caution should be used when prescribing ACEIs or angiotensin receptor blockers to women of childbearing age given their teratogenic risk. It is not clear which antihypertensive drug class should be used as second line. Beta blockers or alpha blockers are preferred for patients with comorbid conditions such as angina or benign prostatic hyperplasia. Calcium channel blockers and diuretics can also be used, but cautiously in ADPKD, because such drugs might play a role in worsening kidney disease progression.

Other cardiovascular risk factors such as hyperlipidemia and smoking should be assessed and treated aggressively. Given that cardiovascular disease is the most common mortality cause among ADPKD patients, low threshold to initiate statins to treat hyperlipidemia seems reasonable. There is emerging evidence that simvastatin improves endothelial dysfunction and could have pleiotropic effects. A randomized trial[17] in 110 children with ADPKD and normal kidney function showed that pravastatin significantly decreased height-adjusted TKV over the 3-year period (23% vs. 31%). This finding has not been confirmed in adults with ADPKD in a post hoc analysis of the HALT-PKD trial looking at the effect of statin therapy on slowing renal cyst growth.[18] Larger randomized trial in young people with ADPKD is still necessary for a more definitive answer.

LIFESTYLE MODIFICATIONS

As previously mentioned, adapting general healthy lifestyle of exercise and normal body weight is beneficial for all the family members with ADPKD to ensure good cardiovascular health. Additional modifications should be implemented given the potential to reduce the renal cyst growth progression. The preclinical and clinical studies assessing lifestyle modifications in ADPKD are summarized in Table 38.1.

Water Intake

Hydration is very essential in ADPKD patients. One of the earliest manifestations in ADPKD is a urinary concentration defect. Vasopressin has a pivotal role in the pathophysiology of the disease progression in ADPKD. Lowering circulating vasopressin concentration by changing lifestyle and diet could be very beneficial. Vasopressin is increased in patients with polycystic kidney disease (PKD), and the concentration of its surrogate copeptin is associated with disease severity when analyzed cross-sectionally,[19] as well as disease progression measured longitudinally as kidney function decline and kidney growth.[20,21] It has been shown that vasopressin directly regulates cyst growth in rats orthologous to human autosomal recessive PKD (ARPKD), which phenotypically resembles human ADPKD. After breeding these rats with vasopressin-deficient Brattleboro rats, it was shown that rats lacking vasopressin had lower levels of cAMP and that cystogenesis was inhibited almost completely. Administration of the vasopressin V2 receptor agonist DDAVP* recovered the full cystic phenotype in these Brattleboro rats.[22]

Lowering the vasopressin effect on the kidney could potentially modify the disease course in ADPKD. This either could be accomplished by blocking the effects of vasopressin in the kidney using a vasopressin V2 receptor–specific antagonist like tolvaptan or could be accomplished by lowering the circulating vasopressin concentration using lifestyle changes such as increased water intake. To suppress efficiently vasopressin, it is essential to drink water throughout the day with short time intervals rather than drinking the same amount of water in prolonged intervals. In a small pilot randomized study, patients with ADPKD who combined low-osmolar diet (low sodium of 1,500 mg/day and low protein of 0.8g/kg body weight) with adjusted water intake has led to a significant reduction in vasopressin secretion and reduction in water required for

vasopressin reduction (from 3.2 to 2.6 L/day).[23] The water prescription was calculated in liters as total solute (mOsm) divided by 280 (mOsm/Kg water) where total solute was equal to 24-hour urine volume (L) × urine osmolality (mOsm/Kg water) with an additional 500 mL of water was added to account for insensible loss. Other small pilot studies have shown similar effect of increasing water intake (average of 3.1 L/day) for 7 days, which led to decline in urine osmolality by 46% to 270 mOsm/L.[24] Another group has performed a study in 34 patients with ADPKD who received either a high or free water intake during 1 year, leading to mean 24-hour urine volumes of 2.6 versus 1.4 liter per day ($p < 0.001$). Plasma arginine vasopressin (AVP) and copeptin were, as expected, lower in the high water intake group (both p = 0.02). However, nonsignificant trends toward faster eGFR decline (–5.6 vs. –1.1 mL/min/1.73 m^2, $p = 0.06$) and TKV growth (9.68%/year vs. 5.28/year, $p = 0.08$), rather than a beneficial effect, were observed in the high compared to the free water intake.[25] Finding no beneficial effects of an increased water intake in this study might have been due to shortcomings of the study design. First, the study had only 34 participants, potentially leading to an underpowered statistical analysis. Second, for assessment of the primary endpoint, historical data were used. Third, participants were not randomized but could enroll in the group they preferred, potentially leading to a selection bias, as is reflected by a significantly higher 24-hour urine volume in the high water intake group at baseline. Finally, the high water intake group was instructed to drink ~50 mL water/kg body weight/day (2.5–3.0 L of water/day) or more, mostly during the first half of the day, which might not be enough to change the disease course and show a beneficial effect.

In another qualitative study, 14 ADPKD patients were assigned dietary intervention for 4 weeks (lower dietary sodium, protein, acid precursors, and supplement with water). Patients had little difficulty with fluid intake and eating less meat and more fruits but had some difficulty reaching the goal amount of fruits and vegetables and tracking the diet daily.[26,27] Raising awareness for both patients and treating clinicians about dietary changes and its potential benefits is important. In a small study interviewing polycystic kidney disease (PKD) patients, not all physicians focused on lifestyle-based treatments, but the majority of PKD patients were motivated and willing to incorporate BP control, exercise,

TABLE 38.1 STUDIES THAT SUGGEST AN ASSOCIATION BETWEEN LIFESTYLE FACTORS AND POLYCYSTIC KIDNEY DISEASE PROGRESSION

Study	Model	Lifestyle	Outcome Measure(s)	Study Type	Main Findings
Nagao et al.[a]	Rats orthologous to human ARPKD	Water intake	Urinary AVP excretion, AVP V2 receptor expression, kidney-to-body weight (%), SUN	Interventional animal study	Urinary AVP excretion decreased 68.3%, AVP V2 receptor expression normalized under high water intake, kidney-to-body-weight decreased 29.8% and 27.0% in male and female rats, respectively, and SUN decreased from 38.7 to 26.3 mg/dL in the male rats.
Hopp et al.[b]	Rats orthologous to human ARPKD and Pkd1[RC]-mice	Water intake	Urine output, plasma AVP, renal cAMP, kidney weight, cyst and fibrosis, plasma urea and creatinine	Interventional animal study	Urine output was increased by 4-fold, and all studied parameters were lower in rats on a high water intake. Despite a more than 7-fold increased urine output in PKD1 mice, no significant differences on any of the markers were observed.
Barash et al.[c]	ADPKD patients	Water intake	24-hour urine volume, urine osmolality	Interventional study	24-hour urine volume increased 64% (to 3.1 L), urine osmolality decreased 46% (to 270±21 mOsm/L).
Higashihara et al.[d]	ADPKD patients	Water intake	Plasma AVP and copeptin, eGFR decline, TKV growth	Interventional study	Plasma AVP and copeptin lower in HW versus LW intake (both $p = 0.02$), whereas no effect on eGFR decline (mL/min/1.73m²), being –5.6 HW vs. –1.1 LW ($p = 0.06$) or TKV growth (9.68 HW vs. 5.28 LW; $p = 0.08$) were observed.
Torres et al.[e]	ADPKD patients	Sodium and protein intake, HDL cholesterol, BSA, BMI	TKV slope and eGFR decline	Multicenter study, case series	Urine osmolality (as marker for AVP activity), urine sodium excretion and low serum HDL-cholesterol were associated with TKV and eGFR slopes. Also baseline BSA, BMI, and estimated protein intake were associated with TKV increase over time.
Torres et al.[f]	ADPKD patients	Sodium intake (as sodium excretion)	TKV growth, eGFR change and risk to reach composite endpoints	Post hoc analysis	Urine sodium excretion was significantly associated with TKV growth ($p < 0.001$), and an non-significant trend for eGFR decline ($p = 0.09$). Averaged urine sodium excretion was significantly associated with eGFR decline ($p < 0.001$) with risk to reach the composite end-point of 50% reduction in eGFR, ESRD, or death.
Amro et al.[g]	ADPKD patients	Low osmolar diet and adjusted water intake	Plasma copeptin, urine osmolality, and total urinary solute	Randomized controlled trial (pilot)	Mean plasma copeptin levels and urine osmolality declined from 6.2±3.05 to 5.3±2.5 pmol/L ($p = 0.02$) and from 426±193 to 258±117 mOsm/kg water ($p = 0.01$), respectively, in the intervention group. Total urinary solute decreased in only the intervention group and significantly differed between groups at week 1 ($p = 0.03$).

Study	Population	Factor	Study type	Outcomes	Results
Vendramini et al.[b]	ADPKD patients	Caffeine	Cross-sectional study	eGFR, TKV, hypertension	Mean caffeine intake was significantly lower in ADPKD patients versus controls (86 vs. 134 mg/day). No significant differences for tertiles of coffee intake and eGFR, TKV, or hypertension.
Ozkok et al.[i]	ADPKD patients	Clinical characteristics like smoking, hypertension and proteinuria	Historical prospective study	Decline in GFR	Rapidly progressing patients had significantly higher history of smoking (36 vs. 18%, $p = 0.01$) and pack-years of smoking. A Cox regression did not confirm that smoking predicted progression of CKD in ADPKD patients ($p = 0.63$), whereas age, presence of hepatic cysts, hypertension, and proteinuria did ($p = 0.01$, $p = 0.001$, $p = 0.04$, and $p = 0.02$, respectively).
Orth et al.[j]	ADPKD patients	Smoking	Case-control study	Progression to ESRD	In smoking men (average pack-years 16.9 ± 20.2), a significant dose-dependent increase of the risk to progress to ESRD compared to controls (average pack-years 8.2 ± 14.9) was found ($p = v0.001$).
Veloso Sousa et al.[k]	Pkd1-deficient mice	Smoking	Interventional animal study	SUN, cystic index, renal fibrosis and cell proliferation	In PKD-1-mice, smoking increased SUN (57.2 ± 32.4 vs. 35.7 ± 6.0 mg/dL, $p < 0.05$), the cystic index (17.4 vs. 4.6%; $p < 0.05$), renal fibrosis (1.1 vs. 0.3%, $p < 0.0001$) and cell proliferation in cystic epithelia (2.1 vs. 1.1%, $p < 0.05$).

[a] Nagao S, Nishii K, Katsuyama M, et al. Increased water intake decreases progression of polycystic kidney disease in the PCK rat. *J Am SocNephrol.* 2006;17:2220–2227.

[b] Hopp K, Wang XF, Ye H, et al. Effects of hydration in rats and mice with polycystic kidney disease. *Am J Physiol-Renal.* 2015;308:F261–F266.

[c] Barash I, Ponda MP, Goldfarb DS, et al. A Pilot Clinical Study to Evaluate Changes in Urine Osmolality and Urine cAMP in Response to Acute and Chronic Water Loading in Autosomal Dominant Polycystic Kidney Disease. *Clin J Am Soc Nephro.* 2010;5:693–697.

[d] Higashihara E, Nutahara K, Tanbo M, et al. Does increased water intake prevent disease progression in autosomal dominant polycystic kidney disease? *Nephrol Dial Transpl.* 2014;29:1710–1719.

[e] Torres VE, Grantham JJ, Chapman AB, et al. Potentially modifiable factors affecting the progression of autosomal dominant polycystic kidney disease. *Clin J Am Soc Nephro.* 2011;6:640–647.

[f] Torres VE, Abebe KZ, Schrier RW, et al. Dietary salt restriction is beneficial to the management of autosomal dominant polycystic kidney disease. *Kidney Int.* 2017;91:493–500.

[g] Amro OW, Paulus JK, Noubary F, et al. Low-osmolar diet and adjusted water intake for vasopressin reduction in autosomal dominant polycystic kidney disease: a pilot randomized controlled trial. *Am J Kidney Dis.* 2016;68:882–891.

[h] Vendramini LC, Nishiura JL, Baxmann AC, et al. Caffeine intake by patients with autosomal dominant polycystic kidney disease. *Braz J Med Bio Res.* 2012;45:834–840.

[i] Ozkok A, Akpinar TS, Tufan F, et al. Clinical characteristics and predictors of progression of chronic kidney disease in autosomal dominant polycystic kidney disease: a single center experience. *Clin Exp Nephrol.* 2013;17:345–351.

[j] Orth SR, Stockmann A, Conradt C, et al. Smoking as a risk factor for end-stage renal failure in men with primary renal disease. *Kidney Int.* 1998;54:926–931.

[k] Veloso Sousa M GAA, Balbo BE, Souza Messias E, de Castro I, Onuchic LF. Smoking worsens the renal phenotype of Pkd1-deficient cystic mice. *J Am Soc Nephrol.* 2016;27:771i.

ARPKD = autosomal recessive polycystic kidney disease. AVP = arginine vasopressin. SUN = serum urea nitrogen. cAMP = cyclic adenosine monophosphate. HW = high water. LW = low water. ADPKD = autosomal dominant polycystic kidney disease. eGFR = estimated glomerular filtration rate. TKV = total kidney volume. HDL = high-density lipoproteins. BSA = body surface area. BMI = body mass index. ESRD = end-stage renal disease.

low-salt diet, and high volume water intake into their daily routines and would like specific recommendations on how to implement these.[28]

Salt Intake

In addition to its beneficial effect on lowering BP, decreasing salt intake would decrease osmolar load thus leading to lower amount of water intake to lower urinary osmolality. In a post hoc analysis of the HALT-PKD trial, urine sodium excretion (a surrogate marker for dietary sodium) in ADPKD patients was significantly associated with TKV growth ($p < 0.001$). Averaged urine sodium excretion was significantly associated with eGFR decline ($p < 0.001$) with risk to reach the composite endpoint of 50% reduction[29] in eGFR, ESRD, or death.[30] These associations suggest a causal relationship between dietary sodium and kidney growth and are consistent with the association between urine sodium excretion and rate of kidney growth observed in the Consortium for Radiologic Imaging Studies of Polycystic Kidney Disease.[31]

Protein Intake

Protein intake could influence osmolar intake and urine osmolality similarly to salt intake. There is some evidence to suggest association of higher protein intake with increased vasopressin concentration.

Caloric Intake

Limiting caloric intake could be a potential therapy to slow down ADPKD progression. Food restriction (FR) effectively slows the course of the disease in mouse models of ADPKD. Mild to moderate (10%–40% reduction of total caloric intake) FR reduced cyst area, renal fibrosis, inflammation, and injury in a dose-dependent manner. Molecular and biochemical studies in these mice indicate that FR ameliorates ADPKD through a mechanism involving suppression of the mammalian target of the rapamycin pathway and activation of the liver kinase B1/AMP-activated protein kinase pathway.[29] Clinical trials will be needed to establish the benefit of caloric restriction in ADPKD patients.

Caffeine Intake

Caffeine intake has been considered as a risk factor in disease progression as it could increase cAMP levels by competitively and nonselectively inhibiting cyclic nucleotide phosphodiesterase. These groups of enzymes degrade the phosphodiester bond in the second messenger cAMP molecules. In vitro studies showed that caffeine activated pro-proliferative signaling pathways and increased transepithelial fluid secretion in murine PKD cells.[32] In a recent clinical prospective study, there was no association between coffee consumption and disease progression in a longitudinal ADPKD cohort (151 patients with median follow up of 4 years). After multivariate adjustment for age, smoking, hypertension, sex, body mass index, and an interaction term (coffee*visit), coffee drinkers did not have a statistically significantly different kidney size compared to noncoffee drinkers (difference of -33.03 cm^3 height adjusted TKV, 95% confidence interval [CI] from -72.41 to 6.34, $p = 0.10$). After the same adjustment, there was no statistically significant difference in eGFR between coffee and noncoffee drinkers (2.03 mL/min/1.73 m^2, 95% CI: -0.31–4.31, $p = 0.089$).[33]

Other Lifestyle Factors

Moderation in alcohol intake is recommended as well. Hard-contact sports such as rugby or American football should be avoided, but individual risk assessment is advised. Exercise is highly recommended. Low high-density lipoprotein (HDL) cholesterol was associated with TKV and eGFR slopes. Increasing HDL by exercise could be beneficial in the renal cystic progression.

NOVEL STRATEGIES FOR NEPHROPROTECTION

There has been great advancement in understanding the pathogenesis of ADPKD, identifying disrupted mechanisms and targets and trying to alleviate the disease by modulating the activity of these targets. These pathways and targets are summarized in Fig. 38.2. Some of these modulators have been used in clinical trials with variable success as summarized in Table 38.2. The following section details the rationale and outcomes of some of these trials.

Tolvaptan (V2R Antagonist)

The increased vasopressin and cAMP concentration associated with PKD formed the rationale for exploring the effects of vasopressin V2 receptor antagonists (V2RA). Administration of V2RA OPC31260 led to a lowered renal cAMP, inhibited disease development, and either halted progression or caused regression of established disease in animal models orthologous to the

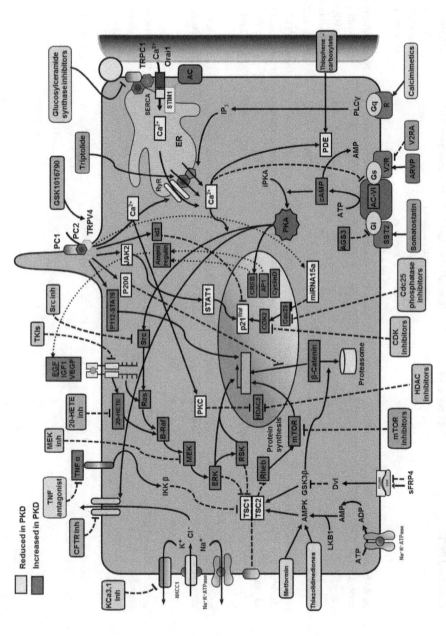

FIGURE 38.2 Pathways and targets involved in the pathogenesis of ADPKD. This figure summarizes the complexity of ADPKD signaling mechanisms. Many targets have been identified and many drugs have been used in vitro and preclinical studies. Few reached clinical trials. ADPKD = autosomal dominant polycystic kidney disease. AC = adenylate cyclase. AMPK = AMP kinase. CDK = cyclin-dependent kinase. ER = endoplasmic reticulum. MAPK = mitogen-activated protein kinase. mTOR = mammalian target of rapamycin. PC1 = polycystin-1. PC2 = polycystin-2. PDE = phosphodiesterase. PKA = protein kinase A. R = somatostatin sst2 receptor. TSC = tuberous sclerosis proteins tuberin (TSC2) and hamartin (TSC1). V2R = vasopressin V2 receptor. V2RA = vasopressin V2 receptor antagonists.

TABLE 38.2 SUMMARY OF CLINICAL TRIALS TREATING ADPKD PATIENTS

Study	Study Design	Population	Intervention	Primary Outcome	Results
HALT-PKD (A) NCT00283686	Double-blinded, placebo-controlled RCT	558 ADPKD patients, 15–49 years old, eGFR >60 mL/min	Standard (120/70–130/80 mmHg) vs. low blood pressure control (95/60–110/75 mmHg) Lisinopril + placebo vs. Lisinopril + telmisartan	Annual percentage change in TKV	Rigorous BP control associated with slower increase in TKV (5.6% vs. 6.6%). No additional benefit if adding ARB to ACEI
HALT PKD (B) NCT01885559	Double-blinded, placebo-controlled RCT	486 ADPKD patients, 18–64 years old, eGFR 25–60 mL/min	Lisinopril + placebo vs. lisinopril + telmisartan	Time to death, ESRD or a 50% reduction from the baseline eGFR.	No significant difference in composite primary outcome (HR with lisinopril-telmisartan = 1.08; 95% CI 0.82 to 1.42)
TEMPO3:4 NCT00428948	Phase 3, placebo-controlled, double-blinded RCT (3 years)	1,445 ADPKD patients, 18–50 years old, eGFR ≥60 mL/min, TKV >750ml	Tolvaptan (V2 receptor antagonist) vs. placebo	Annual rate of change in the TKV	Annual TKV growth lower with treatment (2.8% vs. 5.5%); slower decline in eGFR slope (−2.72 mL/min vs. −3.7 ml/min)
ALADIN NCT00309283	Single-blinded, placebo-controlled RCT, 3 years	79 ADPKD with eGFR >40 mL/min	Octreotide (somatostatin analog) intramuscular injection every 4 weeks vs. placebo	Change in TKV	Favorable trend in halting TKV increase but did not reach statistical significance
Walz et al.[a] (Novartis sponsored) NCT00414440	Double-blinded, placebo-controlled RCT for 2 years	433 ADPKD, stage 2–3 CKD or stage 1 with TKV >1,000 mL	Everolimus (mTOR inhibitor) vs. placebo	Change in TKV	Failed to show benefit despite encouraging animal results
Cadnapaphornchai et al. (University of Colorado)[b]	Double-blinded, placebo-controlled RCT for 3 years	110 ADPKD, 8–22 years old, eGFr >80 mL/min	Pravastatin vs. placebo	≥ 20% change in Ht-TKV, LVMI, or UAE over the study period.	Decrease Ht-TKV over 3-year period (23% vs. 32%)

SWISS	Open-label, randomized, controlled trial for 18 months	100 ADPKD, 18–40 years old, eGFR ≥70 mL/min	Sirolimus (mTOR inhibitor) vs. placebo	TKV at 18 months	18 months of Sirolimus was not effective. TKV in Sirolimus group was 102% of that in the control group at 18 months ($p = 0.26$).
SIRENA NCT00491517	Open-label, randomized, blinded endpoint, parallel group trial	41 ADPKD patients, CKD 3b or 4, proteinuria ≤0.5 g/24 h	Sirolimus vs. placebo	GFR change at 1 and 3 years versus baseline	Unsafe and ineffective. Early trial termination at 1 year due to safety reasons (increased proteinuria, worse decline in GFR) with treatment group
REPRISE NCT02160145	Phase 3, randomized withdrawal, multicenter, placebo-controlled, double-blinded trial for 12 months	1,370 ADPKD, 18–55 years old, eGFR 25–65 mL/min or 56–66 years old, eGFR 25–44 mL/min	Tolvaptan vs placebo	Change in eGFR from baseline to follow-up	Change from baseline in the eGFR was −2.34 mL/min (tolvaptan group) vs. −3.61 mL/min (placebo group), $p < 0.001$.

[a]Walz G, Budde K, Mannaa M, et al. Everolimus in patients with autosomal dominant polycystic kidney disease. *N Engl J Med.* 2010;363:830–840.

[b]Cadnapaphornchai MA, George DM, McFann K, Wang W, Gitomer B, Strain JD, et al. Effect of pravastatin on total kidney volume, left ventricular mass index, and microalbuminuria in pediatric autosomal dominant polycystic kidney disease. *Clin J Am Soc Nephrol.* 2014;9(5):889–896.

RCT = randomized controlled trial. ADPKD = autosomal dominant polycystic kidney disease. BP = blood pressure. TKV = total kidney volume. ARB = angiotensin II receptor blocker. ACEI = angiotensin converting enzyme inhibitor. ESRD = end-stage renal disease. eGFR = estimated glomerular filtration rate HR = hazard ratio. CI = confidence interval. CKD = chronic kidney disease. UAE = uterine artery embolization. LVMI = left ventricular mass index. Ht-TKV = height-adjusted TKV.

human ARPKD and nephronophthisis, as well as in mouse models of ADPKD.[34]

In the TEMPO 3:4 Trial, a large randomized controlled study including 1,445 patients with ADPKD, tolvaptan slowed the disease progression of ADPKD after 3 years of treatment by a lower TKV growth of 2.8% annually versus 5.5% in placebo-treated patients ($p < 0.001$), as well as a decreased slope of the reciprocal of the serum creatinine level, –2.61 mg/mL/year versus –3.81 mg/mL/year, in tolvaptan versus placebo-treated patients, respectively.[35] Patients were eligible if they had an estimated creatinine clearance of ≥60 mL/min. Recent post hoc analyses found similar beneficial effects of tolvaptan in ADPKD across CKD stages 1 to 3[36] and showed that tolvaptan use lowered albuminuria[37] and monocyte chemotactic protein-1 excretion[38] whereas it increased copeptin concentration and significantly lowered the incidence of kidney pain events from 16.8% to 10.1%, with a risk reduction of 36%.[39] A higher albuminuria and a higher copeptin concentration at baseline both predicted renal function decline in placebo- and tolvaptan-treated patients, and both were associated with a stronger tolvaptan treatment effect.[37]

In Japan (March 2014), Canada (February 2015), and the European Union (May 2015), tolvaptan has been approved to delay the progression of ADPKD in patients with a rapid increase in TKV. In the United States, the Food and Drug Administration approval has been deferred until further data are available on potential benefits and risks. The results of the extension of TEMPO 3:4 has been recently revealed in a press release by Otsuka, indicating that primary and key secondary endpoints were positive for tolvaptan versus placebo. The primary endpoint was the change in eGFR from pretreatment baseline levels to posttreatment assessment. In patients treated with tolvaptan, the reduction in eGFR was significantly less than in patients treated with placebo. The difference observed in this study represents a 35% reduction in the loss of kidney function compared to placebo in these patients over the course of one year. The key secondary endpoint was a comparison of the efficacy of tolvaptan treatment versus placebo in reducing the decline of annualized eGFR slope across all measured time points in the study. These data also showed significant benefit from tolvaptan versus placebo ($p < 0.0001$).[35] The details of REPRISE study were published recently, showing that tolvaptan resulted in a slower decline than placebo in the eGFR over a 1-year period in patients with later stage ADPKD.[40]

Drugs With Effects That Are Potentially Synergistic or Additive to Those of Tolvaptan

Tolvaptan has been shown to slow disease progression in ADPKD by antagonizing the vasopressin V2 receptor in the kidney, lowering intracellular cAMP, and inhibiting fluid secretion and cell proliferation. By interfering with aquaporin-2 (AQP2) trafficking, however, it induces aquaresis and enhances vasopressin release. Combining tolvaptan with treatments that lower cAMP or increase AQP2 in the apical membrane of principal cells could increase its efficacy and reduce the side effect of aquaresis.

Long-acting somatostatin analogs acting on somatostatin receptors (SSTR) inhibit adenylyl cyclase and slow renal and hepatic cyst expansion in murine and small clinical trials of ADPKD. Hopp et al.[41] found an additive efficacy of tolvaptan and pasireotide (a SSTR-1, -2, -3 and -5 analogue) compared to either treatment alone, as well as less aquaresis in the combination therapy compared to tolvaptan alone.

Metformin inhibits complex 1 of the mitochondrial respiratory chain thus reducing ATP production and increasing adenosine monophosphate (AMP).[42] AMP, in turn, directly inhibits adenylyl cyclase and activates adenosine monophosphate-activated protein kinase (AMPK). Inhibition of adenylyl cyclase[43] and activation of phosphodiesterase 4B by AMPK-mediated phosphorylation lower cAMP.[44] Furthermore, metformin via AMPK-mediated phosphorylation of AQP2 enhances its accumulation in the apical membrane and reduces the aquaretic effect of tolvaptan.[45] Currently, two phase 2 studies are investigating the effect of metformin treatment on disease progression in ADPKD (Clinicaltrial.gov identifiers: NCT02656017 and NCT02903511).

Statins and tetracycline antibiotics demeclocycline and doxycycline may also have synergistic effects with tolvaptan. Statins may lower cAMP through downregulation of Gαs protein[46] and induce membrane accumulation of AQP2 via inhibition of endocytosis,[47] thus reducing aquaresis. Demeclocycline decreases adenylate cyclase 5/6 expression and, consequently, cAMP generation.[48] In animal studies, doxycycline significantly decreased renal tubule cell proliferation and inhibited cystic disease progression in rats orthologous to human ARPKD.[49] However, the nephrotoxicity of these drugs when used at high doses may limit their potential for the treatment of PKD; for example, doxycycline at a high dose was found to aggravate cyst growth and fibrosis in a mouse model of type 3 nephronophthisis.[50]

Somatostatin Analog

Somatostatin is a peptide hormone that acts on 5 Gi protein-coupled receptors (SSTR1–5), present on cholangiocytes and renal tubular epithelial cells, inhibiting the activity of adenylyl cyclase type 6 and the generation of cAMP. Since somatostatin has a very short half-life, approximately 3 minutes, more stable synthetic peptides (octreotide, lanreotide, and pasireotide) have been developed for clinical use. Octreotide and lanreotide bind mainly to SSTR2 and SSTR3, whereas pasireotide has high affinity SSTR1–3 and SSTR5. In preclinical studies, octreotide halted the expansion of hepatic cysts from PCK rats in vitro and in vivo.[51] Similar effects were observed in the kidneys.

The Long-Acting Somatostatin on Disease Progression in Nephropathy Due to Autosomal Dominant Polycystic Kidney Disease study[52] randomly assigned patients with ADPKD to the somatostatin analogue octreotide or placebo and noted a favorable trend in halting TKV increase. However, statistical significance was not reached in the study, leading the investigators to call for larger trials. DIPAK1 (Developing Interventions to Halt Progression of ADPKD1; NCT01616927) and LIPS (Lanreotide in Polycystic Kidney Disease Study; NCT02127437)are ongoing clinical trials evaluating the effect of the somatostatin analogue lanreotide on disease progression.

mTOR Inhibitors

Sirolimus and everolimus, mTOR-inhibiting rapamycin analogues, failed to show benefit in clinical trials[53,54] despite encouraging results in animal models of PKD[55–57]; this was likely because therapeutic levels could not be reached without inducing systemic toxicity.

CONCLUSION

The natural course and ability to predict and monitor the disease progression makes ADPKD an ideal disease to be targeted for renal protection and delay ESRD onset. Significant advancements in understanding the disease have been accomplished over the past 2 decades. Several therapies showed promise in preclinical trials but were not efficient in patients while others such as tolvaptan were efficient and have been approved in few countries for treatment of subcategories of APDKD patients. Lifestyle modifications such as continuous water intake and low salt, protein, and caloric-count diet should be emphasized as potential disease-modifying measures. The combination of several pharmacotherapies in addition to lifestyle modifications and BP control would likely achieve the best results in halting the disease.

REFERENCES

1. Torres VE, Harris PC, Pirson Y. Autosomal dominant polycystic kidney disease. *Lancet.* 2007;369:1287–1301.
2. Torres VE, Harris PC. Autosomal dominant polycystic kidney disease: the last 3 years. *Kidney Int.* 2009;76:149–168.
3. Chebib FT, Torres VE. Autosomal dominant polycystic kidney disease: core curriculum 2016. *Am J Kidney Dis.* 2016;67:792–810.
4. The polycystic kidney disease 1 gene encodes a 14 kb transcript and lies within a duplicated region on chromosome 16. The European Polycystic Kidney Disease Consortium. *Cell.* 1994;77:881–894.
5. Mochizuki T, Wu G, Hayashi T, et al. PKD2, a gene for polycystic kidney disease that encodes an integral membrane protein. *Science.* 1996;272:1339–1342.
6. Porath B, Gainullin VG, Cornec-Le Gall E, et al. Mutations in GANAB, Encoding the Glucosidase IIalpha Subunit, Cause Autosomal-Dominant Polycystic Kidney and Liver Disease. *Am J Hum Gene.t* 2016;98:1193–1207.
7. Dicks E, Ravani P, Langman D, et al. Incident renal events and risk factors in autosomal dominant polycystic kidney disease: a population and family-based cohort followed for 22 years. *Clin J Am Soc Nephrol.* 2006;1:710–717.
8. Harris PC, Bae KT, Rossetti S, et al. Cyst number but not the rate of cystic growth is associated with the mutated gene in autosomal dominant polycystic kidney disease. *J Am Soc Nephrol.* 2006;17:3013–3019.
9. Hateboer N, v Dijk MA, Bogdanova N, et al.; European PKD1-PKD2 Study Group. Comparison of phenotypes of polycystic kidney disease types 1 and 2. *Lancet.* 1999;353:103–107.
10. Grantham JJ, Torres VE, Chapman AB, et al. Volume progression in polycystic kidney disease. *N Engl J Med.* 2006;354:2122–2130.
11. Harris PC, Torres VE. Genetic mechanisms and signaling pathways in autosomal

dominant polycystic kidney disease. *J Clin Invest.* 2014;124:2315–2324.

12. Torres VE, Harris PC. Strategies targeting cAMP signaling in the treatment of polycystic kidney disease. *J Am Soc Nephrol.* 2014;25:18–32.

13. Pei Y, Obaji J, Dupuis A, et al. Unified criteria for ultrasonographic diagnosis of ADPKD. *J Am Soc Nephrol* .2009;20:205–212.

14. Irazabal MV, Rangel LJ, Bergstralh EJ, et al. Imaging classification of autosomal dominant polycystic kidney disease: a simple model for selecting patients for clinical trials. *J Am Soc Nephrol.* 2015;26:160–172.

15. Schrier RW, Abebe KZ, Perrone RD, et al. Blood pressure in early autosomal dominant polycystic kidney disease. *N Engl J Med.* 2014;371(24):2255–2266.

16. Torres VE, Abebe KZ, Chapman AB, et al. Angiotensin blockade in late autosomal dominant polycystic kidney disease. *N Engl J Med.* 2014;371(24):2267–2276.

17. Cadnapaphornchai MA, George DM, McFann K, et al. Effect of pravastatin on total kidney volume, left ventricular mass index, and microalbuminuria in pediatric autosomal dominant polycystic kidney disease. *Clin J Am Soc Nephrol.* 2014;9:889–896.

18. Brosnahan G, Abebe KZ, Rahbari-Oskoui FF, et al. Effect of statin therapy on the progression of autosomal dominant polycystic kidney disease. A secondary analysis of the HALT PKD trials. *Curr Hypertens Rev.* 2017;13(2):109–120.

19. Meijer E, Bakker SJ, van der Jagt EJ, et al. Copeptin, a surrogate marker of vasopressin, is associated with disease severity in autosomal dominant polycystic kidney disease. *Clin J Am Soc Nephrol.* 2011;6:361–368.

20. Boertien WE, Meijer E, Li J, et al. Relationship of copeptin, a surrogate marker for arginine vasopressin, with change in total kidney volume and GFR decline in autosomal dominant polycystic kidney disease: results from the CRISP cohort. *Am J Kidney Dis.* 2013;61:420–429.

21. Boertien WE, Meijer E, Zittema D, et al. Copeptin, a surrogate marker for vasopressin, is associated with kidney function decline in subjects with autosomal dominant polycystic kidney disease. *Nephrol Dial Transplant.* 2012;27:4131–4137.

22. Wang X, Wu Y, Ward CJ, et al. Vasopressin directly regulates cyst growth in polycystic kidney disease. *J Am Soc Nephrol* 2008;19:102–108.

23. Amro OW, Paulus JK, Noubary F, et al. Low-osmolar diet and adjusted water intake for vasopressin reduction in autosomal dominant polycystic kidney disease: a pilot randomized controlled trial. *Am J Kidney Dis.* 2016;68:882–891.

24. Barash I, Ponda MP, Goldfarb DS, et al. A pilot clinical study to evaluate changes in urine osmolality and urine cAMP in response to acute and chronic water loading in autosomal dominant polycystic kidney disease. *Clin J Am Soc Nephrol.* 2010;5:693–697.

25. Higashihara E, Nutahara K, Tanbo M, et al. Does increased water intake prevent disease progression in autosomal dominant polycystic kidney disease? *Nephrol Dial Transplant.* 2014;29:1710–1719.

26. Taylor JM, Ptomey L, Hamilton-Reeves JM, et al. Experiences and perspectives of polycystic kidney disease patients following a diet of reduced osmoles, protein, and acid precursors supplemented with water: a qualitative Study. *PLoS One* 2016;11:e0161043.

27. Taylor JM, Hamilton-Reeves JM, Sullivan DK, et al. Diet and polycystic kidney disease: a pilot intervention study. *Clin Nutr.* 2017;36:458–466.

28. Tran WC, Huynh D, Chan T, et al. Understanding barriers to medication, dietary, and lifestyle treatments prescribed in polycystic kidney disease. *BMC Nephrol.* 2017;18:214.

29. Warner G, Hein KZ, Nin V, et al. Food restriction ameliorates the development of polycystic kidney disease. *J Am Soc Nephrol.* 2016;27:1437–1447.

30. Torres VE, Abebe KZ, Schrier RW, et al. Dietary salt restriction is beneficial to the management of autosomal dominant polycystic kidney disease. *Kidney Int.* 2017;91:493–500.

31. Torres VE, Grantham JJ, Chapman AB, et al. Potentially modifiable factors affecting the progression of autosomal dominant polycystic kidney disease. *Clin J Am Soc Nephrol.* 2011;6:640–647.

32. Belibi FA, Wallace DP, Yamaguchi T, et al. The effect of caffeine on renal epithelial cells from patients with autosomal dominant polycystic kidney disease. *J Am Soc Nephrol.* 2002;13:2723–2729.

33. Girardat-Rotar L, Puhan MA, Braun J, et al. Long-term effect of coffee consumption on autosomal dominant polycystic kidneys disease progression: results from the Suisse ADPKD, a prospective longitudinal cohort study. *J Nephrol.* 2017.

34. Torres VE. Vasopressin receptor antagonists, heart failure, and polycystic kidney disease. *Annu Rev Med.* 2015;66:195–210.

35. Torres VE, Chapman AB, Devuyst O, et al. Tolvaptan in patients with autosomal dominant polycystic kidney disease. *N Engl J Med.* 2012;367:2407–2418.

36. Torres VE, Higashihara E, Devuyst O, et al. Effect of Tolvaptan in Autosomal Dominant Polycystic Kidney Disease by CKD Stage: Results from the TEMPO 3:4 Trial. *Clin J Am Soc Nephrol.* 2016;11:803–811.

37. Gansevoort RT, Meijer E, Chapman AB, et al. Albuminuria and tolvaptan in autosomal-dominant polycystic kidney disease: results of the TEMPO 3:4 Trial. *Nephrol Dial Transplant.* 2016;31:1887–1894.

38. Grantham JJ, Chapman AB, Blais J, et al. Tolvaptan suppresses monocyte chemotactic protein-1 excretion in autosomal-dominant polycystic kidney disease. *Nephrol Dial Transplant.* 2017;32:969–975.

39. Casteleijn NF, Blais JD, Chapman AB, et al. Tolvaptan and kidney pain in patients with autosomal dominant polycystic kidney disease: secondary analysis from a randomized controlled trial. *Am J Kidney Dis.* 2017;69:210–219.

40. Torres VE, Chapman AB, Devuyst O, et al. Tolvaptan in later-stage autosomal dominant polycystic kidney disease. *N Engl J Med.* 2017;377:1930–1942.

41. Hopp K, Hommerding CJ, Wang X, et al. Tolvaptan plus pasireotide shows enhanced efficacy in a PKD1 model. *J Am Soc Nephrol.* 2015;26:39–47.

42. Owen MR, Doran E, Halestrap AP. Evidence that metformin exerts its anti-diabetic effects through inhibition of complex 1 of the mitochondrial respiratory chain. *Biochem J.* 2000;(348 Pt 3):607–614.

43. Miller RA, Chu Q, Xie J, et al. Biguanides suppress hepatic glucagon signalling by decreasing production of cyclic AMP. *Nature.* 2013;494:256–260.

44. Johanns M, Lai YC, Hsu MF, et al. AMPK antagonizes hepatic glucagon-stimulated cyclic AMP signalling via phosphorylation-induced activation of cyclic nucleotide phosphodiesterase 4B. *Nat Commun.* 2016;7:10856.

45. Efe O, Klein JD, LaRocque LM, et al. Metformin improves urine concentration in rodents with nephrogenic diabetes insipidus. *JCI Insight.* 2016;1(11):e88409.

46. Kou R, Shiroto T, Sartoretto JL, et al. Suppression of galphas synthesis by simvastatin treatment of vascular endothelial cells. *J Biol Chem.* 2012;287:2643–2651.

47. Li W, Zhang Y, Bouley R, et al. Simvastatin enhances aquaporin-2 surface expression and urinary concentration in vasopressin-deficient Brattleboro rats through modulation of Rho GTPase. *Am J Physiol Renal Physiol.* 2011;301:F309–F318.

48. Kortenoeven ML, Sinke AP, Hadrup N, et al. Demeclocycline attenuates hyponatremia by reducing aquaporin-2 expression in the renal inner medulla. *Am J Physiol Renal Physiol.* 2013;305:F1705–F1718.

49. Liu B, Li C, Liu Z, et al. Increasing extracellular matrix collagen level and MMP activity induces cyst development in polycystic kidney disease. *BMC Nephrol.* 2012;13:109.

50. Osten L, Kubitza M, Gallagher AR, et al. Doxycycline accelerates renal cyst growth and fibrosis in the pcy/pcy mouse model of type 3 nephronophthisis, a form of recessive polycystic kidney disease. *Histochem Cell Biol.* 2009;132:199–210.

51. Masyuk TV, Masyuk AI, Torres VE, et al. Octreotide inhibits hepatic cystogenesis in a rodent model of polycystic liver disease by reducing cholangiocyte adenosine 3',5'-cyclic monophosphate. *Gastroenterology.* 2007;132:1104–1116.

52. Caroli A, Perico N, Perna A, et al. Effect of longacting somatostatin analogue on kidney and cyst growth in autosomal dominant polycystic kidney disease (ALADIN): a randomised, placebo-controlled, multicentre trial. *Lancet.* 2013;382:1485–1495.

53. Serra AL, Poster D, Kistler AD, et al. Sirolimus and kidney growth in autosomal dominant polycystic kidney disease. *N Engl J Med.* 2010;363:820–829.

54. Walz G, Budde K, Mannaa M, et al. Everolimus in patients with autosomal dominant polycystic kidney disease. *N Engl J Med.* 2010;363:830–840.

55. Gattone VH, 2nd, Sinders RM, Hornberger TA, et al. Late progression of renal pathology and cyst enlargement is reduced by rapamycin in a mouse model of nephronophthisis. *Kidney Int.* 2009;76:178–182.

56. Shillingford JM, Piontek KB, Germino GG, et al. Rapamycin ameliorates PKD resulting from conditional inactivation of Pkd1. *J Am Soc Nephrol.* 2010;21:489–497.

57. Novalic Z, van der Wal AM, Leonhard WN, et al. Dose-dependent effects of sirolimus on mTOR signaling and polycystic kidney disease. *J Am Soc Nephrol.* 2012;23:842–853.

39

Hepatitis-Associated Glomerulonephritis

JULIE BELLIERE, STANISLAS FAGUER, AND NASSIM KAMAR

It is now acknowledged that chronic infection can lead to autoimmunity. The initial immune response directed against an exogenous agent can develop into an autoimmune response that can lead to kidney injury. In this chapter, we focus on viral hepatitis-associated glomerulonephritis (GN), namely, hepatitis A-, B-, C-, and E-virus–associated GN.

GENERAL PATHOGENESIS OF HEPATITIS-ASSOCIATED GN

Several factors favor a transition from an antiviral response into an autoimmune response. First, heredity (genetic and epigenetic traits) may predispose individuals to elaborate nephritogenic responses after exposure to an environmental trigger. Exposure to the virus is followed by activation of the innate immune system (Toll-like receptors, complement, innate immune cells). An antigen-specific response then develops that is supported by the adaptive immune system (B and T cells). Antibodies directed against viral particles are generated and circulate within the blood stream. Immune complexes, referred to as antigen-antibody complexes, cause the integral binding of an antibody to a soluble antigen. Immune complexes can undergo complement deposition, opsonization, and phagocytosis or be processed by proteases. In some cases, immune complexes can be deposited in organs and can cause great toxicity. As summarized in Fig. 39.1, an immune response that is targeted against a virus may lead to GN through the following 3 main mechanisms.

1. **Immune-complexes deposition**: The host's humoral response is directed toward the viral surface; however, this can lead to the development of pathogenic immune complexes. During viral infections, the presence of immune complexes in the glomerulus is frequent. It can be related to either the deposition of circulating immune complexes or to their in situ formation. Immune complexes are thought to activate Toll-like receptors and the complement component of the innate immune system. Complement activation causes glomerular injury, especially via chemotactic attraction of circulating inflammatory cells (neutrophils, macrophages, basophils, natural cell killers), which release toxic mediators. Resident glomerular cells are also activated by C5b-9 and can perpetuate tissue injury.

2. **Autoimmune processes**: In some cases, the useful primary antigen-specific response is converted into an inappropriate response that is directed against endogen autoantigens. This loss of tolerance can be caused by the following factors:
   - A defect in the regulation of previously existent autoimmunity
   - Molecular mimicry (caused by the similarity between a viral particle and an endogenous protein)
   - Epitope spreading (expansion of reactivity, which increases with worsening of the disease)
   - Epitope conformational changes (exposure of a previously hidden component that then becomes the target of the autoimmune response)
   - Adjuvant/bystander effect (some viruses express superantigens that do not require processing and can directly induce nonspecific T-cell activation)
   - Autoantigen complementarity (antibodies to the antigen-binding region [idiotype] of an antibody can

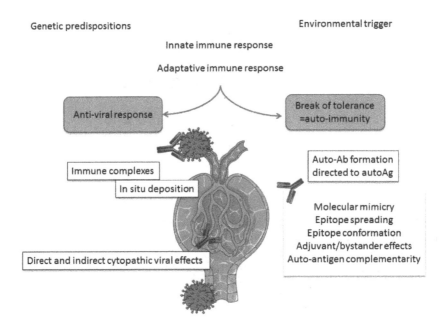

FIGURE 39.1 Mechanisms of glomerular injury in the context of antiviral response.

be generated and lead to the formation of anti-idiotypic antibodies and anti-Fc antibodies, such as immunoglobin M [IgM] cryoglobulins/rheumatoid factors). These autoantibodies may then be deposited in the glomeruli and trigger local immune processes.

3. **Direct and indirect cytopathogenic effects of viruses**. Viral antigens derived from the hepatitis virus have been detected in kidneys, suggesting a possible direct cytopathogenic effect of viral proteins on glomerular cells. For example, it has been shown that hepatitis B virus (HBV) directly induces mesangial cell proliferation and the expression of extracellular matrix proteins. Viral proteins are capable of acting as an indirect transcriptional transactivator and can regulate cell proliferation, trans-differentiation, and apoptosis. Furthermore, the indirect effects of viral infection are also harmful to the kidney environment because viruses induce the release of proinflammatory cytokines, chemokines, adhesion molecules, and growth factors, which can then recruit cell actors that can destroy the glomerular architecture.

In summary, hepatitis infections can initiate GN through several complex pathways that start by activating the immune system and lead to auto-immunity. The broad spectrum of viral properties explains the diversity of kidney injuries that can develop with hepatitis.

HEPATITIS-ASSOCIATED GN

Hepatitis A

The hepatitis A virus (HAV) is a small, nonenveloped, single-stranded RNA virus that is a frequent cause of acute hepatitis worldwide. HAV is fecal-orally transmitted and usually only affects the liver in a self-limiting form; however, extrahepatic manifestations have been reported, such as arthritis, vasculitis, and cryoglobulinemia.[1] Renal impairment is rare (1.5% of patients[2]) and is attributed to several kidney injuries, including acute tubular necrosis, hepatorenal syndrome, and GN. Although acute tubular necrosis is the principal mechanism in HAV-associated kidney failure, very few cases of HAV-related GN have been reported.

In a retrospective study[3] that included 208 patients, 15 patients presented with acute kidney injury (AKI), microscopic hematuria, and proteinuria. Of these, 5 patients underwent a kidney biopsy that revealed acute tubular necrosis in 2 cases, acute interstitial nephritis with immunoglobin A (IgA) nephropathy in 2 cases, and acute tubulointerstitial nephritis in 1 case. IgA deposits consisted of granular deposits showing predominant mesangial and peripheral IgA staining. Ultrastructural examination showed small mesangial deposits. When examined, glomeruli were mildly enlarged, with a mild increase in the mesangial matrix.[3]

In a larger prospective study that included 595 patients, only 9 developed AKI without fulminant hepatitis. Five of the 9 patients had both proteinuria and hematuria. None of the patients had undergone a kidney biopsy. Patients with AKI were predominantly male, were older in age, had a higher body mass index, had a lower serum albumin level, and had higher white blood cell counts compared to patients with healthy kidneys.[2]

Experimental data have revealed several types of HAV-associated glomerular disorders, including membranous nephropathy (MN), mesangial proliferative GN, and membranoproliferative GN (MPGN). There is no specific treatment for HAV infection, including HAV-related GN. The global prognosis for HAV is good with an only a 0.2% risk of fatality and a 0.5% risk of fulminant hepatitis. In a series of 15 patients with kidney injury, reported by Jung and colleagues,[3] 2 patients died from fulminant hepatitis, 1 patient needed a liver transplant, 9 patients required dialysis, and the other 3 had good outcomes. However, no data regarding the long-term outcomes of kidneys were reported.

Hepatitis B

The seroprevalence of HBV occurs in 56% of the world's population. The spectrum of HBV and the natural history of chronic HBV infection are diverse and variable, ranging from a low viremic inactive carrier state to progressive chronic hepatitis, which may evolve to cirrhosis and hepatocellular carcinoma. Extrahepatic manifestations are reported in 16% of HBV carriers. The prevalence of HBV-induced kidney manifestations parallels the geographic patterns of HBV, as suggested by the significant rarefaction of childhood GN observed after national vaccination programs. Overall, GN occurs in a minority of HBV carriers, i.e., those that are Hepatitis B surface antigen positive, with an incidence of ~3%.[4,5] Renal impairment seems to be higher with genotype A (1 of the 8 genotypes of HBV) and with mutations to the HBV X gene in specific locations.[6] The clinical manifestation of HBV-associated GN has been difficult to distinguish from other forms of GN and may present as nephrotic syndrome in 53% cases. Although MN is the most common pathologic type of HBV-associated GN, HBV has also been linked to other types of GN (see following discussion).

HBV-Related Membranous Nephropathy

HBV-related MN is characterized by proteinuria within nephrotic range and microscopic hematuria (rarely macrohematuria), possible hypertension (25% of cases), and preserved kidney function. The usual biological associated abnormalities are the following: elevated transaminases, hypocomplementemia, and an absence of hyperlipidemia caused by liver disease. Circulating immune complexes that contain hepatitis B e-antigen (HBeAg) are small and cationic, thus facilitating their accumulation in subepithelial spaces. Immune complexes that contain HBeAg are known to be correlated with disease severity, and HBeAg is often the predominant antigen in glomerular deposits.[7,8] In contrast to phospholipase A2 receptor–associated primitive MN, where IgG4 is predominant, IgG1 and IgG3 tends to be the predominant IgG subclass in HBV-related MN.

IgG1 and IgG3 are known to generate a greater activation of complement system than IgG4. In HBV-related MN, the subsequent activation of the classical pathway could participate to immune deposits and injury of podocytes. Complement blockade with eculizumab also appears to be a therapeutic option. In a small study, treatment with eculizumab over a 16 weeks period did not lead to a statistically significant reduction of proteinuria compared to the control cohort of untreated patients with HBV-related or non-HBV-related MN.[9] However, eculizumab doses and duration were not optimal, precluding all definitive conclusion. For this reason, to date, the role of eculizumab remains to be established in secondary MN.

HBV-related MN has a better prognosis in children than in adults. HBV-related MN is usually progressive with resolution of proteinuria being relatively uncommon. Development of anti-HBeAg antibodies and HBeAg clearance are associated with remission of proteinuria. However, patients that are not cleared of the virus usually develop progressive kidney failure. Patients with nephrotic syndrome and abnormal liver-function tests have an even worse prognosis, with 50% progressing to end-stage renal disease over the short term.

Membranoproliferative GN

HBV-related MPGN is characterized by nephritic syndrome with or without nephrotic-range proteinuria, frequent hypertension (50% of cases), and altered kidney function in 20% of cases. The usual associated biological abnormalities are C3 and C4 hypocomplementemia and circulating immune complexes. Screening for type 3 cryoglobulinemia (polyclonal IgM and IgG) should be performed. A diagnosis of HBV-related MPGN is suggested by the lobular appearance of the glomerulus with splitting of the basement membrane. Deposits are mesangial or subendothelial or can even be subepithelial. The typical antigen observed in the glomeruli is hepatitis B surface antigen HBsAg. However, hepatitis B core antigen (HBcAg) can also be identified in the mesangium using immunofluorescence.

IgA Nephropathy

Lai and colleagues[10] found a significantly higher prevalence of HBsAg in patients that had IgA nephropathy. Its profile is mesangial proliferative GN with predominant mesangial IgA deposits, with or without co-existing MN and deposits of capillary IgG.

Focal Segmental Glomerulosclerosis

HBV-related focal segmental glomerulosclerosis is a rare form of HBV-related GN, which has been observed in young men who have presented with severe nephrotic syndrome. HBsAg and HBcAg have been identified within glomeruli without immune complexes, suggesting a direct viral effect on podocytes.

Postinfectious Acute GN

Ten cases of patients with HBV and acute GN have been recently reported.[11] Biopsies describe typical diffuse glomerular endocapillary proliferation, but HBV-associated postinfectious acute GN (PIGN) differs from classical PIGN by having much fewer subepithelial glomerular "hump-shaped" immune-complex deposits. Patients exhibit the typical changes associated with acute GN, including glomerular endocapillary proliferation and deposition of immunoglobulin and deposition of complements C3 and C4. The main characteristic of PIGN is the presence of HBsAg in glomerular and tubulointerstitial areas of patients with HBV.

Polyarteritis Nodosa

Another kidney manifestation of HBV is classic polyarteritis nodosa (PAN). HBV-associated PAN is not a GN per se but is a small- and medium-vessel necrotizing vasculitis, where antineutrophil cytoplasmic antibodies are negative. Kidney ischemia and infarction are the main pathological processes. Thanks to vaccination, the prevalence of PAN has dramatically decreased (from 80% in the 1980s to <20% today).

Treatment of HBV-Related GN

Antiviral therapies are effective regimens for patients with HBV-related MN. Interferons (IFNs; conventional interferon-2b and longer-acting peginterferon-2a) and nucleotide analogs (tenofovir, adefovir) or nucleoside analogs (lamivudine, entecavir, telbivudine) can effectively induce remission of proteinuria and the clearance of HBeAg.[12] Lamivudine has been associated with complete resolution of MN lesions in 80% of patients; however, the high rate of resistance has precluded its use as a first-line treatment: nucleotide analogs are used instead. Dose adjustments are required for patients with kidney impairment, and decompensated liver disease contraindicates the use of IFN, which is associated with multiple side effects. A short-term course of steroids may be given in association with an antiviral therapy. However, the indication for the use of steroids is unclear.

Hepatitis C

The seroprevalence of hepatitis C virus (HCV) occurs in 3% of the world's population.[13] Chronic infection develops in up to 90% of patients and extrahepatic manifestations are observed in 40% of individuals.[14] The prevalence of chronic kidney disease among HCV-seropositive patients is about 16.5%.[15] Kidney injury is frequent during HCV infection and may occur after many years or even decades after an HCV infection. HCV-related GN represents a rare cause of renal dysfunction (<10%) and is far less likely than acute tubular necrosis or hepatorenal syndrome.

Cryoglobulinemia as a Hallmark of HCV-Related GN

One hallmark of HCV is its potential to trigger a rapid humoral immune response, secondary to its singular tropism for B-lymphocytes. Repetitive stimulation of B-cells from the production of IgG–HCV complexes triggers the generation of

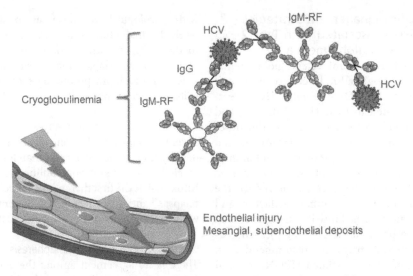

FIGURE 39.2 Hepatitis C virus (HCV) related cryoglobulinemia type III. RF = rheumatoid factor

IgM, which can then react with IgG and also so-called rheumatoid factors.

Cryoglobulins are immunoglobulins that become insoluble at below-body temperature and dissolve when rewarmed. In individuals with HCV infection, these cryoglobulins are immune complexes formed by monoclonal rheumatoid factor IgM, polyclonal IgG, and HCV RNA (Fig 39.2). Cryoglobulins are deposited in the kidney, especially in the mesangium, and form mesangial, subendothelial, dense deposits or filamentous or microtubular structures. The interaction between HCV and lymphocytes seems to affect B-cell function and may induce polyclonal activation and expansion of peripheral CD5+ cells, which are considered to be the major source of IgM rheumatoid factors in type 3 cryoglobulinemia.[16] Thereafter, the emergence of a single dominant clone that produces IgM rheumatoid factor may be responsible for the evolution of type 2 mixed cryoglobulinemia.[17] Cryoglobulinemia is found in most patients that have HCV-related MPGN[18] but is rare in other forms of viral hepatitis.

Varieties of HCV-Associated GN

MPGN associated with type 2 cryoglobulinemia is the predominant type of HCV-related GN.[18-20] Less common forms of GN have also been reported in HCV-infected patients: these include MPGN without cryoglobulinemia, MN,[19] IgA nephropathy, focal segmental glomerulosclerosis, and fibrillary and immunotactoid GN. Cryoglobulinemic thrombotic microangiopathy has been occasionally reported.[21]

MPGN Associated with Type 2 Cryoglobulinemia

Nephrotic syndrome and acute nephritic syndrome with rapid deterioration of kidney function are observed in, respectively, 20% and 25% of patients. Fifty percent of patients have moderate renal insufficiency, and hypertension is present in 80% of patients.[22] Patients with MPGN associated with type 2 cryoglobulinemia often suffer from extrarenal manifestations; those most frequently observed are skin rash (palpable purpura), polyneuropathy, and systemic vasculitis.[23]

Usually, there are only low levels of the complement components, C4 and C1q. Serum C3 level is also moderately and inconstantly decreased. Autoantibodies are also very frequent; 40% and 66% of patients exhibit, respectively, anti-smooth muscle antibodies and anti-nuclear antibodies. A kidney biopsy usually reveals the presence of glomerular infiltration by activated macrophages. The glomerular basement membrane shows double contours, which are caused by the interposition of monocytes between the basement membrane and the endothelium. Immunofluorescence exhibits subendothelial deposits of IgM, IgG, and the complement components. Electron microscopy shows large subendothelial deposits. Vasculitis of the small renal arteries is present in 30% of cases.[24] Cryoglobulin is a pejorative prognosis factor because it is associated with an increased risk of B-cell lymphoma and cardiovascular death.

Specific Management Strategies in MPGN Associated With Type 2 Cryoglobulinemia

The goals of therapy for mixed cryoglobulinemia include immunoglobulin level reduction and antigen elimination. On one hand, HCV treatment is indicated to treat HCV infection and the related kidney injury, and, on the other hand, an immunosuppressive treatment can be necessary to reduce glomerular inflammation (intravenous pulses of steroids), remove cryoglobulins (plasmapheresis), or reduce the production of IgMκ-rheumatoid factor and anti-HCV antibodies (anti-B-cell agents such as cyclophosphamide or rituximab). Whereas isolated antiviral drugs are recommended in mild forms of HCV-associated MPGN, antiviral and immunosuppressive are preferred in severe forms (nephrotic syndrome or rapidly progressive renal failure). To date, whether antiviral and immunosuppressive treatments should be administered simultaneously or sequentially remains to be clarified.

Direct-Acting Antivirals

Direct-acting antivirals (DAAs) against HCV are newly available treatments to achieve sustained viral remissions of >95% of all genotypes.[24] In genotype 1 and 4, the C-SURFER study[25] has shown that the combination of grazoprevir and elbasvir was highly efficient for treating HCV infection in patients with severe renal impairment (CKD stages 4–5) patients. Very recently, in a phase 3 trial, glecaprevir and pibrentasvir, a combination against genotypes 1 to 6, was associated with a high rate of sustained virologic responses in CKD stages 4 and 5 patients.[26] In patients with better kidney function (CKD stage 1–3), sofosbuvir use and consequent HCV cure were associated with a clear improvement in estimated glomerular filtration rate (+ 9 mL/min/1.73 m^2 at 6 months) in a retrospective cohort on 98 patients, suggesting reversibility of lesions and global benefit.[27,38] A few data are now available on DAA impact in HCV-associated cryoglobulinemic vasculitis. In a recent series on 12 patients, the use of DAAs +/– rituximab was associated with an improvement in serum creatinine level and a reduction in proteinuria levels. Cryoglobulin levels decreased in 89% of patients and completely disappeared in 4 of 9 patients who had cryoglobulins measured after treatment.[29] Another study performed on 17 patients treated with DAA revealed that only patients with virological response at posttreatment week 12 had clinical improvement during a median 24 months long-term follow-up.[30] Unfortunately, relapses may occur due to persistent cryoglobulin-producing B-cell clones despite HCV clearance.

Rituximab

Several randomized controlled trials have demonstrated efficacy of rituximab for treatment of HCV-associated cryoglobulinemic vasculitis. Rituximab is the first therapeutic choice in case of relapses[31] and in nonresponders patients or those with contraindications to antiviral treatment.[32]

Efficacy of Plasmapheresis

There is no agreement among the experts concerning treatment intensity, duration, or frequency. The only available recommendations suggest a rhythm of 3 times per week for 2 to 3 weeks (from 6–9 sessions), using the clinical response to guide subsequent therapy. Apheresis, usually combined with other treatments, is usually used in the case of severe, life-threatening cryoglobulinemic manifestations and when other therapies have failed or cannot be used.[32]

Hepatitis E

Hepatitis E virus (HEV) is the most prevalent viral hepatitis worldwide. It causes 3.3 million cases of hepatitis and 56,600 deaths every year. Patients who have pre-existing chronic liver disease and who have genotypes-1 or -3 HEV can develop fulminant hepatitis. In immunosuppressed patients (i.e., organ- or stem-cell-transplant recipients, individuals infected with the human immunodeficiency virus, and hematological patients receiving chemotherapy), genotype-3 and -4 HEV can cause chronic hepatitis and cirrhosis.

Extrahepatic manifestations have been described in patients infected with different genotypes of HEV. The main manifestations are neurological disorders, hematological manifestations, and kidney injuries. HEV-associated GN has been diagnosed in immunocompetent patients and in immunosuppressed patients during acute or chronic phases. Seven cases of HEV-GT3–associated GN have been described.[33-35] Types of renal injury have included MPGN ($n = 4$), IgA GN ($n = 2$), and MN ($n = 1$). Although the underlying mechanisms by which HEV infection induces glomerular disease remain to be established, processes that are similar to the mechanisms of HCV-associated GN could be implicated. Further studies are required to examine the association between HEV and cryoglobulinemia.

HEV clearance can be achieved spontaneously after reducing immunosuppression or after antiviral therapy (IFN and/or ribavirin, with the latter being the first-choice therapy). When HEV RNA becomes undetectable in the serum, proteinuria levels decrease or return to within normal ranges, renal function improves, and cryoglobulinemia disappears.

CONCLUSION

Hepatitis-associated GN is common. Patients presenting with features of glomerular disease should be screened for viral hepatitis, especially if liver enzyme levels are increased and/or there is a history of hepatitis. Viral serologies and/or nuclear acid tests should be performed. Cryoglobulinemia should be assessed, and a kidney biopsy is required to confirm the diagnosis. Viral clearance, using antiviral therapies, when available, is necessary to improve kidney outcomes.

REFERENCES

1. Cuthbert JA. Hepatitis A: old and new. *Clin Microbiol Rev.* 2001;14(1):38–58.
2. Jung YM, Park SJ, Kim JS, et al. Atypical manifestations of hepatitis A infection: a prospective, multicenter study in Korea. *J Med Virol.* 2010;82(8):1318–1326.
3. Jung YJ, Kim W, Jeong JB, et al. Clinical features of acute renal failure associated with hepatitis A virus infection. *J Viral Hepat.* 2010;17(9):611–617.
4. Cacoub P, Saadoun D, Bourlière M, et al. Hepatitis B virus genotypes and extrahepatic manifestations. *J Hepatol.* 2005;43(5):764–770.
5. Zhang X, Liu S, Tang L, et al. Analysis of pathological data of renal biopsy at one single center in China from 1987 to 2012. *Chin Med J (Engl).* 2014;127(9):1715–1720.
6. Hui D, Yan X, Wei J, Ruixia M, Guangju G. Significance of mutations in hepatitis B virus X gene for the pathogenesis of HB-associated glomerulonephritis. *Acta Virol.* 2014;58(3):278–281.
7. Johnson RJ, Couser WG. Hepatitis B infection and renal disease: clinical, immunopathogenetic and therapeutic considerations. *Kidney Int.* 1990;37(2):663–676.
8. Gregorek H, Jung H, Ułanowicz G, Madaliński K. Immune complexes in sera of children with HBV-mediated glomerulonephritis. *Arch Immunol Ther Exp (Warsz).* 1986;34(1):73–83.

9. Ma H, Sandor DG, Beck LH, Jr. The role of complement in membranous nephropathy. *Semin Nephrol.* 2013;33(6):531–542.
10. Lai KN, Lai FM, Tam JS, Vallance-Owen J. Strong association between IgA nephropathy and hepatitis B surface antigenemia in endemic areas. *Clin Nephrol.* 1988;29(5):229–234.
11. Zhang Y, Li J, Peng W, et al. HBV-associated postinfectious acute glomerulonephritis: a report of 10 cases. Leite-de-Moraes M, ed. *PLoS One.* 2016;11(8):e0160626.
12. Yang Y, Ma Y, Chen D, Zhuo L, Li W. A meta-analysis of antiviral therapy for hepatitis b virus-associated membranous nephropathy. Kramvis A, ed. *PLoS One.* 2016;11(9):e0160437.
13. Fabrizi F, Messa P, Martin P. Novel evidence on hepatitis C virus–associated glomerular disease. *Kidney Int.* 2014;86(3):466–469.
14. Cacoub P, Renou C, Rosenthal E, et al.; The GERMIVIC (Groupe d'Etude et de Recherche en Medecine Interne et Maladies Infectieuses sur le Virus de l'Hepatite C). Extrahepatic manifestations associated with hepatitis C virus infection. A prospective multicenter study of 321 patients. *Medicine (Baltimore).* 2000;79(1):47–56.
15. Chen Y-C, Lin H-Y, Li C-Y, Lee M-S, Su Y-C. A nationwide cohort study suggests that hepatitis C virus infection is associated with increased risk of chronic kidney disease. *Kidney Int.* 2014;85(5):1200–1207.
16. Curry MP, Golden-Mason L, Doherty DG, et al. Expansion of innate CD5pos B cells expressing high levels of CD81 in hepatitis C virus infected liver. *J Hepatol.* 2003;38(5):642–650.
17. Morra E. Cryoglobulinemia. *Hematol Am Soc Hematol Educ Progr.* 2005:368–372
18. Roccatello D, Fornasieri A, Giachino O, et al. Multicenter study on Hepatitis C virus–related cryoglobulinemic glomerulonephritis. *Am J Kidney Dis.* 2007;49(1):69–82.
19. Morales JM. Hepatitis C virus infection and renal transplantation. *Transplant Proc.* 1999;31(6):2221–2224.
20. Sabry A, E-Agroudy A, Sheashaa H, et al. HCV associated glomerulopathy in Egyptian patients: clinicopathological analysis. *Virology.* 2005;334(1):10–16.
21. Wu H, Zou H-B, Xu Y, et al. Hepatitis C virus-related heat-insoluble cryoglobulinemia and thrombotic microangiopathy. *Am J Med Sci.* 2013;346(4):345–348.
22. D'Amico G. Renal involvement in hepatitis C infection: cryoglobulinemic glomerulonephritis. *Kidney Int.* 1998;54(2):650–671.
23. Kamar N, Izopet J, Alric L, Guilbeaud-Frugier C, Rostaing L. Hepatitis C virus-related

kidney disease: an overview. *Clin Nephrol.* 2008;69(3):149–160.

24. Li T, Qu Y, Guo Y, Wang Y, Wang L. Efficacy and safety of direct-acting antivirals-based antiviral therapies for hepatitis C virus patients with stage 4-5 chronic kidney disease: a meta-analysis. *Liver Int.* 2017;37(7):974–981.

25. Roth D, Nelson DR, Bruchfeld A, et al. Grazoprevir plus elbasvir in treatment-naive and treatment-experienced patients with hepatitis C virus genotype 1 infection and stage 4-5 chronic kidney disease (the C-SURFER study): a combination phase 3 study. *Lancet.* 2015;386(10003):1537–1545.

26. Gane E, Lawitz E, Pugatch D, et al. Glecaprevir and pibrentasvir in patients with HCV and severe renal impairment. *N Engl J Med.* 2017;377(15):1448–1455.

27. Sise ME, Backman E, Ortiz GA, et al. Effect of sofosbuvir-based hepatitis C virus therapy on kidney function in patients with CKD. *Clin J Am Soc Nephrol.* 2017;12(10):1613–1623.

28. Johnson RJ, Shimada M. Contemporary management of hepatitis C in patients with CKD. *Clin J Am Soc Nephrol.* 2017;12(10):1563–1565.

29. Sise ME, Bloom AK, Wisocky J, et al. Treatment of hepatitis C virus-associated mixed cryoglobulinemia with direct-acting antiviral agents. *Hepatology.* 2016;63(2):408–417.

30. Sollima S, Milazzo L, Antinori S, Galli M. Direct-acting antivirals and mixed cryoglobulinemia vasculitis: long-term outcome of patients achieving HCV eradication. *Am J Gastroenterol.* 2017;112(11):1753–1754.

31. Quartuccio L, Zuliani F, Corazza L, et al. Retreatment regimen of rituximab monotherapy given at the relapse of severe HCV-related cryoglobulinemic vasculitis: long-term follow up data of a randomized controlled multicentre study. *J Autoimmun.* 2015;63:88–93.

32. Pietrogrande M, De Vita S, Zignego AL, et al. Recommendations for the management of mixed cryoglobulinemia syndrome in hepatitis C virus-infected patients. *Autoimmun Rev.* 2011;10(8):444–454.

33. Del Bello A, Guilbeau-Frugier C, Josse A-G, Rostaing L, Izopet J, Kamar N. Successful treatment of hepatitis E virus-associated cryoglobulinemic membranoproliferative glomerulonephritis with ribavirin. *Transpl Infect Dis.* 2015;17(2):279–283.

34. Taton B, Moreau K, Lepreux S, et al. Hepatitis E virus infection as a new probable cause of de novo membranous nephropathy after kidney transplantation. *Transpl Infect Dis.* 2013;15(6):E211–E215.

35. Guinault D, Ribes D, Delas A, et al. Hepatitis E virus–induced cryoglobulinemic glomerulonephritis in a nonimmunocompromised person. *Am J Kidney Dis.* 2016;67(4):660–663.

40

Hepatorenal Syndrome

FRANÇOIS DURAND, CLAIRE FRANCOZ, JOSEPH DINORCIA,
YURI S. GENYK, AND MITRA K. NADIM

INTRODUCTION

Hepatorenal syndrome (HRS) is a severe complication of advanced cirrhosis and constitutes approximately 17% of cases of acute kidney injury (AKI) in hospitalized patients with end-stage liver disease. HRS results in part from arterial vasodilatation, a hyperkinetic state ,and a status of effective hypovolemia that triggers intense renal vasoconstriction. It is associated with a poor prognosis without liver transplantation.[1] HRS is considered to be functional in nature with a potential for complete recovery following liver transplantation. However, in contrast to prerenal azotemia in critically ill patients without cirrhosis, HRS is characterized by the absence of response to volume expansion. Major improvements have been achieved in understanding the mechanisms involved in HRS. Vasoactive agents, especially vasopressin analogues, have proved to be effective at improving outcomes in type 1 HRS, but liver transplantation remains the only definitive cure.

DEFINITION AND CLINICAL PRESENTATION

The definition of AKI in cirrhosis has undergone significant changes over the past several years. In 2012, the Acute Dialysis Quality Initiative[2] recommended adaptation of the Acute Kidney Injury Network criteria to define AKI in patients with cirrhosis instead of the traditional definition using a fixed serum creatinine (SCr) cut-off value of >1.5 mg/dL. These criteria were irrespective of the cause of AKI and as such, type 1 HRS was categorized as a specific type of AKI while type 2 HRS as a form of acute on chronic kidney disease (CKD). Since then, the use of Acute Kidney Injury Network criteria in predicting mortality has been validated in numerous studies of hospitalized patients with cirrhosis, including those in the intensive care unit (ICU).

As a result of the changes in the definition of AKI in patients with cirrhosis, the definition of HRS has also been revised in recent years to be included in a more general entity.[3] The International Ascites Club has defined AKI in cirrhosis based on the Kidney Disease Improving Global Outcomes definition, which is an increase in SCr ≤ 0.3 mg/dL within 48 hours or a $\leq 50\%$ increase in SCr from baseline that is known or presumed to have occurred within the prior 7 days. Once AKI is established, a staging system then defines its severity. Although oliguria is not included in the current definition of AKI in patients with cirrhosis and has yet to be validated, urine output has been found to be a sensitive and early marker for AKI in ICU patients associated with adverse outcomes.[4]

Among patients with cirrhosis and AKI, several criteria define HRS (Table 40.1). The main characteristic of HRS is the absence of response after 2 consecutive days of diuretic withdrawal and plasma volume expansion with albumin (1 g/kg of body weight).[3] Type 1 HRS is frequently triggered by a precipitating factor such as sepsis and is characterized by a rapid decline in urine output, rapid increase in SCr, low urine sodium concentration (<10 mmol/L), absence of significant proteinuria (proteinuria <500 mg/dL), absence of microhematuria, and normal findings on renal ultrasonography. Patients not responding to vasopressors have a mortality rate of 80% to 90% with short life expectancy. Type 2 HRS, which is less common, represents a more chronic phenotype with fluctuations in SCr. The dominant clinical feature of type 2 HRS is refractory ascites. A major limitation of the HRS criteria is that they do not allow for the coexistence of other forms of acute or chronic kidney disease, such as underlying diabetic nephropathy or other glomerular diseases often associated with patients with liver

TABLE 40.1 DIAGNOSTIC CRITERIA FOR HEPATORENAL SYNDROME IN PATIENTS WITH CIRRHOSIS

- **Diagnosis of cirrhosis and ascites**
- **Diagnosis of AKI according to the ICA AKI criteria**
- Increase in serum creatinine (SCr) ≤0.3 mg/dL (≤26.5 µmol/L) within 48 hours or a percentage increase of SCr ≤ from baseline which is known or presumed to have occurred within the prior 7 days
- **No response after 2 consecutive days of diuretic withdrawal and plasma volume expansion with albumin (1 g per kg of body weight)**
- **Absence of shock**
- **No current or recent use of nephrotoxic drugs NSAIDs, aminoglycosides, iodinated contrast media, etc.)**
- **No macroscopic signs of structural kidney injury[a] defined as**
- Absence of proteinuria (>500 mg/d)
- Absence of microhematuria (>50 RBCs per high power field)
- Normal finding on ultrasonography

[a]Patients who fulfill these criteria may still have structural damage such as tubular damage.

ICA = International Club of Ascites. AKI = acute kidney injury. NSAIDs = nonsteroidal anti-inflammatory drugs. RBCs = red blood cells.

Source: Angeli P, Gines P, Wong F, et al. Diagnosis and management of acute kidney injury in patients with cirrhosis: revised consensus recommendations of the International Club of Ascites. *J Hepatol.* Apr 2015;62(4):968–974.

disease (e.g., immunoglobin A, membranous or membranoproliferative disease). However, patients with underlying kidney disease can still develop "hepatorenal physiology." As a result, the Acute Dialysis Quality Initiative[2] proposed that the term "hepatorenal disorders" be used to describe all patients with advanced cirrhosis and concurrent kidney dysfunction. Such a definition would allow patients with cirrhosis and renal dysfunction to be properly classified and treated while maintaining the term "hepatorenal syndrome."

PATHOGENESIS

Arterial Vasodilatation Theory

Arterial vasodilatation, a characteristic feature of advanced cirrhosis, plays a central role in HRS (Fig. 40.1).[1] Cirrhosis is characterized by circulatory changes including portal hypertension, splanchnic arterial vasodilatation, decreased systemic vascular resistance (SVR), and increased cardiac output. In early stages of compensated cirrhosis, arterial vasodilatation and decreased SVR are mild. Mild reduction in arterial pressure is balanced by an increase in cardiac output, and renal perfusion is preserved. In more advanced stages of decompensated cirrhosis, splanchnic arterial vasodilatation increases due to increased synthesis of nitric oxide and other mediators. Neoangiogenesis in mesenteric arteries and impaired response to vasoconstrictors may contribute to reduced SVR. As disease severity progresses, the increase in cardiac output can no longer balance arterial vasodilatation and decreased SVR. A state of arterial under filling or effective hypovolemia develops. Effective hypovolemia activates systems responsible for vasoconstriction and salt and water retention, such as the renin–angiotensin system, the sympathetic nervous system, and arginine vasopressin. While these systems help maintain blood pressure, they cause intense renal vasoconstriction with a decrease in renal perfusion and glomerular filtration rate (GFR). These factors eventually lead to HRS.

Kidney Factors

In the kidney, the vasodilatory effects of prostaglandins are protective against the vasoconstrictive effects of the renin–angiotensin system, the sympathetic system, and arginine vasopressin. The levels of both prostaglandin E1 and E2 are increased in patients with ascites, and administration of medications such as nonsteroidal anti-inflammatory drugs, which inhibit prostaglandin synthesis, frequently induce AKI in cirrhosis. Changes in autoregulation of renal blood flow may also play a role in HRS. For a given level of renal perfusion pressure, renal blood flow tends to be lower in patients with advanced cirrhosis compared to patients with compensated cirrhosis. These changes could be related to sympathetic nervous system activity.

Inflammatory Response

There is now evidence that cirrhosis is associated with a chronic inflammatory state that may play a role in circulatory changes and contribute to the development of HRS.[1] In advanced cirrhosis, there is an increase in circulating levels of protein C and proinflammatory cytokines, which parallels with portal hypertension and a hyperkinetic state. Translocation of bacteria or bacterial

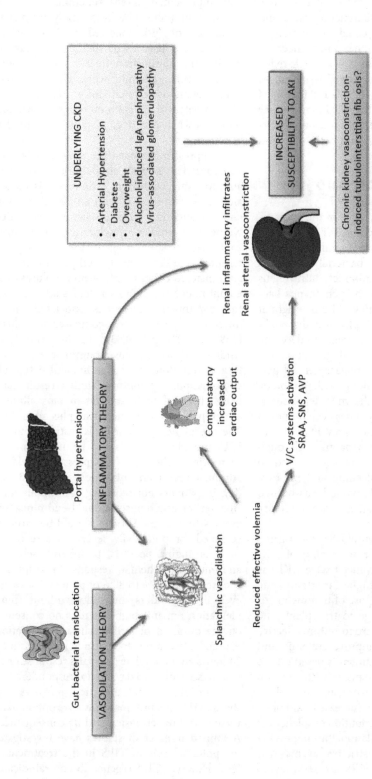

FIGURE 40.1. Mechanisms contributing to impaired kidney function in cirrhosis. In end-stage liver diseases, several factors contribute to increase susceptibility of the kidney to acute kidney injury (AKI). Both vasodilation secondary to portal hypertension and systemic inflammation induced by gut bacterial translocation tend to induce renal arterial vasoconstriction, due to the activation of V/C systems (SRAA, SNS, and AVP) in response to decreased effective blood volume. Intrarenal inflammation induces intrarenal microvascular changes resulting in decreased glomerular filtration rate with an imbalance between preglomerular and postglomerular resistance (which corresponds to both preglomerular and post glomerular vascular tone) as well as impaired renal microcirculation affecting tubular and glomerular function. Underlying CKD due to associated comorbidities eventually increases the risk for AKI. Consequences of prolonged kidney vasoconstriction are not clearly elucidated but may induce tubular interstitial fibrosis and further increase the risk of AKI. AKI = acute kidney injury. CKD = chronic kidney disease. IgA = immunoglobin A. V/C = vasoconstriction. Reproduced with permission from Francoz C, Nadim MK, Durand F. Kidney biomarkers in cirrhosis. *J Hepatol.* 2016;65(4):809–824.

products from the gut lumen to the bloodstream through mesenteric lymph nodes may be one of the mechanisms of inflammatory state and is associated with an increased production of the proinflammatory cytokines tumor necrosis factor-α and interleukin-6 as well as nitric oxide with increased circulatory levels. These changes are associated with decreased SVR and increased cardiac output, suggesting that the inflammatory response may precipitate HRS in advanced cirrhosis by worsening the hyperkinetic state and decreasing renal perfusion.

PREVENTION AND MANAGEMENT

Prevention of HRS is a key issue in the management of patients with end-stage liver disease.[5] Judicious use of diuretics and lactulose to avoid dehydration, spontaneous bacterial peritonitis prophylaxis with daily antibiotics, intravenous albumin use in patients with spontaneous bacterial peritonitis with 1.5 g/kg of body weight at the time of diagnosis and 1 g/kg of body weight at treatment day 3 and in patients undergoing large-volume paracentesis (6–8 g/L of ascitic fluid removed, and prompt replacement of gastrointestinal blood loss, along with antibiotic prophylaxis, have all been shown to decrease the incidence of HRS. Similarly, it has been proposed that N-acetyl-cysteine may prevent HRS in patients with alcoholic hepatitis. Although nonselective beta blockers are widely used to prevent gastrointestinal bleeding and improve survival, they have been shown to be associated with reduced survival in patients with refractory ascites.

The etiology of AKI should be investigated quickly to prevent further worsening of AKI because progression to advanced stage AKI has been associated with a higher mortality rate (Fig. 40.2).[5] The main purpose of treatments for HRS is to provide a bridge to transplant. The first objectives of therapy are to restore effective circulating volume and improve systemic and renal hemodynamics. Treatment is based on the combination of volume expansion with albumin coupled with vasoconstrictive agents. The role of vasoconstrictive agents is to increase blood pressure and to achieve a redistribution of splanchnic blood to the systemic circulation, thus improving renal perfusion. Vasoconstrictive agents that have been used to treat HRS are terlipressin, octreotide plus midodrine, and norepinephrine.[1] Whatever the vasoconstrictive agent that is used,

increasing mean arterial pressure is correlated with improvement in renal function.

Albumin (20%–25%) is generally given at an initial dose of 1 g/kg followed by 20 to 50 g/day. There is no consensus on the optimal duration of albumin administration. It is recommended to discontinue albumin when effective circulating volume is restored and/or SCr decreases. Unfortunately, there is no objective marker that indicates when effective circulating volume has been restored.

Terlipressin has been the most widely used vasoconstrictive agent, although it is not available in some countries. Terlipressin is an analogue of vasopressin with intrinsic systemic and splanchnic vasoconstrictor properties. Numerous studies, including randomized controlled trials, proved the efficacy of terlipressin (Table 40.2). Terlipressin can be administered either as intravenous boluses or as a continuous infusion. A recent study suggests that continuous infusion is associated with a lower rate of side effects compared to boluses (35% vs. 62%, $p < 0.03$).[6] In the majority of studies, terlipressin plus albumin was superior to albumin alone or midodrine and octreotide combination.[7] By contrast, similar results have been observed with terlipressin plus albumin as compared to norepinephrine plus albumin.[8,9] The use of norepinephrine is restricted to the ICU, and adverse events may be more common than with terlipressin. Terlipressin should be administered at an initial dose of 2 to 3 mg/day. In patients not receiving continuous infusion, terlipressin boluses should be administered every 4 to 6 hours. Patients should be carefully screened for potentially severe adverse events such as angina pectoris, peripheral ischemia, and intestinal ischemia. Response to terlipressin is observed in 35% to 80% of patients; however, even in responders, mortality without transplantation remains high. There is no consensus on the duration of terlipressin administration. A practical option is to continue terlipressin for 24 hours after complete or partial response or up to a maximum of 15 days in nonresponders.[6]

Transjugular intrahepatic portosystemic shunt (TIPS) is a minimally invasive option to reverse portal hypertension and its consequences. A limited number of studies have investigated the potential role of TIPS in the treatment of HRS. However, TIPS is generally contraindicated in patients with advanced cirrhosis due to the risk of further deterioration of liver function.

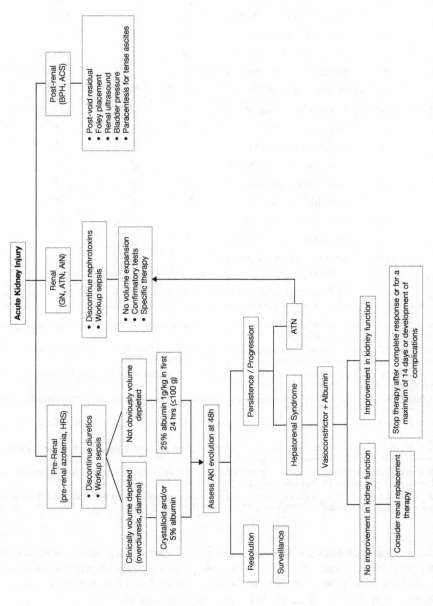

FIGURE 40.2 Algorithm for management of AKI. HRS = hepatorenal syndrome. GN = glomerulonephritis. ATN = acute tubular necrosis. AIN = acute interstitial nephritis. BPH = benign prostatic hypertrophy. ACS = abdominal compartment syndrome. FeNa = fractional excretion of sodium. AKI = acute kidney injury.

Text within figure:

Acute Kidney Injury

Pre-Renal
(pre-renal azotemia, HRS)
- Discontinue diuretics
- Workup sepsis

Renal
(GN, ATN, AIN)
- Discontinue nephrotoxins
- Workup sepsis

- No volume expansion
- Confirmatory tests
- Specific therapy

Post-renal
(BPH, ACS)
- Post-void residual
- Foley placement
- Renal ultrasound
- Bladder pressure
- Paracentesis for tense ascites

Clinically volume depleted
(overdiuresis, diarrhea)

Not obviously volume depleted

Crystalloid and/or
5% albumin

25% albumin 1g/kg in first
24 hrs (≤100 g)

Assess AKI evolution at 48h

Resolution

Surveillance

Persistence / Progression

Hepatorenal Syndrome

ATN

Vasoconstrictor + Albumin

No improvement in kidney function

Improvement in kidney function

Consider renal replacement therapy

Stop therapy after complete response or for a maximum of 14 days or development of complications

TABLE 40.2 RESULTS OF RANDOMIZED STUDIES OF TERLIPRESSIN IN PATIENTS WITH TYPE 1 HEPATORENAL SYNDROME

Author	Year	Treatment	Patients	Hepatorenal Syndrome Reversal (%)	Mortality without Transplantation (%)
Alessandria et al.[a]	2007	Terlipressin + albumin	12	83	90
		Norepinephrine + albumin	10	70	100
Sharma et al.[b]	2008	Terlipressin + albumin	20	50	45
		Norepinephrine + albumin	20	50	45
Sanyal et al.[c]	2008	Terlipressin + albumin	56	34	87
		Placebo + albumin	56	13	91
Martin-Llahi et al.[d]	2008	Terlipressin + albumin	23	43.5	73
		Albumin	23	8.7	81
Singh et al.[e]	2012	Terlipressin + albumin	23	39	61
		Norepinephrine + albumin	23	43	52
Cavallin et al.[f]	2015	Terlipressin + albumin	27	70	41
		Midodrine + albumin	22	29	57
Boyer et al.[g]	2016	Terlipressin + albumin	97	24	42
		Albumin	99	15	46
Cavallin et al.[h]	2016	Terlipressin (continuous) + albumin	37	76	47
		Terlipressin (bolus) + albumin	34	65	31

[a]Alessandria C, Ottobrelli A, Debernardi-Venon W, et al. Noradrenalin vs terlipressin in patients with hepatorenal syndrome: a prospective, randomized, unblinded, pilot study. *J Hepatol.* 2007;47(4):499–505.

[b]Sharma P, Kumar A, Shrama BC, Sarin SK. An open label, pilot, randomized controlled trial of noradrenaline versus terlipressin in the treatment of type 1 hepatorenal syndrome and predictors of response. *Am J Gastroenterol.* 2008;103(7):1689–1697.

[c]Sanyal AJ, Boyer T, Garcia-Tsao G, et al. A randomized, prospective, double-blind, placebo-controlled trial of terlipressin for type 1 hepatorenal syndrome. *Gastroenterology.* 2008;134(5):1360–1368.

[d]Martin-Llahi M, Pepin MN, Guevara M, et al. Terlipressin and albumin vs albumin in patients with cirrhosis and hepatorenal syndrome: a randomized study. *Gastroenterology.* May 2008;134(5):1352–1359.

[e]Singh V, Ghosh S, Singh B, et al. Noradrenaline vs. terlipressin in the treatment of hepatorenal syndrome: a randomized study. *J Hepatol.* 2012;56(6):1293–1298.

[f]Cavallin M, Kamath PS, Merli M, et al. Terlipressin plus albumin versus midodrine and octreotide plus albumin in the treatment of hepatorenal syndrome: A randomized trial. *Hepatology.* 2015;62(2):567–574.

[g]Boyer TD, Sanyal AJ, Wong F, et al. Terlipressin plus albumin is more effective than albumin alone in improving renal function in patients with cirrhosis and hepatorenal syndrome type 1. *Gastroenterology.* 150(7):1579–1589.

[h]Cavallin M, Piano S, Romano A, et al. Terlipressin given by continuous intravenous infusion versus intravenous boluses in the treatment of hepatorenal syndrome: a randomized controlled study. *Hepatology.* Mar 2016;63(3):983–992.

Therefore, most patients with HRS are not suitable candidates for TIPS placement.

Albumin dialysis using the Molecular Adsorbent Recirculating System (MARS®) has been proposed.[1,2,10] It has been suggested that with the addition of albumin in the dialysate, MARS® more efficiently removes substances putatively involved in HRS. In addition, MARS® uses a specific membrane that optimizes removal of circulating toxins and binding to albumin in the dialysate. A very small controlled study[11] has shown a modest survival benefit with MARS® as compared to conventional therapy. In addition, there is no evidence that MARS® is superior to conventional hemofiltration.

The initiation of renal replacement therapy (RRT) should be made on clinical grounds, including electrolyte disturbances (e.g., hyperkalemia or hyponatremia not responding to medical management), metabolic acidosis, oliguria with increasing volume overload, and diuretic resistance or intolerance. The ideal timing for initiation of RRT has not been studied in patients with cirrhosis; however, recent data from AKI studies in critically ill patients without liver disease suggest that early RRT initiation may have a beneficial impact on survival.[12,13] RRT may be required to prevent fluid accumulation and should be considered when patients cannot maintain an even or negative daily fluid balance despite normal urine output. A positive fluid balance is associated with poorer outcomes and may lead to underestimation of the severity of AKI.[14,15] In patients receiving RRT, continuous RRT allows for the slower correction of serum sodium over time and provides greater cardiovascular stability compared to intermittent hemodialysis.

While liver transplantation is the only definitive treatment for HRS, it is clear that patients with renal failure have poorer outcomes than patients without renal failure at the time of transplant. Furthermore, prolonged renal dysfunction pretransplant is associated with worse posttransplant renal recovery, and predicting recovery remains a challenge. Whatever the phenotype of AKI, new tools are needed to facilitate the recovery of renal function after liver transplantation.

PERIOPERATIVE MANAGEMENT OF HRS

The goal of managing HRS in the pretransplant period is to optimize patients for surgery. This optimization often requires RRT to achieve euvolemia and correct electrolyte and metabolic derangements such as hyponatremia, uremia, or acidosis prior to transplant. HRS can worsen the fluid overload and hyponatremia present in patients with advanced cirrhosis, and the uremia and acidosis associated with renal dysfunction can further worsen the hepatic encephalopathy and hemodynamic instability commonly seen in patients with end-stage liver disease. Simultaneous liver–kidney transplantation should be considered when renal failure reflects CKD with GFR $\leq$30 mL/min or AKI with GFR $\leq$25 mL/min with or without dialysis for more than 6 weeks prior to transplant.[16]

The liver transplant operation itself is characterized by major hemodynamic changes, electrolyte and acid-base derangements, and coagulopathy, all of which become even more challenging to manage in patients with HRS who are refractory to standard treatment methods.

Intraoperative RRT offers better control of the patient's physiology by allowing adjustments in intravascular volume, metabolic abnormalities, and body temperature based on hemodynamic changes, biochemistry profiles, and arterial blood gas results. Large-volume fluid resuscitation and blood product administration in response to intraoperative hemodynamic instability, bleeding, and coagulopathy can exacerbate hypervolemia, hyperkalemia, hypothermia, and associated complications, particularly in patients with HRS.[17] Several studies have shown that intraoperative RRT is feasible and safe, suggesting that intraoperative RRT may facilitate the management and recovery of critically ill patients with HRS who undergo liver transplantation.[18,19]

In the posttransplant period, prolonged hypotension, infection, reoperation, and nephrotoxic medications for immunosuppression increase the risk of persistent renal dysfunction in patients with HRS prior to transplant.[20] Any degree of renal dysfunction after liver transplantation portends poor long-term survival and is associated with increased rates of acute rejection and infection, longer ICU stays, greater hospital costs, and increased mortality. Strategies to optimize pretransplant renal function are paramount to ensure favorable postoperative outcomes for patients with HRS undergoing liver transplant.

Predicting the recovery of impaired renal function and the extent of that recovery after liver transplantation is a challenge. The treatment of choice for patients with type 1 HRS is liver transplantation, and, theoretically, renal function is fully reversible posttransplant. However, several reports have shown that the mean SCr after liver transplantation is higher in patients with HRS pretransplant compared to patients without HRS pretransplant. Finding novel ways to identify the etiology of AKI in patients with cirrhosis is important, as the potential for renal recovery and long-term survival depend on the etiology of renal dysfunction. A recent study revealed that renal recovery and patient survival 1 and 5 years after liver transplant were significantly worse for patients with renal dysfunction secondary to acute tubular necrosis (ATN).[21] However, it remains difficult to delineate the relative contributions of pre-existing comorbidities, unrecognized intrinsic renal disease, perioperative events, and posttransplant immunosuppression to renal dysfunction after liver transplant.

ROLE OF BIOMARKERS

In theory, patients with HRS do not have underlying chronic kidney changes. However, a series of cirrhotic patients who had transvenous kidney biopsies has shown that various glomerular, interstitial, or vascular lesions could be observed in patients meeting the diagnostic criteria for HRS. Finally, prolonged vasoconstriction during HRS may promote inflammation and fibrosis as shown in experimental models. Diagnostic tools are needed to differentiate HRS from other phenotypes of AKI in cirrhosis because therapeutic approaches are different. Diagnostic tools are also needed to predict reversibility of HRS after liver transplantation. The diagnosis of HRS is based on simple clinical and laboratory criteria.[3] However, a clinical diagnosis of HRS does not exclude associated structural changes, in particular, ATN. Several studies were aimed at comparing HRS and ATN in cirrhosis. However, none of these studies included a gold standard (histology) for the diagnosis of ATN. A diagnosis of ATN remains difficult to establish in patients with cirrhosis and acutely impaired renal function. Rather than 2 distinct entities, HRS and ATN may be considered a continuum. Several recent studies have shown that some urine biomarkers, such as neutrophil gelatinase-associated lipocalin (NGAL), interleukin-18, urine microalbuminuria, or fractional excretion of sodium may be helpful in the differential diagnosis.[22]

NGAL is secreted into urine by tubular cells. In patients without cirrhosis, ATN is characterized by a higher increase in urinary NGAL as compared to prerenal azotemia or CKD. In patients with cirrhosis, urinary NGAL is also significantly higher in patients with a clinical diagnosis of ATN than in patients with HRS or CKD. Urinary NGAL is higher in patients with persistent AKI than in patients with transient AKI. Finally, urinary NGAL is predictive of early mortality in patients with cirrhosis and AKI. Although novel and interesting, NGAL has some limitations and must be interpreted with caution. Urinary NGAL is increased during acute or chronic inflammation and CKD. Therefore, interpretation of NGAL is more difficult to interpret when HRS is associated with sepsis. Secondly, even if on average, urinary NGAL is higher in ATN, clinical studies have shown a significant overlap in urinary NGAL values between ATN and HRS patients. Finally, measurement of urinary NGAL is obviously impossible in patients with anuria.

In patients with cirrhosis, significantly higher urinary levels of interleukin-18 have been observed in ATN as compared to other phenotypes. However, there is also an important overlap between ATN and non-ATN patients with no threshold value to definitely identify ATN. Other biomarkers including kidney injury molecule 1, liver-type fatty acid binding protein, and osteopontin have also been tested to differentiate ATN from other phenotypes of AKI or CKD. Combinations of biomarkers are possibly more attractive than a single marker. A recent study suggests that the combination of elevated plasma (not urinary) osteopontin and tissue inhibitor of metalloproteinase 1 levels, age <57 years, and absence of diabetes pretransplantation has a good accuracy to differentiate reversible from irreversible AKI posttransplantation.

CONCLUSION

HRS is one phenotype of AKI in patients with end-stage liver disease. Its definition is based on both clinical and laboratory criteria, and early diagnosis is essential to initiate vasopressors in combination with albumin resuscitation. Novel biomarkers may help differentiate HRS from ATN, which does not justify vasopressors. Reversal of HRS can be achieved in more than 50% of patients receiving terlipressin. However, even in responders to terlipressin, life expectancy is limited, and liver transplantation is the only definitive cure for HRS. Impaired renal function may not fully recover after liver transplantation as a consequence of underlying chronic kidney changes or irreversible changes induced by persistent kidney hypoperfusion. Systemic inflammation plays a role in the occurrence of HRS as well as in response to therapy. Therapeutic interventions aimed at controlling the inflammatory response may help prevent the occurrence of HRS.

REFERENCES

1. Durand F, Graupera I, Gines P, Olson JC, Nadim MK. Pathogenesis of Hepatorenal Syndrome: Implications for Therapy. *Am J Kidney Dis.* 2016;67(2):318–328.
2. Nadim MK, Kellum JA, Davenport A, et al. Hepatorenal syndrome: the 8th International Consensus Conference of the Acute Dialysis Quality Initiative (ADQI) Group. *Crit Care.* 2012;16(1):R23.

3. Angeli P, Gines P, Wong F, et al. Diagnosis and management of acute kidney injury in patients with cirrhosis: revised consensus recommendations of the International Club of Ascites. *J Hepatol.* Apr 2015;62(4):968–974.

4. Kellum JA, Sileanu FE, Murugan R, Lucko N, Shaw AD, Clermont G. Classifying AKI by urine output versus serum creatinine level. *J Am Soc Nephrol.* 2015;26(9):2231–2238.

5. O'Leary JG, Levitsky J, Wong F, Nadim MK, Charlton M, Kim WR. Protecting the kidney in liver transplant candidates practice-based recommendations from the American Society of Transplantation Liver and Intestine Community of Practice. *Am J Transplant.* 2016;20:1–16.

6. Cavallin M, Piano S, Romano A, et al. Terlipressin given by continuous intravenous infusion versus intravenous boluses in the treatment of hepatorenal syndrome: a randomized controlled study. *Hepatology.* Mar 2016;63(3):983–992.

7. Cavallin M, Kamath PS, Merli M, et al. Terlipressin plus albumin versus midodrine and octreotide plus albumin in the treatment of hepatorenal syndrome: A randomized trial. *Hepatology.* 2015;62(2):567–574.

8. Sharma P, Kumar A, Shrama BC, Sarin SK. An open label, pilot, randomized controlled trial of noradrenaline versus terlipressin in the treatment of type 1 hepatorenal syndrome and predictors of response. *Am J Gastroenterol.* 2008;103(7):1689–1697.

9. Singh V, Ghosh S, Singh B, et al. Noradrenaline vs. terlipressin in the treatment of hepatorenal syndrome: a randomized study. *J Hepatol.* 2012;56(6):1293–1298.

10. Karvellas CJ, Durand F, Nadim MK. Acute Kidney Injury in Cirrhosis. *Critical Care Clinics.* 2015;31(4):737–750.

11. Mitzner SR, Stange J, Klammt S, et al. Improvement of hepatorenal syndrome with extracorporeal albumin dialysis MARS: results of a prospective, randomized, controlled clinical trial. *Liver Transpl.* 2000;6(3):277–286.

12. Zarbock A, Kellum JA, Schmidt C, et al. Effect of early vs delayed initiation of renal replacement therapy on mortality in critically ill patients with acute kidney injury: The ELAIN randomized clinical trial. *J Am Med Assoc.* 2016;315(20):2190–2199.

13. Gaudry S, Hajage D, Schortgen F, et al. Initiation strategies for renal-replacement therapy in the intensive care unit. *N Engl J Med.* 2016;375:122–133.

14. Liu KD, Thompson BT, Ancukiewicz M, et al. Acute kidney injury in patients with acute lung injury: impact of fluid accumulation on classification of acute kidney injury and associated outcomes. *Crit Care Med.* 2011;39(12):2665–2671.

15. Nadim MK, Durand F, Kellum JA, et al. Management of the critically ill patient with cirrhosis: a multidisciplinary perspective. *J Hepatol.* 2016;64(3):717–735.

16. Formica RN, Aeder M, Boyle G, et al. Simultaneous liver–kidney allocation policy: a proposal to optimize appropriate utilization of scarce resources. *Am J Transplant.* 2016;16(3):758–766.

17. Sedra AH, Strum E. The role of intraoperative hemodialysis in liver transplant patients. *Curr Opin Organ Transplant.* 2011;16(3):323–325.

18. Nadim MK, Annanthapanyasut W, Matsuoka L, et al. Intraoperative hemodialysis during liver transplantation: a decade of experience. *Liver Transplant.* 2014;20(7):756–764.

19. Agopian VG, Dhillon A, Baber J, et al. Liver transplantation in recipients receiving renal replacement therapy: outcomes analysis and the role of intraoperative hemodialysis. *Am J Transplant.* 2014;14(7):1638–1647.

20. Levitsky J, O'Leary JG, Asrani S, et al. Protecting the kidney in liver transplant recipients: practice-based recommendations from the American Society of Transplantation Liver and Intestine Community of Practice. *Am J Transplant.* 2016;16(9):2532–2544.

21. Nadim MK, Genyk YS, Tokin C, et al. Impact of the etiology of acute kidney injury on outcomes following liver transplantation: acute tubular necrosis versus hepatorenal syndrome. *Liver Transplant.* 2012;18(5):539–548.

22. Francoz C, Nadim MK, Durand F. Kidney biomarkers in cirrhosis. *J Hepatol.* 2016;65(4):809–824.

41

Cardiorenal Syndrome

EDWARD A. ROSS, UYANGA BATNYAM, AND ABDO M. ASMAR

INTRODUCTION

Cardiac and renal impairment may coexist, or one may worsen or exacerbate the other's function. When both organs are impaired, it is referred to as cardiorenal syndrome (CRS). Subclassifications were proposed by Ronco et al.[1] based on the primary organ involved and the acuity of onset, which is of relevance in that strategies for renal protection may need to focus on the kidney or system disorders rather than on just the cardiac condition.

Poor cardiac function leads to decreased forward pump, backward pressure build-up, decreased renal perfusion, renal ischemia, and neurohumoral activation, thereby causing worsening of renal function. A vicious cycle occurs in that renal impairment causes activation of neurohumoral and inflammatory pathway and sodium and water retention, thereby causing systemic congestion, hypertension, vascular and myocardial calcification, accelerated atherosclerosis, and, eventually, cardiac dysfunction. Both chronic kidney disease (CKD) and heart failure (HF) are a major public health problem and a global burden. It is associated with poor quality of life, high healthcare expenditures, and high morbidity and mortality rates. In a large meta-analysis[2] that included over 1 million patients with HF, the overall prevalence of CKD was 49%, and it was associated with significantly higher mortality rate (hazard ratio = 2.43%) as compared to patients with HF alone. According to the Acute Decompensated Heart Failure National Registry (ADHERE)[3] data from 118,465 patient with acute decompensated HF (ADHF) hospitalization, only 9% patients had normal renal function, 27.4% had CKD stage 2, 57% had CKD stage 3 or 4, and 7% had ESRD. The mortality rate was also significantly high in patients with concomitant renal impairment. We have much improved understanding of the pathophysiology of this syndrome; however, the exact mechanisms for organ crosstalk are still not completely validated.

PATHOPHYSIOLOGY

Neurohumoral Derangement

The interaction between the kidneys and the heart plays an important role in hemodynamic stability. The underlying pathophysiologic mechanism of CRS differs depending on the acuity and degree of renal impairment and whether there is preserved or reduced ejection fraction (Fig. 41.1). Renal impairment causes salt and water retention with subsequent neurohumoral activation, systemic congestion, arterial hypertension, activation of inflammatory cascades, and vascular and myocardial calcification due to alteration in mineral homeostasis thereby causing cardiac remodeling and accelerated atherosclerosis. HF with reduced ejection fraction (HFrEF) leads to decreased forward flow with subsequent decrease in renal perfusion, renal ischemia and progressive CKD. Angiotensin II (AT II) and aldosterone increase renal tubular sodium and water reabsorption, and with the decreased concentration of sodium and water in distal tubules, aldosterone sensitivity in distal nephrons will further increase. As disease progresses, chronic poor forward flow, sodium and water retention from secondary hyperaldosteronism, and systemic venous congestion progressively worsens, increases preload, and causes more stretch on cardiac myocytes. By Frank-Starling mechanisms, cardiac stroke volume further decreases, and the renin–angiotensin–aldosterone system (RAAS) and sympathetic nervous system (SNS) remain chronically activated. Catecholamines, renin, and angiotensin II cause vasoconstriction and increase systemic vascular resistance and

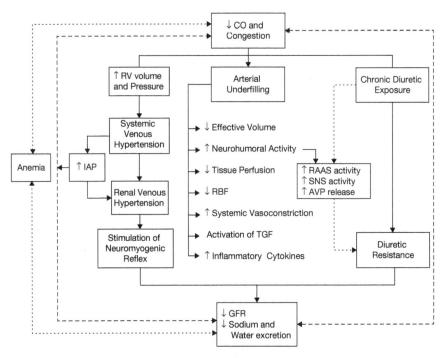

FIGURE 41.1   Pathophysiologic mechanisms of Cardiorenal Syndrome.

CO = carbon dioxide. RV = right ventricle. IAP = intra arterial pressure. RAAS = renal angiotensin aldosterone system. RBF = renal blood flow. TGF = tubuloglomerular feedback. GFR = glomerular filtration rate. SNS = sympathetic nervous system. AVP = arginine vasopressin.

afterload, which is counterproductive in already malfunctioning cardiac pump.

Venous Congestion

Association between renal impairment and venous congestion has increasingly been emphasized, and it is more evident in HF with preserved ejection fraction or right-side predominant HF. Studies have failed to consistently confirm traditionally hypothesized association between forward pump failure and renal dysfunction, highlighting alternate mechanisms. According to the data from ADHERE registry, renal impairment was not associated with decreased left ventricular (LV) function.[4] In the ESCAPE trial,[5] renal dysfunction had a closer relationship with right atrial pressure than cardiac index. Another retrospective analysis demonstrated that renal dysfunction was closely related to elevated central venous pressure but not cardiac index and that central venous pressure was a better mortality predictor.[6] Venous hypertension causes decreased renal arterial flow by affecting renal autoregulation through a myogenic response (vasoconstriction is medicated by increased wall tension in the vascular wall), tubuloglomerular feedback (TGF; increased

delivery of solutes in macula densa causes afferent vasoconstriction), and by neurohumoral mechanisms (RAAS and SNS).[7] Renal venous congestion increases the intracapsular pressure within the kidneys, and without the capacity for further distention, the congestion within the renal capsule causes interstitial hypertension and possible local hypoxia.[8] Congested veins may compress renal tubules, causing decreased transglomerular pressure and collapsed tubules; it may even cause tubulointerstitial fibrosis.

Renal venous congestion and renal arteriolar vasoconstriction results in decreased arterial-to-venous pressure gradient thence decreased glomerular filtration rate (GFR). Decreased renal perfusion and decreased GFR further trigger renal autoregulation and neurohumoral response that is already maladaptive in HF patients. In a recent study,[9] almost one-third of patients with clinical HF had no acute weight gain, and multiple studies have shown clinical improvement of HF without change in weight or net fluid loss.[10] This has been explained by alterations in venous capacitance. Venous system is heavily innervated by adrenergic receptors, has far more compliance than arterial system, and contains approximately 70% of the circulatory volume.[10] Venous compliance is affected by SNS activation, and with venous vasoconstriction, the venous reservoir is shifted to the effective circulatory volume and thus decompensates HF without change in total body fluid. Venous congestion, renal ischemia, neurohumoral activation, and myocardial and venous endothelial stretching triggers the activation of immune cells and increases the levels of circulating cytokines such as tumor necrosis factor, interleukin-6 and fibroblast growth factor-23.[11–14]

Diuretic Resistance

With chronic exposure to diuretics, patients may develop unsatisfactory natriuresis and progressively worsening systemic congestion despite escalading dose of diuretics. Underlying mechanisms include diuretics that stimulate RAAS and SNS and can also upregulate the $Na^+/K^+/2Cl^-$ cotransporter in the loop of Henle. Persistent high concentration of sodium delivery to the distal convoluted tubules from chronic loop diuretic exposure stimulates and causes cellular hypertrophy and hyperplasia, thereby increasing sodium reabsorption in the distal convoluted tubules that can be deleterious to the natriuresis achieved with loop diuretics. With the development of CKD, especially in patients with hypoalbuminemia and proteinuria, the delivery of loop diuretics to the site of action will be decreased due to poor transporter availability (albumin).

Tubuloglomerular Feedback and Adenosine Mediators

TGF is a mechanism to maintain NaCl homeostasis by sensing its concentration at the macula densa and adjust glomerular vasomotor tone to adjust NaCl excretion. There are multiple mediators that are associated with afferent vasoconstriction, and the most potent include adenosine (through the A1 receptor), thromboxane, and superoxide. Vasodilation is mediated by nitric oxide, carbon monoxide, kinins, and adenosine (A2 receptor).[15] The A1 receptor has been well-studied because its antagonism could theoretically cause afferent vasodilation and thereby potentiate diuresis and improve systemic congestion in CRS.

Anemia

Anemia in CRS can be caused by alteration of effective erythropoiesis and iron metabolism due to inflammatory pathways and increased hepcidin production and erythropoietin deficiency/insensitivity and due to hemodilution from systemic congestion. Anemia, cardiac, and renal impairment have close interaction, and the triad causes a vicious cycle, resulting in worsening disease severity, morbidity, and mortality, as well as explaining how iron deficiency was found to be associated with reduced exercise capacity in HF patients.

PREVENTION, TREATMENT, AND MANAGEMENT CONSIDERATIONS

The management of CRS is challenging due to its complex organ interaction; therefore, prevention should start from the early diagnosis of either heart or kidney dysfunction. Outpatient monitoring of HF patients with daily weight and urine output and limiting daily salt and water intake are important measures for preventing CRS and hospitalization. Outpatient wireless pulmonary artery hemodynamic monitoring has shown to be effective to decrease HF hospitalization in CHAMPION trial[16] and also had a good safety profile in renal failure patients. Utilizing natriuretic peptide (B-type natriuretic peptide) levels to screen patients at high risk for HF development is recommended by one of the most recent clinical guidelines[17] and may thus be a good tool to diagnose and treat early HF, thereby preventing CRS.

It is important to identify and treat precipitating events such as myocardial ischemia, arrhythmia, abnormalities of heart valves or pericardium, use of nephrotoxic medications, and urinary tract obstruction and infection. Patients with chronic HF should be optimized using guideline-directed medical therapy, and nephrotoxic medication should be avoided. Drug-induced hypotension or renal dysfunction commonly limit pharmacological treatments, and, hence, close monitoring is needed. Angiotensin converting enzyme inhibitors (ACEIs), angiotensin receptor blockers (ARBs) and beta blockers should be escalated to maximum tolerated evidence based doses. For HF patients with New York Heart Association (NYHA) class >II with estimated GFR >30 mL/min and K^+<5.0 meq/L, aldosterone antagonists should be considered, and if tolerating ACEI or ARB, the clinician may consider switching to combined ARB–neprilysin inhibition.[17] For NYHA classes II to IV African American HF patients, there is evidence that the combination of hydralazine and nitrate offers benefit. If heart rate is >70 bpm despite maximum beta-blockade dosing, then ivabradine, a sinoatrial nodal Na^+-K^+ inward current blocker can be considered.[17]

Loop diuretics are associated with symptomatic improvement but no mortality benefit in chronic settings. However, close hemodynamic monitoring and early escalation of diuretic doses in the case of increased systemic congestion is associated with decreased HF hospitalization. For management of acute decompensated CRS, clinician should consider patients' previous exposure to diuretics and tailor the treatment depending on the degree of fluid overload. Most patients respond to a step-up pharmacological approach, which will be further discussed.

Pharmacological Management
Diuretics

Loop diuretics remain the first-line treatment for ADHF. The intravenous route is usually preferred if possible and early administration of a loop diuretic is associated with better outcome. Depending on the patient's response, the diuretic dose may need to be escalated or administered more frequently, especially true in those who are chronically on high doses. Some patients with diuretic resistance may need additional long-acting thiazide diuretic administration to potentiate and help maintaining natriuresis.[18]

Mild worsening of renal function laboratory parameters is tolerated with aggressive diuresis to achieve clinical cardiac compensation. It can be a reflection of hemoconcentration if intravascular volume loss outpaces refill from the extravascular volume, which results in an elevated serum creatinine concentration. Growing evidence suggest that treatment-induced transient rise in serum creatinine is associated with better outcome.[19,20] In contrast, persistently worsening renal function may suggest poor outcome, and close monitoring is required.

Continuous administration of loop diuretics (such as furosemide 5–40 mg/h) can be used in diuretic resistant patients; however, there was no superiority when it was compared with intermittent bolus dose in the DOSE trial.[21] There was only transient worsening of renal function without long-term poor outcome in higher dose diuretics as compared to lower dose in this study, and no superiority observed in either approach.[21] In contrast, Eshaghian et al.[22] demonstrated direct dose-dependent all-cause mortality (mean diuretic dose 98 mg in survivors vs. 140 mg in nonsurvivors, $p < 0.0001$) in ADHF patients independent of baseline renal function. Stepped up pharmacological intervention was associated with better clinical outcome in HF patients with

concomitant renal dysfunction in CARRES-HF tiral.[23] Stepped pharmacological care for acute decompensation includes an assessment of the clinical response to intravenous diuretics and the addition of vasodilators and inotropes based on a set algorithm.

Renin–Angiotensin–Aldosterone System Antagonist

Mild elevation of serum creatinine (<0.5 mg/dL) after initiation of ACEIs can be a reflection of intrarenal hemodynamic change rather than a true worsening of renal function[24] and not necessarily indicate poor clinical outcome. In multiple clinical studies, a mild rise in serum creatinine level was associated with long-term preservation of renal function and maintenance of the cardiovascular benefit despite an apparent worsening of baseline renal function laboratory parameters.[25,26] ACEIs might also be beneficial by blocking diuretic induced RAAS activation, thereby ameliorating diuretic resistance. Patients with advanced CKD, however, may develop significant worsening of renal function with diuresis; ACEIs/ARBs dosage may need to be temporarily decreased or even stopped. Aldosterone blockade also had mortality benefits despite causing an early decline in GFR.[27,28] As long as there is no persistent worsening renal function or severe hyperkalemia (K >5.6 mmol/L), RAAS-blockades should be continued. Patient should be evaluated for renal artery stenosis if extreme intolerance to ACEI or ARB is observed.

Vasodilators

Vasodilators are commonly used in the treatment of patients with ADHF. They have arterial and venodilatory effects, decrease preload and afterload, and augment cardiac output. Although vasodilators are commonly used in clinical practice, data showing improved renal outcomes are lacking and are conflicting in regard to overall benefit.[29-32] Nesiritide, a recombinant B-type natriuretic peptide, was initially approved for acute, decompensated HF due to its cardiac benefit, but subsequent studies showed poor renal outcomes. A large ($N = 7,141$) multicenter clinical trial—Acute Study of Clinical Effectiveness of Nesiritide in Decompensated Heart Failure,[31] however, failed to show its beneficial effect over placebo. The rates of worsening renal function, defined by more than a 25% decrease in the estimated GFR, were not different between the groups.

Neprilysin Inhibitors

Neprilysin is a neutral endopeptidase that degrades several endogenous vasoactive peptides, including natriuretic peptides, bradykinin, and adrenomedullin. With the goal of increasing the serum level of natriuretic peptide in HF patients, omapatrilat, an inhibitor of both neprilysin and ACEIs was developed. It was associated with improved short-term outcomes and reverse cardiac remodeling as compared with an ACEI alone in the IMPRESS,[33] OVERTURE,[34] and OCTAVE trials.[35] Unfortunately, it was associated with severe angioedema due to related effects on bradykinin degradation. A newer drug was developed to minimize bradykinin effects, and the combination of angioedema and an angiotensin receptor neprilysin inhibitor (sacubitril/valsartan) was compared with an ACEI alone in PARADIGM-HF trial[36] in patients with HFrEF (ejection fraction <35%). The study was terminated early due to the overwhelming benefit with the study drug. Sacubitril/valsartan was associated with 21% reduced risk for hospitalization and decreased symptoms and physical limitations of HF.[37] In patients with chronic symptomatic HFrEF with NYHA class II or III who tolerate ACEIs or ARBs, angiotensin receptor neprilysin inhibitors are recommended to further reduce morbidity and mortality (American College of Cardiology/American Heart Association 2017 update, class IB-R recommendation).[17]

Sympathetic Nervous System Inhibition

Use of beta-adrenergic blockers has proven mortality benefit in multiple large trials in patients with HF and is often well-tolerated even in many patients with renal impairment.[38,39] Notably, in patients with ADHF and low stroke volume, tachycardia acts as a compensatory mechanism to augment cardiac output, and blocking such compensatory system may further deteriorate cardiac output and thus increase the risk of acute cardiogenic shock, which can lead to the worsening of renal function. Initiation of beta blockers is thus not recommended during the acute state.

Adenosine A1 Receptor Inhibitors

Adenosine levels are elevated in HF patients and have shown correlation with the severity of chronic HF.[40] As previously discussed, adenosine A1 receptors (A1R) are associated with afferent arteriolar vasoconstriction, increased sodium reabsorption in proximal tubules, and decreased GFR in HF patients. To block such an effect, a new A1R blocker (BG9719) was developed, and it has shown favorable outcomes by increasing urine output in cardiorenal patients,[41] while another A1R blocker (rolofylline; PROTECT trial)[42] showed no clinical benefit and was associated with more side effects. Currently, another novel adenosine A1R antagonist is under clinical investigation.

Inotropes

Intravenous inotropic agents such as milrinone, dobutamine, and dopamine are mainly used in cardiogenic shock. Inotropic agents might help patients with acute exacerbation of HFrEF. Given the lack of proven clinical benefit, its use should be reserved for patients who have poor clinical response to intravenous diuretics and vasodilators as a stepped up pharmacological approach.[23]

Treatment of Anemia

Definitive data on anemia treatment guidelines in CRS patient is lacking. Although iron supplement and erythropoietin-stimulating agents are broadly used in CKD management, there are inconsistent findings in HF patients. Intravenous iron infusion was associated with improved functional capacity and LV ejection fraction (LVEF) but showed no significant mortality benefit in a meta-analysis[43] that included 5 randomized controlled trials. In contrast, erythropoietin use is a class III recommendation in HF patients[17] due to its lack of benefit and increased adverse events that were seen in a large clinical trial.[44]

Nonpharmacological Approach for Salt and Fluid Removal

Nonpharmacological salt and fluid removal can theoretically possibly be advantageous over pharmacological treatments by virtue of proposed mechanisms of attenuated stimulation of the RAAS or SNS, avoidance of TGF, and the ability to carefully adjust fluid removal; however, the current literature has not shown a consistent benefit from this approach, and there can be serious adverse events from these interventional procedures. Thus, these approaches have not been adopted as a standard of care and are usually reserved for patients who are refractory to pharmacological treatments.

Paracentesis

Patients with fluid overload may have elevated intra-abdominal pressure due to the development of ascites, interstitial edema, splanchnic congestion, and renal venous hypertension, which can contribute to impaired renal function.[45] Mechanical fluid and thus salt removal with paracentesis had favorable renal outcome in HF patients.[46] However, it usually causes significant amount of protein loss and can predispose patients to infection. Paracentesis might be useful in selected patients with ascites and decompensated HF who fail to respond to standard therapy.

Intracorporal Ultrafiltration (Peritoneal Dialysis)

Peritoneal dialysis (PD) is generally used as a chronic treatment while extracorporeal ultrafiltration (UF) and step-up medical management are more commonly applied in acute settings of CRS. PD will not only effectively remove excessive sodium and fluid, it could potentially improve kidney function by decreasing intra-abdominal pressure.[46] Although the current literature describes favorable outcomes with PD in cardiorenal patients, it has confounding factors such as different stages of underlying CKD in the study participants and the use of hemodialysis therapy as an initial care in some patients. PD was associated with significant decreases in hospitalization days (6.30 vs. 1.22 days/year; $p = 0.0001$), improvement in LVEF (34.78 vs. 38.86%; $p = 0.0013$), and significant reduction in body weight (73.37 vs. 69.71 kg; $p = 0.0006$) but no statistically significant difference observed in GFR (24.89 vs. 21.88 mL/min; $p = 0.1065$) in a recent meta-analysis included 673 refractory HF patients,[47] and the mean incidence of peritonitis was 14.5% per year (note that only half of the study population had data on peritonitis). PD has not shown mortality benefit (from a mean mortality rate of 20.3% per year) in the setting of ADHF, but it can be used in refractory decompensated HF to improve the quality of life and to decrease hospitalization duration. Possible adverse outcomes when using PD as an acute therapy includes infection, catheter leakage, and electrolyte disturbances.

Extracorporeal Ultrafiltration

Extracorporeal UF has several proposed advantages over diuretics such as attenuation of neurohumoral activation, potential to remove more sodium (e.g., from fluid that is isotonic not hypotonic as in that from diuresis), and predictable fluid removal. UF was also found to decrease the levels of plasma renin, aldosterone, and norepinephrine soon after the UF as compared with diuretics.[48] Renal benefits of UF are mostly observed in HF patients with low urine output.[48] In patients who have preserved diuretic response and preserved GFR (mean GFR ~ 48 mL/min), there was no significant difference between intravenous diuretics as compared to UF.[49]

Isolated UF or traditional dialysis can be used in cardiorenal patients and temporary catheter access can be achieved in acute settings. During acute decompensation of HF, patients often do not tolerate large amounts or rates of fluid removal (> ~2L) due to low blood pressure. UF causes rapid variation of effective intravascular volume in the absence of proper neurohumoral balance; thus, hypotension or even shock could occur.[50] The rate of UF should not exceed the rate of which the interstitial fluid refills the intravascular component to avoid hypovolemia and hypotension, which can be counterproductive for renal function due to decreased renal perfusion, thereby renal injury. Determining a safe rate is difficult, and a wide range has been used by clinicians and in trials, often the range of 75 to 500 mL/h by the clinician, and the rate commonly used in current practice is approximately 250 mL/h.[51] In one study, UF rates >10 mL/Kg/h were associated with greater mortality among patients on hemodialysis.[52] Advances in technology also allow for the monitoring of hemoconcentration by optic sensor, which may help in guiding the UF therapy.

Despite having extensive experience with UF and the many studies that have been conducted to date, the clinical outcome data for UF in cardiorenal patients are still conflicting. When comparing early UF versus usual care in patients hospitalized for AHDF in the RAPID-CHF trial,[53] the UF group had greater fluid removal yet had no statistically significant difference in weight loss at 24 hours or symptomatic improvement. In contrast, a study by Costanzo et al.[54] used early UF (within 4.7±3.5 hours of hospitalization) before the initiation of intravenous diuretics in ADHF patients, and it showed decreased weight and symptomatic improvement that persisted to 90 days follow-up. Although that preliminary study result was promising, it lacked s randomized cohort. The investigators conducted another randomized controlled trial (UNLOAD),[55] where 200 patients with ADHF were randomized to UF group or intravenous loop diuretic group. The UF group was associated with higher weight (*p* = 0.001) and net fluid loss (*p* = 0.001), fewer rehospitalization for HF (*p* = 0.037), rehospitalization (*p* = 0.022) per patient, and unscheduled visits (*p* = 0.009) at 90 days post hospitalization, but no difference was observed in dyspnea score or serum creatinine levels. CARRESS-HF,[23] a large multicenter, prospective clinical trial, compared continuous venovenous UF versus stepped pharmacological therapy in 188 ADHF patients with worsening renal function. Stepped pharmacological treatment with escalating dose of intravenous diuretics with added vasodilators or inotropes showed a more favorable outcome as compared with UF alone. The UF arm had more adverse events and worsening of kidney function than in the pharmacological group, and there was no difference in weight change at 96 hours.[23] This was followed by the AVOID-HF[56] trial, which was initially designed to enroll 810 hospitalized HF patients to compare adjustable UF versus adjustable intravenous diuretics. The study was terminated early after enrolling 224 patients due to slower than expected enrollment. Adjustable UF group had greater total amount of fluid removed (18.7 vs. 14.0 L, *p* = 0.015) and net fluid loss (12.9 vs. 8.9 L, *p* = 0.006). Despite the fact that the study only enrolled a fourth of the originally planned sample size, it did show a lower rate of a rehospitalization for HF and length of stay for HF rehospitalization, rehospitalization for CV events and length of stay for CV events, and rehospitalization at 30 days of intervention. There was no change in renal function (GFR, serum creatinine, blood urea nitrogen, and its ratio) at 90 days.

The treatment protocols, treatment comparisons, and patient characteristics in the many UF clinical trials had shortcomings in that the pharmacological and nonpharmacological therapies were quite different and there were confounding factors and adverse events from catheter utilization. Thus, the cardiorenal effects from the slow prolonged removal of sodium and fluid by UF are not totally understood, and if utilized after the failure of stepped pharmacological care protocols, the mode and rate of UF would need to be crafted on case-by-case basis.

Treatments Under Development

Finerenone, a novel nonsteroidal mineralocorticoid receptor antagonist showed similar efficacy to eplerenone in chronic CHF patients with diabetes mellitus and/or CKD,[57] and further

investigation is underway. In regard to nervous system control of renal function and kidney–cardiac interaction, a small pilot study[57] tested for the first-time catheter-based renal denervation in human participants. The study was safe and showed symptomatic improvement with improved exercise tolerance. Larger studies are underway to further investigate its safety and efficacy in CRS patients. Lastly, serelaxin, a recombinant human relaxin-2, was tested in HF patients with CKD in the RELAX-AHF trial.[58] Relaxin-2 is a naturally occurring peptide secreted during pregnancy, and by increasing arterial compliance, cardiac output, and renal blood flow, it regulates maternal adaptations during the pregnancy. Serelaxin improved dyspnea at day 5 and had fewer cardiovascular and all-cause deaths at day 180 when compared to placebo but did not affect hospital readmission.

CONSIDERATIONS IN KIDNEY TRANSPLANTATION

Kidney transplantation was associated with improved outcome with improved LVEF, functional status, and survival independent of pretransplantation LVEF.[59,60]

CONCLUSION

Despite advancements in pharmaceuticals and technology, the treatment of CRS remains challenging, and morbidity and mortality rate remains high. It is important to focus on prevention and treating conventional and modifiable risk factors. Medication compliance should be assessed and treatable triggering conditions should be investigated and treated. Current evidence suggests stepped pharmacotherapy with escalating dose of diuretics along with vasodilators as the first approach over UF in acute decompensated states. The efficacy and role of UF remains undetermined. Future trials should aim to design diagnostic and treatment strategies that help with the early identification and prevention of acute kidney injury in patients presenting with HF.

REFERENCES

1. Ronco C, House AA, Haapio M. Cardiorenal syndrome: refining the definition of a complex symbiosis gone wrong. *Intensive Care Med.* 2008;34(5):957–962.
2. Damman K, Valente MA, Voors AA, O'Connor CM, van Veldhuisen DJ, Hillege HL. Renal impairment, worsening renal function, and outcome

in patients with heart failure: an updated meta-analysis. *Eur Heart J*. 2014;35(7):455–469.

3. DeVore AD, Greiner MA, Sharma PP, et al. Development and validation of a risk model for in-hospital worsening heart failure from the Acute Decompensated Heart Failure National Registry (ADHERE). *Am Heart J*. 2016;178:198–205.

4. Heywood JT, Fonarow GC, Costanzo MR, et al. High prevalence of renal dysfunction and its impact on outcome in 118,465 patients hospitalized with acute decompensated heart failure: a report from the ADHERE database. *J Card Fail*. 2007;13(6):422–430.

5. Nohria A, Hasselblad V, Stebbins A, et al. Cardiorenal interactions: insights from the ESCAPE trial. *J Am Coll Cardiol*. 2008;51(13):1268–1274.

6. Damman K, Voors AA, Hillege HL, et al. Congestion in chronic systolic heart failure is related to renal dysfunction and increased mortality. *Eur J Heart Fail*. 2010;12(9):974–982.

7. Braam B, Cupples WA, Joles JA, Gaillard C. Systemic arterial and venous determinants of renal hemodynamics in congestive heart failure. *Heart Fail Rev*. 2012;17(2):161–175.

8. Ross EA. Congestive renal failure: the pathophysiology and treatment of renal venous hypertension. *J Card Fail*. 2012;18(12):930–938.

9. Bourge RC, Abraham WT, Adamson PB, et al. Randomized controlled trial of an implantable continuous hemodynamic monitor in patients with advanced heart failure: the COMPASS-HF study. *J Am Coll Cardiol*. 2008;51(11):1073–1079.

10. Fallick C, Sobotka PA, Dunlap ME. Sympathetically mediated changes in capacitance: redistribution of the venous reservoir as a cause of decompensation. *Circ Heart Fail*. 2011;4(5):669–675.

11. Colombo PC, Ganda A, Lin J, et al. Inflammatory activation: cardiac, renal, and cardio-renal interactions in patients with the cardiorenal syndrome. *Heart Fail Rev*. 2012;17(2):177–190.

12. Kalra D, Sivasubramanian N, Mann DL. Angiotensin II induces tumor necrosis factor biosynthesis in the adult mammalian heart through a protein kinase C-dependent pathway. *Circulation*. 2002;105(18):2198–2205.

13. Moriyama T, Fujibayashi M, Fujiwara Y, et al. Angiotensin II stimulates interleukin-6 release from cultured mouse mesangial cells. *J Am Soc Nephrol*. 1995;6(1):95–101.

14. Kurosu H, Kuro OM. The Klotho gene family as a regulator of endocrine fibroblast growth factors. *Mol Cell Endocrinol*. 2009;299(1):72–78.

15. Schnermann J. Concurrent activation of multiple vasoactive signaling pathways in vasoconstriction caused by tubuloglomerular feedback: a quantitative assessment. *Annu Rev Physiol*. 2015;77:301–322.

16. Abraham WT, Adamson PB, Bourge RC, et al. Wireless pulmonary artery haemodynamic monitoring in chronic heart failure: a randomised controlled trial. *Lancet*. 2011;377(9766):658–666.

17. Yancy CW, Jessup M, Bozkurt B, et al. 2017 ACC/AHA/HFSA focused update of the 2013 ACCF/AHA guideline for the management of heart failure: a report of the American College of Cardiology/American Heart Association Task Force on Clinical Practice Guidelines and the Heart Failure Society of America. *J Card Fail*. 2017;136(6):e137–e161.

18. Rosenberg J, Gustafsson F, Galatius S, Hildebrandt PR. Combination therapy with metolazone and loop diuretics in outpatients with refractory heart failure: an observational study and review of the literature. *Cardiovasc Drugs Ther*. 2005;19(4):301–306.

19. Aronson D, Burger AJ. The relationship between transient and persistent worsening renal function and mortality in patients with acute decompensated heart failure. *J Card Fail*. 2010;16(7):541–547.

20. Testani JM, Chen J, McCauley BD, Kimmel SE, Shannon RP. Potential effects of aggressive decongestion during the treatment of decompensated heart failure on renal function and survival. *Circulation*. 2010;122(3):265–272.

21. Felker GM, Lee KL, Bull DA, et al. Diuretic strategies in patients with acute decompensated heart failure. *N Engl J Med*. 2011;364(9):797–805.

22. Eshaghian S, Horwich TB, Fonarow GC. Relation of loop diuretic dose to mortality in advanced heart failure. *Am J Cardiol*. 2006;97(12):1759–1764.

23. Bart BA, Goldsmith SR, Lee KL, et al. Ultrafiltration in decompensated heart failure with cardiorenal syndrome. *N Engl J Med*. 2012;367(24):2296–2304.

24. Schoolwerth AC, Sica DA, Ballermann BJ, Wilcox CS, Council on the Kidney in Cardiovascular D, the Council for High Blood Pressure Research of the American Heart Association. Renal considerations in angiotensin converting enzyme inhibitor therapy: a statement for healthcare professionals from the Council on the Kidney in Cardiovascular Disease and the Council for High Blood Pressure Research of the American Heart Association. *Circulation*. 2001;104(16):1985–1991.

25. Testani JM, Kimmel SE, Dries DL, Coca SG. Prognostic importance of early worsening renal function after initiation of angiotensin-converting enzyme inhibitor therapy in patients with cardiac dysfunction. *Circ Heart Fail*. 2011;4(6):685–691.

26. Tokmakova MP, Skali H, Kenchaiah S, et al. Chronic kidney disease, cardiovascular risk, and response to angiotensin-converting enzyme inhibition after myocardial infarction: the Survival And Ventricular Enlargement (SAVE) study. *Circulation.* 2004;110(24):3667–3673.

27. Vardeny O, Wu DH, Desai A, et al. Influence of baseline and worsening renal function on efficacy of spironolactone in patients With severe heart failure: insights from RALES (Randomized Aldactone Evaluation Study). *J Am Coll Cardiol.* 2012;60(20):2082–2089.

28. Eschalier R, McMurray JJ, Swedberg K, et al. Safety and efficacy of eplerenone in patients at high risk for hyperkalemia and/ or worsening renal function: analyses of the EMPHASIS-HF study subgroups (Eplerenone in Mild Patients Hospitalization And SurvIval Study in Heart Failure). *J Am Coll Cardiol.* 2013;62(17):1585–1593.

29. Publication Committee for the VMAC Investigators (Vasodilatation in the Management of Acute CHF). Intravenous nesiritide vs nitroglycerin for treatment of decompensated congestive heart failure: a randomized controlled trial. *J Am Med Assoc.* 2002;287(12):1531–1540.

30. Abraham WT, Adams KF, Fonarow GC, et al. In-hospital mortality in patients with acute decompensated heart failure requiring intravenous vasoactive medications: an analysis from the Acute Decompensated Heart Failure National Registry (ADHERE). *J Am Coll Cardiol.* 2005;46(1):57–64.

31. O'Connor CM, Starling RC, Hernandez AF, et al. Effect of nesiritide in patients with acute decompensated heart failure. *N Engl J Med.* 2011;365(1):32–43.

32. Chen HH, Anstrom KJ, Givertz MM, et al. Low-dose dopamine or low-dose nesiritide in acute heart failure with renal dysfunction: the ROSE acute heart failure randomized trial. *J Am Med Assoc.* 2013;310(23):2533–2543.

33. Kostis JB, Packer M, Black HR, Schmieder R, Henry D, Levy E. Omapatrilat and enalapril in patients with hypertension: the Omapatrilat Cardiovascular Treatment vs. Enalapril (OCTAVE) trial. *Am J Hypertens.* 2004;17(2):103–111.

34. Solomon SD, Skali H, Bourgoun M, et al. Effect of angiotensin-converting enzyme or vasopeptidase inhibition on ventricular size and function in patients with heart failure: the Omapatrilat Versus Enalapril Randomized Trial of Utility in Reducing Events (OVERTURE) echocardiographic study. *Am Heart J.* 2005;150(2):257–262.

35. Rouleau JL, Pfeffer MA, Stewart DJ, et al. Comparison of vasopeptidase inhibitor, omapatrilat, and lisinopril on exercise tolerance and morbidity in patients with heart failure: IMPRESS randomised trial. *Lancet.* 2000;356(9230):615–620.

36. McMurray JJ, Packer M, Desai AS, et al. Angiotensin-neprilysin inhibition versus enalapril in heart failure. *N Engl J Med.* 2014;371(11):993–1004.

37. McMurray J, Packer M, Desai A, et al. A putative placebo analysis of the effects of LCZ696 on clinical outcomes in heart failure. *Eur Heart J.* 2015;36(7):434–439.

38. Castagno D, Jhund PS, McMurray JJ, et al. Improved survival with bisoprolol in patients with heart failure and renal impairment: an analysis of the cardiac insufficiency bisoprolol study II (CIBIS-II) trial. *Eur J Heart Fail.* 2010;12(6):607–616.

39. Cohen-Solal A, Kotecha D, van Veldhuisen DJ, et al. Efficacy and safety of nebivolol in elderly heart failure patients with impaired renal function: insights from the SENIORS trial. *Eur J Heart Fail.* 2009;11(9):872–880.

40. Dohadwala MM, Givertz MM. Role of adenosine antagonism in the cardiorenal syndrome. *Cardiovasc Ther.* 2008;26(4):276–286.

41. Gottlieb SS, Brater DC, Thomas I, et al. BG9719 (CVT-124), an A1 adenosine receptor antagonist, protects against the decline in renal function observed with diuretic therapy. *Circulation.* 2002;105(11):1348–1353.

42. Voors AA, Dittrich HC, Massie BM, et al. Effects of the adenosine A1 receptor antagonist rolofylline on renal function in patients with acute heart failure and renal dysfunction: results from PROTECT (Placebo-Controlled Randomized Study of the Selective Adenosine A1 Receptor Antagonist Rolofylline for Patients Hospitalized with Acute Decompensated Heart Failure and Volume Overload to Assess Treatment Effect on Congestion and Renal Function). *J Am Coll Cardiol.* 2011;57(19):1899–1907.

43. Kapoor M, Schleinitz MD, Gemignani A, Wu WC. Outcomes of patients with chronic heart failure and iron deficiency treated with intravenous iron: a meta-analysis. *Cardiovasc Hematol Disord Drug Targets.* 2013;13(1):35–44.

44. Swedberg K, Young JB, Anand IS, et al. Treatment of anemia with darbepoetin alfa in systolic heart failure. *N Engl J Med.* 2013;368(13):1210–1219.

45. Verbrugge FH, Dupont M, Steels P, et al. Abdominal contributions to cardiorenal dysfunction in congestive heart failure. *J Am Coll Cardiol.* 2013;62(6):485–495.

46. Mullens W, Abrahams Z, Francis GS, Taylor DO, Starling RC, Tang WH. Prompt reduction in intra-abdominal pressure following large-volume

mechanical fluid removal improves renal insufficiency in refractory decompensated heart failure. *J Card Fail.* 2008;14(6):508–514.

47. Lu R, Mucino-Bermejo MJ, Ribeiro LC, et al. Peritoneal dialysis in patients with refractory congestive heart failure: a systematic review. *Cardiorenal Med.* 2015;5(2):145–156.

48. Marenzi G, Grazi S, Giraldi F, et al. Interrelation of humoral factors, hemodynamics, and fluid and salt metabolism in congestive heart failure: effects of extracorporeal ultrafiltration. *Am J Med.* 1993;94(1):49–56.

49. Rogers HL, Marshall J, Bock J, et al. A randomized, controlled trial of the renal effects of ultrafiltration as compared to furosemide in patients with acute decompensated heart failure. *J Card Fail.* 2008;14(1):1–5.

50. Marenzi G, Lauri G, Grazi M, Assanelli E, Campodonico J, Agostoni P. Circulatory response to fluid overload removal by extracorporeal ultrafiltration in refractory congestive heart failure. *J Am Coll Cardiol.* 2001;38(4):963–968.

51. Felker GM, Mentz RJ. Diuretics and ultrafiltration in acute decompensated heart failure. *J Am Coll Cardiol.* 2012;59(24):2145–2153.

52. Assimon MM, Wenger JB, Wang L, Flythe JE. Ultrafiltration rate and mortality in maintenance hemodialysis patients. *Am J Kidney Dis.* 2016;68(6):911–922.

53. Bart BA, Boyle A, Bank AJ, et al. Ultrafiltration versus usual care for hospitalized patients with heart failure: the Relief for Acutely Fluid-Overloaded Patients with Decompensated Congestive Heart Failure (RAPID-CHF) trial. *J Am Coll Cardiol.* 2005;46(11):2043–2046.

54. Costanzo MR, Saltzberg M, O'Sullivan J, Sobotka P. Early ultrafiltration in patients with decompensated heart failure and diuretic resistance. *J Am Coll Cardiol.* 2005;46(11):2047–2051.

55. Costanzo MR, Guglin ME, Saltzberg MT, et al. Ultrafiltration versus intravenous diuretics for patients hospitalized for acute decompensated heart failure. *J Am Coll Cardiol.* 2007;49(6):675–683.

56. Costanzo MR, Negoianu D, Jaski BE, et al. Aquapheresis versus intravenous diuretics and hospitalizations for heart failure. *JACC Heart failure.* 2016;4(2):95–105.

57. Filippatos G, Anker SD, Bohm M, et al. A randomized controlled study of finerenone vs. eplerenone in patients with worsening chronic heart failure and diabetes mellitus and/or chronic kidney disease. *Eur Heart J.* 2016;37(27):2105–2114.

42

Cardiac Surgery and the Kidney

ANNETTE L. MAZZONE AND JONATHAN M. GLEADLE

INTRODUCTION

In the United States, coronary artery bypass grafting (CABG) is among the most commonly performed major surgical procedure with over 400,000 operations performed annually.[1] Cardiac procedures vary in complexity from CABG to the repair or replacement of stenotic or regurgitant valves and correction of complex congenital abnormalities. During these procedures cardiopulmonary bypass (CPB) can be used to support the function of the heart and lungs and to allow the surgeon to operate on a still heart in a bloodless operating field. Cardiac surgical procedures expose a variety of organs including the kidney to a significant risk of acute injury.

EPIDEMIOLOGY

Incidence of Acute Kidney Injury With Cardiac Surgery

Acute kidney injury (AKI) is a frequent and serious complication of cardiac surgery with an incidence reported from <1% to > 40%, depending in large part on the definition of AKI used. The Acute Dialysis Quality Initiative Group developed a consensus definition for AKI, the Risk-Injury-Failure-Loss-End Stage kidney disease (RIFLE) classification, and in 2007, the Acute Kidney Injury Network (AKIN) proposed a modification of the RIFLE classification, known as the AKIN classification. Further to this, in 2011, the Kidney Disease: Improving Global Outcomes Clinical Practice Guidelines for AKI was released by the Acute Kidney Injury Workgroup (Table 42.1).

A lack of a uniform definition for AKI has complicated research in this field and made comparisons of results difficult. Of the larger scale studies, one with 4,800 patients by Englberger and others[2] comparing RIFLE and AKIN found that significantly more patients were

diagnosed as AKI according to AKIN (n = 1272; 26.3%) than by RIFLE (n = 915; 18.9%) criteria (p < 0.0001). Of the 1,272 patients who developed AKI according to RIFLE, 14.8% developed RIFLE-R, 3.5% developed RIFLE-I, and 0.64% were classified as RIFLE-F. According to AKIN 23.6% patients were classified as stage 1, 1.2% as stage 2 and 1.5% as stage 3 AKI.

In a study of 1,030 patients, Hansen and others,[3] defining AKI according to AKIN criteria, found that a total of 287 patients (27.9%) had an episode of AKI during the first 5 postoperative days with 23.1% of patients in AKI stage 1 and 4.8% of patients in AKIN stage 2 or 3. Despite the different definition of AKI used, these results were in agreement with a study by Lopez-Delgado et al.[4] of 2,940 patients using the RIFLE criteria to define AKI. Fourteen percent (n = 409) suffered an AKI event with 8% suffering RIFLE-R, 3% patients with RIFLE-I, and 3% with RIFLE-F.

Regardless of the definition used or the incidence of AKI reported, numerous studies highlight that renal function deterioration post cardiac surgery has serious implications, associated with a more complicated hospital course with associated cost implications. AKI is also an independent predictor of in-hospital mortality. A meta-analysis by Pickering[5] concluded that AKI following CPB was associated with a 4-fold increase in early mortality (risk ratio [RR] 4.0; 95% confidence interval [CI]: 3.1–5.2). These adverse effects resulting from an episode of AKI continue into the longer term with even mildly increased creatinine levels following cardiac surgery being associated with significant increased mortality.[6] Furthermore, long-term survival is significantly affected by AKI duration. Duration of an AKI episode after cardiac surgery was directly proportional to long-term mortality.[7] Aside from mortality, there is a paucity of reports of other long-term outcomes

TABLE 42.1 RIFLE, AKIN, AND KDIGO CLASSIFICATION OF AKI

RIFLE	Serum Creatinine/ GFR Criteria	Urine Output Criteria	AKIN	GFR Criteria	Urine Output Criteria
Risk	↑ serum creatinine 150% or ↓ GFR > 25%	<0.5 mL/kg/h for 6 hrs	Stage 1	↑ serum creatinine ≥ 0.3 mg/dL or ↑ serum creatinine 150–200%	<0.5 mL/kg/h for 6 hrs
Injury	↑ serum creatinine 200% or ↓ GFR > 50%	<0.5 mL/kg/h for 12 hrs	Stage 2	↑ serum creatinine 200%–300%	<0.5mL/kg/h for 12 hrs
Failure	↑ serum creatinine 300% or serum creatinine >4mg/dL ↓ GFR 75%	<0.3 mL/kg/h for 24 hrs or anuria for 12 hrs	Stage 3	↑ serum creatinine >300% or serum creatinine >4 mg/dL ↓ GFR 75%	<0.3mL/kg/h for 24 hrs or anuria for 12 hrs
Loss	Persistent ARF— complete loss of kidney function >4 weeks				
ESKD	End stage kidney disease >3 months				

KIDGO	Serum Creatinine	Urine Output Criteria
1	1.5–1.9× baseline OR ≥ 0.3 mg/dL increase	<0.5 mL/kg/h for 6–12 hrs
2	2.0–2.9× baseline	<0.5ml/kg/h ≥ 12 hrs
3	3.0× baseline OR increase in serum creatinine to >4.0 mg/dL OR initiation of RRT	<0.3ml/kg/h for ≥ 24 hrs or anuria ≥ 12 hrs

RIFLE = Risk-Injury-Failure-Loss-End Stage kidney disease classification. AKIN = Acute Kidney Injury Networ. KDIGO = Kidney Disease: Improving Global Outcomes AKI = acute kidney disease. GFR = ARF = acute renal failure. RRT = renal replacement therapy.

following AKI after cardiac surgery, especially in regards to renal outcomes.

Preoperative Risk Factors for AKI

Risk prediction models of AKI following cardiac surgery have been developed in which the major risk factors are age, female gender, preoperative renal insufficiency, low ejection fraction, emergency surgery, and diabetes. Preoperative renal function may be further compromised by diuresis and the use of nonsteroidal anti-inflammatory drugs.

MECHANISMS OF KIDNEY INJURY

Cardiopulmonary Bypass and the Perioperative Period

The perioperative period provides a unique opportunity for testing renoprotective interventions due to the known timing and similarity of the renal insult. Mechanisms of cardiac surgery-associated AKI include renal ischemia, reperfusion injury, hemolysis, oxidative stress, and activation of the systemic inflammatory response.

There are numerous surgical factors, anesthetic considerations, and bypass-related factors that may impact on the incidence of AKI postcardiac surgery.

Surgical risk factors include type of procedure, with aortic surgery carrying a greater risk, emergency surgery, return to theater, cholesterol atheromatous embolization, and calcific debris following manipulation of the aorta for cannulation and cross-clamping. Anesthetic considerations include the delivery of nephrotoxic drugs including vancomycin, gentamycin, and inotrope use.

The management of CPB provides a unique opportunity to examine a variety of factors known to contribute to an increased risk of AKI, potentially providing an opportunity for intervention and prevention of AKI. Contributing factors include the nonphysiological, nonpulsatile flow of CPB; management of adequate mean arterial pressure; pump flow and oxygen delivery; and the fine balance between hemodilution, hematocrit, anemia, and transfusion. The CPB circuit itself poses a risk due to the production of increased plasma free hemoglobin. Increased time on CPB time is a known risk factor for AKI, as duration of CPB compounds the other factors.

CLINICAL PRESENTATION

Establishing an accurate and timely diagnosis of AKI enables proper treatment. As previously described, current guidelines define AKI based on serum creatinine measurements and urine output. Oliguria is common following cardiac surgery and, hence, precedes serum creatinine rises. The measure of creatinine has its limitations as it does not reflect real time changes in glomerular filtration rate (GFR). The serum creatinine response to renal insult is slow and late. However, measurement of levels still constitutes the main measure for assessment of renal function due to the simplicity and ready availability. This delay in recognition, however, may delay appropriate supportive and therapeutic interventions. In practice, the diagnosis of AKI depends on observing an increase in creatinine, and this may not become readily apparent until 24 to 72 hours after a decrease in GFR.[8]

The emergence of numerous renal tubular damage-specific biomarkers offers an opportunity to diagnose AKI in a timelier manner. The markers of renal damage including NGAL, KIM-1, NAG, IL-18, and the marker of renal function cystatin C possess several theoretical advantages over the use of serum creatinine for the diagnosis of AKI. Concentrations of these biomarkers increase in blood and urine within hours of injury may be more specific to determine the site of injury and are more sensitive.

TREATMENT AND MANAGEMENT CONSIDERATIONS

Due to the uncertainty in the development of AKI in the general clinical setting, the unique predictability and timing of CPB and its potential risk of contributing to AKI allows for the testing of potential preoperative protective interventions.

PREOPERATIVE PROTECTIVE THERAPIES

Many patients undergoing cardiac surgery are on an angiotensin-converting enzyme inhibitor (ACEI), angiotensin receptor blocker (ARB), statin, and/or aspirin therapy; however, whether such medications have a protective role or put patients at an increased risk for AKI following surgery remains unclear.

ACEIs are commonly held prior to surgery due to concern of causing perioperative efferent arteriolar vasodilation and reductions in GFR, systemic vasodilatation, and hypotension; however, studies examining ACEI/ARBs in this setting have shown disparate findings. A recent Cochrane review assessed the benefits and harms of administration of preoperative ACEI or ARBs in adults undergoing any type of surgery under general anesthesia including cardiac surgery for the prevention of mortality and morbidity. The risk of death was 2.7% in the ACEI or ARBs group and 1.6% in the placebo group (RR 1.61; 95% CI: 0.44–5.85). Overall, the review did not find evidence to support that perioperative ACEIs/ARBs prevent mortality, morbidity, or complications including hypotension, cerebrovascular complications, and cardiac surgery-related kidney injury.[9]

In meta-analyses[10,11] of the use of statins in patients undergoing cardiac surgery, statin use has been associated with decreased mortality, atrial fibrillation, and stroke; hence, statins are routinely used preoperatively. However, in such studies, no definite influence on the incidence of postoperative AKI has been identified.

Aspirin therapy is common for most patients with coronary artery disease for the prevention of myocardial infarct (MI), stroke, and death. One of the study objectives of the Aspirin and Tranexamic Acid for Coronary Artery Surgery trial[12] was to determine if aspirin should be continued up until the day of CABG surgery. This randomized multicenter controlled trial enrolled 2,100 patients, of which 1,047 received aspirin therapy and 1,047 received a placebo. The study found that in patients undergoing coronary artery surgery the administration of preoperative aspirin until the day of surgery resulted in neither a lower risk of death nor complications including kidney injury.[13]

In an attempt to ameliorate the role of oxidant stress and reactive oxygen stress caused by CPB and potential contributors to the development of AKI, the prophylactic or early therapeutic use of antioxidant therapy has been suggested as having a potential therapeutic role in the prevention and treatment. Medications such as N-acetylcysteine and selenium containing antioxidants have been suggested to protect the kidney from oxidative stress.[14] While experimental and animal studies look promising in regards to decreasing inflammatory biomarkers, the translation to improved renal outcomes and randomized controlled trials is lacking; hence, the administration of antioxidants is not recommended.

PERIOPERATIVE PROTECTIVE THERAPIES

Off-Pump Coronary Artery Bypass Grafting Surgery

The technique of off-pump coronary artery bypass grafting surgery (OPCABG) was developed in attempts to ameliorate the perioperative complications associated with CPB. The OPCABG technique allows the heart to continue beating and maintain systemic circulation, using a device to stabilize the heart during coronary grafting, thus offering more physiological pulsatile renal perfusion and reduced manipulation of the aorta due to the absence of aortic cannulation and cross clamping. However, large multicenter trials and meta-analyses suggest that while there may be benefit in short term outcomes, including reduced cerebrovascular and kidney injury, longer term benefits have not been seen.[15,16] Lamy et al.[17] reported 5-year outcomes after off-pump or on-pump CABG and the rate of the composite outcome of death, stroke, MI, renal failure, or repeat revascularization at 5 years of follow-up was similar among patients who underwent OPCABG and those who underwent on-pump CABG.

OPCABG may potentially be advantageous for patients with pre-existing renal impairment. Chawla et al.[18] retrospectively reviewed data from 742,909 non-emergent, isolated CABG cases and suggested that patients with CKD experienced lower mortality or incident renal replacement therapy (RRT) when treated with off-pump compared with on-pump CABG (odds ratio [OR] 0.20; 95% CI: 0.12–0.27, $p < 0.001$).

Preoperative Prophylactic Intra-Aortic Balloon Pump

Preoperative prophylactic intra-aortic balloon pump insertion for cardiac indications has also been found to improve renal perfusion by decreasing vasoconstriction and acidosis and by optimizing oxygen consumption. A meta-analysis by Wang et al.[19] on preoperative prophylactic intra-aortic balloon pump therapy indicated to primarily support poor left ventricular function demonstrated a significant beneficial effect on renal function in high-risk patients undergoing CABG, with the greatest benefit seen in OPCABG (on pump high-risk patients compared with controls [OR 0.54; 95% CI: 0.36–0.79; $p = 0.002$] vs. off-pump [OR 0.47; 95% CI: 0.27–0.81, $p = 0.006$]).

CARDIOPULMONARY BYPASS CONSIDERATIONS

Conventional Ultrafiltration

Conventional ultrafiltration (CUF) is commonly used during the cardiopulmonary bypass period to correct electrolyte imbalances and to treat the hemodilutional effects of CPB by removing excess plasma water. There are few studies that have reported on the relationship of CUF and postoperative kidney injury. The use of CUF has been explored as a potential intervention to mitigate AKI risk in cardiac surgery; however, CUF may also have adverse consequences on the kidney related to fluid shift imbalances and renal hypoperfusion. A study by Paugh et al.[20] suggested that CUF during CPB was associated with higher adjusted odds of AKI in patients with an impaired creatinine clearance and removing an increased volume of CUF in this cohort was associated with a higher risk of AKI (OR 1.36; 95% CI :1.12–1.16, $p = 0.002$).

Pulsatile Perfusion

Numerous studies have been carried out to determine the effects of pulsatile versus nonpulsatile flow CPB on the kidney. Studies have found that while levels of biomarkers IL-18 and NGAL levels were lower, there were no significant differences in creatinine levels or incidence of AKI post cardiac surgery.

Duration of CPB

A meta-analysis by Kumar et al.[21] in 2012 found that longer duration of CPB was associated with a higher risk of developing AKI, which, in turn, significantly affected overall mortality. Nine studies were identified which examined the association between CPB time and AKIN defined AKI. A subsequent prospective study by Lopez-Delgado et al.[4] of 2,940 consecutive operations identified longer CPB times as in independent intraoperative predictor of AKI. The average time on CPB was 109 + 37 minutes in patients without AKI compared with 135 + 55 minutes ($p \leq 0.001$) in patients who developed AKI.

Biocompatible Circuits

Hemolysis is an important side effect of CPB and may be an important contributor to postoperative kidney injury. Cardiopulmonary bypass related hemolysis is caused by mechanical shear stress within the extracorporeal circuit including roller pumps; turbulent passage through the oxygenator, reservoir, filters, and arterial and venous cannulae; cardiotomy suction; the air-to-blood interface; cell salvage; and transfusion.[22] There is also an increase in red blood cell fragility and aggregability due to contact with the foreign extracorporeal circuit. Despite continued development to improve the biocompatibility of the CPB circuit, design, and flow performance, the release of plasma-free hemoglobin and its potential to contribute to the development of AKI remains.

NATRIURETICS AND DIURETICS

A systematic review by Park et al.[23] of the prevention of AKI in patients undergoing cardiac surgery found that of the 4 randomized controlled trials analyzed atrial natriuretic peptide (ANP) was associated with a reduction in AKI. Further meta-analyses of ANP, however, suggested that there are an insufficient number of high-quality studies to make any definitive statements about the role of ANP in prevention of AKI.

Perioperative infusions of human recombinant brain natriuretic peptide (BNP) have also been reported to reduce AKI, shorten hospital stay, and improve 6-month outcomes. However, a study by Ejaz et al.[24] found no benefit for the prophylactic use of recombinant BNP on the incidence of dialysis or mortality in patients undergoing high risk CABG. Diuretic agents such as furosemide and mannitol were also noted to have no effect.[23]

ANESTHETIC INTERVENTIONS

To improve the balance between renal oxygen supply and consumption, use of vasoactive agents to increase blood flow or decrease oxygen consumption have been tested. Fenoldopam is a selective dopamine receptor D_1 agonist, which induces vasodilation of the renal, mesenteric, peripheral, and coronary arteries. Meta-analyses of randomized trials report a reduction in the incidence and progression of AKI. However, among patients with AKI post cardiac surgery, fenoldopam infusion did not reduce the need for RRT or risk of 30-day mortality.[25]

Numerous other vasodilators including dopamine, noradrenaline, and vasopressin have also been investigated for improving renal perfusion and reducing the incidence of AKI. The potential advantageous effects of low-dose dopamine include an increase in renal blood flow via activation of dopaminergic receptors in the renal vasculature, an increase in GFR and an increase in sodium and water excretion. In a study by Lassnigg et al.,[26] a continuous infusion of low dose dopamine was ineffective and did not prevent postoperative dysfunction after cardiac surgery.

REMOTE ISCHEMIC PRECONDITIONING

Remote ischemic preconditioning (RIPC), in which brief episodes of nonlethal ischemia and reperfusion are created in distant tissue, may provide protection to tissues and organs from subsequent injury. In cardiac surgery, adverse outcomes are mainly linked to perioperative myocardial injury hence most research has focused on RIPC and reducing the incidence of myocardial injury and infarction. Evidence is limited regarding the protective utility of limb RIPC against AKI in patients undergoing cardiac surgery. A meta-analysis of 13 trials and over 1,300 patients by Yang and others[27] described no difference in levels of postoperative kidney biomarkers (serum creatinine and GFR), incidence of RRT, in-hospital mortality, and length of stay between the control group and patients undergoing RIPC.

Other protective measures that have been trialed include a 24-hour continuous sodium bicarbonate infusion. The proposed method of reducing the incidence of AKI by urinary alkalinization using sodium bicarbonate infusion was found not to reduce the incidence of AKI or attenuate tubular damage following cardiac surgery and was potentially associated with increased mortality.[28]

OTHER RECENT AND UPCOMING TRIALS OF NOTE

ABT-719

ABT-719, a novel, synthetic α-melanocyte-stimulating hormone (α-MSH) analog, inhibits inflammatory, cytotoxic, and apoptotic pathways caused by ischemia/reperfusion injury. α-MSH has direct protective effects on the kidney, which may result from stimulation of the melanocortin receptors in the outer renal medulla. However, ABT-719 treatment did not lower AKI incidence as defined by AKIN.[29]

Erythropoietin

A prospective trial evaluated the effectiveness of EPO in the prevention of AKI after CABG. Erythropoietin has been shown to have tissue-protective effects in experimental models; however, clinical investigations have shown no difference in AKI outcomes.[30]

Alkaline Phosphatase

Alkaline phosphatase is an endogenous enzyme that exerts detoxifying effects through dephosphorylation of endotoxins and proinflammatory extracellular adenosine triphosphate overall effect is to attenuate the inflammatory response. A trial is underway to test the hypothesis that a bolus of alkaline phosphatase at induction of anesthesia followed by infusion over 24 hours will reduce numerous composite endpoints including AKI.[31]

Hepatocyte Growth Factor/Scatter Factor Mimetic

BB3, developed by Angion Biomedica Corp, exerts significant nephroprotective effects in preclinical renal injury models. It is being tested as a therapy to prevent and/or treat AKI in patients following cardiac surgical procedures involving cardiopulmonary bypass.[32]

CONCLUSION

To date, few interventions and no pharmacological agents have been clearly proven to be efficacious in preventing cardiac surgery associated perioperative AKI (Table 42.2). Future studies could aim to improve the understanding of the role of CPB and its contribution to the development of AKI. This, in turn, may result in changes in the management of CPB by optimizing CPB parameters of flow, pressure, and oxygen delivery.

TABLE 42.2 SUMMARY OF INTERVENTIONS AND PHARMACOLOGICAL AGENTS ASSESSED FOR THE PREVENTION OF CSA-AKI

	Level of Evidence	Major Findings	Effect on Incidence of AKI	Number of Patients
Preoperative				
ACEIs/ARBs[a]	Cochrane Review	No effect in reducing mortality or morbidity	No effect	571
Statins[b]	Meta-analysis	Decreased mortality, atrial fibrillation and stroke	No effect	91,491
Aspirin[c]	ATACAS trial, multicenter RCT	No effect on mortality, nor thromboembolic complications	No effect	2,100
Antioxidants[d]	RCT	No effect on organ function endpoints, length of stay, mortality	No effect	200

TABLE 42.2 CONTINUED

	Level of Evidence	Major Findings	Effect on Incidence of AKI	Number of Patients
Perioperative				
OPCABG[e]	Meta-analysis Observational study of STS cardiac surgery database	Short term -reduction in cerebrovascular injury. Long term-no effect on mortality, stroke, MI or repeat revascularization CKD patients reduced in-hospital mortality. No effect on patients with normal renal function	Short-term: reduced AKI Long term: no effect CKD patients: reduced need for RRT No effect on patients with normal renal function	4,752 742,909
Prophylactic IABP (high-risk patients with impaired left ventricular ejection function)[f]	Meta-analysis	Decreased short term mortality	Decreased incidence of post op RRT Decreased incidence of post CABG AKI	2,539
Ultrafiltration[g]	Observational	No effect on mortality, death, stroke, bleeding	Increased risk of AKI	6,407
CPB Time	Meta-analysis	Not reported	Increased CPB duration Increased risk of AKI	12,466
Natriuretics/ diuretics				
ANP[h]	Meta-analysis	No effect on mortality	Decreased incidence of AKI	241
BNP[i]	RCT	No effect on mortality	No effect	94
Furosemide[j]	Meta-analysis	Not reported	No effect	132
Mannitol[k]	Meta-analysis	No effect on mortality	No effect	187
Inotropes				
Fenoldopam[l]	RCT	No effect on 30 day mortality, ventilation hours, length of ICU or hospital stay. Increase in hypotension	No effect	667
Dopamine[m]	RCT	Not reported	No effect	132
RIPC[n]	Meta-analysis	No effect on biomarkers. RRT, in-hospital mortality or hospital stay	No effect	1,334
Sodium Bicarbonate[o]	Meta-analysis	Increased ventilation time, ICU stay And risk of alkalemia	No effect	1,079
α-MSH analog[p]	RCT	No effect on ICU stay No effect on MACE	No effect	120
Erythopoietin[q]	Meta-analysis	No effect on mortality	No effect	473

(*continued*)

TABLE 42.2   CONTINUED

	Level of Evidence	Major Findings	Effect on Incidence of AKI	Number of Patients
Alkaline phosphatase[r]		Ongoing		
HGF/SF mimetic[s]		Ongoing		

[a]Zou Z, Yuan HB, Yang B, Xet al. Perioperative angiotensin-converting enzyme inhibitors or angiotensin II type 1 receptor blockers for preventing mortality and morbidity in adults. *Cochrane Db Sys Rev.* 2016;1:CD009210.

[b]Kuhn EW, Liakopoulos, OJ, Stange S, et al. Preoperative statin therapy in cardiac surgery: a meta-analysis of 90 000 patients. Eur J Cardiothorac Surg. 2014;45:17–26.

[c]Myles PS, Smith JA, Forbes A, et al. For the ATACAS Investigators of the ANZCA clinical trials network: stopping vs continuing aspirin before coronary artery surgery. *N Engl J Med.* 2016;374(8):728–737.

[d]Berger MM, Soguel L, Shenkin A, et al. Influence of early antioxidant supplements on clincial evolution and organ function in critically ill cardiac surgery, major trauma and subarachnoid hemorrhage patients. *Crit Care.* 2008;12:R101.

[e]Lamy A, Devereaux PJ, Prabhakaran, D, et al. Five-year outcomes after Off-pump or On-pump coronary artery bypass grafting. *N Engl J Med.* 2016;375:2359–2368; Chawla LS, Zhao Y, Lough FC, et al. Off-pump versus on-pump coronary artery bypass grafting outcomes stratified by preoperative renal function. *J Am Soc Nephrol.* 2012;23:1389–1397.

[f]Wang J, Yu W, Gao M, et al. Preoperative prophylactic intraaortic balloon pump redcues the incidence of postoperative acute kidney injury and short-term death of high-risk patients undergoing coronary artery bypass grafting: a meta-analysis of 17 studies. *Ann Thoraic Surg.* 2016;101:2007–2019.

[g]Paugh TA, Dickinson TA, Martin JR, et al. Impact of ultrafiltration on kidney injury after cardiac surgery: the Michigan experience. *Ann Thoraic Surg.* 2015;100(5):1683–1688.

[h]Kumar AB, Suneja M, Bayman EO, et al. Association between postoperative acute kidney injury and duration of cardiopulmonary bypass: a meta-analysis. *J Cardiovasc Vas An.* 2012;26:64–69.

[i]Ricci Z, Pezzella C, Romagnoli S, et al. High levels of free haemoglobin in neonates and infants undergoing suugery on cardiopulmonary bypass. *Interact Cardiov Th.* 2014;19:183–188.

[j]Park M, Coca SG, Nigwekar, SU, et al. Prevention and treament of acute kidney injury in patients undergoing cardiac surgery: a systematic review. *Am J Nephrol.* 2010;31:408–418.

[k]Ejaz AA, Martin TD, Johnson RJ, et al. Prophylactic nesiritide does not prevent dialysis or all-cause mortality in patients undergoing high-risk surgery. *J Thoracic Cardiovasc Surg.* 2009;138(4):959–964.

[l]Bove T, Zangrillo A, Guarracino F, et al. Effect of fenoldopam on use of renal replacement therapy among patients with acute kidney injury after cardiac surgery. A randomised clinical trial. *J Am Med Assoc.* 2014;312(21):2244–2253.

[m]Lassnigg A, Donner E, Grubhofer G, et al. Lack of renoprotective effects of dopamine and furosemide during cardiac surgery. *J Am Soc Nephrol.* 2000;11:97–104.

[n]Yang Y, Lang X, Zhang P, et al. Remote ischemic preconditioning for prevention of acute kidney injury: a meta-analysis of randomized controlled trials. *Am J Kidney Dis.* 2014;64(4):574–583.

[o]Tie HT, Luo MZ, Luo MJ, et al. Sodium bicarbonate in the prevention of cardiac surgery-associated acute kidney injuty: a systematic reveiw and meta-analysis. *Crit Care.* 2014;18:517.

[p]McCullough PA, Bennett-Guerrero E, Chawla LS, et al. ABT-719 for the prevention of acute kidney injury in patients undergoing high-risk cardiac surgery: a randomised phase 2b clinical trial. *J Am Heart Assoc.* 2016;5(8).

[q]Penny-Dimri JC, Cochrane AD, Epid M, et al. Characterising the role of perioperative erythropoietin for prevent acute kidney injuty after cardiac surgery: systematic review and meta-analysis. *Heart Lung Circ.* 2016;25:1067–1076.

[r]Preventing systemic inflammation after cardiac surgery with alkaline phosphatase (APPIRED-III). NCT 03050476. ClinicalTrials.gov; 2017–. https://clinicaltrials.gov/ct2/show/NCT03050476?term=alkaline+phosphatase+as+AKI&rank=2

[s]Study to prevent acute kidney injury after cardiac surgery involving cardiopulmonary bypass. NCT02771509. ClinicalTrials.gov; 2017–. https://clinicaltrials.gov/ct2/show/NCT02771509?term=aKI+and+BB3&rank=1

ACEIs = angiotensin converting enzyme inhibitors. ARBs = angiotensin II receptor blockers. RCT = randomized controlled trial. CABG = coronary artery bypass graft. OPCABG = off-pump CABG. AKI = acute kidney injury. CKD = chronic kidney disease. RRT = renal replacement therapy. CPB = cardiopulmonary bypass. ANP = atrial natriuretic peptide. BNP = brain natriuretic peptide. IABP = intra-aortic balloon pump. RIPC = remote ischemic preconditioning. HGS/SF = hepatocyte growth factor/scatter factor.

In sum

- Most studies for potential renoprotective interventions are underpowered to demonstrate a beneficial effect on reducing incidence of AKI, acute RRT and mortality.

- No pharmacological interventions have definite benefit in reducing the incidence of AKI following cardiac surgery.
- It is important to limit time on CPB and optimize CPB parameters such as flow, pressure, and oxygen delivery.

- Avoid use of nephrotoxic drugs.
- Consider using OPCABG in patients with pre-existing chronic kidney disease.

REFERENCES

1. Alexander JH, Smith PK. Coronary-Artery Bypass Grafting. *N Engl J Med*. 2016;374:1954–1964.
2. Englberger L, Suri, RM, Li, Z, et al. Clinical accuracy of RIFLE and Acute Kidney Injury Networl (AKIN) criteria for acute kidney injury in patients undergoing cardiac surgery. *Crit Care*. 2011;15:R16.
3. Hansen MK, Gammelager, H, Mikkelsen, MM, et al. Post-operative acute kidney injury and five-year risk of death, myocardial infarction and stroke among elective cardiac surgical patients: a cohort study. *Crit Care*. 2013;17(6):R292.
4. Lopez-Delgado JC, Esteve, F, Torrado, H, et al. Influence of acute kidney injury on short and long term outcomes in patients undergoing cardiac surgery: risk factors and prognostic value of a modified RIFLE classification. *Crit Care*. 2013;17:R293.
5. Pickering JW, James, MT, Palmer, SC. Acute kidney injury and prognosis after cardiopulmonary bypass: a meta-analysis of cohort studies. *Am J Kidney Dis*. 2015;65(2):283–293.
6. Lassnigg A, Schmidlin, D, Mouhieddine, M, et al. Minimal changes of serum creatinine predict prognosis in patients after cardiothoracic surgery: a prospective cohort study. *J Am Soc Nephrol*. 2004;15:1597–1605.
7. Brown JR, Kramer, RS. Coca, SG, et al. Duration of acute kidney injury impacts long-term survival after cardiac surgery. *Ann Thoraic Surg*. 2010;90:1142–1149.
8. Endre ZH, Pickering, JW, Walker, RJ. Clearance and beyond: the complementary roles of GFR measurement and injury biomarkers in acute kidney injury (AKI). *Am J Physiol Renal Physiol*. 2011;301:F697–F707.
9. Zou Z, Yuan HB, Yang B, Xet al. Perioperative angiotensin-converting enzyme inhibitors or angiotensin II type 1 receptor blockers for preventing mortality and morbidity in adults. *Cochrane Db Sys Rev*. 2016;1:CD009210.
10. Arora P, Kolli H, Nainani N, et al. Preventable risk factors for acute kidney injury in patients undergoing cardiac surgery. *J Cardiovasc Vas An*. 2012;26(4):687–697.
11. Kuhn EW, Liakopoulos, OJ, Stange S, et al. Preoperative statin therapy in cardiac surgery: a meta-analysis of 90 000 patients. *Eur J Cardiothorac Surg*. 2014;45:17–26.
12. Myles PS, Smith J, Knight J, et al. Aspirin and Tranexamic Acid for Coronary Artery Surgery (ATACAS) trial: rationale and design. *Am Heart J*. 2008;155:224–230.
13. Myles PS, Smith JA, Forbes A, et al. For the ATACAS Investigators of the ANZCA clinical trials network: stopping vs continuing aspirin before coronary artery surgery. *N Engl J Med*. 2016;374(8):728–737.
14. Berger MM, Soguel L, Shenkin A, et al. Influence of early antioxidant supplements on clincial evolution and organ function in critically ill cardiac surgery, major trauma and subarachnoid hemorrhage patients. *Crit Care*. 2008;12:R:101.
15. Kowalewski M, Pawliszak W, Malvindi PG, et al. Off-pump coronary artery bypass grafting improves short-term outcomes in high-risk patients compared with on-pump coronary artery bypass grafting: meta-analysis. *J Thorac Cardiovasc Surg*. 2016;151(1):60–77.
16. Puskas JD, Martin J, Cheng DC, et al. ISMICS consensus conference and statement of randmonised controlled trials of off-pump versus conventional coronary artery bypass grafting. *Innovations (Phila)*. 2015;10(4):219–229.
17. Lamy A, Devereaux PJ, Prabhakaran, D, et al. Five-year outcomes after Off-pump or On-pump coronary artery bypass grafting. *N Engl J Med*. 2016;375:2359–2368.
18. Chawla LS, Zhao Y, Lough FC, et al. Off-pump versus on-pump coronary artery bypass grafting outcomes stratified by preoperative renal function. *J Am Soc Nephrol*. 2012;23:1389–1397.
19. Wang J, Yu W, Gao M, et al. Preoperative prophylactic intraaortic balloon pump redcues the incidence of postoperative acute kidney injury and short-term death of high-risk patients undergoing coronary artery bypass grafting: a meta-analysis of 17 studies. *Ann Thoraic Surg*. 2016;101:2007–2019.
20. Paugh TA, Dickinson TA, Martin JR, et al. Impact of ultrafiltration on kidney injury after cardiac surgery: the Michigan experience. *Ann Thoraic Surg*. 2015;100(5):1683–1688.
21. Kumar AB, Suneja M, Bayman EO, et al. Association between postoperative acute kidney injury and duration of cardiopulmonary bypass: a meta-analysis. *J Cardiovasc Vas An*. 2012;26:64–69.
22. Ricci Z, Pezzella C, Romagnoli S, et al. High levels of free haemoglobin in neonates and infants undergoing suugery on cardiopulmonary bypass. *Interact Cardiov Th*. 2014;19:183–188.
23. Park M, Coca SG, Nigwekar, SU, et al. Prevention and treament of acute kidney injury in patients undergoing cardiac surgery: a systematic review. *Am J Nephrol*. 2010;31:408–418.

24. Ejaz AA, Martin TD, Johnson RJ, et al. Prophylactic nesiritide does not prevent dialysis or all-cause mortality in patients undergoing high-risk surgery. *J Thoracic Cardiovasc Surg.* 2009;138(4):959–964.

25. Bove T, Zangrillo A, Guarracino F, et al. Effect of fenoldopam on use of renal replacement therapy among patients with acute kidney injury after cardiac surgery. A randomised clinical trial. *J Am Med Assoc.* 2014;312(21):2244–2253.

26. Lassnigg A, Donner E, Grubhofer G, et al. Lack of renoprotective effects of dopamine and furosemide during cardiac surgery. *J Am Soc Nephrol.* 2000;11:97–104.

27. Yang Y, Lang X, Zhang P, et al. Remote ischemic preconditioning for prevention of acute kidney injury: a meta-analysis of randomized controlled trials. *Am J Kidney Dis.* 2014;64(4):574–583.

28. Tie HT, Luo MZ, Luo MJ, et al. Sodium bicarbonate in the prevention of cardiac surgery-associated acute kidney injuty: a systematic reveiw and meta-analysis. *Crit Care.* 2014;18:517.

29. McCullough PA, Bennett-Guerrero E, Chawla LS, et al. ABT-719 for the prevention of acute kidney injury in patients undergoing high-risk cardiac surgery: a randomised phase 2b clinical trial. *J Am Heart Assoc.* 2016;5(8).

30. Penny-Dimri JC, Cochrane AD, Epid M, et al. Characterising the role of perioperative erythropoietin for prevent acute kidney injuty after cardiac surgery: systematic review and meta-analysis. *Heart Lung Circ.* 2016;25:1067–1076.

31. Preventing systemic inflammation after cardiac surgery with alkaline phosphatase (APPIRED-III). NCT 03050476. ClinicalTrials.gov; 2017–. https://clinicaltrials.gov/ct2/show/NCT03050 476?term=alkaline+phosphatase+as+AKI&rank=2

32. Study to prevent acute kidney injury after cardiac surgery involving cardiopulmonary bypass. NCT02771509. ClinicalTrials.gov; 2017–. https://clinicaltrials.gov/ct2/show/NCT02771509?term=aKI+and+BB3&rank=1

43

Tubulointerstitial Nephropathies

ABHILASH KORATALA, GIRISH SINGHANIA, AND A. AHSAN EJAZ

INTRODUCTION

Diseases of the tubulointerstitium is generally termed tubulointerstitial nephritis (TIN), irrespective of the underlying pathology. Acute TIN typically manifests clinically as an unexplained (i.e., without a preceding hypotension episode) rise in serum creatinine in a nonoliguric patient. Blood pressure and urine output are usually maintained; laboratory findings of abnormalities in potassium, hyperchloremic metabolic acidosis, elevated blood urea nitrogen and creatinine, and decreased urine concentration capacity reflect impairment of tubular function. Urine pH can be helpful in localizing the anatomical site of tubular injury. The mechanism for urinary acidification is tightly regulated in the distal part of the nephron, and injury to this section can result in urine pH >5.5. Eosinophiluria >10% has sensitivity and specificity of 67% and 83%, respectively, to detect acute TIN. Once the clinico-laboratory diagnosis of tubulointerstitial disease is made, unveiling its etiology requires careful history-taking, physical examination, and additional testing including kidney biopsy. The histological hallmark of TIN is the presence of inflammatory infiltrates within the interstitium, associated with interstitial edema that separates the tubules. Tubulitis, associated with infiltration of inflammatory cells (primarily lymphocytes) is present, but the blood vessels and glomeruli are not typically involved. Fibrosis becomes the dominant component as the process progresses to chronic TIN. The first step in the management of TIN is establishing the clinical diagnosis. This chapter assumes that the clinical diagnosis of TIN has been established. Hereafter, the focus is on pathomechanisms as the basis for renoprotection in nontransplant patients.

CLASSIFICATION OF TUBULOINTERSTITIAL NEPHRITIS

The tubulointerstium may be the primary or secondary target of pathogenetic processes and the accurate determination is often complicated by the chronicity of events as sustained tubulointerstitial inflammation results in tissue fibrosis. Classification of acute interstitial nephritis (AIN) is based on etiology, histology, and clinical features (Table 43.1) and provides guidance for treatment and prognosis. A summary of TIN classification, highlighting select entities, is presented.

Infection-Associated Tubulointerstitial Nephritis

Renal lesions of bacterial, viral, fungal, and protozoal infections are classified according to their clinical and pathologic characteristics that range from AIN to thrombotic microangiopathy. In Puumala hanta virus-induced hemorrhagic fever with renal syndrome, the typical renal histologic lesion is acute TIN, interstitial hemorrhages, cortical peritubular capillaritis, medullary vasa recta inflammation, and acute tubular necrosis. In addition to TIN, Influenza A H1N1 infection can manifest as membranoproliferative glomerulonephritis in children, and hepatitis A can present as virus-associated hemophagocytic syndrome. Additionally, medications used to treat these conditions can also contribute to TIN. Therefore, a high index of clinical suspicion is required for diagnosis. Symptom-appropriate microbiology tests, viral antibody titers, special stains, ribonucleic acid sequence by polymerase chain reaction, and renal biopsies are often required to identify the pathogens. Treatment consists of antimicrobial therapy and supportive care.

TABLE 43.1 CLASSIFICATION OF TIN WITH CHARACTERISTIC FEATURES OF SELECT ENTITIES

Class	Entity	Characteristic Features
Infection	HIV	TDF: prominent eosinophilic intracytoplasmic inclusions within proximal tubular epithelial cells, tubular cysts; giant dysmorphic mitochondria.
	TB	Caseating granulomatous interstitial nephritis.
	HVN	Microvascular inflammation, interstitial hemorrhages.
Drugs	General	Interstitial eosinophilic aggregates.
	Lithium	Distal and collecting duct tubular cysts.
	CPI	Long latency period (21–245 days) from exposure to diagnosis.
Immune	IC-TIN	Hypocomplentemia, granular TBM staining for IgGs and complements, electron-dense TBM deposits.
	IgG4-TIN	Elevated plasma IgG4, dense lymphoplasmacytic tubulointerstial infiltrate, storiform fibrosis, increased IgG4 plasma cells.
Hereditary familial	ADTKD	Family history of CKD, early onset gout, hyperuricemia, progressive tubulointerstitial fibrosis and progression to ESRD, genetic testing.
	TINU	Proximal renal tubular acidosis, visual and neurological symptoms.
	Alagille	Elfin facies, jaundice, renovascular hypertension, renal agenesis.
	ApoA-1	Medullary amyloid deposits, APOA1 gene mutation.
Glomerular and vascular		Coexisting features of underlying glomerular and vascular diseases.
Heavy metals		Anemia, hypertension, kidney failure, developing countries.
Emerging entities	MEN	Tropical agricultural workers in Central America, Sri Lanka
	Balkan	Endemic areas of the Danube river, China
	Crystallopathy	Hyperuricemia.
Miscellaneous	Obstructive nephropathy	Urinary symptoms.
	Ischemic/toxic ATN	Patchy or diffuse denudation of the renal tubular cells, loss of brush border, tubular dilatation, intratubular casts, inflammatory infiltrate.

TB = tuberculosis. HVN = hantavirus nephropathy. TDF = Tenofovir. CPI = check point inhibitors. IC-TIN = immune complex tubulointerstitial nephritis. TBM = tubular basement membrane. ADTKD = autosomal dominant tubulointerstitial kidney disease. NBCe1 = electrogenic sodium bicarbonate cotransporter ESRD: end-stage kidney disease. ApoA-I = Apolipoprotein A-I amyloidosis. MEN = Mesoamerican Nephropathy; GN = glomerulonephritis. ATN = acute tubular necrosis.

Selected Entities

HIV/AIDS

Human immunodeficiency virus infection and acquired immune deficiency syndrome (HIV/AIDS) is a global pandemic and deserves mention. Renal lesions associated with HIV/AIDS include HIV-associated nephropathy (considered a subtype of primary focal and segmental glomerulosclerosis), HIV-associated immune complex kidney disease and TIN. HIV infection itself is very rare direct cause of AIN and is a diagnosis of exclusion. Antiretroviral drugs actively accumulate in tubular cells and are the major contributors to tubulopathy (75%–80%) and TIN (10%–15%). The proportion of tubular damage in patients taking tenofovir disoproxil fumarate (TDF), other high activity antiretroviral therapy regimens, and drug-naive groups were reported to be 22%, 6%, and 12%, respectively.[1] Tubulopathy can manifest as Fanconi's syndrome (proximal tubulopathy characterized by aminoaciduria, glucosuria with normal serum glucose, and phosphate wasting), renal tubular acidosis, and nephrogenic diabetes insipidus. TDF causes Fanconi's syndrome by down-regulating mitochondrial chaperone TRAP1 and succinate dehydrogenase subunit B to metabolically reprogram glucose metabolism and induce nephrotoxicity. A distinct feature of TDF nephrotoxicity is prominent eosinophilic intracytoplasmic inclusions within proximal tubular epithelial cells and dysmorphic mitochondria—small to markedly enlarged, swollen with irregular contours, prominent clumping, and loss and disorientation of cristae—on a background of diffuse TIN accompanied by cyst formations surrounded by multinuclear giant cells.[2,3] In contrast, AIN is associated with a broader spectrum of pathologic lesions and etiologies. Female gender, age, and protease inhibitors are independent risk factors for nephrotoxicity. Prophylactic strategies for the prevention of protease inhibitor nephrotoxicity consist of adequate hydration after each dose, monitoring of renal function at least semiannually, and more frequently as appropriate, with blood and urine chemistries in stable asymptomatic patients on antiretroviral therapy. Decline in glomerular filtration rate by >25% from baseline and to a level <60 mL/minute/1.73m^2 that fails to resolve after potential nephrotoxic drugs are removed, albuminuria >300/mg/day, hematuria combined with either albuminuria/proteinuria, or increasing blood pressure should prompt further evaluation. If significant renal insufficiency persists, temporary protease inhibitor withdrawal or switching to another protease inhibitor should be considered. The new prodrug tenofovir alafenamide maybe an option as it has equal efficacy but with decreased renal injury and bone mineral density loss compared with TDF. Caution is advocated with other novel antiretroviral drugs (e.g., the integrase inhibitors), which have also been linked to tubulopathy and TIN by inhibition of tubular secretion of serum creatinine by organic cation transporters. An evolving entity in untreated or uncontrolled HIV infection is diffuse infiltrative lymphocytosis syndrome that is associated with bilateral parotitis, lymphadenopathy, and involvement of the lungs, nervous system, liver, kidneys, and digestive tract. The hallmark feature is polyclonal CD8+ T-cell lymphocytosis and polyclonal CD8+ T-cell organ infiltration. Distal renal tubular acidosis, mild proteinuria, hematuria, and polyuria can occur. Renal biopsy shows acute TIN with interstitial infiltrates of lymphocytes, plasmocytes, and monocytes. Treatment with antiretroviral agents is the mainstay of therapy. Steroids may be required in severe cases.[4] Immune reconstitution inflammatory syndrome is another entity that develops in the most immunosuppressed patients 3 to 4 months after starting treatment with the most potent regimens—the highly active antiretroviral therapy. Treatment with steroids remains problematic.

Tuberculosis-Associated TIN

The incidence of tuberculosis is increasing. Genitourinary tuberculosis may present with sterile pyuria, pelvicalyceal deformities, and systemic symptoms. Primary renal manifestation, without pulmonary involvement, is less common and is difficult to diagnose as staining for the pathogen and culture are often negative. The characteristic histological findings are interstitial inflammation with eosinophilia and caseating granulomas. The classic granuloma is seen only in ~20% of the cases.[5] Molecular tests for the detection of tubercular DNA have a higher sensitivity and specificity for the diagnosis of tubercular infection. Antituberculosis medication is the mainstay of therapy.

Drug-Induced Tubulointerstitial Nephritis

Nonsteroidal anti-inflammatory drugs, proton pump inhibitors, and antibiotics are commonly implicated in TIN, but many others are also potential inducers. Chronological relationship exist between exposure and effect in drug-induced TIN. The latency period is generally shorter with antibiotics than with nonsteroidal anti-inflammatory drugs. The proposed mechanisms of acute TIN involve binding of the drug to a normal component of the tubular basement membrane and acting as a hapten, or it can mimic an antigen normally present within the tubular basement membrane or the interstitium and induce an immune response directed against this antigen. Drugs can also bind to the tubular basement membrane or deposit within the interstitium and act as a planted antigen, or it can elicit the production of antibodies and deposit in the interstitium as circulating immune complexes.[6] Another important mechanism of acute TIN is crystalluria, by either

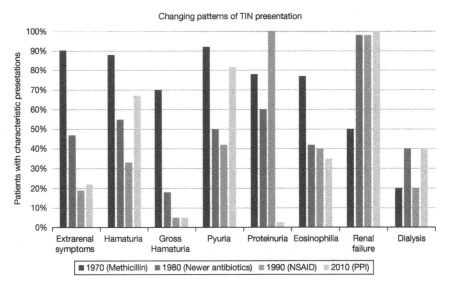

FIGURE 43.1 Changing pattern of clinical presentation of acute TIN. TIN = tubulointerstitial nephritis. NSAID = nonsteroidal anti-inflammatory drug. PPI = proton pump inhibitor.

tubular obstruction, direct cytotoxic effects, or inflammation. The clinical presentation varies depending on risk factors, but there has been a distinct change in the spectrum of presentation over time (Fig. 43.1). Histologically, the coexistence of significant interstitial eosinophilic aggregates with the predominantly lymphocytic infiltration favor drug-induced processes. However, interstitial eosinophilic aggregates are also common in diabetic nephropathy and are not diagnostic of drug-induced allergic TIN. Rarely, drug-induced TIN can be associated with granulomas consisting of loose appearing aggregates of epithelioid macrophages.

Select Entities

Lithium

Dose and duration of treatment are risk factors for lithium-associated kidney diseases that range from urinary concentrating defect to nephrogenic diabetes insipidus (NDI) and chronic TIN. Lithium causes NDI in 40% of patients by several mechanisms including inhibition of arginine vasopressin–stimulated translocation of cytoplasmic urinary aquaporin 2 (AQP2) to the apical membrane via inactivation of adenylyl cyclase and subsequent inhibition of protein kinase A-induced phosphorylation of cytoplasmic AQP2, dysregulation of renal prostaglandins, altered purinergic signaling, and

changes in renal architecture.[7] Usually reversible in the early phase of therapy, NDI can become permanent with prolonged exposure to lithium. Treatment of NDI include discontinuation of lithium, administration of amiloride to block the entry of lithium into collecting duct principals cell via epithelial sodium channels and thiazides, which produce mild sodium depletion and decreased distal tubule delivery of sodium and therefore increase water reabsorption in the collecting ducts. Lithium-induced chronic TIN is characterized by the insidious development over 5 to 30 years of drug exposure, with little or no proteinuria. Fifty percent of patients treated with lithium for >20 years had estimated glomerular filtration rate <60 mL/min/1.73m². Progression to end-stage kidney disease is rare, and contribution of lithium nephrotoxicity to dialysis population is 0.22%. Characteristic histological findings are TIN and tubular cysts originating mainly from the distal tubule and collecting duct, a result of lithium-induced inhibition of glycogen synthase kinase-3β isoform, a central regulator of the microtubule dynamics.[8] Additional complicating factor in long-term lithium therapy is the reported increased incidence of solid renal tumors. Conservative dosing, combination drug therapies, regular clinical observation, pharmacovigilance, and educating patients and caregivers to recognize early signs of intoxication remain the mainstay for renoprotection.

Immune Checkpoint Inhibitors

Immune checkpoint inhibitors (CPIs) are an emerging class of immunotherapy used in treating solid organ and hematologic malignancies. CPIs, such as cytotoxic T-lymphocyte antigen 4 (CTLA4), programmed cell death 1 (PD-1), and programmed cell death ligand 1 (PD-L1) are expressed on immune cells and tumor cells. They regulate immune responses to prevent tissue injury and autoimmunity. Combination therapy (e.g., CTLA-4 antagonist ipilimumab and PD-1 antagonist nivolumab) is a risk factors for acute kidney injury that occurred in 2.2% of patients. On renal biopsy, the primary lesion was TIN. However, unlike other drugs, the median time from initiation of a CPI to acute TIN was long (median, 91 days; range, 21–245 days). Most patients responded to corticosteroids; however, long-term outcomes are not known.[9]

Immune Complex Tubulointerstitial Nephritis

Immune complex TIN (IC-TIN) is induced by antibodies reacting with tubular basement membrane or brush border antigens, autologous or exogenous immune complexes, cell-mediated hypersensitivity, or by immediate hypersensitivity. Patients present with advanced kidney injury in the setting of severe hypocomplementemia without extrarenal manifestations, proteinuria, or active urinary sediments. Antibrush border autoantibodies can cause direct epithelial injury, accumulate in the tubular basement membrane, and elicit an interstitial inflammatory response.[10] Characteristic histologic features are mononuclear inflammatory interstitial infiltrate, tubular atrophy, and normal-looking glomerulus; granular tubular basement membrane staining for immunoglobin (Ig) Gs and complements and electron-dense deposits along the tubular basement membrane. IC-TIN has also been associated with lupus nephritis, postinfectious glomerulonephritis, cryoglobulinemia, IgG4-related systemic diseases, polyomavirus, and drugs. Rarely, it can be associated with autoimmune polyglandular syndrome type 1 because of an autoimmune insult on the kidney collecting duct cells. IC-TIN are generally responsive to immunosuppression (exception polyomavirus).

Select Entities

Sjögren's Syndrome

Renal diseases associated with Sjogren's syndrome can present as distal renal tubular acidosis and less frequently as proximal renal tubular acidosis. TIN accounts for one-third of renal involvement with Sjögren's syndrome. Patients with TIN have a more favorable prognosis than those with glomerular lesions. Affected patients are at increased risk of developing non-Hodgkin's lymphoma, in particular, lymphomas of B-cell origin. Characteristic renal lesions are acute or chronic TIN with lymphoplasmacytic infiltrate and edema, interstitial fibrosis, and tubular atrophy. The infiltrate consists of CD4/CD8 T-cells, B-cells, and plasma cells with scattered tubulitis. Rarely, noncaseating, multifocal granulomas containing giant cells and eosinophils are present. Chronic, especially long-standing, TIN can lead to secondary amyloidosis. Corticosteroids are the first line of therapy in Sjögrens-related TIN. In steroid-intolerant, resistant, or dependent TIN, mycophenolate mofetil is favored.[11,12]

Tubulointerstitial Nephritis and Uveitis Syndrome

The characteristic renal histologic findings in tubulointerstitial nephritis and uveitis syndrome (TINU) syndrome is T-cell-dominant tubulointerstitial infiltration of marked immune cells including CD54-positive non-B lymphocytes. Eosinophils can be present in about one-third of the patients. The cross-reactive antigens of TINU syndrome from renal tubulointerstitial and ocular tissue remain unidentified. Recent reports suggest that the modified C-reactive protein is a candidate antigen. TIN resolves spontaneously, and long-term prognosis is good. Uveitis, however, has frequent relapses. Systemic steroids may be required for uveitis but not for TIN.[13]

IgG4-Related Tubulointerstitial Nephritis

IgG4-related disease is a fibro-inflammatory condition that has a tendency to form tumefactive (swelling) lesions in multiple sites. IgG4 has been linked to TIN and membranous nephropathy. It is estimated that approximately 30% of patients with pancreatic involvement show evidence of TIN.[14] The consensus diagnosis of IgG4-related

TIN is based on the combined presence of the characteristic histopathological appearance of dense lymphoplasmacytic tubulointerstial infiltrate, a storiform pattern (matted, irregularly whorled pattern, somewhat resembling that of a straw mat) of fibrosis, and increased numbers of IgG4 plasma cells. Although tissue IgG4 counts and IgG4/IgG ratios are considered secondary in importance, the finding of >30 IgG4 plasma cells/high power field has been reported to have acceptable specificity and >50/high power field highly specific. In Japan, IgG4/IgG plasma cell ratio >40% is considered a histological diagnostic criterion for IgG4-related disease. Most patients with IgG4-related TIN have increased serum total IgG or IgG4 levels or hypergammaglobulinemia. Detection of tuberculous meningitis (TBM) immune complex deposits on electron microscope is a key feature and is important in diagnosing renal-limited cases of IgG4-related systemic diseases. Initial treatment consists of prednisone at a dose of 0.6 mg/kg/day for 2 to 4 weeks, then taper over 3 to 6 months to 5 mg/day, and then continue 2.5 to 5 mg/day for up to 3 years.[15] While most patients respond to glucocorticoid therapy, flares are common. Azathioprine, mycophenolate mofetil, and methotrexate have been used as steroid-sparing agents. For patients with recurrent or refractory disease, B-cell depletion therapy with rituximab may be beneficial.

Heredofamilial Renal Tubulointerstitial Disorder
Autosomal Dominant Tubulointerstitial Kidney Disease

Gene mutations causing renal tubular dysfunction and interstitial nephritis is a rare but emerging entity encompassing diseases caused by mutations in the genes encoding for uromodulin, hepatocyte nuclear factor-1B, renin, and mucin-1. The group of diseases formerly known as medullary cystic kidney disease, familial juvenile hyperuricemic nephropathy, and uromodulin-associated kidney disease are now termed autosomal dominant tubulointerstitial kidney disease (ADTKD). ADTKD is characterized by progressive tubulointerstitial fibrosis and progression to end-stage kidney disease between the ages of 25 and 70 years of age or even earlier (3–51 years) in those with hyperuricemia. The clinical findings are usually nonspecific—normal blood pressure, bland urine sediment, minimal proteinuria, and normal or small kidneys—and make detection difficult. Early onset of gout, hyperuricemia,

hypokalemia, and hypomagnesemia (due to reduced potassium channel Kir5.1 activity in patients with hepatocyte nuclear factor-1B mutations), and anemia can occur. Histology reveals interstitial fibrosis; tubular atrophy; thickening and lamellation of tubular basement membrane; microcysts; and, depending on the underlying genetic defect, intracellular uromodulin deposits in the thick ascending limb; mucin-1 deposits in the distal tubules; and reduced renin staining in the juxtamedullary apparatus. More dramatic renal presentations can be seen in hepatocyte nuclear factor-1B mutations and include multicystic renal dysplasia, renal hypoplasia, unilateral renal agenesis, microcystic dysplasia, horseshoe kidney, atypical familial juvenile hyperuricemic nephropathy, and urinary tract malformations. Kidney Disease: Improving Global Outcomes recommends that ADTKD should be suspected when autosomal dominant inheritance suspected in conjunction with nonspecific clinical and histological manifestations and the absence of evidence for kidney disease of other etiology.[16] Definitive diagnosis requires fulfilling the clinical characteristics or demonstration of a mutation in 1 of the 4 genes in an affected individual or at least 1 family member. Genetic testing of minors is not recommended at this time due to lack of specific treatments.

Tubular Dysfunction Associated With Mutations in NBCe1

In the proximal tubule, bicarbonate is transported into the peritubular space by a basolateral electrogenic sodium-bicarbonate cotransporter (NBCe1; encoded by SLC4A4), and H+ reenters the tubular lumen via a sodium-hydrogen exchanger and, to a lesser extent, via H+-ATPase-driven H+ secretion. Autosomal recessive mutations in NBCe1 have been linked to proximal renal tubular acidosis.[17] NBCe1 is also expressed in other organs, including the eye and brain, resulting in extrarenal manifestations such as speech and gait abnormalities, short stature, and marked corneal opacities. Diagnosis is confirmed by genetic analysis of SLC4A4 (homozygous deletion, c.2211_2213delCCT; p.L738del).[18] Alkali therapy can ameliorate the acidosis and improve growth but not the extrarenal manifestations. Other causes of proximal renal tubular acidosis with additional proximal tubule transport abnormalities include Dent's disease, Wilson's disease, galactosemia, hereditary fructose intolerance, cystinosis, tyrosinemia,

Lowe's syndrome, Fanconi-Bickel syndrome, methylmalonic academia, pyruvate carboxylase deficiency, metachromatic leukodystrophy, and cytochrome C oxidase deficiency.

Alagille Syndrome

Alagille syndrome is an autosomal dominant, multisystem disease due to mutation in the Notch signaling pathway that is crucial for cell differentiation in embryonic life. Children present with at least 3 of the following 5 abnormalities: chronic cholestasis, peripheral pulmonary artery stenosis, vertebral arch defects, embryotoxon, and typical facies. Renal anomalies including renal agenesis, renovascular hypertension, cystic renal disease, TIN, and renal tubular acidosis occur in 20% to 70% of patients. The heart, eye, and vertebrae can also be involved. Adults with Alagille syndrome can present with renovascular hypertension and chronic TIN. Dialysis access placement, if required, can be complicated due to vascular stenosis.[19]

Hereditary Apolipoprotein A-I Amyloidosis

Apolipoprotein A-I is the main protein of high-density lipoprotein particles, that promotes efflux of cholesterol from cells. Gain-of-function mutations of APOA 1 gene is associated with autosomal dominant hereditary systemic amyloidosis, which can cause renal dysfunction and tubular proteinuria. The primary renal lesion is TIN with variable degrees of tubular atrophy, interstitial fibrosis, and glomerular sclerosis and medullary amyloid deposits and absence of light chains and protein AA. Apo AI amyloidosis is a slowly progressive renal disease, and end-stage renal disease occurs approximately 3 to 15 years from initial diagnosis.[20] Renal transplantation offers an acceptable graft survival in these patients. Simultaneous liver and kidney transplantation could be considered in hepatorenal involvement.

Glomerular and Vascular Diseases

TIN is caused by glomerular injury both by a glomerulonephritis dependent and independent mechanism. Although injury may originate in the glomerulus, resulting proteinuria and complement activation within the tubular lumen may lead to tubulointerstitial damage and progressive renal disease. MPO-ANCA-associated glomerulonephritis is an example of glomerulonephritis independent mechanism of TIN. In this entity, NLRP3 inflammasome-dependent processing in macrophages releases the mature active form of IL-1β, which may lead to the development and deterioration of TIN. Secondary TIN (e.g., in lupus nephritis) correlates with advanced class of glomerular involvement and can be mediated by lupus-related immunologic mechanism or by a nonimmunologic injury as in any type of advanced nonlupus glomerular disease. A rare entity is primary lupus TIN, which manifests as acute kidney injury with no or mild proteinuria. Histology shows immunoglobulin/complement deposits along the tubular basement membrane. Primary lupus TIN responds well to steroid and has a good prognosis. TIN on renal biopsy without an apparent etiology should prompt further evaluation, including for glomerular pathology. Vascular diseases can be caused by any factors—congenital to metabolic—but invariably with a common result of tissue ischemia. Glomerular injury and vasoconstriction of efferent arterioles decrease postglomerular peritubular capillary blood flow. The relative chronic hypoxia from decreased oxygen delivery and increased metabolic demand in tubular cells induces inflammatory pathways that leads to tubulointerstitial injury. Renoprotection involves prevention and treatment of the underlying conditions utilizing statins, renin–angiotensin system blockade, anemia, and metabolic and blood pressure controls.

Heavy Metals

Acute or chronic exposure to heavy metals can induce renal tubulointerstitial injuries, including acute tubular necrosis, chronic TIN, Fanconi syndrome, renal tubular acidosis, and renal tubular dysfunction without morphological changes. Simultaneous exposure to multiple heavy metals and glyphosate have been linked to TIN in Sri Lanka. Lead exposure can cause hypertension, anemia, lead line, hyperuricemia, and acute or chronic TIN. Mesangioproliferative glomerulonephritis can also be seen, but immune deposits are absent on immunofluorescence.[21] Cadmium, inorganic germanium, copper, gold, and gadolinium have been linked to kidney injury. The main actions of these metals are to increase free radical production and oxidative stress and stimulation of angiotensin I-converting enzyme activity, thereby affecting vascular reactivity. The risk of heavy metal related toxicities, including TIN, remain high in underdeveloped parts of the world.

Emerging/Endemic Nephropathies

Global epidemics of chronic kidney disease, unexplained by conventional theories, have spurred interest in nontraditional pathomechanisms. Mesoamerican nephropathy Balkan endemic nephropathy, crystalline-related TIN, and Balkan endemic nephropathy are discussed here.

Mesoamerican Nephropathy

An epidemic of chronic kidney disease in young male agricultural workers working in hot environments and subject to recurrent dehydration in Central America and Sri Lanka has been termed Mesoamerican nephropathy. The postulated mechanism is heat stress related to repeated subclinical or clinical acute kidney injury that eventually manifests as chronic kidney disease. It can manifest as subclinical rhabdomyolysis with release of nucleotides and a rise in serum uric acid. Dehydration results in high urinary uric acid concentrations that can exceed solubility, which ultimately leads to crystal-induced renal injury.[22] The characteristic histologic feature of this slowly progressive disease is TIN, sometimes with a component of global glomerulosclerosis. Others have implicated lead and silica (India), multiple heavy metals, and herbicides such as glyphosate (Sri Lanka) in this entity.

Crystalline-Related Tubulointerstitial Disease

Crystallopathies encompass organ injuries caused by deposits of crystals, misfolded proteins, or aggregation of atoms and ions into amorphous crystals. In addition to mechanical obstruction, crystals can elicit direct cytotoxicity, inflammation, and inflammation-driven necrosis. Crystal-induced renal entities include acute kidney injury, nephrocalcinosis, fibrillary glomerulonephritis, amyloidosis, and nephrolithiasis. Uric acid crystal-induced chronic TIN is known for decades, although the immunostimulatory effects of uric acid microparticles are only being recognized. Crystals cause cell stress, apoptosis, inflammation, necrosis, granuloma, and fibrosis. The pathway involves NLRP3 inflammasome, which is a central primary and secondary driver of crystal-related inflammation.

Balkan Endemic Nephropathy

Balkan endemic nephropathy is caused by aristolochic acid and the characteristic renal lesion is chronic TIN. Urothelial carcinoma is found in up to 50% of the patients. Initially diagnosed in the rural areas along the Danube River, it has also been found in China. Contamination of wheat with seeds from the plant producing aristolochic acid and certain herbal remedies were implicated in Balkan nephropathy. A 2-year follow-up study[23] indicated that metals and metalloids did not play a role in the etiology of Balkan endemic nephropathy. Patients present with tubular proteinuria, impaired concentrating capacity, and reduced glomerular filtration rate in their sixth decade with slow progression to end-stage kidney disease. Treatment is supportive therapy. Against the assumption in the literature, selenium was not protective but a risk factor.

Miscellaneous

TIN is also classified according to their existence with ischemic or toxic acute kidney or obstructive nephropathy. Acute tubular necrosis and acute or chronic TIN are probably secondary processes of each other, mediated by downstream inflammatory pathways. Obstructive nephropathy is a common cause of TIN and, untreated, can lead to irreversible kidney injury. Treatment is directed at relieving underlying pathology. Secondary malignancies involving the kidney are uncommon. In 1 series, only 75 (5%) of 1,572 renal biopsies identified a secondary malignancy.[24] The majority of the renal infiltrates were metastases from solid tumors, and hematological malignancies accounted for 27% of cases. TIN is often reported with cancer agents and increased vigilance is required with newer agents. BRAF-targeted and MEK-targeted therapy have been linked to TIN.

APPROACH TO RENOPROTECTION IN TIN

The first step in the management of TIN is clinical suspicion, followed by clinical diagnosis and identification and removal of offending factors. Fig. 43.2 suggests a practical approach to diagnosis and treatment. The most difficult decision point is what to do when biopsy is relatively contraindicated (solitary kidney, coagulation disorders), and the patient remains unresponsive to empiric treatment with steroids. Gallium-67 scan is often helpful in differentiating acute TIN from acute tubular necrosis and normal kidneys; however, its sensitivity and specificity is 58% to 69% and 50% to 60%, respectively. There are little data on the utility of 2-[18F] fluoro-2-deoxy-D glucose-positron emission tomography (FDG-PET). The treatment of TIN is based on

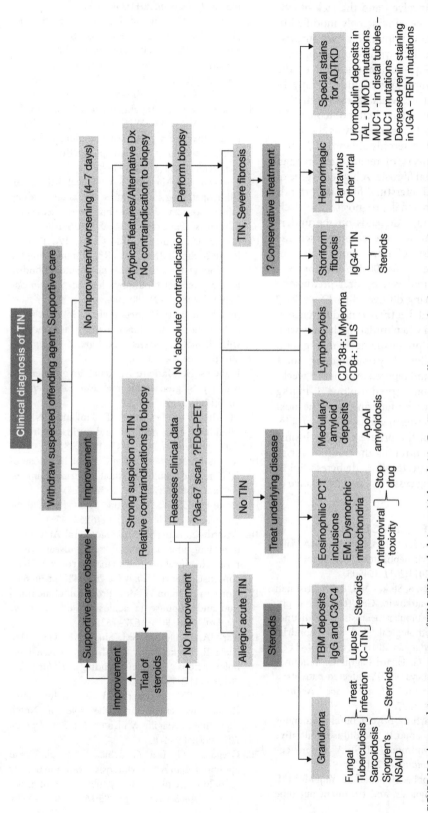

FIGURE 43.2 Approach to management of TIN. TIN = tubulointerstitial nephritis. Ga-67 scan = gallium-67 radiopharmaceutical scan. FDG-PET = fluorodeoxyglucose-positron emission tomography. NSAID = nonsteroidal anti-inflammatory drug. IC-TIN = Immune complex tubulointerstitial nephritis. PCT = proximal convoluted tubule. ApoAI = Apolipoprotein A-I. DILS = diffuse infiltrative lymphocytosis syndrome. ADTKD = Autosomal Dominant Tubulointerstitial Kidney Disease. TAL = thick ascending limb of Henle loop. UMOD = uromodulin. MUC 1 = mucin 1. JGA = juxtaglomerular apparatus. REN = gene encoding renin.

immunosuppression despite the multiplicity of pathomechanisms involved and the lack of evidence that TIN can be convincingly modified in patients by immune manipulation. Not surprisingly, treatment for TIN with immunosuppression remains inadequate. Identification of the causative factor is important to guide therapy. In the limited data that are available, early initiation of treatments appear to have better outcomes.[25,26] Acute TIN precedes fibrogenesis by as short as 7 to 14 days and corticosteroids are more effective in accelerating recovery of renal function than preventing interstitial fibrosis. A higher degree of tubular atrophy and interstitial fibrosis portends a poorer long-term renal prognosis. The decision to initiate therapy depends on the underlying pathomechanisms. The common scheme of treatment consists of intravenous pulses of methylprednisolone (250–500 mg/day for 3–4 consecutive days) followed by oral prednisone (1 mg/kg/day) tapering off over 8 to 12 weeks.[26] Others have reported that there is no difference in achieving remission when initiating therapy with intravenous (methylprednisolone 30 mg/kg for 3 consecutive days followed by oral prednisolone 1 mg/kg for 2 weeks and tapered over next 3 week) or oral corticosteroids (prednisolone 1 mg/kg for 3 weeks followed by tapering over the next 3 weeks).[27] The long-term management of TIN is the retardation of the progression of chronic kidney disease by controlling the traditional risk factors such as hypertension, diabetes, lipids, proteinuria, smoking cessation, and avoidance of nephrotoxic agents.

REFERENCES

1. Fernandez-Fernandez B, Montoya-Ferrer A, Sanz AB, et al. Tenofovir nephrotoxicity: 2011 update. *AIDS Res Treat.* 2011;2011:354908.

2. Herlitz LC, Mohan S, Stokes MB, Radhakrishnan J, D'Agati VD, Markowitz GS. Tenofovir nephrotoxicity: acute tubular necrosis with distinctive clinical, pathological, and mitochondrial abnormalities. *Kidney Int.* 2010;78(11):1171–1177.

3. Tourret J, Deray G, Isnard-Bagnis C. Tenofovir effect on the kidneys of HIV-infected patients: a double-edged sword? *J Am Soc Nephrol.* 2013;24(10):1519–1527.

4. Ghrenassia E, Martis N, Boyer J, Burel-Vandenbos F, Mekinian A, Coppo P. The diffuse infiltrative lymphocytosis syndrome (DILS). A comprehensive review. *J Autoimmun.* 2015;59:19–25.

5. Chapagain A, Dobbie H, Sheaff M, Yaqoob MM. Presentation, diagnosis, and treatment outcome of tuberculous-mediated tubulointerstitial nephritis. *Kidney Int.* 2011;79(6):671.

6. Rossert J. Drug-induced acute interstitial nephritis. *Kidney Int.* 2001;60(2):804–817.

7. Kishore BK, Ecelbarger CM. Lithium: a versatile tool for understanding renal physiology. *Am J Physiol Renal Physiol.* 2013;304(9):F1139–F1149.

8. Markowitz GS, Radhakrishnan J, Kambham N, Valeri AM, Hines WH, D'Agati VD. Lithium nephrotoxicity: a progressive combined glomerular and tubulointerstitial nephropathy. *J Am Soc Nephrol.* 2000;11(8):1439–1448.

9. Cortazar FB, Marrone KA, Troxell ML, et al. Clinicopathological features of acute kidney injury associated with immune checkpoint inhibitors. *Kidney Int.* 2016;90(3):638–647.

10. Rosales IA, Collins AB, do Carmo PA, Tolkoff-Rubin N, Smith RN, Colvin RB. Immune complex tubulointerstitial nephritis due to autoantibodies to the proximal tubule brush border. *J Am Soc Nephrol.* 2016;27(2):380–384.

11. Bitik B, Gonul II, Haznedaroglu S, Goker B, Tufan A. Granulomatous interstitial nephritis associated with Primary Sjögren's syndrome. *Z Rheumatol.* 2017;76(5):458–460.

12. François H, Mariette X. Renal involvement in primary Sjögren syndrome. *Nat Rev Nephrol.* 2016;12(2):82–93.

13. Mandeville JT, Levinson RD, Holland GN. The tubulointerstitial nephritis and uveitis syndrome. *Surv Ophthalmol.* 2001;46(3):195–208.

14. Raissian Y, Nasr SH, Larsen CP, et al. Diagnosis of IgG4-related tubulointerstitial nephritis. *J Am Soc Nephrol.* 2011;22(7):1343–1352.

15. Stone JH, Zen Y, Deshpande V. IgG4-related disease. *N Engl J Med.* 2012;366(6):539–551.

16. Eckardt KU, Alper SL, Antignac C, et al. Autosomal dominant tubulointerstitial kidney disease: diagnosis, classification, and management–a KDIGO consensus report. *Kidney Int.* 2015;88(4):676–683.

17. Norman P, Orson W. Moe. Proximal tubule function and response to acidosis. *Clin J Am Soc Nephrol.* 2014; 9(9): 1627–1638.

18. Kari JA, El Desoky SM, Singh AK, Gari MA, Kleta R, Bockenhauer D. The case | Renal tubular acidosis and eye findings. *Kidney Int.* 2014;86(1):217–218.

19. Kamath BM, Spinner NB, Rosenblum ND. Renal involvement and the role of Notch signalling in Alagille syndrome. *Nat Rev Nephrol.* 2013;9(7):409–418.

20. Gregorini G, Izzi C, Obici L, et al. Renal apolipoprotein A-I amyloidosis: a rare and usually ignored cause of hereditary tubulointerstitial nephritis. *J Am Soc Nephrol.* 2005;16(12):3680–3686.

21. Kute VB, Shrimali JD, Balwani MR, et al. Lead nephropathy due to Sindoor in India. *Ren Fail.* 2013;35(6):885–887.

22. Roncal-Jimenez CA, García-Trabanino R, Wesseling C, Johnson RJ. Mesoamerican nephropathy or global warming nephropathy? *Blood Purif.* 2016;41(1–3):135–138.

23. Karmaus W, Dimitrov P, Simeonov V, Tsolova S, Bonev A, Georgieva R. Metals and kidney markers in adult offspring of endemic nephropathy patients and controls: a two-year follow-up study. *Environ Health.* 2008;7:11.

24. Huang H, Tamboli P, Karam JA, Vikram R, Zhang M. Secondary malignancies diagnosed using kidney needle core biopsies: a clinical and pathological study of 75 cases. *Human Pathology Hum Pathol.* 2016;52:55–60.

25. Clarkson MR, Giblin L, O'Connell FP, et al. Acute interstitial nephritis: clinical features and response to corticosteroid therapy. *Nephrol Dial Transplant.* 2004; 19:2778–2783.

26. González E, Gutiérrez E, Galeano C, et al.; Grupo Madrileño De Nefritis Intersticiales. Early steroid treatment improves the recovery of renal function in patients with drug-induced acute interstitial nephritis. *Kidney Int.* 2008; 73:940–946.

27. Ramachandran R, Kumar K, Nada R, Jha V, Gupta KL, Kohli HS. Drug-induced acute interstitial nephritis: A clinicopathological study and comparative trial of steroid regimens. *Indian J Nephrol.* 2015; 25:281–286.

44

Cholesterol Crystal Embolism

ALAIN MEYRIER

INTRODUCTION

Cholesterol crystal embolism (CCE), also known as atheroembolic disease or multiple cholesterol embolization syndrome, was first mentioned as an anecdotal postmortem finding in the second half of the 19th century.[1] It remained a complication of atherosclerosis chiefly found at autopsy, until the practice of vascular surgery in the 1950s,[2] followed some decades later by interventional radiology[3] that shed a distressing light on an iatrogenic complication of aortic atherosclerotic plaques.[4] This complication affects the kidneys in more than 80% of cases. Renal involvement spans a spectrum, from acute kidney injury (AKI) in fulminant forms to relatively mild progressive renal disease that can be mistaken for hypertensive nephrosclerosis.[5] The source of emboli is the aortic wall[6] and in a majority of cases cholesterol crystal emboli originate from the aortic arch (Fig. 44.1).[7] This explains the great variability of signs and symptoms, a variability that makes CCE ("the great masquerader") a multiorgan systemic disease that can be considered as a disseminated small-vessel angiitis resulting from crystal foreign bodies.

EPIDEMIOLOGY

In all cases, CCE complicates widespread atherosclerosis with disseminated plaques covering the aortic wall and the inner aspect of the main visceral arteries. The epidemiology of CCE parallels that of atherosclerosis in terms of age, background, and geographic and ethnic factors. While atherosclerotic disease, hypertension, history of smoking, and the elevation of baseline plasma C-reactive protein are risk factors, race is not in the majority of studies. The typical patient is a hypertensive male (the male/female ratio is ~70%), older than 50, lean, dyslipidemic, and a cigarette smoker. Two localizations of atheroma are significantly associated with CCE: plaques involving the aortic arch and an abdominal aortic aneurysm (97% and 67%, respectively, in Belenfant et al.[7]). In unselected autopsy series, the frequency of finding atheroemboli is low, from 0.31% to 2.4%.[8] In a geriatric study of 334 kidney biopsy in patients ≥65 years of age, the prevalence was 4% to 6.5%.[9] Studies focused on kidney biopsy reported a frequency of 1%. This mostly reflects the low incidence of spontaneous CCE. Conversely autopsy studies performed in patients who died after aortic surgery or angiography revealed a high prevalence of 12% to 77%.[1] In fact, the frequency of CCE is variably estimated, depending on systematic search on autopsy material as opposed to clinical diagnosis. Fine et al.[10] reviewed 221 histologically proven cases. Among 75 cases, clinical diagnosis of gastrointestinal and pancreatic involvement was made in 26.7%, of renal involvement in 22.7%, and of spleen, liver, and adrenal involvement in 1.33%. At autopsy, among 92 cases, the respective figures were 95.6%, 83.7%, and 100%.

ETIOPATHOGENESIS

The source of cholesterol crystal emboli is a ruptured or denuded atherosclerotic plaque.[5,6] Atherosclerotic plaques are made of a fibrous cap overlying a soft atheromatous core containing necrotic cellular debris, macrophages, foam cells, and cholesterol crystals (Fig. 44.2). The fibrous cap is often calcified. It may be cracked by mechanical trauma, such as clamping during vascular surgery, dislodgement by a Seldinger catheter, or crush by angioplasty maneuvers. Plaques frequently undergo spontaneous ulceration. The denuded core is covered with a clot that separates the cholesterol crystals from the bloodstream. This last barrier against crystal migration may undergo spontaneous lysis—the usual cause

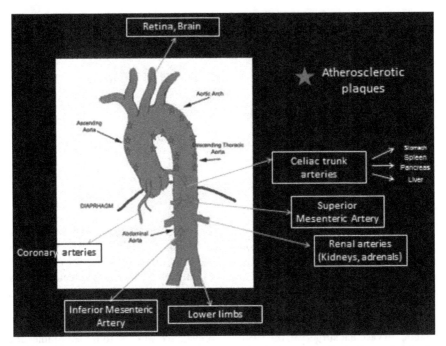

FIGURE 44.1 A majority—but not all cases—of cholesterol crystal emboli originate from atherosclerotic plaques in the aortic arch. Crystals follow the bloodstream and may reach every organ system, from coronary arteries, retina, and central nervous system to the lower extremities.

of noniatrogenic CCE—or thrombolysis may be precipitated by anticoagulant or by fibrinolytic treatment. The foregoing mechanisms explain well the fact that CCE is in a majority of cases an iatrogenic complication of vascular surgery, interventional radiology and/or anticoagulation in a patient with aortic atherosclerosis. In fact, the hazard of CCE ranks among the main concerns

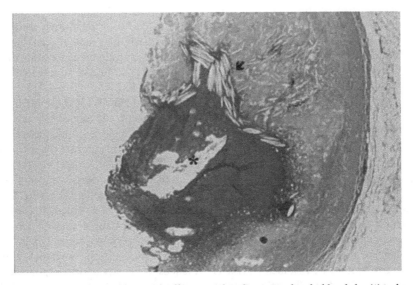

FIGURE 44.2 Ulcerated atherosclerotic plaque. The fibrous cap has disappeared and a blood clot (*) isolates the underlying soft atheromatous material and cholesterol crystals (→) from the blood stream. Lysis of the clot from anticoagulant or fibrinolytic treatment, or dislodgement by a Seldinger catheter, angioplasty material, or by a surgical clamp are common mechanisms of crystal migration.

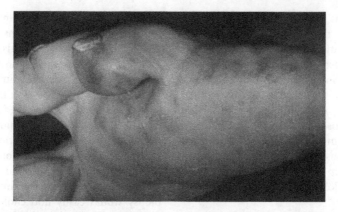

FIGURE 44.3 A typical appearance of blue toes (arrow) and livedo reticularis (arrowhead) in a patient with cholesterol crystal embolism. From Meyrier A. Atherosclerosis and the kidney. Encycl Med Chir (Elsevier SAS) Paris, *Néphrologie* 18-046-A-10: 2003, 1–13. with permission from the publisher.

of vascular surgeons[11] and of interventional radiologists and may tip the risk–benefit ratio toward a contraindication to an otherwise fully indicated surgical or radiologic procedure.

Crystals lodge in small arteries with a lumen diameter of 150 to 200 μm. They are too small to clog up these arteries, and vessel obstruction results from a delayed inflammatory endothelial reaction as addressed in the following discussion (Fig. 44.3). Crystals may progress further to capillaries, especially within the skin but also to visceral small vessels such as afferent glomerular arteries and even glomerular tuft capillaries. By light microscopy, crystals that are dissolved by the fixation process appear as transparent double-convex, spindle-shaped ghosts of the original solid material.

MECHANISMS OF KIDNEY INJURY

Animal experiments have been based on the injection of cholesterol crystals into the renal artery followed by serial observations of the vascular lesions.[12] Shortly after lodging in the lumens, crystals induce platelet aggregation and thrombosis. Thereafter, the thrombus undergoes lysis. Subsequently, from 5 days to 1 month onwards, progressive fibrous endarteritis leads to complete arterial obstruction. The fate of cholesterol crystals is to persist indefinitely. These findings help understand the course of the human disease: massive CCE complicated with early AKI is induced by widespread thrombosis of the renal arterial tree with scattered multifocal infarction, whereas milder forms progress to a delayed, obstructive inflammatory reaction to foreign bodies. In the latter subset, the delay between the inciting event and the onset of renal insufficiency may be a deceptive feature of the disease, especially for an unsuspecting mind.

CLINICAL PRESENTATION

Cholesterol crystal embolism is not an isolated renal disease. Kidney involvement is part of a generalized atheroembolic process that may involve most organs, viscera, and tissues of the body, from coronary arteries to feet and toes.

Renal Involvement

Renal complications of CCE cover 3 scenarios: acute, subacute, and chronic kidney disease.[1,5]

AKI occurring within 2 to 7 days following the inciting event is observed in about one-third of the cases. It is often fulminant, following massive migration of crystals. Ischemic AKI is painless and is not accompanied by hematuria. Oliguria appears rapidly and is accompanied with severe hypertension or the abrupt aggravation of previous hypertension. Half of 129 patients reported by Lye et al.[13] were hypertensive, most of them severely. Left ventricular failure and pulmonary edema complicate AKI in two-thirds of these cases (41 of 67 patients in Belenfant et al.[7]).

The subacute subset may represent some diagnostic challenges as renal manifestations appear weeks or even months after the inciting event. Frock et al.[14] in 17 patients with CCE observed that acute kidney insufficiency occurred 5.3±0.9 weeks after angiography. Renal function impairment often develops in a stepwise fashion over the following weeks. Each aggravation follows a triggering event eliciting another shower of crystals, such as repeat angiography, vascular surgery, and/or anticoagulation.

In most cases of CCE, proteinuria is nonsignificant. Some cases, however, may be accompanied by nephrotic proteinuria. Greenberg et al.[15] found 10 cases of focal segmental glomerulosclerosis in 24 patients with CCE whose proteinuria reached nephrotic levels. These observations have fostered speculations on the relationship between renal ischemia and focal segmental glomerulosclerosis, including its collapsing variant.[16]

The chronic subset is frequent and underdiagnosed, understandably if one considers the patients' vascular and hypertensive background. It manifests by a slowly progressive form of renal disease with bouts of aggravation. In an atherosclerotic patient in his 60s, suffering from hypertension and renal insufficiency, and in whom renal artery plaques are common, renal insufficiency complicating low-grade cholesterol crystal embolism to the kidneys is usually ascribed to nephrosclerosis.[17] However, careful examination of the feet, funduscopy, and high blood eosinophil counts may lead to the diagnosis of chronic renal CCE.

Extrarenal Cholesterol Crystal Embolism

The kidney is not the sole organ involved. Depending on the site of ruptured or denuded plaques, multiple vital organ damage has been described, including—in a downstream progression from the aortic arch to the abdominal aorta—the coronary arteries, the retina, the central nervous system, the spinal cord artery, the lungs, the mesenteric blood supply, the pancreas, and the adrenal glands. Virtually all organs may be involved by cholesterol crystals that can be found by the pathologists in various tissue specimens following surgical removal or at autopsy, such as adrenals, testes, prostate, thyroid, and lymph nodes. These localizations are anecdotal and of little interest to the clinician nephrologist. However—this is a personal opinion—atheroembolism to the adrenal glands might have bearing on the initial clinical manifestations and explain the benefit of corticosteroids on the patient's management.

We describe the main localizations of CCE and especially those that lead to the diagnosis without having recourse to invasive procedures and especially to a kidney biopsy.

First and foremost, CCE involves the dermal capillaries. Cutaneous lesions are observed in 75% to 96% of cases,[1,5] and this easily visible skin localization is of major diagnostic interest. Areas of skin ischemia translate clinically into lesions of *livedo reticularis,* that is, a mottled discoloration of the skin. It is described as being reticular (net-like, lace-like) and cyanotic (reddish blue discoloration). The discoloration surrounds pale central skin. Livedo may involve the lumbar region, the thighs, the knees and/or the feet. It may be more apparent in the standing position. A skin biopsy would easily find cholesterol crystals in dermal small vessels and rule out another cause of livedo.

Distal ischemic lesions affect the toes. Their microvascular nature is confirmed by persistence of distal artery pulses. "Blue toes" may evolve to necrosis that is usually painful. (Fig. 44.4). Pain can be excruciating and require major analgesics. Painful, complete gangrene of toes may necessitate amputation.

Massive CCE usually involves lower limb muscles and bone marrow. Muscle ischemia contributes to wasting. In some instances, bone biopsy revealed cholesterol crystals in the bone marrow.

Cholesterol emboli may be seen at funduscopy.[18] This should be a systematic investigation oriented by specific information to the ophthalmologist as there may be only 1 or 2 crystals per fundus. Retinal involvement is present in 6% to 25% of cases. The latter figure is probably closer to reality as not all published papers mention systematic ocular examination in their patients. Finding retinal cholesterol crystals suffices to avoid invasive diagnostic procedures. It points to the ascending aorta as source of emboli. It helps explain some neurological disorders complicating embolization to the central nervous system, such as *amaurosis fugax,* mental confusion, transient ischemic attack, and/or focal neurological deficits.

Gastrointestinal involvement is frequent as atheroembolism to the celiac and the mesenteric arteries occurs commonly in acute and subacute forms. Abdominal pain and is due to intestinal and pancreatic ischemia. Splenic infarcts are commonly discovered at autopsy but do not entail clinical manifestations.

The patients complain of abdominal pain, anorexia, and rapidly lose weight. Stomach and colon biopsies rank among the mildly invasive procedures that often reveal cholesterol

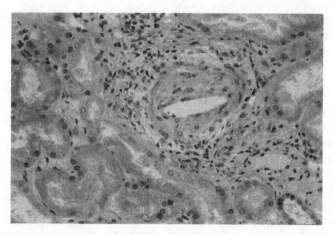

FIGURE 44.4 Kidney biopsy. A typical "ghost" of cholesterol crystal is lodged within an interlobular artery. The crystal was too small to totally suppress the blood flow, but this foreign body caused a delayed inflammatory reaction with progressive obstruction. Note the perivascular reaction with inflammatory cells.

crystals in the mucosa (Fig. 44.5). Migration of crystals to the pancreas adds to abdominal pain and wasting. The diagnosis is rarely made clinically, although pancreatic involvement is found at autopsy in virtually all cases.[10] That adrenal gland involvement is constant[10] could imply that patients with massive CCE are often in a state of adrenal insufficiency and explain the favorable effect of corticosteroids at the initial phase.

Moolenaar and Lamers[19] retrospectively studied the clinical and histopathologic features of CCE to the gastrointestinal tract in 96 patients (70 men, 26 women, mean age 73.8 [range 58–95] years) from 1973 to 1992; 130 CCE sites were found throughout the alimentary tract, mostly in the colon (42.3%). Most patients had a history of atherosclerotic disease and presented with

abdominal pain, diarrhea, or gastrointestinal bleeding, sometimes after surgical or radiological vascular procedures. A number were taking oral anticoagulant treatment. The diagnosis of CCE had been considered before the histological diagnosis in only 11 patients. In the remaining cases, ischemic colitis, tumor, and inflammatory bowel disease were suggested in the differential diagnosis. A premortem diagnosis of CCE was made in 70.8% of the cases. In 24 of the 35 necropsy examinations, CCE seemed to be directly or indirectly related to the cause of death. In this unselected, homogenous group of patients, emboli were most frequently found in the colon. Gastrointestinal visceral ischemia may explain such laboratory changes as rise of hepatic enzymes or elevations in amylase and lipase levels.

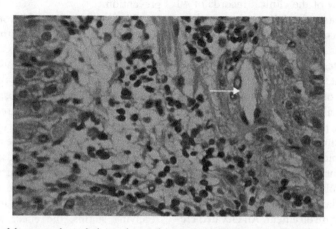

FIGURE 44.5 Biopsy of the stomach. A cholesterol crystal (arrow) is lodged in a small vessel.

Other Visceral Manifestations

Emboli that emanate from the ascending aorta or the proximal segments of the coronary arteries may be associated with angina and sudden cardiac death. Pulmonary involvement, characterized by diffuse alveolar hemorrhage mimicking systemic vasculitis, has been described in a few case reports. Finally, a number of nonspecific findings can accompany the course of CCE, including fever, weight loss, myalgias, and headache—that, along with elevated markers of inflammation and eosinophilia, demonstrate the systemic nature of the disease and explain possible confusion with other systemic diseases, especially vasculitis.

Laboratory Findings

Some laboratory test findings are nonspecific. They may include anemia, leukocytosis, thrombocytopenia, and elevation of inflammatory markers (erythrocyte sedimentary rate or C-reactive protein). Urinalysis is a poorly contributive to the diagnosis, with few cells and minimal proteinuria. Low complement levels are not of diagnostic interest.

Conversely, blood eosinophilia, commonly occurring during the acute phase of the disease and in case of relapses, is of great diagnostic interest. In the first report on 6 cases of eosinophilia in patients with atheroembolic disease, Kasinath et al.[20] found, by examination of biopsy of kidney or skin, extensive atheroembolic lesions in the vasculature. No evidence of vascular or tubulointerstitial inflammation was observed. Eosinophil count ranged from 540 to 2,000 cells/mm³. Upon review of the literature, 80% (29 out of 36) of patients with adequately reported total and differential leukocyte counts had eosinophilia in association with atheroembolic disease. In contrast, review of the clinical records of 40 consecutive patients with AKI seen during an 18-month period uncovered only 1 case of eosinophilia (2.5%). This latter patient was established as having acute interstitial nephritis. Eosinophilia is usually transient, ranging from 6% to 18%. In a larger study, 67% of 354 patients had an eosinophil count >500 cells/μl.[22] Eosinophilia is helpful in establishing the diagnosis of CCE, and in case of recurrence, rising eosinophil counts entail a high index of suspicion.

Some laboratory abnormalities reflect specific organ involvement. Increased hepatic enzymes or amylase and lipase levels suggest liver or pancreatic involvement. An elevated creatinine phosphokinase level accompanies muscle ischemia. An increase in serum aspartate aminotransferase and lactate dehydrogenase levels may point to kidney infarction.[21]

TREATMENT AND MANAGEMENT CONSIDERATIONS

Preventive Measures

CCE is in most cases a complication of widespread atherosclerosis. It is outside the scope of this review to consider the lifelong prevention of this arterial disease. From this standpoint, however, abstaining of smoking and cholesterol-lowering drugs should in the long term reduce the incidence of spontaneous low-grade embolization.

Considering the frequency of iatrogenic, life-threatening acute and subacute forms, prevention is the mainstay in treatment consideration. In a patient with widespread atherosclerotic plaques radiologists must carefully consider the pros and cons of endovascular procedures for diagnostic and therapeutic purposes. The risk of severe CCE following Seldinger-catheter angiography or angioplasty and stenting may justify abstention of such maneuvers by fear of plaque crushing and dislodgement, and vascular surgeons may refuse to operate a high-risk patient. Thrombolytic therapy has been published as a possible triggering factor. In the same line anticoagulation is a frequent cause of CCE in patients with atherosclerotic plaques and in this setting the indication of antivitamin K treatment should be poised in terms of risk/benefit. Aspirin associated with clopidogrel may be substituted to antivitamin Ks without documented risk of triggering cholesterol-crystal migration.

In addition to the previously discussed measures, statins play a major role in secondary prevention.

Occasional cases of atheroembolic renal disease have responded to statins. In a prospective study, Scolari et al.[22] assigned patients to statin therapy and found a lowered risk of progression to end-stage renal disease. The same group carried out a large prospective study that confirmed this finding. Three hundred fifty-four patients were followed up for an average of 2 years. They tended to be elderly males and to have cardiovascular diseases and abnormal renal function at baseline. During the study, 116 patients required dialysis, and 102 died. The risk of dialysis and death was 50% lower among those receiving statins; the effect was evident even when statin therapy was started after diagnosis of atheroembolic renal disease. The protective effect of statins is attributable to plaque stabilization and even plaque regression through lipid-lowering and anti-inflammatory mechanisms.[23]

CONSIDERATION IN RENAL REPLACEMENT THERAPY

Fulminant forms with extensive pancreatic, intestinal, and often central nervous system ischemia associated with gangrene of the toes do not die of AKI but of multivisceral compromise.

Supportive treatment must be analyzed in the setting of dialysis in the intensive care unit.

Belenfant and co-authors[7] presented the results of a protocol based on the usual causes of death in patients with severe forms of CCE. This protocol consisted in stopping any form of anticoagulation and forbidding any new radiologic and/or vascular surgery procedure; treating hypertension drastically with renin–angiotensin antagonists and vasodilators; achieving a strict fluid balance by loop diuretics and dialysis/ultrafiltration; implementing parenteral nutrition; and giving ~1 mg/kg/d of prednisone to improve appetite and relieve abdominal discomfort. In-hospital mortality was 16%. Survival at 1 year was 87% and 52% at 4 years, which compared favorably with corresponding figures published earlier. However, some form of bias might have influenced these figures as Ravani et al.,[24] using a conservative regimen, obtained roughly similar results and did not observe untoward effects of peritoneal dialysis compared with hemodialysis.[1]

The issue of corticosteroid treatment advocated by Belenfant et al.[7] has been debated. The Scolari group, in a prospective study of 354 patients with atheroembolic renal disease, concluded that steroids were not associated with improved renal or patient outcomes.[24] Nevertheless, a Medline search at the time of this writing yields a majority of papers in favor of early corticosteroid treatment of atheroembolic disease.[25]

CONSIDERATIONS IN KIDNEY TRANSPLANTATION

Atheroembolic renal disease in renal allografts is rare, with a frequency ranging from 0 to less than 0.50%. In 2010, 45 cases of CCE in renal transplants had been published,[1] too scarce a number to reflect the real incidence of this complication.

The source of crystals can be ascribed to the donor at the time of procurement, to recipient's atherosclerosis, to invasive radiology, or to anticoagulation/fibrinolytic treatment.[5] The time course to the graft compromise (when specified) is short (6–18 days) when emboli emanate from the donor's artery and apparently long, in the order of years, when the recipient is the victim of his own underlying atherosclerosis.[25] In fact, CCE may be triggered several years and even decades after grafting by angioplasty, anticoagulation, or fibrinolytic therapy. CCE occurring at the time of transplantation leads to rapid graft loss in one-third of cases and recovery in about 50%. CCE due to the recipient's atherosclerosis has a better prognosis with recovery in two-thirds of cases. One may postulate that CCE is more common in renal transplantation than presumed and often misinterpreted as acute or chronic rejection or resulting from calcineurin inhibitor toxicity. Outside the case of rapid graft failure followed by thorough pathologic examination of a surgically removed transplant, many cases fail to be diagnosed on the limited amount of tissue yielded by a thin needle renal biopsy.

CONCLUSION

- Cholesterol crystal embolism originates from ulcerated atherosclerotic plaques of the aorta, essentially the aortic arch, and affects multiple organ systems, including the kidneys in >80% of cases. It may be considered as a form of foreign body–induced microscopic angiitis.
- Lower extremity skin involvement with livedo reticularis and blue toes is found in the majority of patients.
- Atheroembolization can be spontaneous but is increasingly recognized as a iatrogenic complication of invasive vascular procedures, including angiography, peripheral and coronary angioplasty, vascular surgery, and anticoagulant or fibrinolytic therapy. These triggering factors list the rationale of primary preventive measures for reducing the incidence of the disease.
- Diagnosis may be overlooked in the frequent, deceptive cases where a time lag of 1 to several weeks separates the triggering event from the onset of kidney insufficiency.
- Among the laboratory features, the best clue is the presence of eosinophilia.
- Kidney biopsy is rarely indicated for diagnosing acute and subacute forms as, in

a patient with widespread atherosclerosis, a triggering event + typical skin lesions + retinal emboli at funduscopy + eosinophilia is diagnostic in > 80% of cases.

- When a kidney biopsy is deemed indicated, cholesterol crystals, dissolved by the fixation process, appear as elongated, spindle-shaped, biconvex, clear bodies within small arteries and in capillaries. They induce an endothelial inflammatory reaction that leads to progressive, irreversible vascular obstruction.
- In fulminant and acute forms, death is not due to kidney involvement but to visceral ischemia, especially gastrointestinal and pancreatic. In less severe forms, those who survive with supportive therapy do not recover renal function, and >50% are fated to remain on renal replacement therapy.
- Cholesterol crystal embolization may complicate kidney transplantation and be misinterpreted as rejection or drug toxicity.
- Treatment with statins significantly reduces the mortality and the progression to end-stage renal failure.

REFERENCES

1. Scolari F, Ravani P. Atheroembolic renal disease. *Lancet.* 2010;375(9726):1650–1660.
2. Thurlbeck WM, Castleman B. Atheromatous emboli to the kidneys after aortic surgery. *N Engl J Med.* 1957;257(10):442–447.
3. Ramirez G, O'Neill WM Jr, Lambert R, Bloomer HA. Cholesterol embolization: a complication of angiography. *Arch Intern Med.* 1978;138(9):1430–1432.
4. Thadhani R, Camargo C, Xavier R, Fang L, Bazari H. Atheroembolic renal failure after invasive procedures: natural history based on 52 biopsy-proven cases. *Medicine.* 1995;74:350–358.
5. Meyrier A. Cholesterol crystal embolism: diagnosis and treatment. *Kidney Int.* 2006;69:1308–1312.
6. Flory CM. Arterial occlusions produced by emboli from eroded aortic atheromatous plaques. *Am J Pathol.* 1945;21:549–565.
7. Belenfant X, Meyrier A, Jacquot C. Supportive treatment improves survival in multivisceral cholesterol crystal embolism. *Am J Kidney Dis.* 1999;33:840–850.
8. Cross SS. How common is cholesterol embolism? *J Clin Pathol.* 1991; 44:859–861.
9. Preston RA, Stemmer CL, Materson BJ, Perez-Stable E, Pardo V. Renal biopsy in patients 65 years of age or older: an analysis of the results of 334 biopsies. *J Am Geriatr Soc.* 1990;38(6):669–674.
10. Fine MJ, Kapoor W, Falanga V. Cholesterol crystal embolization: a review of 221 cases in the English literature. *Angiology.* 1987; 42:769–784.
11. Krishnamurthi V, Novick AC, Myles JL. Atheroembolic renal disease: effect on morbidity and survival after revascularization for atherosclerotic renal artery stenosis. *J Urol.* 1999;161:1093–1096.
12. Warren BA, Vanes O. The ultrastructure of the stages of atheroembolic occlusion of renal arteries. *Br J Exp Pathol.* 1973;54:469–478.
13. Lye WC, Cheah JS, Sinniah R. Renal cholesterol embolic disease. *Am J Nephrol.* 1993;13:489–493.
14. Frock J, Bierman M, Hammeke M, Reyes A. Atheroembolic renal disease: experience with 22 patients. *Nebr Med J.* 1994;79:317–321.
15. Greenberg A, Bastacky SI, Iqbal A, Borochovitz D, Johnson JP. Focal segmental glomerulosclerosis associated with nephrotic syndrome in cholesterol atheroembolism. *Am J Kidney Dis.* 1987;29:334–344.
16. Thadhani R, Pascual M, Nickeleit V, Tolkoff-Rubin N, Colvin R. Preliminary description of focal segmental glomerulosclerosis in patients with renovascular disease. *Lancet.* 1996;347:231–233.
17. Zucchelli P, Zuccala A. The diagnostic dilemma of hypertensive nephrosclerosis: the nephrologist's view. *Am J Kidney Dis.* 1993;21:87–91.
18. Graff-Radford J, Boes CJ, Brown RD Jr. History of Hollenhorst plaques. *Stroke.* 2015;46:e82–e84.
19. Moolenaar W, Lamers CB. Cholesterol crystal embolisation to the alimentary tract. *Gut.* 1996;38(2):196–200.
20. Kasinath BS, Corwin HL, Bidani AK, Korbet SM, Schwartz MM, Lewis EJ. Eosinophilia in the diagnosis of atheroembolic renal disease. *Am J Nephrol.* 1987;7:173–177.
21. Scolari F, Ravani P, Gaggi R, et al. The challenge of diagnosing atheroembolic renal disease: clinical features and prognostic factors. *Circulation.* 2007;116(3):298–304.
22. Corti R, Fuster V, Fayad ZA, et al. Lipid lowering by simvastatin induces regression of human atherosclerotic lesions: two years' follow-up by high resolution noninvasive magnetic resonance imaging. *Circulation.* 2002;106:2884–2887.
23. Ravani P, Gaggi R, Rollino C. Lack of association between dialysis modality and outcomes in atheroembolic renal disease. *Clin J Am Soc Nephrol.* 2010;5(3):454–459.
24. Nakayama M, Izumaru K, Nagata M, et al. The effect of low-dose corticosteroids on short- and long-term renal outcome in patients with cholesterol crystal embolism. *Ren Fail.* 2011;33(3):298–306.
25. Scolari F, Tardanico R, Pola A, et al. Cholesterol crystal embolic disease in renal allografts. *J Nephrol.* 2003;16:139–143.

SECTION VI

Kidney Protection in Transplantation

45

High-Risk Kidney Transplantation

ILIAS P. GOMATOS, SUSAN LERNER, AND MADHAV C. MENON

INTRODUCTION

Kidney transplantation is the most common solid organ transplant performed, with ~17,000 kidney transplants performed in the United States in 2016. In most circumstances, kidney transplantation offers improved patient survival and a superior quality of life at reduced healthcare cost than other modalities of renal replacement therapy. For instance, based on data from the 2016 US Renal Data System annual data report, in 2013, the adjusted 2-year survival rate on hemodialysis patients was 824.6/1,000 patient-years while the 2-year survival probabilities in the same era were 95% and 98% for recipients of deceased-donor and live-donor kidneys, respectively.[1] A study estimated the average annual cost of hemodialysis, peritoneal dialysis, and transplantation as around 90,000, 60,000 and 20,000 Canadian dollars after the first year of transplantation.[2] Hence, transplantation is the treatment of choice for advanced chronic kidney disease (CKD). The increased prevalence of diabetes and hypertension (HTN) causing end-stage renal disease (ESRD), improved survival on dialysis, increased numbers of previous transplant recipients with allograft failure requiring retransplantation, and an aging population have ensured an expanding kidney transplant waitlist. Most high-volume centers in the United States including ours routinely encounter ESRD patients with increasing comorbidities on the transplant waitlist. In this chapter, we outline the major pretransplant recipient comorbidities that we as a high-volume transplant center encounter, namely, hepatitis C virus (HVC), HIV, cardiovascular disease (CVD), and pretransplant tumor history. We outline our strategies for triage or candidate selection and specific posttransplant management of these high-risk kidney recipients.

HCV and Renal Transplantation

The prevalence of HCV infection in patients with ESRD (8.1%) is very high, and, as such, it has implications not only for dialysis patients but also for transplant patients.[3] The natural history of HCV in the ESRD population remains incompletely understood. A meta-analysis[4] demonstrated that HCV-positive patients on dialysis have an increased risk of mortality compared with HCV negative patients. Knoll et al.,[5] examined survival in the transplant population versus wait-listed patients and demonstrated that HCV-positive renal transplant recipients had a better survival than similar HCV-positive patients awaiting transplant. Fabrizi et al.[6] analyzed HCV disease progression after renal transplantation, observing that HCV-positive recipients have an increased risk of mortality and graft failure than HCV-negative patients, in part related to an increase in liver-related deaths due to hepatocellular carcinoma and/or cirrhosis. Newer studies,[7] however, suggest that infection (not HCV) is the most common cause of death among HCV-positive recipients. Since HCV-positive recipients have also been shown to be at increased risk for new-onset diabetes after transplantation (NODAT),[8] in our institution we employ steroid-sparing strategies for all HCV-positive recipients. The effect on NODAT may reflect direct pancreatic infection and viral cytopathy, contributing to overall survival. Given this impact of HCV disease on recipient and all-cause graft survival, proper patient selection is imperative. Of note, it is unclear at this point whether the new antiviral regimens will impact this long-term survival.

It is recommended that all potential kidney transplant recipients be evaluated for HCV infection. In addition, given the evidence of decreased patient and graft survival, all HCV-positive patients should be informed and counseled about the associated hepatic and extrahepatic risks and the need for additional diagnostic studies and therapeutic interventions before and after transplantation.[9] The Kidney Disease: Improving Global Outcomes Work Group suggests that all persistently viremic HCV-infected kidney transplant candidates should undergo pretransplant liver biopsy to assess the severity of liver disease and, therefore, the prognosis/management of these patients before and after transplant. There are no definitive studies that have examined whether the histologic stage of the biopsy predicts posttransplant outcome; however, the presence of cirrhosis on the biopsy has been associated with a 10-year survival of only 26%.[9] The liver biopsy may show advanced fibrosis or cirrhosis, and these patients should be cautiously considered for kidney transplant alone. For instance, in those cases without evidence of portal HTN despite fibrosis on biopsy, at our center we give consideration to kidney transplant alone. However, for the majority of advanced histologic fibrosis, for all patients with obvious portal HTN, and for those with decompensated liver disease, consideration should be given for simultaneous liver kidney transplantation (i.e., liver transplant listing).

The waiting list for kidney transplantation has increased at a higher rate than the number of donors and organs. Therefore, the use of expanded-criteria organs (now kidney donor profile index >85%) and donors with potentially transmissible diseases has been explored as a way to expand the donor pool. In 2004, Abbott et al.[10] conducted a retrospective study of the US Renal Data System. Their objective was to determine whether transplantation of HCV-positive donor kidneys for HCV-positive recipients was associated with a survival advantage or disadvantage for chronic kidney disease CKD patients receiving a transplant, compared with wait-listed patients remaining on dialysis. Although the use of HCV-positive donor kidneys was associated with an increased risk of mortality compared with HCV-negative donor kidneys, their study found that the use of HCV-positive donor kidneys was associated with improved survival compared with dialysis. An analysis of HCV-positive kidney transplant recipients undergoing deceased donor kidney transplantation in the United States,[11] found that recipients of HCV-positive renal allografts had shorter waiting times for transplantation. On average, patients who received kidneys from HCV-positive donors underwent transplantation 9±3 months after being placed on the waiting list, compared with 29±3 months for patients who received a kidney from an HCV-negative donor. Shorter waiting times were noted in every blood group without differences in rejection episodes, infectious complications, renal function, liver function, graft survival, or patient survival.

The risks and effects of superinfection with an HCV genotype from the donor that is different from the genotype of the potential HCV-infected recipient are unknown. There is usually insufficient time to do genotype testing in the donor, which would make requiring this information impractical. Prospective studies would be needed to examine further the effect of superinfection and its clinical impact on transplantation. But with the arrival of the newest antiviral agents that are effective against all genotypes, this issue may become less relevant.

Finally, whether to treat HCV infection prior to or after a successful kidney transplant is controversial. In most patients the renal impairment limits the safety and efficacy of the drugs. In addition, the advantage of a shorter waiting time for an HCV-positive donor kidney must be considered. The safety of delaying treatment needs to be balanced, however, with the expected waiting time, the degree of liver disease, the rate of progression, and the presence of extrahepatic HCV manifestations. All patients with HCV infection who have received a kidney transplant should be treated with antiviral therapy under the guidance of a hepatologist. We delay the start of treatment for 3 to 6 months after transplant when the kidney function as well as the immunosuppressive drug dosing is stable.

HIV-POSITIVE KIDNEY TRANSPLANT

Over the last 35 years, HIV has transformed from a syndrome with devastatingly high mortality to a chronic condition, largely due to the development of combination antiretroviral therapy (ART). While the mortality attributable directly to HIV has declined sharply since then, the epidemic remains an important risk to public health with an estimated 2.1 million new infections and 36.7 million persons living with HIV infection worldwide at the end of 2015.[12] In the early years of the AIDS epidemic, a rapidly progressive form of focal segmental glomerular sclerosis termed HIV-associated nephropathy was driving 10% of HIV patients to rapidly progressive ESRD through direct infection of renal epithelial cells by HIV.[13,14] Moreover, there are well-known associations between certain antiretrovirals (tenofovir, ritonavir-boosted atazanavir, or ritonavir-boosted lopinavir) and renal dysfunction.[15] HIV-positive patients are a unique subgroup of the ESRD population, since their remaining on dialysis is associated with morbidity and mortality worse than that observed in HIV-negative patients.

The National Institutes of Health multicenter trial of solid organ transplantation in HIV[16] was the first large prospective study to clearly demonstrate positive outcomes of kidney transplantation in this population. At 19 US centers, 150 HIV-positive patients received a transplant between 2003 and 2009. After a median follow-up of 1.7 years, patient survival rates at 1 and 3 years were 94.6% and 88.2%, and graft survival rates were 90.4% and 73.7%, respectively. These survival rates were better than a comparator cohort of HIV-negative but older recipients (>65 years old), yet slightly lower than the overall transplant population. Similar results have been reported elsewhere,[17] as well as a survival benefit over those HIV monoinfected patient remaining on dialysis.[18] HIV–HCV co-infected patients have demonstrated inferior transplant outcomes compared to HIV monoinfected patients,[17,19] something that will probably change in the era of direct-acting antiviral medication against HCV. Growing experience with HIV-positive recipients has revealed a number of complications unique to this population, including higher than expected rates of acute rejection (31% in the first year, compared to the expected US Scientific Registry of Transplant Recipients 1-year rejection rate of 12.3%),[16] delayed graft function (42.5% vs. 30.4% without effect on graft failure),[20] and challenging drug–drug interactions between highly active antiretroviral therapy and calcineurin inhibitors. In an effort to diminish drug–drug interactions, many centers have transitioned patients to protease inhibitor-free regimens, whenever possible, replacing them with integrase inhibitor-based regimens[21] as well as adding fusion inhibitors and CCR5 inhibitors.

In addition to meeting the qualifying standards set for all potential recipients, HIV-infected potential recipients need to present undetectable viral load (<50 copies/mL), and CD4 count >200/mm³, while on a stable ART regimen for at least 6 months. Referral rates of HIV-positive patients with ESRD for transplantation remain unknown. However, increased rate of failure to complete the preoperative evaluation has been reported in this group of patients (80% vs. 27% in uninfected individuals) with lower CD4 counts, substance abuse history, and black race being associated with failure to achieve listing.[22]

To expand the donor pool for HIV-positive and, indirectly, all ESRD patients, the landmark HIV Organ Equity (HOPE) Act was passed by the US Congress in late 2013, following the example of HIV to HIV Transplant in South Africa. This allows for transplantation of HIV-positive organs to HIV-positive recipients in a research setting. The inclusion criteria include the absence of invasive opportunistic infections in deceased donors; negative history of primary central nervous system lymphoma or progressive multifocal leukoencephalopathy, and, especially for living donors, CD4 count >500/mm³ for 6 months prior to donation; undetectable viral load (<50 copies/mL); complete ART history and viral resistance profile; and predonation kidney biopsy.

Currently, only transplant centers with established programs for HIV-positive recipients are allowed to transplant HIV-positive organs under the HOPE Act. HIV-to-HIV donation is still in its infancy in the United States, with many questions remaining to be answered, including the potential for superinfection with a second HIV strain and the actual population effect on the expansion of the donor pool by transplanting HIV-positive organs accounting for the ESRD HIV-positive transplant recipients as well. In South Africa, 27 patients were transplanted between 2008 and 2014 with 84% 3-year patient and graft survival rates, while the 1-year rejection rate was found to be comparable to that of HIV-positive recipients of HIV-negative kidneys in the United States.[23] However, questions exist regarding the quality of these organs. Richterman et al.[24] concluded that only 13 out of 508 examined in-depth HIV-positive patients could be accounted for as potentially suitable deceased HIV-positive donors. The median kidney donor risk index for these donors was 1.8, corresponding with a kidney donor profile index of 95%. Although, most of the potential HIV-positive donors in the study were older, more likely to be African American, and had a higher prevalence of diabetes and higher likelihood to be HCV co-infected compared to the actual HIV-negative donor group, still organ quality from HIV-positive donors is of great concern. Further, recent data[25] suggest the role of the allograft as a reservoir for HIV-infection, even in the absence of viremia, the long-term implications of which are currently unknown.

In our center, all HIV patients who complete their generic kidney specific evaluation are evaluated for candidacy at the HIV-specific recipient review committee meeting to assess listing criteria. Once the decision is made that the HIV patient is eligible for listing, the option to receive an HIV-positive donor organ and participate in the institutional review board–approved research protocol is discussed with the patient. Our immunosuppressive protocol for HIV monoinfected and HIV–HCV co-infected recipients includes induction with basiliximab (Simulect®) 20 mg during transplantation and on postoperative day 3 (thymoglobulin should be avoided). Initial reports suggested profound CD4 T cell depletion and increased risk of opportunistic infections in HIV-positive recipients receiving thymoglobulin[26]; however, recent retrospective data suggest safety and lowered rejection rates with thymoglobulin in these patients.[27] Standard triple drug maintenance immunosuppression is usually achieved with a calcineurin inhibitor using the same target levels as in a non-HIV-positive patient, an antimetabolite, and prednisone. Among living donor HIV-positive recipients, calcineurin inhibitor (CNI) therapy 2 weeks prior to the scheduled transplantation may be provided to determine CNI interactions while prophylaxis is also begun at the same time. Posttransplant prophylaxis includes trimethoprim-sulfamethoxazole for life and other chemoprophylactic agents as in non-HIV recipients. In our center, all HIV-positive recipients are managed in close collaboration with infectious disease specialists, often with their pretransplant HIV physicians. Only with an increasing number of HIV-to-HIV transplants under the HOPE act will we get adequate information of how to optimally utilize HIV-positive organs in the United States. Notwithstanding this, the sum of data obtained so far suggests relative safety and benefit for HIV-positive patients who receive kidney transplants, not dissimilar to the general population, and represents a true modern breakthrough.

CARDIOVASCULAR DISEASE AND KIDNEY TRANSPLANT

Despite improvements in overall graft and patient survival rates as well as the advances in cardiovascular health maintenance posttransplantation, CVD remains the leading cause of posttransplant mortality and a leading cause of graft loss accounting for 40% to 50% of all deaths.[28,29] The increased prevalence of CVD among kidney transplant recipients has been attributed to a number of causes including metabolic and systemic derangements related to ESRD (kidney disease and azotemia), immunosuppression, and increased infection and rejection rates. CVD can be categorized into atherosclerotic/ischemic heart disease and cardiac systolic/or diastolic dysfunction, which typically manifests as congestive heart failure or cardiac arrhythmia.

CVD risk remains significantly greater in transplant recipients when compared with age- and sex-matched general population.[30,31] The American College of Cardiology/American Health Association has proposed guidelines for the evaluation and management of patients with CVD on the kidney and liver transplant wait lists.[32,33] These guidelines have been endorsed by the American Society of Transplantation, American Society of Transplant Surgeons, and the National Kidney Foundation and have been discussed elsewhere in this chapter. These guidelines generally encompass all types of CVD, which are addressed in the following discussion. For instance, "active cardiac conditions" from any cardiac/vascular disease in candidates would need urgent management before listing can proceed (level of evidence 1A). The presence of 1 or more of these conditions confers high rates of perioperative cardiovascular morbidity and mortality and may require delay or cancellation of surgery. These include severe, symptomatic coronary heart disease and congestive heart failure. We actively screen transplant candidates for severe coronary artery disease (CAD), severe congestive heart failure (ejection fraction <20%), and severe peripheral vascular disease, which are all considered relative contraindications for transplantation. The general rationale for preoperative testing is to identify risk factors that are amenable to modification and to exclude patients whose operative risk exceeds any likely benefit, targeting to achieve <1% perioperative mortality following transplant. All listing and delisting decisions are made in concert with a cardiologist at our center.

Atherosclerotic Vascular Disease

Traditional risk factors for CAD and CVD morbidity[33,34] are more prevalent in the transplant population compared with the general population even after adjusting for age and sex. In the preoperative setting, all patients prior to renal transplantation require an electrocardiogram and a transthoracic echocardiogram. Patients aged >40, patients on dialysis for more than 5 years, patients with diabetes mellitus (DM) or poor exercise tolerance and those with history/findings of atherosclerotic disease require additional pharmacologic cardiac stress testing.[35] Patients with high-risk stress test, moderate degree of ischemia on imaging, or increased cardiac risk with any degree of ischemia on imaging should be scheduled for cardiac catheterization. Reported outcomes after coronary revascularization in selected cohorts of potential transplant candidates range from nonsignificant through survival benefit (in patients with 3-vessel CAD) to excellent survival in transplant recipients receiving preemptive revascularization.[36-38] Current guidelines stipulate that transplant recipients with significant CAD (constituting one-third of the entire group of transplant candidates) should be offered the potential benefit of myocardial revascularization.[39] Considering the higher early and 30-day mortality following coronary artery bypass grafting, percutaneous coronary intervention is currently the most popular mode of revascularization in these fragile and compromised patients. Newer generation drug-eluting stents should be preferred over bare-metal stents because of the lower risk of restenosis and stent thrombosis. Moreover, everolimus-eluting stents allow discontinuing dual antiplatelet therapy before 12 months, which is a further advantage. Given the prolonged periods that patients can await transplantation, physicians must be extremely judicious in the use of contrast angiography in ESRD individuals with residual kidney function not yet requiring dialysis.

Additional imaging with computed tomography angiography is required in patients with (i) evidence of significant aortic aneurysm, (ii) restrictive or constrictive cardiomyopathy, (iii) incidentally discovered intracardiac masses or valvular disease, or (iv) when there is a contraindication to cardiac catheterization.

Pulmonary Hypertension

Pulmonary HTN ranges from 9% to 39% in patients with stage 5 CKD and between 18.8%

and 68.8% in hemodialysis patients.[40] Correcting volume overload and treating left ventricular disorders is of paramount importance, while for the accurate assessment of pulmonary pressures, a repeat echocardiogram after optimization of fluid status is done. Right heart catheterization for accurate evaluation of pulmonary pressures and assessment for valvular heart disease or cardiomyopathy may also be indicated in the majority of such patients prior to listing. Any patient with moderate pulmonary HTN (not deemed to be related to volume overload) or symptomatic pulmonary HTN and/or evidence of right ventricular dysfunction/cor pulmonale will need evaluation by a specialized pulmonary HTN service, followed by initiation of appropriate pharmacologic management. Based on the increased risk of all-cause mortality with pulmonary HTN post transplant,[41] uncorrected moderate or severe pulmonary HTN or the need for specific pharmacotherapy is considered a relative contraindication to transplantation.

Left Ventricular Hypertrophy

Left ventricular hypertrophy (LVH) is present in 40% to 60% of transplant recipients representing together with DM, the strongest predictor of all-cause mortality following transplant.[42] Following renal transplant, LVH regression has been observed until 2 years following transplantation, after which the effect plateaued.[43] However, in a study examining cardiac MRI findings,[44] there was no difference in left ventricular (LV) measurements between transplant recipients and those who remained on dialysis. Potential interventions to improve LVH include administration of angiotensin converting enzyme inhibitors and calcium channel blockers with no overall difference when directly compared, with both reducing LV mass index by 15%.[45] Conversion from CNIs to mechanistic target of rapamycin (mTOR) inhibitors such as sirolimus has also been shown to result in a regression of LVH within 1 year after conversion by reducing LV wall thickness.[46]

Effect of Kidney Transplantation on CVD Risk

Overall, although transplantation has been shown to reduce cardiovascular events compared to dialysis, kidney recipients continue to be at higher risk for CVD complications when compared to the general population. Management of all recipients should therefore include focus on (i) precise preoperative screening as described, (ii) close posttransplant follow-up for graft dysfunction and CVD complications, and (iii) identifying modifiable risk factors, such as HTN, DM including NODAT and hyperlipidemia. The occurrence of allograft dysfunction, especially when associated with proteinuria, can contribute to the development or worsening of CAD, similar to native kidney CKD.[47] Graft dysfunction also causes HTN, as do CNIs, by means of volume overload, sodium retention, and activation of the renin–angiotensin–aldosterone system.[48] HTN, in turn, further exacerbates the worsening estimated glomerular filtration rate, creating a negative spiral. Worsening graft function can cause insulin resistance and affect lipase function, resulting in hyperglycemia and abnormal lipid profile, particularly reducing high-density lipoprotein levels[49] and increasing the risk of CVD. Corticosteroids, CNIs, and the mTOR inhibitors (sirolimus and everolimus) all exert unfavorable effects on serum lipid levels, with mTOR inhibitors associated with the most negative effects. Hence, CNI dose reduction or withdrawal, corticosteroid dose reduction, or steroid-sparing regimens are clinically acceptable regimens for selected candidates to minimize CVD risks/complications of NODAT and HTN.[50] Newer non-nephrotoxic agents that allow CNI avoidance or minimization, such as belatacept, have been associated with improved graft function with reduced metabolic risk.[51–53] Early detection and management of new-onset posttransplant DM and good glycemic control (specifically in the first few weeks after transplantation) appear to have long-standing effects.[54] The Collaborative Transplant study showed that patients with systolic blood pressure in the range of 120 mmHg have better outcomes than those with 130 mmHg.[55,56] The ALERT trial[57] demonstrated reduced cardiovascular events in the statin arm, which was further increased with earlier institution of statin therapy.[58] Our recipients with pre-existing CVD continue cardiology follow-up and optimal posttransplant stress testing (1–2 yearly). Acknowledging that immunosuppression plays a pivotal role in preserving the graft while contributing to CVD risk factors and progression implies the need to optimize these medications to prevent toxicity causing a worsening of CVD.

PRETRANSPLANT CANCER AND KIDNEY TRANSPLANT

Malignancy is known to be the second most common cause of death in kidney transplant recipients after CVD, being responsible for about one-third of deaths after transplantation.[59,60] In a recent meta-analysis,[61] pretransplant malignancy (PTM) was associated with increased risk of all-cause and cancer-specific mortality and of developing de novo malignancies after transplantation compared with those without PTM. Detailed discussion of all individual pretransplant cancers and posttransplant outcomes is beyond the scope of this chapter. Skin cancer is the most common type of malignancy in humans, and a history of non-melanoma skin cancer alone is usually not considered to be a contraindication to organ transplant. However, using United Network for Organ Sharing data from 2005 to 2013, Kang et al.[62] showed that pretransplant skin cancer was associated with an increased risk of posttransplant skin cancer (hazard ratio [HR] 2.92; 95% confidence interval [CI]: 2.52–3.39), posttransplant lymphoproliferative disorder (HR 1.93; 95% CI: 1.01–3.66), solid organ cancer (HR 2.60; 95% CI: 2.27–2.98), death (HR 1.20; 95% CI: 1.07–1.34), and graft failure (HR 1.17; 95% CI: 1.05–1.30). In addition, patients with a history of skin cancer treated before transplantation seem to be at increased risk of metastasis after transplantation.[63] In a historical study, Penn[64] detailed the outcomes of the Cincinnati Tumor Transplant Registry for patients who had skin cancer before transplantation. After transplantation, 30% of patients with melanoma experienced metastasis, and all died of their disease while in patients with a history of nonmelanoma skin cancer before transplantation, 62% developed nonmelanoma skin cancer or melanoma after transplantation. These results reaffirm the need for careful screening, detailed counseling, close follow-up, and tailored management of transplant recipients with PTM. Especially in kidney transplant recipients with previous cutaneous squamous-cell carcinomas, switching from calcineurin inhibitors to sirolimus appears to provide an antitumoral effect.[65]

In summary, prudent candidate selection, optimal pre- and posttransplant testing and follow-up in close collaboration with specialists can ensure that high-risk kidney transplant candidates obtain the benefit of kidney transplantation without exposing them to undue risk and improve patient and allograft survival.

REFERENCES

1. 2017 annual data report. US Renal Data System; 2017. https://www.usrds.org/adr.aspx
2. Klarenbach SW, Tonelli M, Chui B, Manns BJ. Economic evaluation of dialysis therapies. *Nat Rev Nephrol*. 2014;10:644–652.
3. Pereira BJ, Levey, AS. Hepatitis C virus infection in dialysis and renal transplantation. *Kidney Int*. 1997;51:981–999.
4. Fabrizi F, Martin P, Dixit V, Bunnapradist S, Dulai G. Meta-analysis: effect of hepatitis C virus infection on mortality in dialysis. *Aliment Pharmacol Ther*. 2004;20:1271–1277.
5. Knoll GA, Tankersley MR, Lee JY, Julian BA, Curtis JJ. The impact of renal transplantation on survival in hepatitis C positive end stage renal disease patients. *Am J Kidney Dis*. 199729:608–614.
6. Fabrizi F, Martin P, Dixit V, Bunnapradist S, Dulai G. Hepatitis C virus antibody status and survival after renal transplantation: meta-analysis of observational studies. *Am J Transplant*. 2005;5:1452–1461.
7. Heo NY, Mannalithara A, Kim D, Udompap P, Tan JC, Kim WR. Long-term patient and graft survival of kidney transplant recipients with hepatitis C virus infection in the United States. *Transplantation*. 2017;102(3):454–460
8. Morales JM, Bloom R, Roth D. Kidney transplantation in the patient with hepatitis C virus infection. *Contrib Nephrol*. 2012;176:77–86.
9. Kidney Disease: Improving Global Outcomes (KDIGO). KDIGO clinical practice guidelines for the prevention, diagnosis, evaluation, and treatment of hepatitis C in chronic kidney disease. *Kidney Int Suppl*. 2008;109:S1–S99.
10. Abbott KC, Lentine KL, Bucci JF, Agodoa LY, Peters TG, Schnitzler MA. The impact of transplantation with deceased donor hepatitis c positive kidneys on survival in wait-listed long-term dialysis patients. *Am J Transplant*. 2004;4:2032–2037.
11. Mandal AK, Kraus ES, Samaniego M, et al. Shorter waiting times for hepatitis C virus seropositive recipients of cadaveric renal allografts from hepatitis C virus seropositive donors. *Clin Transplant*. 2000;14:391–396.
12. Global statistics. HIV.gov; 2018. https://www.aids.gov/hiv-aids-basics/hiv-aids-101/global-statistics/
13. Wyatt CM, Klotman PE. HIV-1 and HIV-associated nephropathy 25 years later. *Clin J Am Soc Nephrol*. 2007;2(Suppl 1):S20–S24.
14. Ross MJ. Advances in the pathogenesis of HIV-associated kidney diseases. *Kidney Int*. 2014;86:266–274.
15. Mocroft A, Lundgren JD, Ross M, et al.; Data Collection on Adverse Events of Anti-HIV Drugs (D:A:D) Study. Cumulative and current exposure to potentially nephrotoxic antiretrovirals and development of chronic kidney disease in HIV-positive individuals with a normal baseline estimated glomerular filtration rate: a prospective international cohort study. *Lancet HIV*. 2016;3:e23–e32.
16. Stock PG, Barin B, Murphy B, et al. Outcomes of kidney transplantation in HIV-infected recipients. *N Engl J Med*. 2010;363:2004–2014.
17. Locke JE, Mehta S, Reed RD, et al. A national study of outcomes among HIV-infected kidney transplant recipients. *J Am Soc Nephrol*. 2015;26:2222–2229.
18. Locke JE, Gustafson S, Mehta S, et al. Survival benefit of kidney transplantation in HIV-infected patients. *Ann Surg*. 2017;265:604–608.
19. Sawinski D, Forde KA, Eddinger K, et al. Superior outcomes in HIV-positive kidney transplant patients compared with HCV-infected or HIV/HCV-coinfected recipients. *Kidney Int*. 2015;88:341–349.
20. Malat G, Jindal RM, Mehta K, Gracely E, Ranganna K, Doyle A. Kidney donor risk index (KDRI) fails to predict kidney allograft survival in HIV (+) recipients. *Transplantation*. 2014;98:436–442.
21. Tricot L, Teicher E, Peytavin G, et al. Safety and efficacy of raltegravir in HIV-infected transplant patients cotreated with immunosuppressive drugs. *Am J Transplant*. 2009;9:1946–1952.
22. Sawinski D, Wyatt CM, Casagrande L, et al. Factors associated with failure to list HIV-positive kidney transplant candidates. *Am J Transplant*. 2009;9:1467–1471.
23. Muller E, Barday Z, Kahn D. HIV-positive-to-HIV-positive kidney transplantation. *N Engl J Med*. 2015;372:2070–2071.
24. Richterman A, Sawinski D, Reese PP, et al. An assessment of HIV-infected patients dying in care for deceased organ donation in a United states urban center. *Am J Transplant*. 2015;15:2105–2116.
25. Canaud G, Dejucq-Rainsford N, Avettand-Fenoël V, et al. The kidney as a reservoir for HIV-1 after renal transplantation. *J Am Soc Nephrol*. 2014;25:407–419.
26. Carter JT, Melcher ML, Carlson LL, Roland ME, Stock PG. Thymoglobulin-associated Cd4+ T-cell depletion and infection risk in HIV-infected renal transplant recipients. *Am J Transplant*. 2006;6:753–760.
27. Kucirka LM, Durand CM, Bae S, et al. Induction immunosuppression and clinical outcomes in kidney transplant recipients infected with human immunodeficiency virus. *Am J Transplant*. 2016;16:2368–2376.
28. Wolfe RA, Ashby VB, Milford EL, et al. Comparison of mortality in all patients on

dialysis, patients on dialysis awaiting transplantation, and recipients of a first cadaveric transplant. *N Engl J Med.* 1999;341:1725–1730.

29. Ojo AO, Hanson JA, Wolfe RA, Leichtman AB, Agodoa LY, Port FK. Long-term survival in renal transplant recipients with graft function. *Kidney Int.* 2000;57:307–313.

30. Kasiske BL, Chakkera HA, Roel J. Explained and unexplained ischemic heart disease risk after renal transplantation. *J Am Soc Nephrol.* 2000;11:1735–1743.

31. Ducloux D, Kazory A, Chalopin JM. Predicting coronary heart disease in renal transplant recipients: a prospective study. *Kidney Int.* 2004;66:441–447.

32. Lentine KL, Costa SP, Weir MR, et al.; American Heart Association Council on the Kidney in Cardiovascular Disease and Council on Peripheral Vascular Disease; American Heart Association; American College of Cardiology Foundation. Cardiac disease evaluation and management among kidney and liver transplantation candidates: a scientific statement from the American Heart Association and the American College of Cardiology Foundation: endorsed by the American Society of Transplant Surgeons, American Society of Transplantation, and National Kidney Foundation. *Circulation.* 2012;126:617–663.

33. Grundy SM, Pasternak R, Greenland P, Smith S Jr, Fuster V. AHA/ACC scientific statement: assessment of cardiovascular risk by use of multiple-risk-factor assessment equations: a statement for healthcare professionals from the American Heart Association and the American College of Cardiology. *J Am Coll Cardiol.* 1999;34:1348–1359.

34. Vanrenterghem YF, Claes K, Montagnino G, et al. Risk factors for cardiovascular events after successful renal transplantation. *Transplantation.* 2008;85:209–216.

35. European Renal Best Practice Transplantation Guideline Development Group. ERBP guideline on the management and evaluation of the kidney donor and recipient. *Nephrol Dial Transplant.* 2013;28(Suppl 2):ii1–ii71.

36. Kumar N, Baker CS, Chan K, et al. Cardiac survival after pre-emptive coronary angiography in transplant patients and those awaiting transplantation. *Clin J Am Soc Nephrol.* 2011;6:1912–1919.

37. Herzog CA, Ma JZ, Collins AJ. Long-term outcome of renal transplant recipients in the United States after coronary revascularization procedures. *Circulation.* 2004;109:2866–2871.

38. Garcia S, Moritz TE, Ward HB, et al. Usefulness of revascularization of patients with multivessel coronary artery disease before elective vascular surgery for abdominal aortic and peripheral occlusive disease. *Am J Cardiol.* 2008;102:809–813.

39. Windecker S, Kolh P, Alfonso F, et al. 2014 ESC/EACTS guidelines on myocardial revascularization: The Task Force on Myocardial Revascularization of the European Society of Cardiology (ESC) and the European Association for Cardio-Thoracic Surgery (EACTS) developed with the special contribution of the European Association of Percutaneous Cardiovascular Interventions (EAPCI). *Eur Heart J.* 2014;35:2541–2619.

40. Bolignano D, Rastelli S, Agarwal R, et al. Pulmonary hypertension in CKD. *Am J Kidney Dis.* 2013;61:612–622.

41. Sise ME, Courtwright AM, Channick RN. Pulmonary hypertension in patients with chronic and end-stage kidney disease. *Kidney Int.* 2013;84:682–692.

42. Rigatto C, Foley R, Jeffery J, Negrijn C, Tribula C, Parfrey P. Electrocardiographic left ventricular hypertrophy in renal transplant recipients: prognostic value and impact of blood pressure and anemia. *J Am Soc Nephrol.* 2003;14:462–468.

43. Rigatto C, Foley RN, Kent GM, Guttmann R, Parfrey PS. Long-term changes in left ventricular hypertrophy after renal transplantation. *Transplantation.* 2000;70:570–575.

44. Patel RK, Mark PB, Johnston N, McGregor E, Dargie HJ, Jardine AG. Renal transplantation is not associated with regression of left ventricular hypertrophy: a magnetic resonance study. *Clin J Am Soc Nephrol.* 2008;3:1807–1811.

45. Midtvedt K, Ihlen H, Hartmann A, et al. Reduction of left ventricular mass by lisinopril and nifedipine in hypertensive renal transplant recipients: a prospective randomized double-blind study. *Transplantation.* 2001;72:107–111.

46. Paoletti E, Amidone M, Cassottana P, Gherzi M, Marsano L, Cannella G. Effect of sirolimus on left ventricular hypertrophy in kidney transplant recipients: a 1-year nonrandomized controlled trial. *Am J Kidney Dis.* 2008;52:324–330.

47. Fernández-Fresnedo G, Escallada R, Rodrigo E, et al. The risk of cardiovascular disease associated with proteinuria in renal transplant patients. *Transplantation.* 2002;73:1345–1348.

48. Edmunds M, Russell G, Swales J. Hypertension in renal failure. In: Swales J *Textbook of Hypertension.* London, Blackwell, 1994: 798–810.

49. Ardhanari S, Alpert MA, Aggarwal K. Cardiovascular disease in chronic kidney disease: risk factors, pathogenesis, and prevention. *Adv Perit Dial.* 2014;30:40–53.

50. Pascual J, Zamora J, Galeano C, Royuela A, Quereda C. Steroid avoidance or withdrawal for

kidney transplant recipients. *Cochrane Db Sys Rev.* 2009;1:CD005632.

51. Oberbauer R, Segoloni G, Campistol JM, et al.; Rapamune Maintenance Regimen Study Group. Early cyclosporine withdrawal from a sirolimus-based regimen results in better renal allograft survival and renal function at 48 months after transplantation. *Transpl Int.* 2005;18:22–28.

52. Vincenti F, Charpentier B, Vanrenterghem Y, et al. A phase III study of belatacept-based immunosuppression regimens versus cyclosporine in renal transplant recipients (BENEFIT study). *Am J Transplant.* 2010;10:535–546.

53. Vitko S, Tedesco H, Eris J, et al. Everolimus with optimized cyclosporine dosing in renal transplant recipients: 6-month safety and efficacy results of two randomized studies. *Am J Transplant.* 2004;4:626–635.

54. Joss N, Staatz CE, Thomson AH, Jardine AG. Predictors of new onset diabetes after renal transplantation. *Clin Transplant.* 2007;21:136–143.

55. Opelz G, Wujciak T, Ritz E.; Collaborative Transplant Study. Association of chronic kidney graft failure with recipient blood pressure. *Kidney Int.* 1998;53:217–222.

56. Midtvedt K, Neumayer HH. Management strategies for posttransplant hypertension. *Transplantation.* 2000;70(11 Suppl): SS64–SS69.

57. Holdaas H, Fellström B, Jardine AG, et al.; Assessment of LEscol in Renal Transplantation (ALERT) Study Investigators. Effect of fluvastatin on cardiac outcomes in renal transplant recipients: a multicentre, randomised, placebo-controlled trial. *Lancet.* 2003;361:2024–2031.

58. Holdaas H, Fellström B, Cole E, et al.; Assessment of LEscol in Renal Transplantation (ALERT) Study Investigators. Long-term cardiac outcomes in renal transplant recipients receiving fluvastatin: the ALERT extension study. *Am J Transplant.* 2005;5:2929–2936.

59. Kauffman HM, Cherikh WS, Cheng Y, Hanto DW, Kahan BD. Maintenance immunosuppression with target-of-rapamycin inhibitors is associated with a reduced incidence of de novo malignancies. *Transplantation.* 2005;80(7):883–889.

60. Pruthi R, Casula A, MacPhee I. UK Renal Registry 15th annual report: chapter 3. Demographic and biochemistry profile of kidney transplant recipients in the UK in 2011: national and centre-specific analyses. *Nephron Clin Pract.* 2013;123(Suppl 1):55–80.

61. Acuna SA, Huang JW, Daly C, Shah PS, Kim SJ, Baxter NN. Outcomes of solid organ transplant recipients with preexisting malignancies in remission: a systematic review and meta-analysis. *Transplantation.* 2017;101:471–481.

62. Kang W, Sampaio MS, Huang E, Bunnapradist S. Association of pretransplant skin cancer with posttransplant malignancy, graft failure and death in kidney transplant recipients. *Transplantation.* 2017;101:1303–1309.

63. Penn I. The effect of immunosuppression on pre-existing cancers. *Transplantation.* 1993;55:742–747.

64. Penn I. Malignant melanoma in organ allograft recipients. *Transplantation.* 1996;61:274–278.

65. Euvrard S, Morelon E, Rostaing L, et al.; TUMORAPA Study Group. Sirolimus and secondary skin-cancer prevention in kidney transplantation. *N Engl J Med.* 2012;367:329–339.

46

Recurrence of Primary Glomerular Diseases Post Kidney Transplantation

JOHN MANLLO-DIECK AND NADA ALACHKAR

INTRODUCTION

Although not a cure for end-stage renal disease (ESRD), kidney transplantation remains the best modality of renal replacement therapy. However, the culprit disease causing the patient's renal failure may recur in the transplanted organ, leading to allograft failure and ESRD.

Glomerulonephritis (GN) is the third most common cause of ESRD in the United States, behind diabetes and hypertension according to the US Renal Data System 2016 report.[1] In other countries such as Australia and New Zealand, where the incidence of diabetes and hypertension is not as high, 50% of patients undergoing kidney transplant due to a primary glomerular disease.[2] Prevalence of primary glomerular disease is probably higher than reported as many patients do not undergo kidney biopsy before transplantation, and renal disease is assumed to be in many cases due to diabetes or hypertension or simply remained undiagnosed.

Therefore, having a definite renal diagnosis prior to transplantation is crucial, given that most of primary glomerular diseases recur after transplantation, and having a diagnosis may assist with the disease and management of recurrence.

The incidence of allograft GN increases with time post transplantation. Reported incidence varies in the literature due to several factors depending on the inclusion of patients with recurrent GN versus allograft GN and wide variations in observation time and due to studies based on protocol or clinical biopsies. Researchers evaluated protocol biopsies of 1965 kidney recipients between 1998 and 2011 in a single center and found that the cumulative incidence of allograft GN was 5.2%, 18.2%, 21.7%, 35.8%, and 42.3% at 1, 3, 5, 8, and 10 years, respectively.[3]

It is difficult in some cases to differentiate recurrent versus de novo GN. By definition, the diagnosis of recurrent disease requires histologic diagnosis of same disease in the native kidneys. Distinction is likely not precise because pretransplant native kidney biopsies are often not performed. Incidence of allograft GN, as expected, is higher and is diagnosed earlier in patients with a pretransplant diagnoses of GN. There are some cases of de novo GN that are diagnosed in the early posttransplant period, likely suggesting that these are actually recurrent disease given that de novo disease typically develops later.[4] In some cases, clinical diagnoses of recurrent GN can be made late as recurrence can remain clinically silent for several months to years.

It is important to point out that histology of early GN is often different from advanced GN diagnosed in native kidney biopsies. For example, in primary focal segmental glomerulosclerosis (FSGS), where the characteristic histological finding on light microscopy is segmental areas of mesangial collapse and sclerosis in some glomeruli, in recurrent FSGS light microscopy may be normal and an early sign of recurrence is diffuse podocyte effacement under electron microscopy.[5]

Essentially, all GN's may recur after transplant; nonetheless, the rate of recurrence and the impact on allograft survival varies immensely depending on the disease.[2,4] Immunosuppression may also play a role in the rate of recurrence. Retrospective observational studies have shown a reduction in the incidence of recurrence in patient who received thymoglobulin induction.[6] Using steroid-free or rapid discontinuation of steroid protocols for maintenance immunosuppression may be associated with increase rate of recurrent GN.[7]

In this review, we will discuss the recurrence rate, clinical manifestations, and management of recurrent primary glomerular diseases post kidney transplantation.

IGA NEPHROPATHY

Primary immunoglobulin A (IgA) nephropathy (IgAN) is the most common type of GN in the world.[8,9] It progresses to ESRD in approximately 20% to 40% of patients.[9-11] IgAN can occur at any age, but it presents most commonly during the second and third decade of life. IgAN is caused by deposition of IgA1 immune complex in the renal parenchyma. Mechanism of injury is thought to be due to 4 processes. There is aberrant glycosylation of IgA1, synthesis of antibodies directed against galactose deficient IgA1, binding of galactose deficient IgA1 by antibodies to form immune complexes, and accumulation of these immune complexes in the mesangium of the glomeruli.

The incidence of recurrent IgAN has been reported anywhere from 13% to 65%.[9] This wide variation in the literature is attributed to studies having different indications for allograft biopsies (protocol biopsy vs. clinical indication) and also on the follow-up time of the patients. Some studies have shown that clinical evidence of recurrence is present in 30% of patients, but it is rare to see clinical evidence of disease during the first 3 to 5 years post transplant.[4,12] Whereas histological recurrent IgAN is more common and presents earlier in the posttransplant period, and it can be present without any clinical symptoms.

In kidney allografts, the natural course of IgAN is likely altered due to the use of immunosuppressions, and with the introduction of newer immunosuppressants, especially mycophenolate and the use of triple immunosuppressant therapy, the incidence of recurrent IgAN has decreased over the recent years.[11]

Risk factors for IgA recurrence include younger age, rapid progression of disease to ESRD,[4,12] elevated levels of IgA in serum,[13] and previous graft loss due to IgA recurrence. Specific HLA antigens (HLA-B8, HLA-B35, HLA-DR3, HLA-DR4) have been associated with recurrence and worst prognosis[4,10,12-14] whereas other HLA antigens present in the transplant recipient (HLA-A2, HLA-B46) may be protective against developing recurrence.[13] Receiving a living related kidney versus a deceased donor has also been associated with increased incidence of recurrence, but this has not been consistent in all published literature.[4,12-14] Regardless, it is not recommended to avoid living donor transplant in IgA nephropathy. Studies have shown an increase incidence of recurrence in patient on a steroid-free maintenance immunosuppressive regimen.[15]

In patients with recurrent disease, factors associated with progression and poor outcome are proteinuria of >1 g/day and glomerular sclerosis >30% on a kidney biopsy, which was associated with increased risk of graft loss within 6 years.

Allograft survival for primary IgA nephropathy is better than other glomerulopathies.[4,11] Allograft loss within the first 3 years after transplant is rare; it is probable mainly in patients whose disease progressed rapidly to ESRD or in patients who lost a prior kidney transplant due to recurrence.[16] Some studies report that graft survival in patients with IgA recurrent disease compared to patients whose cause of renal disease is IgA nephropathy but without recurrence in the allograft was similar within the first 10 years post transplant.[10,11,14]

Recurrence can be immunopathological only when it is found during a protocol biopsy in asymptomatic patients. Clinical manifestations of IgA recurrence vary as patients can present with persistent microscopic hematuria; new or worsening proteinuria, usually below nephrotic range; elevation in serum creatinine; or a combination of any of the 3.

There are limited options for the treatment of recurrent IgA. Some studies have shown decrease incidence in recurrence when antithymocyte globulin is used as induction.[6,17] The use of angiotensin converting enzyme inhibitors (ACEI) has been shown to reduce proteinuria is patients with recurrent IgA nephropathy. The use of fish oil has been studied in the treatment for IgA nephropathy, but this has not been studied in detailed in transplant patients. Given reports of increased recurrence while using steroid-free protocol as maintenance immunosuppression, it is reasonable to add prednisone back to the regimen. It is our opinion that a steroid-free protocol should be avoided in this group of patients. In patients with clinical evident disease that does not respond to optimization of maintenance immunosuppression, tight blood pressure control or ACEIs and pulse dose of steroids with a prolonged taper has shown benefits. In patients with aggressive disease (crescentic IgA) or rapidly progressive disease, cyclophosphamide can be used. If cyclophosphamide is used, immunosuppression needs to be adjusted and the antimetabolite discontinued.

FOCAL SEGMENTAL GLOMERULOSCLEROSIS

FSGS is a common cause of ESRD that highly recurs post kidney transplant. FSGS is a histologic lesion characterized by segmental areas of mesangial collapse and sclerosis in some glomeruli. FSGS histological pattern is thought to be the result of adaptive changes to glomerular hyperfiltration. FSGS can be divided into primary and secondary FSGS.

Primary FSGS is thought to be due to loss of podocyte structural integrity and function. Pathogenesis is not well understood; it is thought to be due to circulating permeability factors, which bind to the podocyte cell membrane, leading to alteration in the podocyte morphology and function.[4,5,18]

Secondary causes of FSGS include loss of renal mass (e.g., unilateral renal agenesis) due to compensatory intraglomerular hypertension, and hypertrophy in the remaining glomeruli causes an increase in filtration rate to maintain glomerular filtration rate (GFR); over the years, this will lead to FSGS. Other causes include obesity; viral infections like HIV or parvovirus; drugs including bisphosphonates, interferon, anabolic steroids, or sirolimus; and illegal drugs like heroin.

Secondary FSGS does not recur in the renal allograft assuming etiology leading to FSGS is modified. There are also genetic causes of FSGS, which are associated to APOL1 gene; this population has a very low risk of recurrence.[4]

Primary FSGS commonly recurs after kidney transplant. It has been reported as high as 30% to 40% despite the use of immunosuppressive therapy. In high-risk patients, which include younger age at time of diagnoses, patients with rapid progression to ESRD (<3 years), white race, and high level of proteinuria, recurrence can be as high as 60%; the incidence of recurrence increases to 80% with a second transplant if the graft was lost due to recurrence.[4,5,18,19]

Primary FSGS may recur very early post transplant, in some cases within days. The initial presentation is usually nephrotic range of proteinuria; some patients may present with nephrotic syndrome. In patients who still make urine before transplant, it can be difficult to determine if proteinuria is from the native kidneys or from the renal allograft; therefore, it is recommended to have a baseline urine protein-to-creatinine ratio prior to transplant. It is also recommended to perform urine protein-to-creatinine ratio screening post transplant to detect early recurrence, especially in patients who are at high risk.

Diagnosis of recurrent FSGS is challenging as histological characteristics of FSGS take time to develop; therefore, light microscopy may be normal, and the only finding is diffuse podocyte effacement under electron microscopy, which can be seen as early as hours after transplant.[5]

The cause of FSGS recurrence is thought to be due to one or a number of circulating factors that may cause podocyte injury, leading to FSGS. Identifying the circulating factor or factors has been the focus of an extensive research work for more than 30 years. Although several factors were claimed to be the circulating factors, there has been no agreement among researchers about the right factor. Therefore, treatment of recurrent FSGS is still very challenging and has been relying on removing the plasma that possibly contain the circulating factor or factors. Although, not approved by the Food and Drug Administration, plasmapheresis is considered the treatment of choice for recurrent FSGS. It has been shown to reduce protein excretion and induce complete or partial remission in patients with recurrent disease with variable outcome.[20,21] The typical plasmapheresis regimen used is 1 plasma volume exchange for 3 consecutive days followed by every other day to complete a total of 9 to 10 treatments. Patients also receive intravenous immunoglobulin (100 mg/kg) after plasmapheresis.[5] However, the duration and frequency of the plasmapheresis therapy vary, depending on patients' response.

There is an emerging literature in the use of rituximab, a monoclonal antibody directed against CD-20 expressed in B-lymphocytes, as a potential treatment for recurrent FSGS. Rituximab was first described as a potential treatment for recurrent FSGS in 2006 on a patient with posttransplant lymphoproliferative disorder; the patient was treated with rituximab, and an improvement in proteinuria was noticed. It is thought that rituximab reduces circulating permeability factors by direct depletion of CD-20 positive B cells or via indirect suppression of T cells that interact with B cells, but rituximab has also been shown to have direct podocyte interaction via preserving sphingomyelin-phosphodiesterase-acid-like-3b expression and acid-sphingomyelinase activity, which are important in maintaining podocyte integrity. A retrospective study of patients with recurrent FSGS treated with plasmapheresis and rituximab showed improvement in proteinuria compared to plasmapheresis alone.[5,18,20,22,23]

MEMBRANOUS NEPHROPATHY

Membranous nephropathy (MN) is one of the most common causes of nephrotic syndrome in adults. The characteristic histological lesion seen on light microscopy is diffuse thickening of the glomerular basement membrane (GBM) throughout the glomeruli without hypercellularity. Immunofluorescence microscopy shows a diffuse granular pattern of IgG and C3 staining along the GBM. Electron microscopy shows subepithelial electro-dense deposits on the outer aspect of the GBM, effacement of the foot processes, and expansion of the GBM.

MN can be idiopathic, an autoimmune disorder, or secondary, resulting from a variety of conditions, including (i) infections like hepatitis B and C and syphilis; (ii) autoimmune diseases such as systemic lupus erythematous and sarcoidosis; (iii) solid organ malignancies especially prostate, lung, or gastrointestinal tract; and (iv) drugs like nonsteroidal anti-inflammatory drugs, gold, penicillamine, and antitumor necrosis factor agents. Secondary causes of MN does not recur in the renal allograft if underlying etiology is treated.

Idiopathic MN (iMN) can present in the kidney allograft as recurrent disease or de novo. iMN recurrence in the renal allograft has been reported as high as 40% to 50%.[4,24,25] The risk of recurrence is higher in patients with higher levels of proteinuria pretransplant.[25] It has been described that 70% of patients with iMN have autoantibodies against podocyte antigen phospholipase A2 receptor (PLA2R)[26,27] Patients with anti-PLA2R antibodies present pretransplant have a higher incidence of recurrence versus patients without antibodies pretransplant.[4,25,27] Anti-PLA2R antibodies decline in 50% of the patients post transplant.[4] A decline in PLA2R antibodies has been associated with a reduced risk of recurrence.

Clinical manifestations of recurrent MN typically present between 13 and 15 months after transplant. Most common presentation is new-onset proteinuria at variable degrees, which is progressive. Patients can develop nephrotic syndrome. Renal function is often normal at time of presentation. Studies of protocol biopsies show that histologic recurrence without any clinical evidence of disease occurs most often during the first year post transplant.[24]

Treatment of recurrent MN with ACEIs or angiotensin II receptor blockers in patients with minimal clinical evidence of disease (normal estimated GFR and proteinuria <1 g/day) and only histologic evidence of recurrent MN, in addition to tight blood pressure control and close monitoring. Ensure patient is on a triple immunosuppressive regimen that includes calcineurin inhibitor if patient is not on it, as it been shown to be beneficial in the treatment of MN in native kidneys. If patients develop worsening proteinuria and/or decreasing estimated GFR, pulse dose of steroids with a slow taper alone or in combination with cyclophosphamide is recommended. If cyclophosphamide is used, antimetabolite needs to be discontinued due to high risk of bone marrow suppression. Recent data show that adding a course of rituximab to current immunosuppressive regimen may achieve over 80% of partial or complete remission at 24 months and partial resolution of histologic changes with resorption of electron-dense immune deposits.[4,28,29]

MEMBRANOPROLIFERATIVE GLOMERULONEPHRITIS

Membranoproliferative GN (MPGN) is a glomerular injury pattern characterized by mesangial hypercellularity, endocapillary proliferation and capillary-wall remodeling. These glomerular changes are due to deposition of immunoglobulins, complement or both in the mesangium or capillary walls of the glomeruli. MPGN injury pattern can be caused by systemic diseases like chronic hepatitis C or hepatitis B infections, plasma cell dyscrasias, or autoimmune disease like lupus, Sjögren's syndrome, or rheumatoid arthritis. In rare instances, it can be caused by non-Hodgkin lymphoma, renal cell carcinoma, or melanoma. In most patients, a secondary cause of MPGN can be identified; there is also an idiopathic form of MPGN, which is a diagnosis of exclusion.

In recent years, a new classification has emerged given our understanding of the pathophysiology of MPGN and the role of the alternative complement pathway. This classification is based on the mechanism involved in the glomerular injury rather than location of the immune deposits. Under this new classification, MPGN is divided into immune complex–mediated GN, where immune complex deposition leads to activation of complement deposition of both immunoglobulin and complement protein in glomeruli. The second type of MPGN is complement-mediated GN, which results from dysregulation of the alternative complement pathway, leading to constant complement activation that deposit without immunoglobulin in the glomeruli. These deposits can be distinguished by immunofluorescence techniques under microscopy. Complement-mediated MPGN includes C3 glomerulopathy (C3GN) and dense deposit disease (DDD) both have the same immunofluorescence characteristics and result from dysregulation of complement alternative pathway. They can be differentiated by electron microscopy findings, where DDD is characterized by dense intramembranous deposits.

Studies on the recurrence of idiopathic MPGN are very limited due to the low incidence of MPGN, which accounts for approximately 7% to 10% of all cases of biopsy-proven GN,[30] and most available studies are based on the old classification. The reported range of recurrence in MPGN is widespread ranging from 20% to 80% or even 90%.[4,12,30,31] This wide range is, in part, due to great differences in the rate of recurrence depending on the subtype of MPGN. Complement-mediated MPGN has a higher risk of recurrence.[4,30,31] The recurrence of C3GN is approximately 70%,[4] and DDD recurrence is also quite high with reports fluctuating from 70% to 100%.[4,12,31] Immune-complex GN risk of recurrence varies depending on the type of the depositions. If the immunoglobin is monoclonal, the recurrence rate is approximate 66%, but if the deposition is polyclonal, the recurrence is 30% to 35%.[4,30]

Recurrence in all subtypes is associated with reduced graft survival at variable degrees; C3GN is associated with the highest degree of graft failure.[4,12,31]

Recurrence occurs early post transplant, usually within the first year,[4,31] mainly in patients with C3GN and MPGN with monoclonal immunoglobulin deposition. DDD and MPGN with polyclonal immunoglobulins deposition recur in late post transplant and have a slower rate of progression.

Factors that have been associated with recurrence of idiopathic MPGN are young age, aggressive disease in the native kidneys (crescents present on biopsy), low serum complement levels, presence of monoclonal immunoglobulins,

higher levels of proteinuria, and specific HLA antigens (B8, B49, DR3, DR4).[30,31]

Clinical presentation of recurrent idiopathic MPGN is variable and depends on the subtype. It can range from asymptomatic proteinuria, most of the time >1 g/day, asymptomatic hematuria, or a combination of both with or without elevation in serum creatinine to rapidly progressive GN.

There is limited information regarding treatment of recurrent idiopathic MPGN. Historically, ACEIs or angiotensin II receptor blockers can be used with a goal to decrease proteinuria to <1 g/day, given known benefit in proteinuric kidney disease. In patients with nephrotic range proteinuria or declining of renal function, increasing prednisone to 1 mg/kg for 3 to 4 months followed by a slow taper and increasing antimetabolite (i.e., mycophenolate mofetil to 1,500 mg 2× daily) can be considered. Cyclophosphamide has also been used in recurrent disease that is refractory to initial treatment or in patients with rapidly progressive disease with the addition of pulse dose steroids, followed by a slow taper. In some cases of immune-complex GN, plasma exchange showed some benefit.[30]

With our new understanding of the pathophysiology of MPGN, uncontrolled studies have emerged using rituximab in immune-complex GN with the aim to reduce antibody production.[4,30,32] Eculizumab, a monoclonal IgG antibody against complement protein C5, which prevents formation of C5b and subsequent formation of membrane attack complex, has been reported to be effective in case reports and small uncontrolled studies in the treatment of recurrent C3 glomerulopathy.[30,33]

CONCLUSION

Recurrence of primary glomerular disease post kidney transplantation is common and varies depending of type of glomerular disease (Table 46.1). Its impact on the renal allograft is also variable and depends of many factors. Treatment for recurrent glomerular disease is limited; because of this, early diagnosis with closely monitoring and prompt intervention is key to attempt slowing progression and subsequent allograft lost. On occasion, a pathological diagnosis of the cause of native kidney ESRD is lacking, but if clinical course leading to ESRD is suspicious for glomerular disease, close monitoring may be also recommended. It is also important to keep patients on an optimal regimen of immunosuppression including a CNI, an antimetabolite, and

TABLE 46.1 SUMMARY OF RECURRENT PRIMARY GLOMERULONEPHRITIS

Primary GN	Recurrence Rate	Risk Factors	Treatment
IgA nephropathy	Clinical recurrence: 30% Immunopathological recurrence: 65%	• Young age • Rapid progression to ESRD • Previous graft loss due to IgA recurrence • Specific HLA Antigens • Steroid free IS protocol	• Avoid steroid free IS protocol • ACEI/ARB • Pulse dose steroids if proteinuria >1gram • CYC in crescentic disease or RPGN
FSGS	30%–40%. Up to 80% if first allograft is lost due to recurrence	• Young age • Rapid progression to ESRD • Caucasians • Previous graft loss due to FSGS recurrence	• Avoid steroids free protocol • Plasmapheresis/IVIG • Rituximab
Membranous	40%–50%	• Nephrotic range proteinuria prior to Transplant. • - Anti-PLA2R Antibodies present prior to Transplant.	• ACEI/ARB • Ensure Patient is on a CNI • Pulse dose of Steroids if Proteinuria >1 gram • Steroids/CYC if declined GFR • Adding rituximab to IS regimen
MPGN	Immune-Complex GN ~65% Monoclonal Ig ~30–35% Polyclonal Ig Comp-Mediated GN ~70% in C3GN 70%–100% in DDD	• Young age • Rapid progression to ESRD • Low serum complement levels • Presence of monoclonal immunoglobulins • Higher levels of Proteinuria • Specific HLA antigens	• ACEI/ARB • Increase dose of Steroids (1mg/kg for 3 months followed by a taper) • CYC in refractory disease or RPGN • Rituximab for immune-complex GN • Eculizumab for complement mediated GN (C3GN)

IS = immunosuppression. ESRD = end-stage renal disease. RPGN = rapidly progressive glomerulonephritis. IgA = immunoglobulin A. FSGS = focal segmental glomerulosclerosis. MPGN = membranoproliferative glomerulonephritis. CNI = calcineurin inhibitors. CYC = cyclophosphamide. IVIG = intravenous immunoglobulin. GFR = glomerular filtration rate. GN = glomerulonephritis. DDD = dense deposit disease. Anti-PLA2R = autoantibodies against podocyte antigen phospholipase A2 receptor. RPGN = rapidly progressive glomerulonephritis. ACEI = angiotensin converting enzyme inhibitors. ARB = angiotensin receptor blockers. HLA = human leukocyte antigen.

low-dose steroid as well as avoiding steroid-free protocols.

Kidney allograft loss due to recurrent glomerular disease is not a contraindication for retransplantation. If retransplantation is being considered, referral to a transplant center with experience and infrastructure in managing recurrent glomerular disease is highly recommended.

Additional studies are necessary to have a better understanding of the incidence, prevention, and management of recurrent primary glomerular diseases to improve the short- and long-term impact on the renal allograft.

REFERENCES

1. United States Renal Data System. 2016 USRDS annual data report: epidemiology of kidney disease in the United States. National Institutes of Health, National Institute of Diabetes and Digestive and Kidney Diseases, Bethesda, MD; 2016.

2. Briganti E, Russ GR, McNeil JJ, Atkins RC, Chadban SJ. Risk of renal allograft loss from

recurrent glomerulonephritis. *N Engl J Med.* 2002;347(2):103–109.

3. Cosio FG, El Ters M, Cornell LD, Schinstock CA, Stegall MD. changing kidney allograft histology early posttransplant: prognostic implications of 1-year protocol biopsies. *Am J Transplant.* 2016;16(1):194–203.

4. Cosio FG, Cattran DC. Recent advances in our understanding of recurrent primary glomerulonephritis after kidney transplantation. *Kidney Int.* 2017;91(2):304–314.

5. Alachkar N, Wei C, Arend LJ, et al. Podocyte effacement closely links to suPAR levels at time of posttransplantation focal segmental glomerulosclerosis occurrence and improves with therapy. *Transplantation.* 2013;96(7):649–656.

6. Pascual J, Mezrich JD, Djamali A, et al. Alemtuzumab induction and recurrence of glomerular disease after kidney transplantation. *Transplantation* 2007;83(11):1429–1434.

7. Kukla A, Chen E, Spong R, et al. Recurrent glomerulonephritis under rapid discontinuation of steroids. *Transplantation* 2011;91(12):1386–1391.

8. Floege J. Recurrent IgA nephropathy after renal transplantation. *Sem Nephrol.* 2004;24(3):287–291.

9. Lionaki S, Panagiotellis K, Melexopoulou C, Boletis JN. The clinical course of IgA nephropathy after kidney transplantation and its management. *Transplant. Rev (Orlando, FL).* 2017;31(2):106–114.

10. Nijim S, Vujjini V, Alasfar S, et al. Recurrent IgA nephropathy after kidney transplantation. *Transplant Proc.* 2016;48(8):2689–2694.

11. Moroni G, Longhi S, Quaglini S, et al. The long-term outcome of renal transplantation of IgA nephropathy and the impact of recurrence on graft survival. *Nephrol Dial Transplant.* 2013;28(5):1305–1314.

12. Ponticelli C, Glassock RJ. Posttransplant recurrence of primary glomerulonephritis. *Clin J Am Soc Nephrol.* 2010;5(12):2363–2372.

13. Wang AY, Lai FM, Yu AW, et al. Recurrent IgA nephropathy in renal transplant allografts. *Am J Kidney Dis.* 2001;38(3):588–596.

14. Ponticelli C, Traversi L, Banfi G. Renal transplantation in patients with IgA mesangial glomerulonephritis. *Ped Transplant.* 2004;8(4):334–438.

15. Clayton P, McDonald S, Chadban S. Steroids and recurrent IgA nephropathy after kidney transplantation. *Am J Transplant.* 2011;11(8):1645–1649.

16. Ohmacht C, Kliem V, Burg M, et al. Recurrent immunoglobulin A nephropathy after renal transplantation: a significant contributor to graft loss. *Transplantation.* 1997;64(10):1493–1496.

17. Berthoux F, El Deeb S, Mariat C, Diconne E, Laurent B, Thibaudin L. Antithymocyte globulin (ATG) induction therapy and disease recurrence in renal transplant recipients with primary IgA nephropathy. *Transplantation.* 2008;85(10):1505–1507.

18. Fornoni A, Sageshima J, Wei C, et al. Rituximab targets podocytes in recurrent focal segmental glomerulosclerosis. *Sci Transl Med.* 2011;3(85):85ra46.

19. Artero M, Biava C, Amend W, Tomlanovich S, Vincenti F. Recurrent focal glomerulosclerosis: natural history and response to therapy. *Am J Med.* 1992;92(4):375–383.

20. Hickson LJ, Gera M, Amer H, et al. Kidney transplantation for primary focal segmental glomerulosclerosis: outcomes and response to therapy for recurrence. *Transplantation.* 2009;87(8):1232–1239.

21. Artero ML, Sharma R, Savin VJ, Vincenti F. Plasmapheresis reduces proteinuria and serum capacity to injure glomeruli in patients with recurrent focal glomerulosclerosis. *Am J Kidney Dis.* 1994;23(4):574–581.

22. Pescovitz MD, Book BK, Sidner RA. Resolution of recurrent focal segmental glomerulosclerosis proteinuria after rituximab treatment. *N Engl J Med.* 2006;354(18):1961–1963.

23. Pescovitz MD. Rituximab, an anti-cd20 monoclonal antibody: history and mechanism of action. *Am J Transplant.* 2006;6(5 Pt 1):859–866.

24. Dabade TS, Grande JP, Norby SM, Fervenza FC, Cosio FG. Recurrent idiopathic membranous nephropathy after kidney transplantation: a surveillance biopsy study. *Am J Transplant.* 2008;8(6):1318–1322.

25. Grupper A, Cornell LD, Fervenza FC, Beck LH Jr, Lorenz E, Cosio FG. Recurrent membranous nephropathy after kidney transplantation: treatment and long-term implications. *Transplantation.* 2016;100(12):2710–2716.

26. Beck LH, Bonegio RGB, Lambeau G, et al. M-type phospholipase a2 receptor as target antigen in idiopathic membranous nephropathy. *N Eng J Med.* 2009;361(1):11–21.

27. Kattah A, Ayalon R, Beck LH, et al. Antiphospholipase a$_2$ receptor antibodies in recurrent membranous nephropathy. *Am J Transplant.* 2015;15(5):1349–1359.

28. El-Zoghby ZM, Grande JP, Fraile MG, Norby SM, Fervenza FC, Cosio FG. Recurrent idiopathic membranous nephropathy: early diagnosis by protocol biopsies and treatment with anti-CD20 monoclonal antibodies. *Am J Transplant.* 2009;9(12):2800–2807.

29. Rodriguez EF, Cosio FG, Nasr SH, et al. The pathology and clinical features of early recurrent membranous glomerulonephritis. *Am J Transplant.* 2012;12(4):1029–38.

30. Alasfar S, Carter-Monroe N, Rosenberg AZ, Montgomery RA, Alachkar N. Membranoproliferative glomerulonephritis recurrence after kidney transplantation: using the new classification. *BMC Nephrol.* 2016:17:7.

31. Marinaki S, Lionaki S, Boletis JN. Glomerular disease recurrence in the renal allograft: a hurdle but not a barrier for successful kidney transplantation. *Transplant Proc.* 2013;45(1):3–9.

32. Guiard E, Karras A, Plaisier E, et al. Patterns of noncryoglobulinemic glomerulonephritis with monoclonal Ig deposits: correlation with igg subclass and response to rituximab. *Clin J Am Soc Nephrol.* 2011;6(7):1609–1616.

33. Bomback AS, Smith RJ, Barile GR, et al. Eculizumab for dense deposit disease and C3 glomerulonephritis. *Clin J Am Soc Nephrol.* 2012;7(5):748–756.

INDEX

Tables, figures, and boxes are indicated by an italic *t*, *f*, and *b*, respectively, following the page number.